EXAMINATION IN PHYSICAL THERAPY PRACTICE

Screening for Medical Disease

SECOND EDITION

EXAMINATION IN PHYSICAL THERAPY PRACTICE

Screening for Medical Disease

SECOND EDITION

Edited by

William G. Boissonnault, M.S., P.T.
Director, Spine Center Physical Therapy
University of Wisconsin Hospital/Clinics
Associate Lecturer
University of Wisconsin-Madison Physical Therapy Program
Madison, Wisconsin
Assistant Professor, Institute of Physical Therapy
St. Augustine, Florida
Clinical Assistant Professor, Department of Rehabilitation Sciences
University of Tennessee-Memphis College of Allied Health Sciences
Memphis, Tennessee
Adjunct Faculty, Massachusetts General Hospital
Institute of Health Professions
Boston, Massachusetts
Instructor, Krannert Graduate School of Physical Therapy
University of Indianapolis, Indianapolis, Indiana

CHURCHILL LIVINGSTONE
New York, London, Edinburgh, Melbourne, Tokyo

Library of Congress Cataloging-in-Publication Data

Examination in physical therapy practice : screening for medical disease / edited by William G. Boissonnault. – 2nd ed.

p. cm.

Includes bibliographical references and index.

ISBN 0-443-08956-6

1. Physical therapy. 2. Diagnosis, Differential.

I. Boissonnault, William G.

[DNLM: 1. Physical Therapy. 2. Physical Examination. WB 460 E96 1995]

RM701.E9 1995

615.8′2–dc20

DNLM/DLC

for Library of Congress 95-17807

CIP

Distributed in the United Kingdom by Churchill Livingstone, Robert Stevenson House, 1–3 Baxter's Place, Leith Walk, Edinburgh EH1 3AF, and by associated companies, branches, and representatives throughout the world.

Accurate indications, adverse reactions, and dosage schedules for drugs are provided in this book, but it is possible that they may change. The reader is urged to review the package information data of the manufacturers of the medications mentioned.

The Publishers have made every effort to trace the copyright holders for borrowed material. If they have inadvertently overlooked any, they will be pleased to make the necessary arrangements at the first opportunity.

Acquisitions Editor: *Carol Bader*
Production Editor: *Elizabeth Bowman-Schulman*
Production Supervisor: *Laura Mosberg Cohen*
Desktop Coordinator: *Jo-Ann Demas*
Cover Design: *Jeannette Jacobs*

Printed in the United States of America

First published in 1995 7 6 5 4 3 2 1

To my wife, Jill, and my children Joshua and Eliya, who are my heart and soul, and to my parents, Gregory and Geneva Boissonnault, whose love and support have been a continuing source of strength.

To my son Jacob, the newest addition to my family, and to my grandfather Peter Boissonnault, whose presence continually rekindles some of my warmest memories.

Contributors

David Arnall, Ph.D., P.T.
Assistant Professor, Program in Physical Therapy, Northern Arizona University, Flagstaff, Arizona

Susan Barker, M.S., P.T., N.C.S.
Assistant Professor, Department of Physical Therapy, Philadelphia College of Pharmacy and Science, Philadelphia, Pennsylvania; Partner, Motion Physical Therapy and Sports Rehab Center, Medford, New Jersey

Warren J. Bilkey, M.D.
Clinical Assistant Professor, Department of Physical Medicine and Rehabilitation, University of Minnesota Medical School–Minneapolis; Associate Medical Director, Chronic Pain Rehabilitation Program, Sister Kenny Institute, Minneapolis, Minnesota

Jill S. Boissonnault, M.S., P.T.
Physical Therapy Program Coordinator, Meriter Hospital, Madison, Wisconsin

William G. Boissonnault, M.S., P.T.
Director, Spine Center Physical Therapy, University of Wisconsin Hospital/Clinics; Associate Lecturer, University of Wisconsin–Madison Physical Therapy Program, Madison, Wisconsin; Assistant Professor, Institute of Physical Therapy, St. Augustine, Florida; Clinical Assistant Professor, Department of Rehabilitation Sciences, University of Tennessee–Memphis College of Allied Health Sciences, Memphis, Tennessee; Adjunct Faculty, Massachusetts General Hospital Institute of Health Professions, Boston, Massachusetts; Instructor, Krannert Graduate School of Physical Therapy, University of Indianapolis, Indianapolis, Indiana

Mark R. Bookhout, M.S., P.T.
Instructor, Office of Continuing Medical Education, Michigan State University College of Osteopathic Medicine, East Lansing, Michigan; President, Physical Therapy Orthopaedic Specialists, Inc., Minneapolis, Minnesota

Stephen D. Cain, Pharm.D.
Pharmacist, Boynton Health Service, University of Minnesota, Minneapolis, Minnesota

Paul H. Caldron, D.O., F.A.C.P., F.A.C.R.
Staff Rheumatologist, Arthritis and Rheumatology Associates, P.C., Paradise Valley, Arizona

Jill Downing, M.D.
Instructor, Department of Preventive Medicine, Harvard Medical School; Assistant in Medicine, and Program Director, Cardiac Rehabilitation, Massachusetts General Hospital, Boston, Massachusetts

Jill A. Floberg, P.T.
Regional Manager, Pacific Northwest Region, Physiotherapy Associates, Olympia, Washington

Tim Harbst, M.D.
Chairman, Department of Rehabilitation Medicine, the Gunderson Clinic; Adjunct Faculty, University of Wisconsin–LaCrosse School of Physical Therapy, LaCrosse, Wisconsin

Edward R. Isaacs, M.D., F.A.A.N.
Associate Professor, Department of Neurology, Virginia Commonwealth University Medical College of Virginia School of Medicine, Richmond, Virginia; Associate Clinical Professor, Office of Continuing Medical Education, Michigan State University College of Osteopathic Medicine, East Lansing, Michigan

Steven C. Janos, M.S., P.T.

Assistant Professor, Department of Physical Therapy, University of Central Florida College of Health and Public Affairs, Orlando, Florida

Robert D. Karl, Jr., M.D.

Associate Clinical Professor, Department of Radiology, University of Washington School of Medicine, Seattle, Washington; Chief, Radiology, South Region, Department of Radiology, Group Health Cooperative of Puget Sound, Tacoma, Washington

Patricia M. King, M.A., P.T.

Director, Division of Graduate Studies, Institute of Physical Therapy, St. Augustine, Florida

Michael B. Koopmeiners, M.D.

Associate Professor, Institute of Physical Therapy, St. Augustine, Florida; Family Practice Physician, Maplewood Medical Center—A Group Health Clinic, Maplewood, Minnesota

James Leonard, D.O., P.T.

Assistant Professor, Department of Rehabilitation Medicine, University of Wisconsin Hospital and Clinics, Madison, Wisconsin

Frank W. Ling, M.D.

Associate Professor and Director, Division of Gynecology, Department of Obstetrics and Gynecology, University of Tennessee, Memphis, College of Medicine, Memphis, Tennessee

Diane Madlon–Kay, M.D.

Clinical Assistant Professor, Department of Family and Community Medicine, St. Paul–Ramsey Medical Center, St. Paul, Minnesota

Dudley M. McLinn, M.D.

Specialists in Internal Medicine, P.A., Abbott Northwestern Hospital, Minneapolis, Minnesota

Kevin McMahon, M.D., F.A.A.O.S., F.A.C.S.

Clinical Instructor in Orthopaedics, Uniformed Services University of Health Sciences, Bethesda, Maryland; Team Physician, American University, Washington, D.C.; Potomac Valley Orthopaedic Associates, Montgomery General Hospital, Olney, Maryland

Theresa Hoskins Michel, M.S., P.T., C.C.S.

Assistant Professor, Graduate Program in Physical Therapy, Massachusetts General Hospital Institute of Health Professions; Cardiopulmonary Clinical Specialist, Department of Cardiopulmonary Physical Therapy, Massachusetts General Hospital, Boston, Massachusetts

Craig A. Myers, P.T., M.D.

Department of Obstetrics and Gynecology, University of Tennessee, Memphis, College of Medicine, Memphis, Tennessee

Terry Randall, M.S., P.T., O.C.S., A.T.C.

Clinical Instructor in Physical Therapy, University of Oklahoma, Oklahoma City, Oklahoma; Assistant Chief of Physical Therapy, Reynolds Army Hospital, Fort Sill, Oklahoma

Michael Ryan, M.D., F.A.C.P.

Adjunct Professor, Department of Health, Physical Education, and Recreation, Northern Arizona University; Medical Director, Cardiopulmonary Rehabilitation Program, Phase I, Flagstaff Medical Center, Flagstaff, Arizona

Charles Shapiro, M.Ed., P.T.

Assistant Professor, Program in Physical Therapy, Health Sciences Division, Nova Southeastern University, North Miami Beach, Florida; Private Physical Therapy Practice, The S–P–O–R–T Clinic, Hollywood, Florida; Doctorate of Physical Therapy Candidate, Institute of Physical Therapy, St. Augustine, Florida

Stanley Skopit, D.O.

Associate Clinical Professor of Dermatology, Health Sciences Division, Nova Southeastern University, North Miami Beach, Florida; Private Clinical Dermatology Practice, Hollywood, Florida; Director, Dermatology Residency Training Program, Nova Southeastern University/Universal Medical Center, Ft. Lauderdale, Florida

Foreword to the First Edition

Heraclitus, the Greek philosopher, stated, "There is nothing permanent except change." The profession of physical therapy exemplifies this bit of ancient wisdom. Since the beginning of the profession in 1921 in response to the needs of injured World War I veterans, physical therapists have developed from mere technicians who followed the prescriptions of physicians into increasingly autonomous professionals with a distinct body of knowledge and specialized diagnostic procedures.

This change is illustrated by comparing the Physical Therapy Code of Ethics in 1935 with the latest edition in 1981. In the earlier version, the professional scope of physical therapists was severely limited by the statement, "Diagnosing and stating the prognosis of the case and prescribing treatment shall be entirely the responsibility of the physician. Any assumption of this responsibility by one of our members shall be considered unethical." In the 1981 edition, the only restriction relating to providing services is in the clause, "Physical therapists [will] comply with the laws and regulations governing the practice of physical therapy." The updated laws have allowed physical therapists increasing autonomy in all areas relating to the provision of physical therapy services, while still clearly leaving the area of differential diagnosis to physicians.

Examination in Physical Therapy Practice acknowledges that medical care is a partnership among providers. All but one chapter is written by a physician and either co–authored by or written with input from a physical therapist to take advantage of both perspectives. This is what makes this book unique. I have never read a text that so thoroughly merges the minds of physicians and physical therapists. In this book, both disciplines work as equal partners in the process of healing the patient.

This long overdue text is an effort to give physical therapists the knowledge necessary to make them full partners in the differential diagnostic process. Physical therapists are educated thoroughly in the area of treating problems with the musculoskeletal system, but our education is understandably lacking in the area of differential diagnosis. By contrast, in medical school, physicians often spend little time learning about physical therapy treatment and a great deal of time on differential diagnosis. Therefore, physicians and physical therapists must work in concert to fill the gaps in one another's expertise. This book is an effort to expand the awareness of physical therapists so that we may be informed partners in the diagnostic process.

Differential diagnosis is defined by *Dorland's Illustrated Medical Dictionary* as "the determination of which one of several diseases may be producing the symptoms." Differential diagnosis of the neuromusculoskeletal system is a complex process, particularly for the many physicians who specialize in the diagnosis of systemic disease. These physicians will typically conduct a clinical examination, collecting signs and symptoms to develop an impression or a hierarchical problem list. Based on the results of certain differential tests and measurements, they may decide to send the patient for physical therapy treatment. It is my experience that these physicians do not expect the physical therapist to assist them in gathering data or developing a clinical impression. Although we may be asked to evaluate and treat a patient while the physician is developing his or her diagnostic impression or problem list, we are not asked to provide information regarding our findings or the patient's responses that would facilitate the differential diagnostic process. It is my contention that we need to provide important qualitative and quantitative information that can assist the physician in completing the differential diagnosis. The physical therapist must be accountable for accurate, timely communication with the physician, and must be sensitive to the physician's role and responsibilities. The issue of legal accountability is critical; physical therapists must be able to substantiate their findings and conclusions on a sound, scientific basis.

Theories of medical treatment are separated into two broad categories: those that are focused on pathology and those that are focused on signs, symptoms, and the patient. Before Hippocrates, the Cnidian school of medicine rested on the notion that for every illness there existed one specific cause and one specific treatment. Modern medicine, or at least one aspect of it, is very Cnidian in its approach: for every infection there is a specific antibiotic for treatment; for every injury there is a specific routine of exercises. One can view this Cnidian approach as a pathology–focused treatment in which the medical practitioner focuses on the diagnosis that the patient's condition has been given, and offers whatever the standard treatment is for this diagnosis. The problem with the pathology–focused or single–cause, single–treatment approach is that it fails to appreciate the broader picture of the disorder. This approach also ignores the fact that the physical body that houses the ailment also houses an emotional and intellectual being—the human patient.

An injury invariably affects a patient intellectually and emotionally as well as physically, and an essential aspect of effective treatment is that the whole person must be acknowledged and ministered to for treatment to progress optimally. In short, the foundation of treatment should rest on the signs, symptoms, and patient–focused treatment model of medicine, the roots of which can be traced to Hippocrates. In this approach, the practitioner looks at the total wellness of the patient and focuses on strengthening the body's defenses against illness or injury, as well as treating the signs and symptoms with a foreign agent or set of physical treatments. Treatment is a living process. It is growth. Knowledge can guide but not totally direct treatment. The patient and his or her response guide treatment in the final analysis. Therefore the successful physical therapist must have a broad background of knowledge to determine when things fit and when they do not.

In the signs, symptoms, and patient–focused model of treatment, when patients are referred to physical therapists by physicians, we first perform an evaluation to diagnose the movement dysfunction and to assess the functional profile. As treatment is provided, the therapist carefully monitors the patient's response and communicates with the physician about the patient's progress. When we are approached directly by the patient, we must be aware of the origin of the complaint; if it resides in a system other than the musculoskeletal system, it will require a diagnosis from a physician. We also must be aware of whether the musculoskeletal complaint requires diagnostic tests, measures, and treatment other than what can be provided by the physical therapist.

Pathology is not a fixed set of signs and symptoms. It is a living, changing condition. The position of the physical therapist as a member of the health care team is unique. The nature of treatment allows the therapist to spend more time with the patient than almost any other practitioner. Therefore, the change in pathology can be carefully monitored by the therapist. As a result, more detailed knowledge about pathology in other body systems can assist the therapist in evaluating situations in which changes indicate other factors that need to be addressed by the physician. The knowledge of medical diagnostics helps the therapist to make better–informed decisions. Only time can tell what effect this expanding knowledge will have on health care. If it helps us to better function as members of the medical team, then I feel it will advance the cause. However, if we use this knowledge to become more independent of other practitioners in the treatment of patients, then I feel it is detrimental to both the profession and the patients.

In our society, it is more acceptable to acknowledge a physical problem than it is to attribute emotional stress as a precursor or cause of disease. Physical therapists are in an ideal position to question and listen to a patient to help uncover emotional concomitants to the presenting physical problem. This information may be communicated to the physician by the patient only if he or she acknowledges its relevance. Therefore the physical therapist must inform the physician of a patient's emotional stress, especially in situations in which lack of progress suggests that the stress may be of a magnitude requiring intervention by a psychologist or psychiatrist.

Too often the question of why a physical therapist should know more about medical diagnosis rests on arguments surrounding the issue of direct access. However, there is a far broader issue that concerns the therapist's accountability for the wellness of the patient. Since the physical therapist spends more time with the patient and is in a position to question the patient more often than the physician, the therapist is in an ideal position to assist in the often difficult process of differential diagnosis. Physicians do not often consider physical therapists resources to them in this process. Therapists need a broader view of pathology to communicate with physicians at a more appropriate level. By filling a major gap in the literature that is available to physical therapists, this text meets that need.

Peter I. Edgelow, M.A., P.T.
Faculty, Physical Therapy Residency Program in
Advanced Orthopedic Manual Therapy
Kaiser Permanente Medical Center
Hayward, California

FOREWORD

In the second edition, Bill Boissonnault has brought together a distinguished group of contributors who have built on the first edition by clarifying and expanding it with a thoughtful response to the current needs of their audiences. Those audiences come from a wide variety of professions, not just the major group—practitioners of physical therapy. For physical therapists, the book qualifies without question as a textbook for everyone from the student to the experienced clinician.

Each chapter is must reading for all teachers and students of practical therapy. Never preaching dogma, the book also should be read by all related professions and by representatives of funding agencies. Just as it guides individual hands-on practitioners, the book's clarity, thoroughness, common sense, and wisdom combine to form an excellent guide for problem solving and decision making at the administrative and fiscal levels. On a personal note, I am delighted to have had the honor to be a "godfather" to this book. It has a bright future and will bring me pleasure for years. All who have had a role in producing it deserve sincere thanks and congratulations.

J.V. Basmajian, O.C., O.Ont, M.D., F.R.C.P.C., F.R.C.P.S. (Glasg), F.A.C.A., F.S.B.M., F.A.B.M.R., F.A.F.R.M.-R.A.C.P. (Australia), Hon Dip (St L C)
Professor Emeritus in Rehabilitation Medicine and Anatomy, McMaster University,
Hamilton, Ontario, Canada

Preface

As with the first edition of *Examination in Physical Therapy Practice*, the primary goal of this edition is to provide therapists with the knowledge and clinical tools to medically screen patients for the presence of symptoms and signs that require the expertise of a physician. Having the ability to medically screen patients is an absolute complement to the skills required for the assessment and treatment of movement dysfunction. Medical screening by the therapist involves ruling out the involvement of a body system (e.g., cardiovascular, gastrointestinal systems) rather than ruling out specific diseases (e.g., pleurisy, osteomyelitis, or prostate cancer). I believe screening on a systems versus disease level is what differentiates the therapist's responsibility from that of the physician's.

Written for the clinician and student, *Examination in Physical Therapy Practice* provides information to help ensure that patients receive appropriate and timely medical care. Chapter 1 presents the foundation of this screening process, reviewing examination and treatment principles that assist with the differentiation of physical therapy versus non-physical therapy conditions. Since Chapter 1 contains information that will help the therapist decide which body systems to screen, the reader is advised to read this chapter before other components of the text. Chapters 2 through 13 provide detailed information regarding screening the various body systems. Chapters covering screening of the skin and nervous system have been added to this section. Skin cancer is on the rise, and therapists are in a unique position to detect suspicious lesions and refer the patient to the appropriate physician.

For each body system an overview of anatomy and physiology, relevant to the screening process or to the understanding of the pathologies discussed, is presented. Symptoms and signs that suggest the system may be malfunctioning are presented. Certain specific diseases are reviewed in each chapter, but the list of diseases reviewed is not all inclusive. The emphasis is on those entities therapists are more likely to encounter clinically or those that significantly affect the evaluative and rehabilitative process.

Staying within the mission of this textbook, Chapter 14, Clinical Pharmacology for the Physical Therapist, remains an important chapter. Commonly prescribed groups of medications are discussed with the emphasis on potential side effects, which if noted during the clinical examination would warrant communication between the therapist and physician. Another important addition to this edition is Chapter 15, Emergency Medical Situations in the Clinic. Therapists face situations that require quick, appropriate action to safeguard the patient or themselves. Topics such as onset of chest pain, syncope, suicide ideation, and confronting an abusive, belligerent patient are covered with the focus being appropriate action and communication with the physician. Chapter 16, Radiologic Assessment of the Musculoskeletal System, provides information that should enhance understanding of certain disease entities as well as communication with physicians. Lastly, the appendices have been expanded, providing a quick reference source for a review of systems and upper and lower quarter physical examination screening summaries. Illustrations have been included for many of the "non-musculoskeletal" physical examination techniques. The glossary of terms has been updated to accommodate the new information provided in this edition.

Passage of direct-access legislation appears to have been the wake-up call for our profession regarding medical screening responsibilities. Yet, we have always had this responsibility and for decades have incorporated a screening component into our examination scheme. The question we need to ask is: "Is our screening component adequate?" I believe often we fall short of our responsibilities. The ultimate goal of this textbook is to enhance professional communication between therapists and physicians, facilitating the referral of patients from therapists to physicians. In the spirit of this collaboration most of the chapters were co-authored by a therapist and a physician. Those chapters not co-authored were written with significant input from the other profession. This arrangement allows for the book content to be accurate and applicable to the physical therapy profession. The patient will be the winner as our knowledge base and skills develop and grow in this area.

William G. Boissonnault, M.S., P.T.

Contents

1. Screening for Medical Disease: Physical Therapy Assessment and Treatment Principles / 1
   William G. Boissonnault and Steven C. Janos
2. Screening for Cardiovascular System Disease / 31
   Theresa Hoskins Michel and Jill Downing
3. Screening for Pulmonary System Disease / 69
   David Arnall and Michael Ryan
4. Screening for Gastrointestinal System Disease / 101
   Michael B. Koopmeiners
5. Screening for Male Urogenital System Disease / 117
   Dudley M. McLinn and William G. Boissonnault
6. Screening for Female Urogenital System Disease / 133
   Patricia M. King, Frank W. Ling, and Craig A. Myers
7. Screening for Endocrine System Disease / 155
   Jill S. Boissonnault and Diane Madlon-Kay
8. Screening for Pathologic Origins of Head and Facial Pain / 175
   Edward R. Isaacs and Mark R. Bookhout
9. Screening for Nervous System Disease / 191
   Susan Barker
10. Screening for Musculoskeletal System Disease / 223
    Terry Randall and Kevin McMahon
11. Screening for Rheumatic Disease / 257
    Paul H. Caldron
12. Screening for Psychological Disorders / 277
    Warren J. Bilkey and Michael B. Koopmeiners
13. Screening for Skin Disorders / 303
    Charles Shapiro and Stanley Skopit
14. Clinical Pharmacology for the Physical Therapist / 321
    Stephen D. Cain and Steven C. Janos
15. Medical Emergencies in Physical Therapy / 353
    James Leonard and Tim Harbst
16. Radiologic Assessment of the Musculoskeletal System / 365
    Robert D. Karl, Jr. and Jill A. Floberg

Appendix

I Examination—Review of Systems Summary / 399

II Objective Examination—Upper-Quarter Screening Examination / 401

III Objective Examination—Lower-Quarter Screening Examination / 409

IV Glossary of Terms / 415

Index / 427

1 Screening for Medical Disease: Physical Therapy Assessment and Treatment Principles

William G. Boissonnault, M.S., P.T.
Steven C. Janos, M.S., P.T.

The Challenge of Patient Examination

If there is something you have not studied,
or, having studied it you are unable to do it,
do not file it away; if there is a question
that you have not asked or to which
you have been unable to find the answer,
do not consider the matter closed;
if you have not thought of a problem,
or, having thought of it,
you have not resolved it,
do not think the matter settled;
if you have tried to make a distinction
but have not made it clear,
do not sink into contentment;
if there is a principle which
you have been able to put into practice,
do not let up.
If one man gets there with one try,
try ten times.
If another succeeds with a hundred tries,
make a thousand.
Proceeding in this manner, even one
who is a bit slow will find the light,
even a weak man will find energy.[47]

Numerous challenges face the clinician responsible for patient management. The ultimate challenge is the development of a comprehensive treatment program designed to meet the patient's individual needs. Inherent in the development of such a program is screening for conditions that require the intervention of other health care practitioners. Physical therapists are well trained to treat patients conservatively who present with mechanical musculoskeletal system dysfunction. For the purposes of this book, mechanical musculoskeletal dysfunction is defined as impaired or altered function of skeletal, arthrodial, and myofascial structures resulting from either trauma or abnormal postures.[1] To help develop the appropriate treatment program, the therapist relies on the examination process to identify the anatomic source(s) of the patient's symptoms, to determine the stage of wound healing of the lesion (acute, subacute, or chronic condition), and to identify dysfunction of the neuromusculoskeletal system that may be directly or indirectly influencing the patient's symptoms and functional limitations. Inherent in the attempt to identify the source of a patient's symptoms is ruling out certain structures that could be responsible for the complaints. This process should include screening visceral systems, which if malfunctioning could be responsible for symptoms but would not respond to physical therapy management. In addition, screening the musculoskeletal system for the presence of diseases such as cancer or infections that, if present, would require immediate medical intervention, is also necessary. For the therapist to answer the question "Does this patient present with a condition that will respond to physical therapy treatment?" the patient must be screened for the presence of medical diseases. Answering this question must be one of the primary goals of the therapist's examination process. Screening for these conditions on a systems level (i.e., urogenital, cardiovascular) as opposed to a disease level (i.e., prostatitis, mitral valve prolapse) is what differentiates the role of the therapist from that of the physician.

Differentiating between mechanical musculoskeletal dysfunction and pathologic conditions as the source of a patient's symptoms can be extremely difficult. Pathologic conditions such as gastric ulcers, prostate cancer, kidney infection, and pathologic fracture secondary to a metastatic tumor may be manifested primarily as a mechanical musculoskeletal dysfunction (e.g., joint hypomobility, abnormal muscle tonus), with the sole symptom being pelvic, thoracic, or cervical pain. Most patients with medical disease are prompted to consult a physician because of the overt nature of the medical symptoms, but patients with certain chronic visceral diseases and serious conditions, such as cancer, may not experience the expected medical symptoms. These patients may arrive at the physical therapy clinic with a diagnosis of thoracic outlet syndrome, mechanical low back pain syndrome, or cervical strain. The physical therapist must be aware of the symptoms and signs suggestive of the presence of medical disease that may be responsible for symptoms and must have a working knowledge of the disease entities most likely to be primarily manifested as pain complaints. This knowledge will facilitate the process of referral of the patient to the appropriate physician for medical examination and subsequent diagnosis.

Ruling out pathologic conditions as responsible for all or a portion of a patient's complaints is not the only reason a therapist should screen for medical disease. Assuming that a patient's symptoms are arising from mechanical dysfunction, a medical condition may be present that will influence the outcome of the treatment deemed appropriate by the evaluation findings. For example, certain cardiovascular or endocrine system disorders may have an impact on the wound-healing process of the lesion, delaying or preventing the expected changes from occurring. Certain psychological disorders may prevent a patient from responding as expected to physical therapy procedures seemingly appropriate based on the physical examination. In addition, the presence of certain medical conditions may influence the choice of treatment intervention. For example, a metabolic bone disease such as osteoporosis may influence the type of passive stretching exercise the therapist will use or the position in which the stretching is carried out to increase range of motion (ROM). Patients often arrive at the physical therapy clinic already having been diagnosed as having a medical condition. In these cases, the therapist must ask the appropriate questions regarding the patient's past and current medical history to obtain this information. In other cases, symptoms may not have progressed to the point where they have been brought to the physician's attention. The physical therapist carrying out a detailed evaluation may pick up enough clues to lead to suspicion of the presence of a medical condition. Referral of the patient to a physician would then be appropriate either to rule out the presence of a medical disease or to formulate the specific diagnosis.

The purposes of this chapter are to

1. Review evaluation principles that will assist the therapist in the differentiation of mechanical musculoskeletal dysfunction versus disease entities as the source of a patient's complaints—a process that will include a detailed review of the history and physical examination findings that could be considered clinical red flags regarding the presence of medical disease
2. Discuss examination findings that will aid the therapist in determining the presence of medical conditions that may have an impact on the patient's response to therapeutic intervention but that are not necessarily involved in the patient's symptomatic presentation
3. Present an examination scheme that incorporates the specific questions and physical examination techniques that a therapist can use to assist in screening for the presence of medical conditions
4. Review the principles of how a patient does or does not respond to treatment that may raise suspicion regarding the etiology of the patient's complaints and the appropriateness of continued physical therapy

EXAMINATION PRINCIPLES

History and physical examination findings that may suggest the presence of medical disease are discussed in the following sections. Figure 1-1 is a schematic representation of how components of the history and physical examination can help guide the therapist toward either implementing physical therapy treatment or referring a patient to a physician for a medical consult, or both, if some of the symptoms are believed to be related to mechanical dysfunction and others possibly to disease. No single question or examination procedure definitively

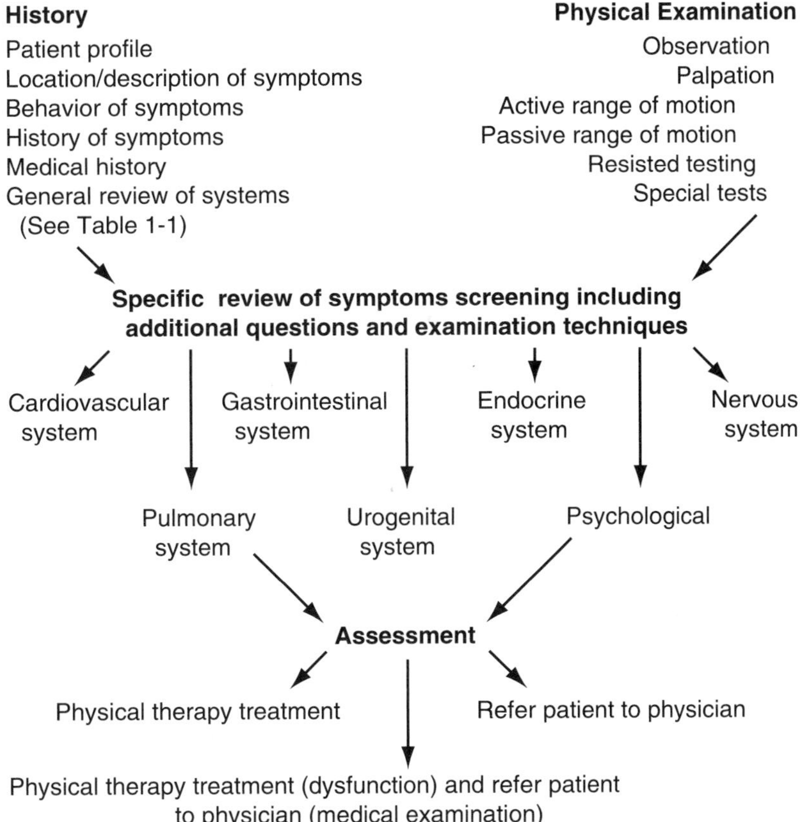

Fig. 1-1. Components of physical therapy evalutation that may provide the clinical information that leads to referring the patient to a physician.

rules out or confirms the presence of a pathologic disorder, but certain symptoms and signs, if noted, should raise suspicion in the therapist's mind of the presence of such conditions. Ultimately correlation of all history and physical examination findings will guide the therapist toward the proper clinical course. This section presents specific questions designed to screen a patient's general health and the various organ systems for disease. Also discussed is the interpretation of specific patient responses to questions that may direct the therapist to ask additional questions or implement specific physical examination techniques to provide more information regarding the patient's health status. Physical examination techniques that specifically assess the status of nonmusculoskeletal system structures are described. Finally, interpretation of physical examination findings that suggest the presence of a condition that may not be amenable to physical therapy care is presented.

History

Performing a complete and thorough history in a timely fashion can be difficult. A history that is carried out in an organized and effective fashion can greatly facilitate the decision-making process in determining how to structure and organize the physical examination, differentiating between mechanical dysfunction and pathologic origins of symptoms, and developing an effective treatment regimen.

The history can be broken down into six parts: patient profile, location and description of symptoms, symptom behavior, symptom history, medical history, and review of systems. The location and description of symptoms will usually provide the therapist with the reason the patient has come to the clinic—that is, the patient's chief complaint. Symptom behavior refers to changes in symptoms over a 24-hour period. This information will reflect the severity (symptoms affecting function) and irritability (how easily the symptoms are provoked and then subsequently alleviated) of the patient's condition. Also, if multiple symptoms are present, this information will help determine whether the symptoms are related to a single lesion. The history of the patient's condition includes a chronologic description of the symptoms, including onset of symptoms, symptom change since onset, and treatment received for the condition. Investigating a patient's medical history includes questions regarding current and past illnesses and hospitalizations, family medical history, medications, and so forth. Review of systems provides additional information regarding the status of body systems (such as cardiovascular or pulmonary). The following section focuses on the information obtained in the history that should raise suspicion in the therapist's mind regarding the presence of a medical condition that would not respond to physical therapy management or that would have an impact on the outcome of physical therapy treatment.

General Patient Profile

For the history, the therapist should record general patient information. This information could include the patient's age, sex, race, marital status, leisure activities, and occupation. Certain disease entities are more common within specific age groups. For example, prostate cancer is more common in men over the age of 50,[2] and the onset of ankylosing spondylitis often occurs between the ages of 15 and 35.[3] The incidence of certain disease processes is much higher in one sex than in the other. For example, ankylosing spondylitis appears predominantly in males,[3] while breast cancer appears predominantly in females. Bladder cancer is much more common in men.[4] Migraine headaches[5] and rheumatoid arthritis[6] are of higher incidence in women than in men. Race may also predispose certain groups to a higher incidence of specific diseases. An example would be sickle cell disease, which is more prevalent in the black population.[7] There is a higher incidence of cancers of the skin such as basal and squamous cell carcinoma and melanoma in the white population.[8] Finally, a patient's occupation may facilitate the development of certain disease processes. Exposure to extremes of hot or cold temperatures; to industrial toxins, such as lead, arsenic, and asbestos; or to extreme levels of mental or emotional pressures may contribute to the patient's clinical presentation.[5] For example, air pollutants such as coal or flour dust and fibrous substances such as asbestos can contribute to lung disease.

When appropriate, age, sex, race and occupation are noted as they relate to specific disease entities described in the remaining chapters of this book. This information can be easily gathered by the physical therapist during the examination process and may provide valuable clues regarding the presence of a suspicious condition.

Location and Description of Symptoms

The patient's chief complaint provides important initial information for the clinician. Documenting the chief complaint includes noting the location of the symptom and how the patient describes the symptoms. This information can be effectively illustrated with the use of a body diagram. Once the chief complaint has been described by the patient, the therapist should screen the remainder of the body for the presence of other symptoms. For example, let us say the patient's chief complaint is a deep, dull, aching sensation in the central low lumbar spine and right buttock, the therapist should then follow with the specific questions: Do you have any symptoms in the pelvic region, lower extremities, middle or upper back, abdominal region, chest, upper extremities, neck and head, or facial areas? Affirmative answers can then be documented on the body diagram, while asymptomatic regions can be noted with a symbol such as a check mark (Fig. 1-2). Patients may be so preoccupied with their low back pain that they forget to inform the physician that they also are experiencing headaches or right shoulder pain, neither of which is interfering with function. Patients may not volunteer to the therapist that they have abdominal or facial pain. Their rationale may be "Why does my therapist need to know if my stomach or head hurts when I am here because of my low back pain?" Yet these "other symptoms" may be related to the low back pain, possibly the result of a mechanical musculoskeletal dysfunction condition, or could be related to a disease process that is affecting a number of body parts simultaneously. Even if these "other symptoms" are not directly related to the low back pain complaints,

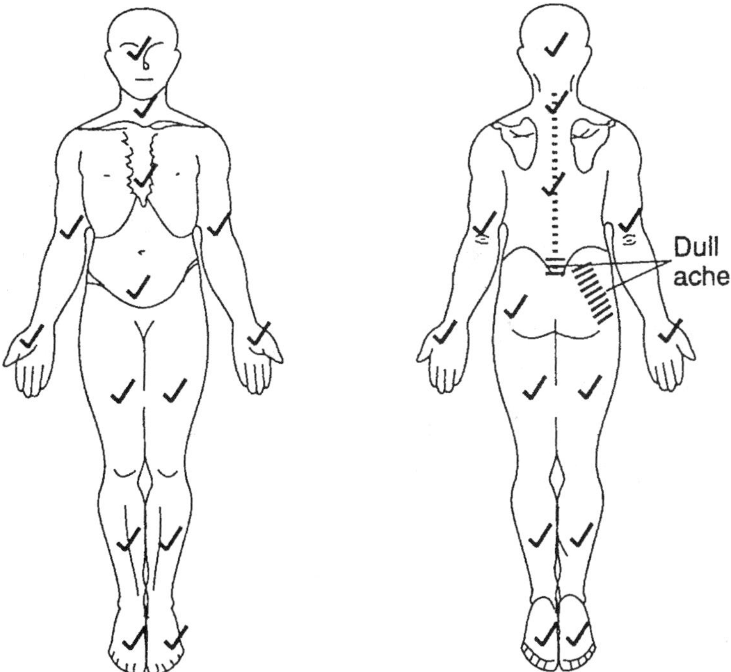

Fig. 1-2. Example of a body diagram used to illustrate symptomatic and asymptomatic body regions.

the presence of the dysfunction or disease process responsible for the symptoms may interfere with the patient's progress during physical therapy for the low back pain. Appropriate treatment, including medical care by a physician, may enhance the therapist's chances of helping the patient. The therapist should periodically repeat the process of screening the patient for location of symptoms. New symptoms may develop while the patient is under the care of the therapist, and it may be weeks or months before the patient is scheduled to see the physician. These new symptoms could be representative of the development of a pathologic condition. Again, the patient may not volunteer that these symptoms have appeared, under the misconception that they have nothing to do with what the patient is being treated for by the physical therapist.

Clinically, the location of symptoms helps little with the differentiation between mechanical dysfunction and visceral disease as the origin of symptoms. Typically, pain from visceral structures would be thought to be located in the chest or abdomen, but a number of visceri are retroperitoneal. These structures include the duodenum, pancreas, kidneys, and ascending and descending colon and, if diseased, may be manifested as back pain as opposed to abdominal pain. Other visceral structures may refer pain to the shoulder girdle or back regions (Fig. 1-3). Conversely, structures other than visceri may account for abdominal pain. Simons and Travell[9] demonstrated that numerous muscles can be the source of abdominal pain. Other structures such as ligaments and facet joints can also refer pain to the abdomen.[10,11] Not until the behavior and history of these symptoms are investigated can one begin to differentiate symptoms resulting from dysfunction versus disease.

Although symptom location helps little in differentiating symptoms, dysfunction versus disease, this information still plays an important role in medical screening. Knowledge of visceral anatomy and potential pain referral patterns of visceral structures can guide the therapist in deciding which organ systems to screen. The cardiovascular, pulmonary, and gastrointestinal systems should be screened in patients complaining of pain in the shoulder girdle and upper/midthoracic regions. The above systems and the urogenital system should be screened in patients with thoracolumbar symptoms. The cardiovascular, gastrointestinal, and urogenital systems should be screened in patients with lumbar or pelvic pain. The reader is

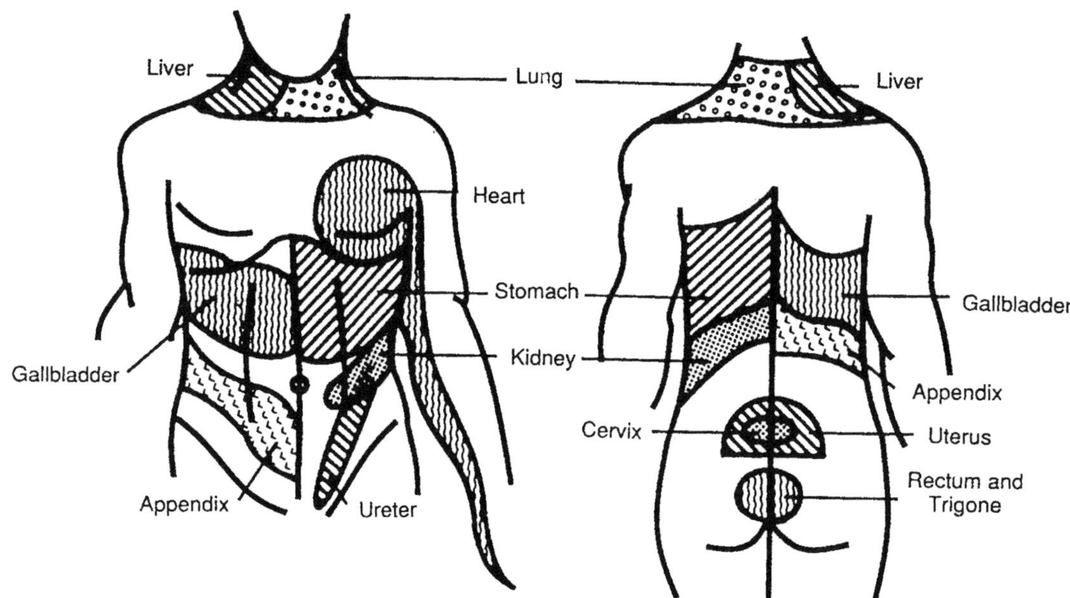

Fig. 1-3. Possible local and referred pain patterns of visceral structures.

directed to the corresponding chapter for each of these organ systems for a checklist of items to be used to help screen the system.

Investigating the chief complaint also includes the interpretation of the terms the patient uses when describing symptoms. Certain descriptors may be indicators of the presence of disease. Visceral pain has generally been described as ranging from sharp, severe, localized pain to poorly localized dull and vague sensations. The problem is that these same descriptors are also used by patients when describing symptoms from mechanical musculoskeletal dysfunction conditions. Therefore, the clinician is helped little by the presence of these particular complaints regarding the origin of symptoms. Other descriptors used by patients can be helpful, however. Sensations of cramping, colicky pain have been attributed to spasm of the smooth muscle wall of a hollow viscus. The intensity of the cramping sensation varies as the smooth muscle wall rhythmically contracts and relaxes. This contraction–relaxation cycle may last up to a few minutes. Gastroenteritis, constipation, menstruation, gallbladder disease, and ureteral obstruction have all been implicated in the cramping pain experienced in the abdomen or referred to the back.[12] Complaints of a throbbing, cramping, or aching type of pain could be suggestive of cardiovascular system involvement. Symptom descriptors such as pressure, tightness, or heaviness in the thoracic, cervical, facial, or upper extremities as well as complaints of restless legs, weakness, and the sensation of pins and needles should also prompt screening of the cardiovascular system. Weakness, poor balance, numbness, and pins-and-needles sensations should also direct the therapist to clear the patient for nervous system involvement.

At times, patients have difficulty in pinpointing the location of their symptoms and in describing exactly what their symptoms feel like. Therapists must do all they can to facilitate this information-gathering process of important clues that may raise suspicion of a disease entity. The next important category of information in the history (behavior of symptoms) is closely related to the chief complaints.

Symptom Behavior

Symptom behavior is described as a change in the location, intensity, and/or quality (e.g., pins-and-needles sensation progressing to numbness) of the patient's complaints as related to activity, cessation of activity (i.e., rest), and assumption of specific body positions.[13] A common descriptor of pain from a visceral structure is a diffuse poorly localized dull sensation. Kellgren[10,14] and Inman and Saunders[15] also described a similar pain sensation that results from irritation of deep ligamentous and musculature structures of the spine. Therefore, the chief complaint may provide minimal insight regarding whether the source of the patient's pain is a visceral or a musculoskeletal structure.

Questions regarding the behavior of the patient's complaints may help the therapist considerably with this differentiation, when faced with this clinical problem. Classically, a change in the location and/or intensity of the symptoms from mechanical musculoskeletal dysfunction can be associated with either an alteration in body posture or specific physical activities. Therefore, if the patient's complaints do not vary with movement or rest, the therapist should be suspicious of a pathologic disorder as the cause of the symptoms. Often patients state that their symptoms are constant, but further questioning indicates that the intensity of the complaint does vary during a 24-hour period. Relating the increase or decrease in symptoms to specific postures, movements, or activities is an important process for the therapist to undertake. Therapists should have expectations of how a dysfunction condition should present: increased symptoms associated with weight-bearing postures, specific movements or physical activities and alleviation of symptoms with assumption of specific nonweight-bearing postures, or other movements or physical activities. If this pattern is not offered by the patient, suspicion should be raised regarding the cause of the complaints.

Investigating symptom behavior over a 24-hour period includes questions regarding the presence of night pain. Night pain (pain waking the patient) has been associated with the presence of serious disease,[16–18] but patients with symptoms secondary to joint dysfunction and degeneration may also experience night pain.[19–21] The presence of night pain should raise considerable concern if the patient cannot fall back to sleep or considerable effort is needed to fall back to sleep. Patients waking secondary to dysfunction often need simply to change positions in bed to go back to sleep. While patients reporting needing considerable walking, pacing, sitting in a recliner, and so forth to get comfortable enough to attempt falling asleep is not typical. Concern should also be raised if the night pain is the most intense, severe pain episode the patient experiences during a 24-hour period. Pain associated with dysfunction is typically most intense and severe during weight-bearing activities and postures as opposed to when the patient is recumbent. An exception to the above scenerio is the severe, acute pain patient for whom even minimal comfort is not achieved in any position.

The therapist must be aware that the presence of symptoms that vary with movement or change in posture does not rule out the possibility of disease. For example, if a pathologic fracture secondary to a metastatic lesion is responsible for the patient's hip pain, certain activities such as standing and walking may increase the intensity of the pain significantly, while positions such as supine or side lying may not eliminate the pain but could decrease the intensity of the symptoms. Another example is occlusive arterial disease. A classic symptom is intermittent claudication, often marked by pain in the buttocks, thighs, or calves, associated with physical activity and relieved with rest. In both examples, other information obtained during the history and the physical examination hopefully will provide clues raising suspicion of the possible presence of a disease process despite symptom behavior findings that are classically representative of a mechanical dysfunction condition.

The behavior of symptoms from visceral organs will vary depending on the function of the structure. Therefore, a patient report of intermittent symptoms does not rule out the possibility of the presence of disease. If the patient's central, mid-thoracic spine pain was the result of a duodenal ulcer, gastrointestinal system activity may alter the pain complaints. For example, the pain from the ulcer may begin a couple of hours after eating and then be relieved when the patient eats. Careful questioning related to the change of symptoms experienced over a 24-hour period may reveal important information patients would not normally have volunteered, as they may not have made the connection between their symptoms and gastrointestinal system function.

Each symptom noted when documenting a patient's complaints should be fully investigated regarding its behavior. This includes noting whether the symptoms are constant or intermittently present. If intermittent, what is the change in symptoms related to activities over a 24-hour period? If multiple symptom locations are noted, as in the patient with low back, buttock, and calf pain, the therapist should not assume that one lesion is responsible for the symptoms in all three locations. The low back and buttock pain may be a result of mechanical musculoskeletal dysfunction at L5–S1, while the calf pain may be due to peripheral vascular disease. The physical therapist must pay careful attention to the behavior of each symptom to avoid being fooled, delaying the provision of appropriate medical care to the patient.

Symptom History

The onset of symptoms may also be an important factor in the differentiation between disease and dysfunction. Classically symptoms related to a mechanical musculoskeletal dysfunction are thought to be the result of a traumatic accident or incident or of an event marked by repetitive microtrauma or sustained postural strains. These events may include lifting an object, falling, or taking an extended car ride or plane trip, or the patient may report awakening with shoulder or low back pain after a day of heavy yard work. Often patients cannot relate the onset of their symptoms to a particular accident or incident. Careful questioning by the therapist regarding the activities the patient engaged in before the initial perception of symptoms often pinpoints the problem. For example, the patient may have had a change in activity level, such as beginning to run after not running for 6 months; being promoted to an administrative position on the job, involving sitting for 8 hours a day; or beginning gardening and doing yard work after a winter of relative inactivity. The therapist should consider a pathologic lesion if the onset of the patient's complaints is truly insidious, if new symptoms occur insidiously during the course of treatment, or if resolved symptoms return during the course of treatment for no apparent mechanical reason.

If the patient relates the onset of symptoms to a specific incident, such as lifting an object, the physical therapist should not rule out the prospect of a disease process as responsible for the complaints. For example, in the presence of a bony neoplastic lesion, a lifting or bending activity may sufficiently load the weakened structure so as to produce a fracture and pain. The symptoms may not be severe enough to present as a medical emergency or to warrant radiographic study, and the patient could arrive at the physical therapy clinic with complaints of low back or hip pain. Another example could be a child with no previous history of knee pain who falls and hurts her knee. Persistent knee pain precipitates a visit to the clinic. It is possible that a previously asymptomatic and undiagnosed tumor could now be responsible for the inordinate duration of the pain, considering the degree of trauma. It is hoped that other examination findings besides the onset of symptoms or lack of response to treatment will make evident the possible presence of a pathologic condition and subsequent referral to a physician. As with behavior of symptoms, each symptomatic area should be investigated regarding onset as this will help determine which complaints are related and which are not.

Medical History

At this point in the history-taking process the emphasis shifts away from pain investigation. Questions regarding current and past illnesses and subsequent treatment, including medications and surgery, family medical history, diet, and tobacco, alcohol and drug usage, can provide important information for the therapist. A self-administered questionnaire could be completed by patients to facilitate collection of this information. Figure 1-4 is one example of such a questionnaire. The therapist can use the answers provided by the patient as the basis for further discussion. For example: A patient referred to physical therapy with a diagnosis of low back pain notes on the questionnaire she has heart problems. The therapist should follow with additional questions investigating the heart condition. The patient should describe the presenting symptoms (i.e., chest pain, neck or shoulder pain, dyspnea). Noting the onset of symptoms is also important. Are they associated with walking a specific distance or climbing a flight of stairs? Once present, what does the patient do to alleviate the symptoms? Does merely stopping the activity relieve the symptoms, or must the patient take nitroglycerin? If nitroglycerin is necessary, does the patient have the medication with her? If so, is the medication easily accessible? The above information provides a therapist with a baseline from which the patient's status can be monitored while she is participating in a rehabilitation program. If the angina complaints occur the therapist also knows what the initial plan of action should be. The history of heart problems would also direct the therapist to assess pulse rate and blood pressure to obtain a baseline. If the patient later develops symptoms, necessitating assessment of vital signs, the therapist now has a basis for comparison.

If the patient denies having been treated for any of the diseases listed, the therapist should ask if the patient has been seen by a health professional for any reason other than a physical examination. Also providing a list of other diseases not included on the questionnaire to the patient is useful. Patients may forget about a particular condition, may not volunteer information they perceive

To ensure you receive a complete and thorough evaluation, please provide us with the important background information on the following form. If you do not understand a question, your therapist will assist you. Thank you!

NAME: ______________________________ AGE : ________

SS #: ______________________ OCCUPATION: ______________

LEISURE ACTIVITIES: ______________________________

Are you currently seeing any of the following?:

A. Medical doctor (M.D.)	YES	NO
B. Osteopath	YES	NO
C. Dentist	YES	NO
D. Psychiatrist/Psychologist	YES	NO
E. Physical therapist	YES	NO
F. Chiropractor	YES	NO

If you have been seen by any of the above during the past three months, please describe for what reason (illness, medical condition, physical examination, etc.):

____

____

____

Have you EVER been diagnosed as having any of the following conditions?

A. Cancer If YES, describe what kind: ______________	YES	NO
B. Heart problems	YES	NO
C. High blood pressure	YES	NO
D. Asthma	YES	NO
E. Emphysema	YES	NO
F. Chemical dependency (e.g., alcoholism)	YES	NO
G. Thyroid problems	YES	NO
H. Diabetes	YES	NO
I. Multiple sclerosis	YES	NO
J. Rheumatoid arthritis	YES	NO
K. Other arthritic conditions	YES	NO
L. Depression	YES	NO
M. Hepatitis	YES	NO
N. Tuberculosis	YES	NO
O. Stroke	YES	NO
P. Kidney disease	YES	NO
Q. Anemia	YES	NO
R. Epilepsy	YES	NO
S. Other ______________		

Fig. 1-4. An example of a self-administered form to collect patient medical history information. (From Boissonnault and Koopmeiners,[22] with permission.) (*Figure continues.*)

Please list any surgeries or other conditions for which you have been hospitalized, including the approximate date and reason for the surgery or hospitalization:

DATE	SURGERY / HOSPITALIZATION / REASON
________	________________________________
________	________________________________
________	________________________________
________	________________________________

Please describe any injuries for which you have been treated (including fractures, dislocations, sprains) and the approximate date of injury:

DATE	INJURY
________	________________________________
________	________________________________
________	________________________________
________	________________________________

Has anyone in your immediate family (parents, brothers, sisters) ever been treated for any of the following?

A. Diabetes	YES	NO
B. Tuberculosis	YES	NO
C. Heart disease	YES	NO
D. High blood pressure	YES	NO
E. Stroke	YES	NO
F. Kidney disease	YES	NO
G. Cancer	YES	NO
H. Arthritis	YES	NO
I. Anemia	YES	NO
J. Headaches	YES	NO
K. Epilepsy	YES	NO
L. Mental illness	YES	NO
M. Alcoholism (chemical dependency)	YES	NO

Which of the following OVER-THE-COUNTER medications have you taken in the last week?

A. Aspirin	YES	NO
B. Tylenol	YES	NO
C. Advil / Motrin / Ibuprofen	YES	NO
D. Laxatives	YES	NO
E. Decongestants	YES	NO
F. Antihistamines	YES	NO
G. Antacids	YES	NO
H. Vitamins / mineral supplements	YES	NO

I. Other ________________________________

Fig. 1-4. *(Continued).*

Please list any PRESCRIPTION medication you are currently taking (INCLUDING pills, injections, and/or skin patches?):

____

____

____

____

____

____

____

How much caffeinated coffee or other caffeine containing beverages do you drink per day? ________

How many packs of cigarettes do you smoke a day?

0	________
1/2	________
1/2 – 1	________
1 – 1 1/2	________
1 1/2 – 2	________
More than 2	________

How many days per week do you drink alcohol?

0 days	________		
0 – 1 days	________	4 days	________
1 day	________	5 days	________
2 days	________	6 days	________
3 days	________	7 days	________

If one drink equals one beer or glass of wine, how much do you drink at an average sitting? ________

How many days per week do you use marijuana?

0 days	________		
0 – 1 days	________	4 days	________
1 day	________	5 days	________
2 days	________	6 days	________
3 days	________	7 days	________

How many days per week do you use drugs such as cocaine, crack, acid, etc.?

0 days	________		
0 – 1 days	________	4 days	________
1 day	________	5 days	________
2 days	________	6 days	________
3 days	________	7 days	________

Fig. 1-4. *(Continued).*

to be unimportant, or may not volunteer sensitive information such as having cancer or being treated for a psychological condition. If the patient has noted having undergone surgery, investigating the reason for the surgery may reveal the presence of a condition not previously mentioned.

The medical history information collected may have a significant impact on physical management of the patient.

Example 1

A low back pain patient is referred to physical therapy with a diagnosis of degenerative disc disease. One of the treatment goals is to establish a conditioning exercise program for the patient. Investigating the medical history reveals the patient is taking β–blockers for high blood pressure. If while the patient is exercising the therapist is monitoring cardiovascular system status solely by assessing pulse rate, the patient is at risk due to the hypertensive medication affecting heart rate response to exercise.[23]

Example 2

A patient is referred to physical therapy with the diagnosis of acute rotator cuff strain/bursitis. Investigating the medical history reveals the patient has been taking nonsteroidal anti-inflammatory medication (NSAID) as prescribed by a physician 3 weeks and on his own has been taking over-the-counter Motrin. The shoulder condition begins to improve, and the patient stops taking the medication. A few physical therapy visits later the patient describes the onset of mid-thoracic pain. The therapist may theorize that the shoulder function has improved, that the mechanical stresses on the thorax have changed, resulting in "compensatory" symptoms. While this is a possibility, the therapist should also consider the role of the NSAIDs related to the thoracic pain. The association of NSAIDs and peptic ulcer disease is well documented.[24,25] While peptic ulcer disease, can be clinically silent, pain is often a presenting complaint.[26–28] But some patients with NSAID-induced peptic ulcer disease may not present with pain as long as they are taking the medication, since NSAIDs are prescribed for inflammation and pain. The perception of pain begins after the patient stops taking the medication, and, if the ulcer develops in the duodenum, a retroperitoneal structure, the patient may experience thoracic pain instead of abdominal pain. We recommend the *Drug Use Education Tips* published by the American Academy of Family Physicians, Kansas City, Missouri, as a resource for information on the most commonly used medications. Familiarity with potential side effects of medications may help the physical therapist explain some of the patient's complaints, including malaise, lightheadedness, headaches, and constipation. Asking patients why they are taking certain medications may also reveal the presence of a medical condition the patient has not mentioned (see Ch. 14 for a detailed description of how to investigate the medication aspect of the medical history).

The patient's family medical history can provide important screening. Certain disease entities, such as rheumatoid arthritis, diabetes, cardiovascular disorders, kidney disease, and cancer have familial tendencies. If family members are deceased, the therapist should inquire as to the causes of death and major illnesses for which they had been treated before death. This chapter discusses in detail the disease entities with significant familial tendencies commonly encountered by physical therapists. Positive family history alone would not warrant the therapist's referring a patient to a physician, but adding this information to the list of other concerns the therapist may have strengthens the reason for a referral when communicating with the physician.

Investigating the patient's caffeine intake, smoking, drinking, and drug use may also provide the therapist with useful information. Symptoms associated with caffeine withdrawal syndrome include headache, lethargy, and muscle pain and stiffness.[29–32] Therapists working with headache patients should be aware of the association, as it may explain a sudden change in a patient's clinical presentation. Collecting caffeine intake data during the initial evaluation will give the therapist a baseline from which intake comparisons can be made. Also, studies have associated delayed bone and soft tissue healing with cigarette smoking,[33–36] which may account for a delayed response to seemingly appropriate physical therapy. Questioning a patient regarding alcohol and drug usage is also important but can be awkward and difficult for therapists (see Ch. 12 for suggestions regarding the investigation of a history of substance abuse).

Review of Systems

The final part of the history includes a review of systems. These questions investigate the presence of symptoms in each of the major body systems, possibly identifying conditions the patient has yet to mention or which have yet to be diagnosed.[36] Figure 1-5 presents a checklist of items that reviews the patient's general health and provides initial information about each of the organ systems. Positive patient responses to any of the items should direct the therapist to ask additional specific questions and/or include physical examination tests that will provide more information about the system (see pertinent chapters for comprehensive screening checklists for each organ system). As stated, other history information that would also direct the therapist to screen a particular system includes location of symptoms and positive medical history for disease of a particular system. A discussion of the suggested checklist illustrated in Figure 1-5 follows.

The first item on the checklist, *fever/chills/sweats*, is associated with common ailments, such as "the flu," but these complaints are also associated with the presence of occult infections and cancer. *Unexplained weight change*, especially weight loss (5% of body weight over a 4-week period) is a potential symptom of a variety of ailments, including gastrointestinal disorders (e.g., ulcers or cancer), diabetes mellitus, hyperthyroidism, adrenal insufficiency, common infections and malignancies, and depression.[36] If the patient has noted weight loss, questions should follow regarding a change in diet or activity level that might explain it. The complaint of *malaise*, *fatigue*, or *loss of energy* is not an uncommon complaint offered by many patients, especially those with a long history of symptoms. This nonspecific complaint can be a result of a number of different disease entities, including depression, infections (e.g., hepatitis or tuberculosis), hypothyroidism, diabetes mellitus, anemia, cancer, nutritional deficits, and rheumatoid arthritis.[37] Certain medications may also produce malaise as a side effect.

Nausea and *vomiting* are most directly related to involvement of the gastrointestinal system. These com-

Review of Systems: General Health

Item	Yes	No	Comments
1. Fever/chills/sweats	______	______	____________________
2. Unexplained weight change	______	______	____________________
3. Malaise	______	______	____________________
4. Nausea/vomiting	______	______	____________________
5. Bowel dysfunction	______	______	____________________
6. Numbness	______	______	____________________
7. Weakness	______	______	____________________
8. Syncope	______	______	____________________
9. Dizziness/lightheadedness	______	______	____________________
10. Night pain	______	______	____________________
11. Dyspnea	______	______	____________________
12. Dysuria	______	______	____________________
13. Urinary frequency changes	______	______	____________________
14. Sexual dysfunction	______	______	____________________

Fig. 1-5. Checklist designed to review the patient's general health status, as part of the history taking process. (Modified from Boissonnault and Bass,[45] with permission.)

plaints also may denote either pregnancy or cancer or may be a side effect of certain medications. Complaints of *numbness* or *weakness* should direct the therapist to investigate the status of the nervous system. *Syncope*, the sudden but temporary loss of consciousness, is a condition associated with inadequate blood flow to the brain. Patients may also describe dizziness and lightheadedness. These symptoms may be associated with side effects of medications for cardiovascular system diseases (e.g., blood pressure problems) or may be a result of hypoglycemia in a diabetic patient. The significance of *night pain* is described under Symptom Behavior. This complaint may indicate the presence of serious pathology such as cancer. Complaints of *dyspnea* or shortness of breath could be an indicator of cardiovascular or pulmonary system disease. If this complaint is present, additional questions and objective tests should follow for further assessment of the status of these two systems. Complaints of *dysuria*, *urinary frequency changes*, and *sexual dysfunction* should direct the therapist to specific screening of the urogenital system.

Summary

Questions related to the patient's health status just before the onset of symptoms can also provide valuable information, especially if the mechanism of the onset of symptoms is unclear or vague. The same questions designed to investigate the patient's current general health status can be used. Treatment for a medical condition just before, or simultaneous with, the onset of symptoms could be significant. For example, the presence of an infectious process before the onset of symptoms could have produced infection elsewhere in the body. Patients who had a bladder infection, but who thought they had recovered from it, may have developed a kidney infection, manifested primarily as low back pain. Osteomyelitis, a condition that may result in a deep, dull, central low back pain complaint, may be precipitated by other infectious diseases, including urinary tract infections. Certain cardiovascular conditions have a history of recurrence or progressing to a point where new symptoms develop. Therefore, a history of treatment for cardiovascular problems should lead the therapist to screen the cardiovascular system during the examination.

Investigating a patient's current and past medical history is an important component of the history portion of the patient examination. These questions will help provide the therapist with information regarding the presence of medical conditions that may not be responsible for symptoms but could have an impact on how well the patient tolerates or responds to therapeutic intervention. These medical conditions could also be directly related to the patient's complaints. Therefore, the patient's report of treatment for certain medical conditions may direct the therapist to more detailed screening of visceral organ systems.

A complete history can provide helpful insight as to the presence of conditions that could interfere with a patient's response to what may be perceived as appropriate physical therapy. The preceding sections emphasized the history components related to ruling out the presence of disease that could be responsible for symptoms and to detecting the presence of disease entities that could interfere with a patient's appropriate progress while receiving treatment by a physical therapist. The history findings can also guide the therapist regarding when to implement special physical examination procedures for the purpose of gathering additional information regarding the patient's health status.

Physical Examination

Many of the physical tests used to provide information regarding the presence of disease fall outside the realm of the physical therapy profession. Examples of these tests include urinalysis, blood tests, and radiologic testing. Nevertheless, physical therapists can obtain important information if they have the knowledge and skills to implement test procedures such as assessment of blood pressure and arterial pulses and can carry out a thorough neurologic evaluation. In addition, having the knowledge to interpret the clinical findings from tests that do fall within the realm of the physical therapy profession, such as observation, palpation, and active, passive, and resisted testing, will provide invaluable clues regarding the nature of the lesion. The clinical findings most suggestive of the presence of a pathologic disorder are emphasized in this section.

General Examination Principles

Important screening information can be collected from the following examination components: observation, palpation, active (AROM) and passive (PROM) motion testing, resisted testing, and special tests. Two of the objectives of these maneuvers are alteration of symptoms and detection of dysfunction. Equally important to the screening process are both the positive findings (symptoms provoked or altered and/or dysfunction noted) and the negative findings (symptoms unchanged or not provoked and/or dysfunction not noted). Concern raised regarding the patient's status is based on the assumption of how a physical therapy condition should present clinically. Examples of this principle and exceptions to the rules follow.

Alteration of Symptoms

Alteration of symptoms from mechanical musculoskeletal dysfunction should be related to a change in the patient's posture or movement. Therefore, if the symptoms cannot be provoked or altered by the examination procedures listed above, the therapist should be suspicious of a functional (psychological) or pathologic condition. Before concluding that this patient should be examined by a physician, though, the therapist needs to consider the following: the lesion may not be irritable,[13] requiring considerable activity on the patient's part to provoke the symptoms, and the therapist may be unable to stress the tissue(s) sufficiently to bring on or increase the complaints. The therapist should be aware of this possibility, though, from information collected while investigating the behavior of symptoms. The therapist may also not have examined the appropriate body region. For example, a patient with lower extremity (bilateral) symptoms resulting from a thoracic spine lesion may have been diagnosed as a lumbar spine condition. Screening the lumbar spine, pelvis, and lower extremities alone may not have revealed the source of the symptoms. Despite the above scenarios, if the therapist is confident that the appropriate body regions have been examined, the condition "sounds" irritable, and the symptoms have not been altered, suspicion should be raised regarding the source of the symptoms.

Adding to the complexity of the clinical decision-making process, the therapist also needs to understand that alteration of symptoms during the physical examination does not absolutely rule out the presence of pathologic disorders. For example, intervertebral disc space infection may cause severe pain that varies in intensity with movement and postural changes. A pathologic fracture of a vertebral body or neck of the femur secondary to metastatic disease may also present in a similar fashion. Active or passive movement testing may stress the structural defect sufficiently to increase the patient's pain, while other movements or special tests may decrease the mechanical stress on the defect with a resultant decrease in pain complaints. In these cases, other findings from the history and physical examination, such as insufficient relief of symptoms when the patient is at rest, should help the therapist reach the conclusion that concern is warranted regarding the nature of the patient's symptoms.

Detection of Dysfunction

A physical therapy condition is marked by the presence of dysfunction. Dysfunction may be represented by abnormal soft tissue or bony palpatory findings, including abnormal skin temperature, muscle tone, bony and soft tissue contour, and texture, as well as edema. With AROM testing, both quantity and quality of movement must be considered. Abnormal quantity of movement can include decreased or excessive ROM. Assessing quality of motion includes the patient's willingness to move, the speed and smoothness of movement, and deviations from the desired, requested motion. It is feasible to have normal quantity but abnormal quality of movement.

As with AROM assessment, quantity and quality of motion need to be considered with PROM assessment. Abnormal quantity of PROM again includes decreased or excessive motion when compared with the expected ROM. Besides the patient's willingness to allow the body part to be moved, the smoothness of the motion, and deviations from the desired motion, the end feel is an important aspect of quality of PROM assessment. Cyriax[38] describes end feel as the different sensations imparted to the clinician's hand at the extreme of the possible PROM. Each movement at each joint has a characteristic end feel. Of the end feels described by Cyriax, the empty end feel is the one not typically associated with mechanical dysfunction. The empty end feel is described as the movement causes considerable pain before the end of the available ROM is reached and before the clinician senses any resistance to the force imparted.[38] Dysfunction may also be noted during resisted testing of the musculotendinous unit, marked by strength deficits.

If the therapist completes the examination and does not detect significant dysfunction related to the patient's functional limitations or symptoms, suspicion of a functional or pathologic condition is again raised. Conversely, the presence of dysfunction does not necessarily rule out disease being present. For example, the pain associated with visceral disease may be sufficient to result in muscle guarding or altered posture, affecting the patient's ability to move. Referral of a patient to a physician is rarely based on a single clinical finding. Correlation of all the data collected from the history and physical examination will help the therapist weigh the importance of an unexpected or atypical finding.

Additional test procedures that can provide important information for the therapist can be grouped under the general categories of observation, palpation, percussion, auscultation, and neurologic examination.

Observation

Observation can provide important information regarding the possible presence of disease processes. A key item to include in the examination scheme is the assessment of skin condition. This assessment includes not only the skin itself but the hair and nails as well. Most abnormalities are benign entities, but certain skin lesions are suggestive of serious pathology, including melanoma and squamous basal cell carcinoma. Characteristics of these serious lesions include variation in color within the noted area or structure, an irregular perimeter or border, a raised and irregular surface, assymetrical shape, a firm to hard consistency, and ulceration or crusting of the lesion. If the therapist notes a lesion or area of skin presenting with any combination of the above characteristics during the postural assessment or during a detailed regional examination, the patient should be asked whether the physician has noted this "spot" on the skin. Questioning the patient regarding noting a change in size, shape, or color of this area would also be appropriate. If the patient states that the physician is not aware of the area of skin involved, a recommendation that a visit to the physician would be advisable should be made in an unalarming fashion. It would then be appropriate for the therapist to telephone the physician regarding why the patient is being sent for examination (see Ch. 13 for a detailed description of screening for diseases of the skin).

Assessment of skin color can also be easily carried out during the postural or regional examination. Cyanosis, a dark bluish coloration of skin, including nails and/or the mucous membranes secondary to poor oxygenation of the blood, can be a sign of advanced lung disease or cardiovascular system involvement. Centrally, the lips, buccal mucosa, or tongue are usually the best structures to assess for the presence of cyanosis, whereas the skin and nails of the upper and lower extremities are the best areas for peripheral assessment. Jaundice, the yellowish coloration of structures, including the skin, tongue, and lips, can be representative of a liver disease or a blood disorder. The scleras of the eyes may also show the color change associated with jaundice. Pallor or paleness of skin can be suggestive of cardiovascular system disorders, including arterial insufficiency and anemia. Abnormal redness may also be indicative of the presence of a disease process. Skin marked by the presence of red streaks can be suggestive of the presence of an infectious process.[36]

Assessment of skin condition also includes observation of body hair and nails. Hair loss of distal extremity parts, such as hands and forearms or feet and lower legs, can be indicative of a peripheral vascular disease. More general hair loss may also be associated with anemia and hypopituitarism, while increased hair patterns can be seen in Cushing syndrome and with certain cancers, such as of the adrenals and gonads. Deformities of the nails can also be markers of disease. Clubbing of the nails can be indicative of pulmonary system disease including lung cancer. Clubbing of the nails is described as the angle between the fingernail and nail base exceeding 180 degrees, with the nail base being swollen and soft.[36] Transverse sulci running perpendicular to the longitudinal axis of the nail (Beau's lines) may accompany anemia, malnutrition, and the acute stage of infectious diseases. Pitting of the nails have been associated with psoriasis, diabetes, and peripheral vascular disease. Nails that are spoon shaped (concave) can be associated with anemia, chronic infection, malnutrition, and Raynaud syndrome.[38]

Palpation

Palpation is another important component of the objective examination that can indicate signs of the presence of disease. Palpation can be used for skin temperature, lymph nodes, vascular pulses, and abnormal soft tissue or bony masses. Besides observation, assessment of the skin and associated structures includes palpation for skin temperature. General decreased skin temperature is one sign of hypothyroidism, while general increased skin temperature is one sign of hyperthyroidism.[36] Localized increased temperature is associated with the presence of an inflammatory process, but, if the tissue temperature is very warm to hot, an infectious process must also be considered.

Palpable lymph nodes may suggest the presence of infection or neoplasm. Although palpable lymph nodes are not easily found in healthy people, lymph nodes of up to 1 cm are considered normal. The presence of palpable lymph nodes that seem to be fixed or immovable from underlying tissues should raise concern. Normal lymph nodes should not be tender to touch, but nodes that are not tender are not necessarily normal. Lymph nodes to which malignancy has spread are usually not tender.[8] Areas that should be palpated for lymph nodes include the submandibular, supraclavicular, anterior and posterior cervical regions, and the axilla. Another important region of the lower quarter to be palpated is the femoral triangle, especially around the inguinal ligament. Generally lymph nodes are also found in close proximity to all the major peripheral joints, including the elbow, wrist, knee, and ankles.

Palpation of peripheral arterial pulses may reveal important information regarding the status of the cardiovascular system. An absent or diminished pulse suggests vascular obstruction that may be related to the patient's complaints. Lower-extremity pulses to be assessed include the femoral artery in the femoral triangle, the popliteal artery, and the dorsal pedis and posterior tibial arteries. In the upper extremity, the brachial artery in the cubital fossa and the radial and ulnar arteries at the wrist should be assessed. Central pulses that can be palpated include the aorta and iliac arteries. The carotid artery can be used, but the therapist must consider that even light pressure on the vessel may stimulate the carotid pressure receptors, resulting in a drop in the heart rate (see Ch. 2 for the parameters of a normal versus abnormal pulse).

When assessing the abdomen, and especially before doing soft tissue mobilization techniques for the abdominal region, the therapist should palpate for the presence of an aortic aneurysm. Most aortic aneurysms occur caudal to the renal arteries and produce a pulsation that is more prominent and distinct within a confined region than in a normal aorta. A palpable pulse greater than 2 to 3 inches wide should raise suspicion of the presence of aneurysm.

Palpation for the presence of abnormal soft tissue and bony masses is an ongoing process during the examination. The clinician must have in-depth knowledge of normal anatomy to be able to detect abnormalities. Many therapists lack familiarity of the normal anatomy of the abdomen, yet the abdomen is an area that often needs manual treatment to improve extensibility of scar tissue, to treat trigger points in the abdominal muscle wall or iliopsoas muscle groups, and to decrease tone in musculature accessible through the abdominal wall, including the abdominals, respiratory diaphragm, and iliopsoas groups (see Ch. 4 for a detailed description of normal abdominal anatomy).

Percussion

Applying a vibratory force to bone tissue may provide information regarding the presence of a disease state or fracture. In the spine, the spinous processus is percussed with a reflex hammer or with fingertips with the patient in a forward-flexed posture. The presence of infection or tumor may be marked by provocation of either severe pain and tenderness or a deep, dull, throbbing pain that does not decrease in intensity immediately after completion of the technique (see Ch. 10 for more information regarding the use of percussion as an examination procedure).[39]

Percussing other body regions, such as the thorax and abdomen, can also give important information regarding the health and location of soft tissue structures. Percussing over solid organs, such as the liver or spleen, should produce a decreased resonance or dullness to the sound. Assuming that there are no abnormal masses in the abdomen, percussing over most of the abdominal cavity will usually produce a tympanic sound (low-pitched, drumlike noise). Exceptions may occur if percussing over the suprapubic region when the bladder or uterus are distended. Normal fluid and fecal material may also produce a duller sound. Physical therapists can use percussion to locate structures such as the liver or spleen and take the appropriate precautions when doing deep soft tissue mobilization techniques in the upper abdominal region (see Ch. 4 for further information regarding assessment of the abdomen).

Auscultation

Listening for body sounds to help assess the status of an organ system is a common evaluation tool used by therapists working in a hospital setting. In certain situations in an outpatient setting, auscultation may provide valuable information to the therapist regarding a patient's health status (see Chs. 2 and 3 for more detailed guidelines regarding the use of auscultation and interpretation of auscultatory findings).

Neurologic Examination

This section provides an overview of neurologic examination principles with emphasis on reflex, sensory, and motor testing (see Chs. 8 and 9 for a detailed description of assessment of the neurocranium and other components of the central and peripheral nervous system).

An argument could be made for performing a neurologic examination on all patients to obtain a baseline of normal regarding the status of their nervous system. There are times, however, when inadequate time to complete the initial evaluation prevents the therapist from including the neurologic examination in the initial visit, or the patient's complaints might not warrant including the neurologic examination within the initial assessment scheme. A neurologic examination should be carried out during the initial evaluation for any patient who describes such symptoms as radicular pain (pain that follows the path of a nerve), weakness, numbness, and/or paresthesias. Some patients may note that they have been dropping objects, stubbing their toes, or tripping over their feet, indicating possible weakness. Others may describe a hand that feels heavy or dead or as though it is falling asleep or hypersensitivity or irritability of the skin, indicating possible sensory changes. Any of the above complaints should direct the therapist to carry out a neurologic examination during the initial assessment. If positive neurologic signs are detected during the evaluation, retesting the status of the nervous system should be a part of each subsequent visit (before and after treatment) to monitor the patient's status closely. This should be done even if the patient reports significant reduction in pain complaints or possibly being pain free. It is possible in this situation that the compression on the nerve has progressed to complete occlusion. The patient's perception is that the problem has subsided because of the reduction in pain, but in fact the condition has worsened. Progressive worsening of neurologic signs should be brought to the physician's attention immediately.

The three most commonly used components of the neurologic examination are reflex, sensory, and motor testing. Appendices II and III list specific tests that can be performed in weight-bearing (standing, sitting) and nonweight-bearing (prone, supine) positions. To provide more valid and reliable information, the tests should be performed with the patient positioned in a consistent fashion. For example, if during a lower-quarter screening examination a portion of the neurologic assessment is done with the patient sitting and the remainder with the patient supine, inconsistent or false-negative findings may occur because of the change in pressure exerted on the nerve or the change in the degree of stretch placed on the nerve as the lumbar spine assumes a different position. False-negative findings may occur, however, even if all the tests are done with the patient remaining in a single position. Patients with a lumbar spinal nerve root compression secondary to lateral foraminal stenosis may be sitting with the lumbar spine in a kyphotic posture or may be supporting the trunk weight on their hands (propping themselves up, unweighting the lumbar spine). These positions may sufficiently relieve the compressive forces on the nerve so all the neurologic tests are negative. Another example would be a patient with cervical radiculopathy. The test results may be altered or influenced by inconsistencies in the patient's head and neck posture. While sitting, the patient may be watching the therapist perform the different tests, placing the neck in a variety of forward-bent, side-bent, and rotated positions. This altered head and neck posture would again alter the environment of the nerve root. The therapist must closely monitor the patient's trunk, head, and neck positions while carrying out neurologic assessment. Consistent spine positioning and considering weight-bearing versus nonweight-bearing postures can greatly enhance the gathering of this important clinical information.

Testing for the status of deep tendon reflexes can be carried out for selected upper- and lower-extremity muscles and selected facial and trunk musculature. The reflex response can be graded using a 0 to 4 scale. A 2+ grade represents a normal response, a 0+ represents an absent response, while 1+ represents a diminished response. A 3+ grade indicates a brisk response and a 4+ grade indicates a very brisk response. Grieve[40] recommends repetitive testing, tapping the tendon up to six times in order to detect the possible presence of a fading reflex response indicating a developing nerve root lesion.

When assessing the abdominal reflexes, instead of being tapping, the skin is stroked with the end of the reflex hammer. Each of the four abdominal quadrants (see Fig. 4-5) is gently stroked, noting movement of the umbilicus. If the reflex is intact, the umbilicus will move toward the stimulus. The upper abdominal quadrants represent the T7–T10 segments, while the lower abdominal quadrants represent the T10–L1 segments.[41]

The most commonly used sensory tests are light touch and pinprick. The clinician notes hyperesthesia, hypoesthesia, numbness, and/or paresthesia as indicators of involvement of the sensory component of the nervous system. Careful comparison of left versus right corresponding body parts can help the therapist detect these sensory changes. If the patient notes a difference in the quality of pinprick or light touch stimulus (i.e., "I don't feel as much on the left side"), the therapist can then compare different regions within the same extremity to help determine whether the left side is hypoesthetic or if the right side is hyperesthetic. The location of the sensory changes will help the therapist differentiate between a peripheral nerve lesion and a spinal nerve root lesion (see Figs. 9-9 and 9-10 for the sensory fields—dermatome versus peripheral nerve supply).

Testing the motor component (myotome) of the nervous system consists of assessing strength of a selected muscle or muscle group that primarily represents a single neurologic segment of the spinal cord. The process of strength assessment usually begins with observation of active ROM of the joint the muscle crosses, against gravity. Active ROM, gravity eliminated, can be implemented if indicated. Assuming the patient can move the joint against gravity, either an isometric contraction against manual resistance or applied resistance throughout the active ROM can then be incorporated into the testing process. A 0 to 5 grading scale can be used to document the test findings. A 0 grade indicates no contraction noted, 1 indicates a flicker/trace of contraction, 2 indicates active movement with gravity eliminated, 3 implies that active movement can occur against gravity, 4 indicates active movement against gravity plus against manual resistance, while a grade 5 indicates normal strength with manual resistance applied.[42]

Applying these test procedures should allow the clinician to detect many of the patient's neurologic motor deficits, but to avoid false-negative findings the therapist should also incorporate repeated contractions or sustained isometric contractions of the muscle or muscle group. Cailliet[43] states that minor compromise of a nerve may be manifested by muscle fatigue rather than by frank weakness. The sign, fatiguability, is more likely to be present in the early stages of nerve root compromise. Detecting muscle fatigue could easily be missed if the myotome test consisted only of a "break" strength test. Even using sustained manual isometric contraction for large, powerful muscles such as quadriceps or the gastrocnemius/soleus may not reveal the muscle fatigue. Cailliet recommends using repetitive unilateral heel raising to assess the gastrocnemius/soleus group as a more delicate method of testing for minor impairment of the S1 nerve. Repetitive unilateral standing deep knee bends could be used for assessing the quadricep muscle group. Careful monitoring of the patient's posture while performing these movements would be extremely important. For the smaller muscle groups (e.g., anterior tibialis, extensor hallucis longus, and biceps), a sustained isometric contraction should be sufficient to screen the upper- and lower-extremity myotomes adequately for the onset of fatigue.[43]

If weakness is noted, the therapist must consider other sources of the deficit besides spinal nerve root involvement. A peripheral nerve lesion or a local muscle condition may also produce the weakness discovered. For example, if the patient presents with shoulder abduction weakness (C5–C6, axillary nerve), the therapist must consider: Does the lesion lie in the C5–C6 nerve roots, in the axillary nerve, or in the shoulder abductor muscle (supraspinatous will be considered)? Other C5–C6 muscles (elbow flexors, musculocutaneous nerve) that are not innervated by the axillary nerve can be tested. If the elbow flexors are also weak, a spinal nerve root lesion as the source of the weakness is supported. If the elbow flexors are strong, an axillary nerve lesion or structural muscle weakness may be responsible for the abduction weakness. A local supraspinatous muscle lesion would be marked by clinical findings, such as absence of other neurologic signs and observable or palpable changes in the muscle. Appendices II and III list the upper- and lower-extremity muscles and their central and peripheral innervations, which can be used for these testing purposes. In addition, correlation of other neurologic signs, such as location of sensory changes and deep tendon reflex findings, may help with this differentiation.

Monitoring the status of a patient's nervous system is an important responsibility of the physical therapist. Progressive worsening of neurologic signs warrants an immediate phone call to the physician. Immediate medical intervention may be necessary to prevent irreversible damage to the nerve tissue.

Summary

Incorporating the above principles and items of the history and physical examination into the evaluation scheme should not add inordinate time to the patient's initial visit. To keep the examination time efficient, the therapist must develop a well-organized history and physical examination format that begins with questions and techniques aimed at providing general information regarding the patient's status. The information obtained during the history will help the therapist decide (1) which body region(s) to assess objectively; (2) which specific examination techniques to use or omit; (3) the sequence of physical examination including patient positioning; and (4) the degree of aggressiveness of the various techniques. The history will also provide valuable information regarding the origin of symptoms, mechanical versus pathologic. Starting the physical examination with an upper- or lower-quarter screening examination can also save the therapist valuable time. These general clearing tests help direct the therapist to examine specific body regions in detail and determine areas of mechanical dysfunction that are directly or indirectly related to the patient's symptoms. In addition, tests are included that help screen the patient for the presence of medical disease. Figure 1-6 presents a general

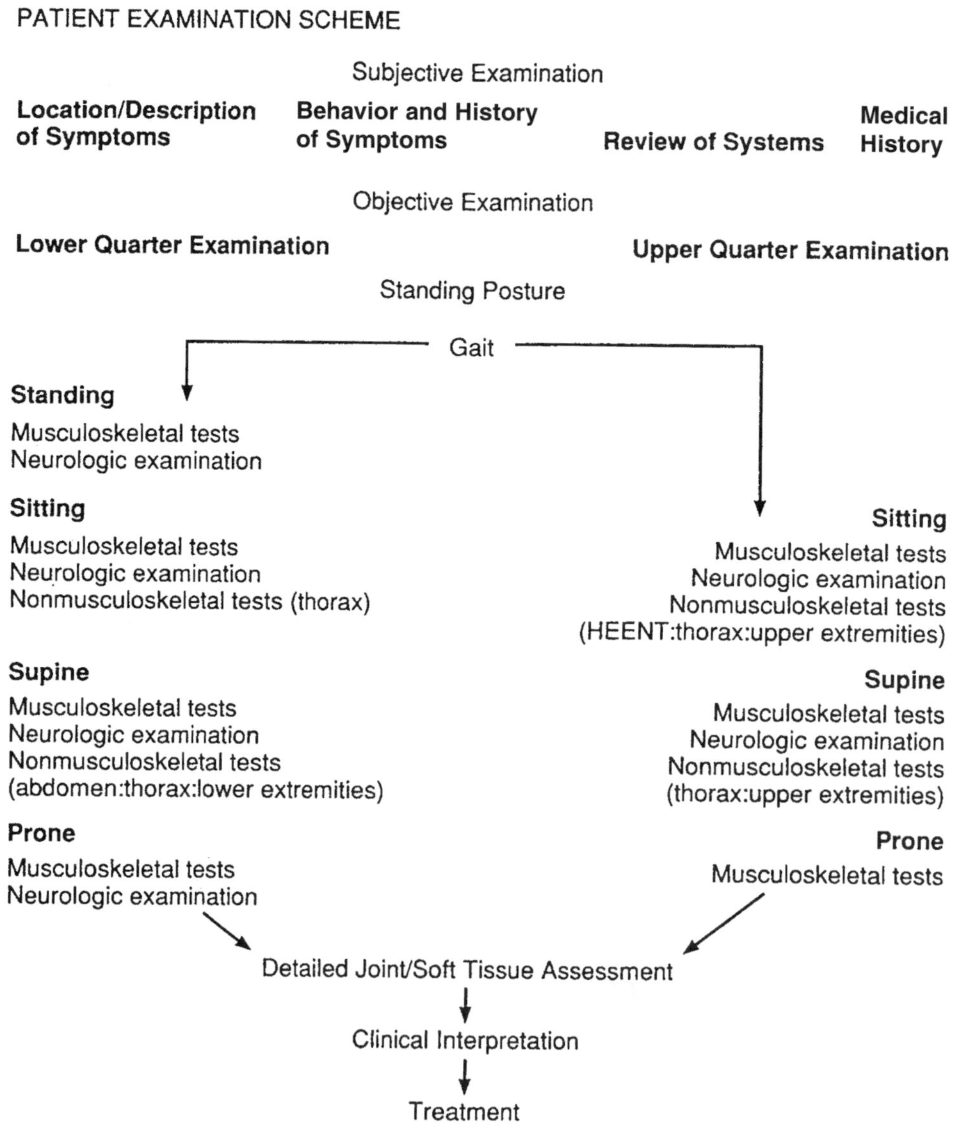

PATIENT EXAMINATION SCHEME

Subjective Examination

Location/Description of Symptoms — **Behavior and History of Symptoms** — **Review of Systems** — **Medical History**

Objective Examination

Lower Quarter Examination — **Upper Quarter Examination**

Standing Posture

Gait

Lower Quarter Examination

Standing
Musculoskeletal tests
Neurologic examination

Sitting
Musculoskeletal tests
Neurologic examination
Nonmusculoskeletal tests (thorax)

Supine
Musculoskeletal tests
Neurologic examination
Nonmusculoskeletal tests
(abdomen:thorax:lower extremities)

Prone
Musculoskeletal tests
Neurologic examination

Upper Quarter Examination

Sitting
Musculoskeletal tests
Neurologic examination
Nonmusculoskeletal tests
(HEENT:thorax:upper extremities)

Supine
Musculoskeletal tests
Neurologic examination
Nonmusculoskeletal tests
(thorax:upper extremities)

Prone
Musculoskeletal tests

Detailed Joint/Soft Tissue Assessment
↓
Clinical Interpretation
↓
Treatment

Fig. 1-6. General patient examination scheme leading to detailed assessment of specific body regions.

examination scheme; Appendices II and III detail the components of suggested upper- and lower-quarter screening examinations.

Owing to time constraints, normally only one of the two screening examinations will be performed during the initial evaluation. Generally, the location and description of symptoms from the history will determine which quadrant examination will be used. Structuring these examinations by position is usually physically easier for the patient and more time efficient for the therapist. The sequence of positioning suggested is standing, sitting, supine, and then prone, although the acuteness of the patient's condition and behavior of the symptoms could alter this sequence. Specific approaches to carrying out and interpreting the tests designed to screen the patient for medical conditions (see Appendices II and III) are described throughout this book. Numerous textbooks are available that describe other tests designed to screen for mechanical dysfunction.

Once the therapist has gathered information from the history and physical examination, analysis and interpretation of findings follow. A problem list is generated from the examination. This is then followed by devising a hypothesis as to what the underlying pathologic process may be giving rise to the patient's signs and symptoms and what possibly precipitated their onset. Relative to diagnosis and treatment of mechanical dysfunction, Maitland[44] uses the term *assessment* in two ways. The first meaning includes interpreting the history of the patient's disorder and the symptoms and signs, so that a diagnosis can be made; determining the stage in the natural history of the disorder; and determining the psychological effect the disorder is having on the patient, taking into account such factors as ethnic background, home, and job situation. The second meaning refers to determining the effect the treatment has had, by checking the patient's symptoms and signs after each application of every technique. This assessment is used to prove the value of the technique used at that particular stage of the disorder. From this information, goals and a prognosis are developed for the patient's treatment program.

Response to Treatment

Prognosis is very important in guiding the therapist. The therapist should have expectations as to how the patient should respond to treatment, both subjectively and objectively. It may not be until noting how the patient responds to treatment that the therapist begins to question the underlying condition responsible for the symptoms. Any deviation from the expected should raise a question as to why the patient is not responding appropriately.

Take the case of a patient with a complaint of headaches. During the physical examination significant joint and soft tissue dysfunction with a moderate loss of cervical ROM are noted. Treatment is initiated and the patient returns for the second visit. The patient notes a marked improvement in the headache, but when the therapist reassesses the patient, the physical examination findings are similar to those noted initially. Treatment is again administered and the patient returns for the third visit. This time the patient describes a marked worsening of the headaches. Yet reassessment of cervical ROM reveals similar findings to the second visit when the patient was doing so well. At this point the therapist needs to question the relevance of the dysfunction to the patient's complaints. During the course of treatment, the physical therapist must continually correlate the subjective and physical examination findings. If the symptoms are related to dysfunction, when symptoms improve, corresponding observable or palpable functional improvement should be noted. Conversely, if marked worsening of symptoms are described, corresponding observable or palpable regression should be noted. If the above-described correlation of changes is not found, the therapist should be suspicious of the presence of a functional (psychological) or pathologic condition.

What can confuse the issue is that it is not uncommon for a patient to have more than one condition responsible for the complaints. Patients may have both musculoskeletal and nonmusculoskeletal conditions simultaneously, making differential diagnosis difficult. A number of patient cases are described to illustrate the above points.

PATIENT CASE STUDY 1

A patient saw her internist with primary complaint of left-sided frontal headaches, as well as left-sided neck and shoulder symptoms. Her physician did a physical examination, ordered a computed tomography (CT) scan, and a benign meningioma was found. Subsequent surgery alleviated the problem. Several months later, the headaches were gone, but the left-sided neck and shoulder symptoms persisted. The patient was referred to an orthopaedic surgeon and subsequently to physical therapy, and clinical signs of a grade II strain of the left supraspinatous were found. Subsequent treatment alleviated the symptoms.

PATIENT CASE STUDY 2

A therapist asked a colleague from the same clinical facility, on an informal basis, to treat her lower back, which was painful as of late. Symptoms were local central pain, not accompanied by neurologic signs or symptoms or by radicular symptoms, but with some decrease in active ROM of trunk, with pain provoked during these movements. The symptomatic therapist was treated twice with heat and passive mobilization exercise. After the second treatment, ROM had markedly improved; however, subjectively there was not a concurrent improvement in pain; in fact, the symptoms were now more constant and intense in nature. At that time, the treating therapist began a more thorough review of the history and review of systems and found she had had surgery several years earlier for pancreatic cancer. The patient offered that she had regular physical examinations and a recent CT scan 1 month before that was negative. She was advised to return to her physician, who ordered repeat scans that revealed metastatic lesions in the abdomen and anterior lumbar spine. Although secondary to abnormal circumstances regarding the abbreviated initial examination, it was the incongruous change in signs versus symptoms that stimulated the treating therapist to perform a more thorough examination and to refer this patient back to the physician.

PATIENT CASE STUDY 3

A 54-year-old woman was referred by a physician who reported a diagnosis of C4–C5 nerve root impingement secondary to an osteophyte in the right intervertebral foramen. She had insidious onset of 1-month duration of intermittent right posterolateral cervical aching with intermittent radiation of the aching to the right side of her head, "through the head" to the right eye (Fig. 1-7). Behavior of symptoms revealed that looking over the right shoulder increased the cervical pain. The patient also noted gross loss of motion in all directions. The primary complaint was that of increased pain and headaches with lying, especially at night before sleep. The pain also woke her two to three

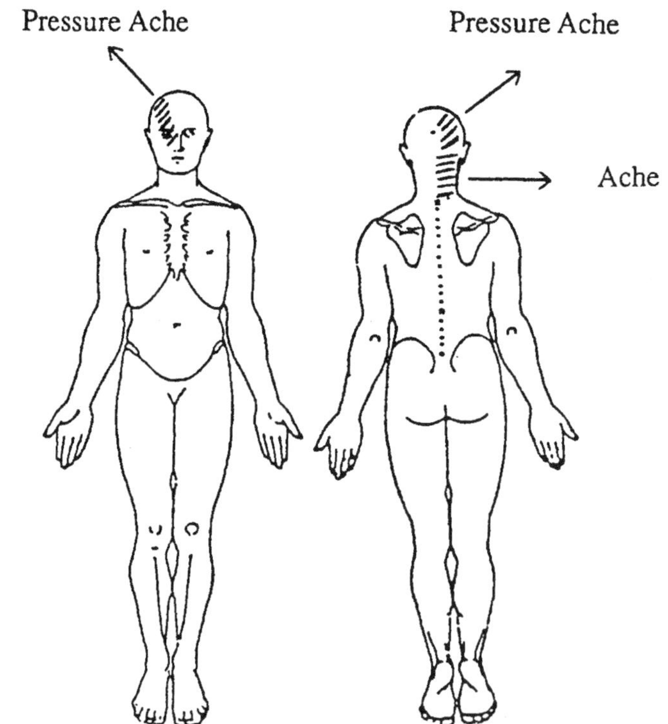

Fig. 1-7. Symptom location for a 54-year-old woman. Intermittent ache, right posterolateral cervical region, and pressurelike ache in the right side of cranium.

times each night. The patient relieved her symptoms temporarily with deep pressure in the right occipital area and with massage and heat.

Review of systems revealed that the patient is currently undergoing chemotherapy for inoperable breast cancer. There are active metastases in her lungs. A bone scan and CT scan of the cervical region were performed 2 weeks before physical therapy examination, and these were unremarkable. The patient had undergone a mastectomy on the right 1 year ago, after which she claimed complete return to function of the right upper extremity without complaint of symptoms. She complained concurrently of some shortness of breath, depression, and nausea but had experienced these since starting chemotherapy. She denied dizziness, syncope, or changes in vision.

Objective Examination

Active ROM of the shoulders into abduction and flexion was 140 degrees bilaterally without pain. Active cervical ROM revealed that chin to chest caused minimal ache in the neck, extension 45 degrees with increase in strain in the mid-cervical area, side bending right 20 degrees with an increase in right-sided neck pain with radiation into the head, and side bending left 40 degrees and pain free. Left rotation 70 degrees produced a slight increase in right-sided neck symptoms, and right rotation 10 degrees produced a marked increase in neck symptoms with radiation to the head. General passive ROM essentially showed the same pattern of restriction of movement and provocation of symptoms as active ROM.

Passive accessory intervertebral movement testing of the cervical spine demonstrated hypomobility throughout the upper cervical region, but without reproduction of symptoms. Passive physiologic intervertebral movement testing also revealed a decrease in mobility throughout the cervical region, especially with a decrease in right passive rotation of C1, which when tested appeared to diminish the patient's symptoms. There was minimal tenderness to palpation in the cervical spine, especially in the upper cervical area, with some spasm noted here bilaterally. Radiologic findings were reported as moderate cervical spondylosis.

The therapist's assessment at this time was (1) primary dysfunction at C1–C2 into right rotation as most limited, but both directions restricted; (2) pain severe relative to functional level (the patient was slightly hysterical, using many descriptors, such as "miserable" and "incredible," to describe her pain); and (3) her medical history is positive for cancer, but this apparently has been ruled out recently. A trial of manual therapy to improve rotation right at C1–C2 was initiated. The patient did not appear irritable to this movement and was thought to tolerate treatment well. Given that symptoms are decreased with this technique, the patient should show short-term improvement.

Treatment and Response

On day 1, manual therapy to increase right rotation resulted in a slight decrease in symptoms and a 5-degree increase in right rotation. On day 2, the patient reported a significant decrease in headaches since her first visit, especially immediately after treatment. ROM and right rotation were worse at this time; treatment continued with heat and manual treatment to C1, which afforded the patient some relief and slight increase in right rotation.

On day 3, pain was now intense and sleeping very difficult. The patient was now hysterical. She came to the clinic 4 hours before her appointment time crying. On reassessment she was noted to be in a right side bent and left rotated head posture, more so than previously. Some relief of symptoms was afforded simply by assuming a supine position. Manual treatment techniques gradually allowed her to increase her right rotation and extension, but after sitting or standing after treatment, her pain and antalgic cervical posture returned within several minutes. Subsequently, the patient's physician was called and her response to treatment was explained. She was referred back to her physician for reexamination. She was then referred to an orthopaedic surgeon and sent for magnetic resonance (MR) imaging to the upper cervical spine. Approximately 5 days later, the patient called with information concerning the diagnosis as metastatic disease to the right C2 vertebra with extension into the right epidural space and right C2–C3 neural foramen (Figs. 1-8 and 1-9).

PATIENT CASE STUDY 4

A 29-year-old flight attendant was referred with a diagnosis of supraspinatus strain and bursitis of the left

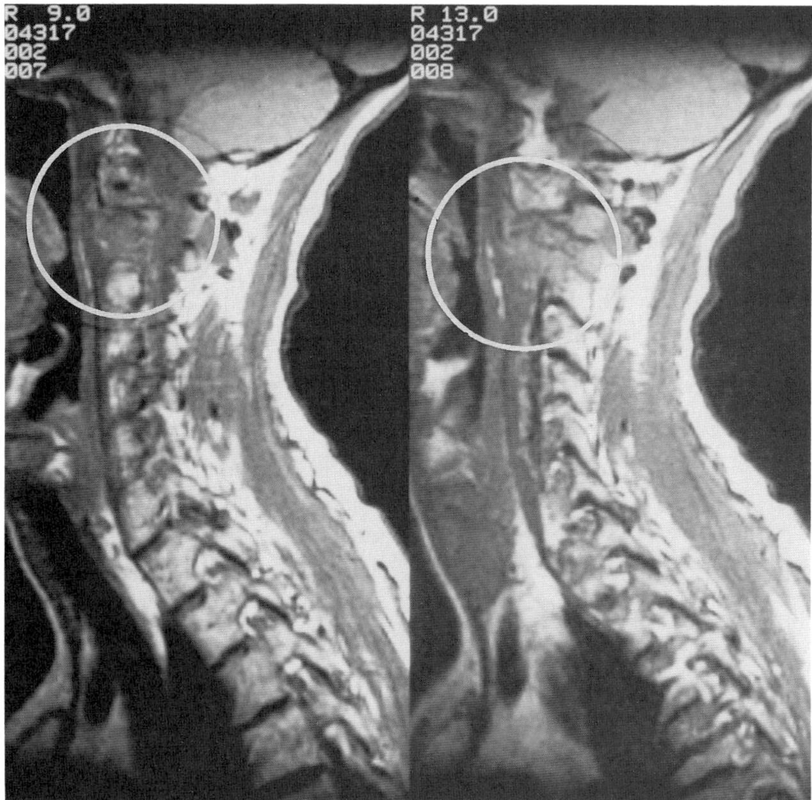

Fig. 1-8. Sagittal view, magnetic resonance imaging. The metastatic lesion is circled.

shoulder. She presented with complaints of left-sided anterolateral shoulder pain and of an occasional sharp but more often burning sensation with occasional grinding and snapping into the shoulder; she also had left-sided cervical spine stiffness, left interscapular aching, and tightness. She had a history of occasional symptoms in the right shoulder in the same location. The patient related that her left shoulder was irritated by overhead movements after several repetitions, especially lifting overhead, lifting her flight bag during work, and lying on her left side. She obtained relief with medications, heating pad, hot shower, and deep massage. Medication included ibuprofen several times a day.

Review of systems revealed little; she was in good health. A history of endometriosis 1 year earlier in 1989 was noted. Previous surgeries included thyroid surgery 10 years earlier secondary to Graves disease. The patient stated that she was right handed. The patient believed that her mother was diagnosed as having rheumatoid arthritis.

History

Two years earlier, while pulling a garment bag from the overhead compartment in an airplane, she had felt a quick jolt of pain in the left shoulder; she felt a pop, and her arm dropped down to her side. The pain was eased immediately afterward but again was painful later that night, primarily at the top of the shoulder. She later saw a physician for this problem and, over the course of a year, had radiographs taken and several subsequent injections into the left subacromial bursa. This afforded minimal relief of symptoms for a short period of time. Upon physical examination, palpation demonstrated tenderness and some thickening of the subdeltoid bursa, more so on her left. Active elevation was slightly hypermobile at the shoulders bilaterally, with pain on the left from 150 degrees until the end of ROM. Internal rotation was slightly limited with slight pain at the end range. Passive physiologic movement demonstrated a

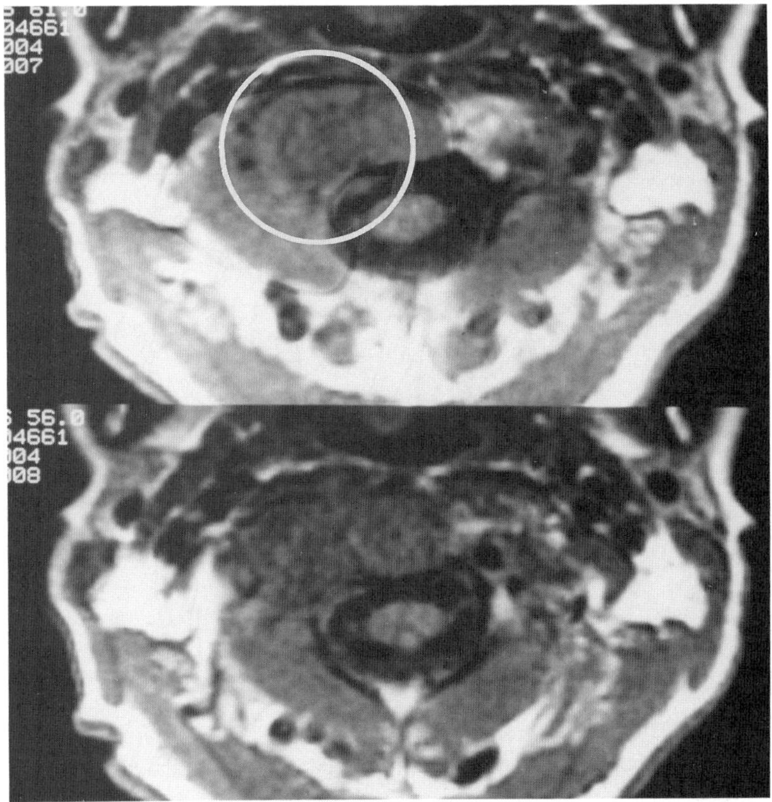

Fig. 1-9. Axial view, magnetic resonance imaging. The metastatic lesion is circled.

similar pattern of movement and pain complaints. Muscle testing revealed 4/5 strength and complaint of pain with resisted abduction and external rotation of the left shoulder.

The patient demonstrated an apparent subdeltoid bursitis/strain of the rotator cuff on the left with generalized hypermobility of both glenohumeral joints, postural dysfunction through the upper quarter facilitating anterior positioning of the humeral head bilaterally secondary to decreased muscle tone, and protraction of the shoulders, generalized weakness in the shoulder girdles bilaterally, and localized stiffness in the cervical and thoracic spine. She had no other complaints or problems of the joints of the upper or lower extremities at that time.

Treatment and Response

The initial treatment course consisted of ultrasound, massage, and passive mobilization exercise followed by resistive exercise/home program for the shoulder girdles. Over the next several visits, she responded very well to treatment with decreased pain, increased ROM, and increased strength of the left shoulder girdle. She continued to work full-time as a flight attendant during her physical therapy treatment course. There were several episodes of exacerbation of symptoms during this time, but each episode was directly related to increased physical exertion of the upper extremities while at work. Overall she continued to improve. The patient was seen for several months, for a total of 12 visits. Several of these sessions emphasized an exercise training class for strengthening of the shoulder girdles, head, neck, and upper extremities. She returned to physical therapy for reassessment and for manual treatment after a 2-week layoff. At this time she had increased complaints of generalized soreness and achiness in several of her joints, including increased pain in both shoulders (Figs. 1–10 and 1–11). On physical examination, she was noted to have an increase in synovial thickening, swelling,

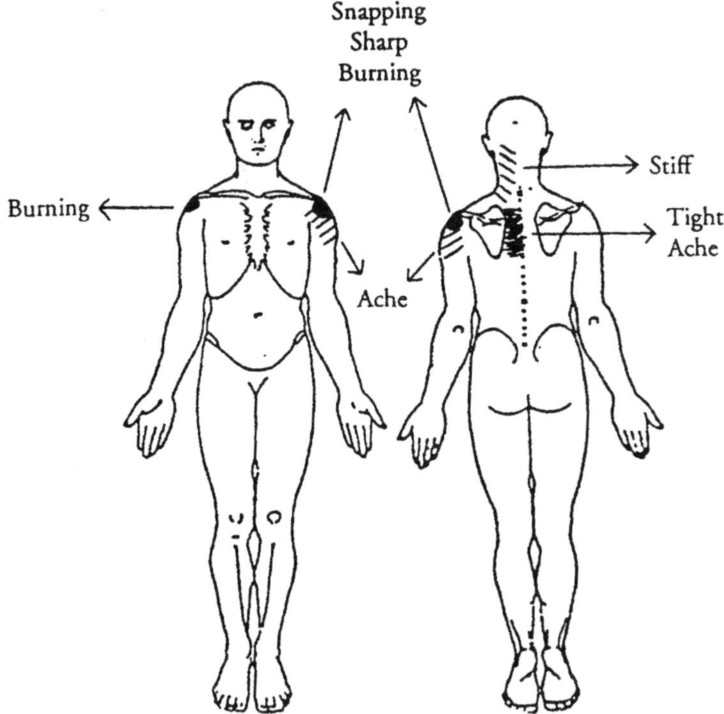

Fig. 1-10. Symptomatic complaints at the initial visit.

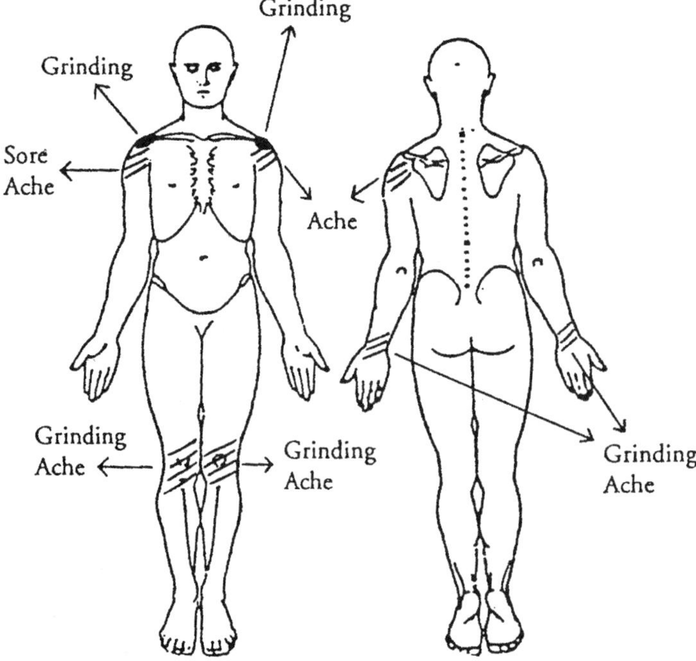

Fig. 1-11. Symptomatic complaints several months after the initial evaluation.

and pain upon palpation of both glenohumeral joints and associated bursae, with decreased abduction and increased crepitation of the shoulders bilaterally.

Secondary to exacerbation of left shoulder symptoms, onset of right shoulder symptoms similar to the left, and multiple other joint complaints (wrists and knees), the patient was asked to seek consultation from a rheumatologist. It was approximately 1 month before she could see this physician, at which time she returned for physical therapy and stated that she had been diagnosed as having systemic lupus erythematosus.

PATIENT CASE STUDY 5*

History

The patient was a 47-year-old highway maintenance worker who was referred to the clinic with a diagnosis of mechanical low back pain syndrome. His chief complaints were constant sharp pain across the lumbosacral junction accompanied by a numb feeling in both buttocks and intermittent numbness in the right anterior thigh. He also complained of intermittent cramping and throbbing pain in the calves bilaterally (Fig. 1–12). The low back and buttocks symptoms were aggravated by sitting for more than 30 to 45 minutes and standing in one place for more than 5 to 10 minutes and by transitional movements such as sit to stand. The intensity of these symptoms decreased by assuming a recumbent position or by constantly changing positions. The right anterior thigh and calf symptoms were specifically provoked by walking a distance of 3 to 4 blocks. The symptoms were then relieved by sitting for short periods of time. The patient described his low back condition as originating in 1978 when reaching out of the cab of his truck to pull a rope; he had felt a sharp tug in the low lumbar region. He had had constant low back and buttock symptoms since the incident, despite receiving four to five separate series of physical therapy sessions. The calf symptoms began in 1985 during the patient's involvement in a fitness program, with just the left calf symptomatic. This problem was diagnosed as a vascular condition and was subsequently treated by angioplasty. The patient felt partial relief of the left calf pain after the procedure but had noted an increased left calf pain and insidious onset of right calf pain during the past year.

The patient's medical history included undergoing three left knee surgeries and bilateral elbow surgery. He suffered a myocardial infarction in 1986. He had a 26-year history of smoking 1 to 2 packs of cigarettes per day. His family medical history showed that his mother had died of a cardiac condition at age 62 and his father of a myocardial infarction at age 58. Radiologic tests of the lumbar spine revealed degenerative facet joint disease from L3 to S1.

Objective Examination

Observation demonstrated a decreased lumbar lordosis and slight lateral shift of the trunk to the right. There appeared to be hair loss of the lower legs and feet. Slight increase in paraspinal muscle tone was noted from L4 to S1 bilaterally with palpation. Also, weak dorsalis pedis and posterior tibial artery pulses were noted bilaterally. These low lumbar and buttock symptoms were provoked with active forward and backward bending in standing. All active movements were moderately restricted. Sharp local low back pain was provoked with passive stress on the L5–S1 segment. Significant hypomobility was noted at L5–S1 and at the thoracolumbar junction. The calf and right anterior thigh symptoms were not provoked with active movements or passive overpressures of the trunk and joints of the lower extremities. When the patient was asked to ambulate, these symptoms were provoked by the time he had walked 100 to 150 feet. Sitting down quickly relieved the thigh and calf symptoms. The low back and buttock symptoms did not change during the ambulation or subsequent sitting. The patient was then asked to ride a stationary bike; within 1 to 2 minutes, the right thigh and calf symptoms returned. Shortly after the patient stopped pedaling, the symptoms disappeared. Again, as with the ambulation, the low back and buttock symptoms did not change with the bike riding.

Assessment and Outcome

The presentation of multiple symptomatic areas is especially challenging when trying to determine the origin of symptoms. Is a local lesion responsible for each symptomatic area? Is one lesion responsible for all the symptoms? Answering these questions requires a detailed his-

*(From Boissonnault and Bass,[46] with permission.)

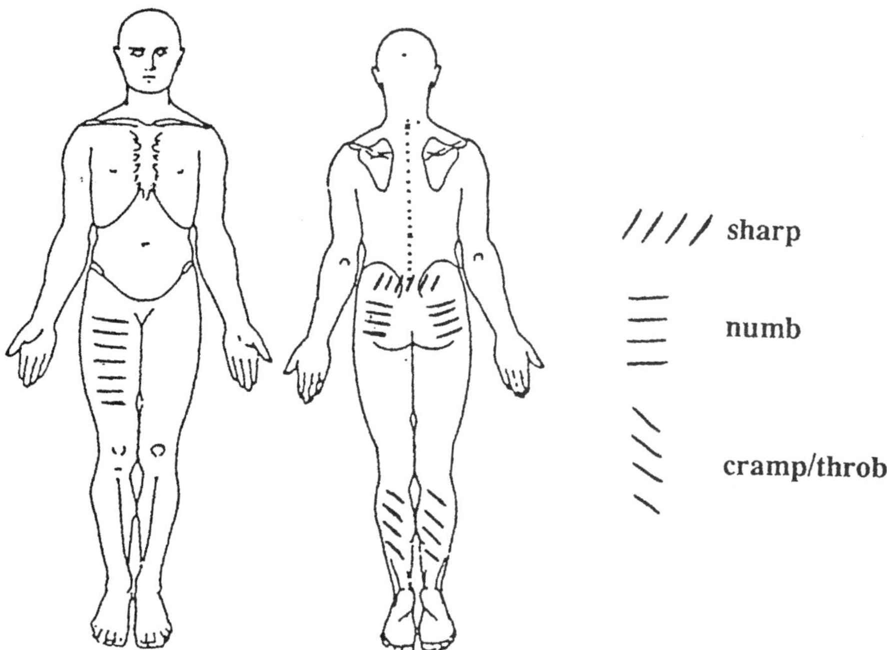

Fig. 1-12. Symptom location for a 47-year-old man. Constant lumbosacral junction and buttock complaints with intermittent right thigh and calf complaints. (From Boissonnault and Bass,[46] with permission.)

tory regarding the behavior and chronologic history of each of the symptoms described by the patient. Also, a careful screening of the appropriate body regions with palpation, active and passive movements, resisted testing, and special tests can provide valuable information regarding the source of the various symptoms.

It was apparent, after the evaluation, that this patient's low back and buttock symptoms were related and that the right anterior thigh and bilateral calf symptoms were related as well. The evaluation findings also suggested that the lumbar and buttock symptoms were the result of mechanical musculoskeletal system dysfunction, while the right thigh and calf symptoms might be related to peripheral vascular system disorder. The lumbar and buttock symptoms were consistently aggravated by sitting, standing, and transitional movements and alleviated by assuming a recumbent position. There was a common precipitating incident for the lumbar and buttock complaints.

Both symptoms were provoked with active movements of the trunk and passive stress on the L5–S1 segment. The anterior thigh and calf symptoms presented with a different behavior pattern; they were only provoked with a specific amount of activity, walking, or biking, then subsequently relieved with sitting. This is the classic pattern of clinical findings associated with intermittent vascular claudication. This finding led to detailed questions regarding the cardiovascular system. These questions revealed the 26-year history of smoking, the myocardial infarction in 1986, past treatment for peripheral vascular disease, and the significant family history of cardiovascular system disease. In addition, careful assessment of the lower-extremity pulses and observation of skin condition had revealed additional signs suggesting possible involvement of the cardiovascular system causing a portion of this patient's complaints.

All this information was communicated to the referring physician. Further medical testing was carried out revealing the presence of significant peripheral vascular disease. While these medical tests and subsequent treatments were being implemented, the patient received physical therapy for the dysfunction related to the lumbar and buttock complaints.

SUMMARY

This chapter emphasized the information obtained during the history and physical examination that would direct the therapist to a more detailed screening of the various organ systems. A general health screening list was presented that could easily be incorporated into the history. These items should be screened in all patients. An upper- and lower-quarter screening examination scheme was also presented. This examination format illustrates how tests that screen for the presence of mechanical dysfunction and medical disease can be clinically integrated.

The information provided is not intended to prepare the therapist to make a medical diagnosis and suggest medical treatment. Rather it is to assist the therapist in screening for the presence of medical disease and to be able to communicate with the physician as to why the patient is being referred.

REFERENCES

1. 1990 Yearbook and Directory of Osteopathic Physicians. 1981 Ed. p. 675 American Osteopathic Association, Chicago, 1990
2. Badalament RA, Drago JR: Prostate cancer. Postgrad Med J 87:65, 1990
3. D'Ambrosia RD: Musculoskeletal Disorders, Regional Examination and Differential Diagnosis. 2nd Ed. JB Lippincott, Philadelphia, 1986
4. Schrier RW, Gottschalk CW (eds): Diseases of the Kidney. Vol. 1. 5th Ed. Little, Brown, Boston, 1992
5. Seidel HM, Ball JW, Dains JE, Benedict GW: Mosby's Guide to Physical Examination. CV Mosby, St. Louis, 1987
6. Kelley WN, Harris ED Jr, Ruddy S, Sledge CB: Textbook of Rheumatology. 4th Ed. Vol. 1. WB Saunders, Philadelphia, 1993
7. Kelly WN, Harris ED Jr, Ruddy S, Sledge CB: Textbook of Rheumatology. 4th Ed. Vol. 2. WB Saunders, Philadelphia, 1993
8. Schwartz MH: Textbook of Physical Diagnosis, History, and Examination. WB Saunders, Philadelphia, 1989
9. Simons DG, Travell JG: Myofascial origins of low back pain. 2. Torso muscles. Postgrad Med 73:66, 1983
10. Kellgren JH: On the distribution of pain arising from deep somatic structures with charts of segmental pain areas. Clin Sci 4:35, 1939
11. McCall IW, Park WM, O'Brien JP: Induced pain referral from posterior lumbar elements in normal subjects. Spine 4:441, 1979
12. Raj PP: Prognostic and therapeutic local anesthetic block. p. 908. In Cousins MJ, Bridenbaugh PO (eds): Neural Blockade in Clinical Anesthesia and Management of Pain. 2nd Ed. JB Lippincott, Philadelphia, 1988
13. Maitland GD: Vertebral Manipulation. 5th Ed. Buttersworth, London, 1986
14. Kellgren JH: Observations of referred pain arising from muscle. Clin Sci 3–4:175, 1938
15. Inman VT, Saunders JB: Referred pain from skeletal structures. J Neurol Ment Dis 99:660, 1944
16. Weinstein JN, McLain RF: Primary tumors of the spine. Spine 12:843, 1987
17. Bianco AJ: Low back pain and sciatica: diagnosis and indications for treatment. J Bone Joint Surg AM 508:170, 1968
18. Sim FH, Dahlin DC, Stauffer RN, Laws ER: Primary bone tumors simulating lumbar disc syndrome. Spine 2:65, 1977
19. Földes K, Bálint P, Gaál M et al: Nocturnal pain correlates with effusions in diseased hips. J Rheum 19:11, 1756, 1992
20. Jönsson B, Strömquist B: Symptoms and signs in degeneration of the lumbar spine: a prospective, consecutive study of 300 operated patients. J Bone Joint Surg 75-B:381, 1993
21. Siegmeth W, Noyelle RM: Night pain and morning stiffness in osteoarthritis: a crossover study of flurbiprofen and diclofenac sodium. J Intern Med Res 16:182, 1988
22. Boissonnault WG, Koopmeiners MB: Medical history profile: orthopaedic physical therapy outpatients. J Orthop Sports Phys Ther 20:2, 1984
23. McArdle W, Katch F, Katch V: Exercise Physiology, Energy Nutrition and Human Performance. 3rd Ed. Lea & Febiger, Philadelphia, 1993
24. Agrawal N: Risk factors for gastrointestinal ulcers caused by non-steroidal anti-inflammatory drugs (NSAIDS). J Fam Pract 32:619, 1991
25. Hazleman BL: Incidence of gastropathy in destructive arthropathies. Scand J Rheumatol 78:1, 1989
26. Miller DK, Burton FR, Burton MS, Ireland GA: Acute upper gastrointestinal bleeding in elderly persons. J Am Geriatr Soc 39:409, 1991
27. Nunes D, Kennedy NP, Weir DG: Treatment of peptic ulcer disease in the arthritic patient. Drugs 38:451, 1989
28. Aabakken L, Weberg R, Lygren I, et al: Gastrointestinal bleeding associated with the use of nonsteroidal anti-flammatory drugs—symptomatology and clinical course. Agents Actions Spec No. C86–87, 1992
29. Couturier EGM, Hering R, Steiner TJ: Weekend attacks in migraine patients: caused by caffeine withdrawal? Cephalalgia 12:99, 1992
30. Griffiths RR, Evans SM, Heishman SJ et al: Low-dose caffeine physical dependence in humans. J Pharmacol Exp Ther 255:1123, 1990

31. Hughes JR, Higgins ST, Bickel WK et al: Caffeine self-administration, withdrawal, and adverse effects among coffee drinkers. Arch Gen Psychiatry 48:611, 1991
32. Silverman K, Evans SM, Strain EC, Griffiths RR: Withdrawal syndrome after the double-blind cessation of caffeine consumption. N Engl J Med 327:1109, 1992
33. Brown CS, Orune TJ, Richardson HD: The rate of pseudoarthrosis (surgical nonunion) in patients who are smokers and patients who are nonsmokers: a comparison study. Spine 11:942, 1998
34. Lind J, Kramhoft M, Bodtker S: The influence of smoking on complications after primary amputations of the lower extremity. Clin Orthop 267:211, 1991
35. Jones, J, Triplett R: The relationship of cigarette smoking to impaired intraoral wound healing: a review of evidence and implications for patient care. J Oral Maxillofac Surg 50:237, 1992
36. Bates B: A Guide to Physical Examination and History Taking. 5th Ed. JB Lippincott, Philadelphia, 1991
37. Malasanos L, Barkauskas V, Stoltensberg-Allen K: Health Assessment. 4th Ed. CV Mosby, St. Louis, 1990
38. Cyriax J: Textbook of Orthopaedic Medicine: Diagnosis of Soft Tissue Lesions. 8th Ed. Vol. 1. Bailliere-Tindall, London, 1982
39. Zohn DA, Mennell J: Musculoskeletal Pain, Diagnosis, and Physical Treatment. 2nd Ed. Little, Brown, Boston, 1987
40. Grieve GP: Common Vertebral Joint Problems. 2nd Ed. Churchill Livingstone, Edinburgh, 1988
41. Hoppenfeld S: Physical Examination of the Spine and Extremities. Appleton and Lange, East Norwalk, CT, 1976
42. Devinsky O, Feldmann E: Examination of the Cranial and Peripheral Nerves. Churchill Livingstone, New York, 1988
43. Cailliet R: Low Back Pain Syndrome. 2nd Ed. FA Davis, Philadelphia, 1968
44. Maitland GD: Peripheral Manipulation. 3rd Ed. Butterworth-Heinemann, London, 1991
45. Boissonnault B, Bass C: Pathological origins of trunk and neck pain: part I–pelvic and visceral disorders. J Orthop Sports Phys Ther 12:192, 1990
46. Boissonnault B, Bass C: Pathological origins of trunk and neck pain: part II—disorders of the cardiovascular and pulmonary systems. J Orthop Sports Phys Ther 12:208, 1990
47. Kei-Hua, E: Kung-Fu Meditations and Chinese Proverbial Wisdom, Farout Press, Thor Publishing, Ventura, CA, 1994

2 Screening for Cardiovascular System Disease

Theresa Hoskins Michel, M.S., P.T., C.C.S.
Jill Downing, M.D.

Physical therapists have always had an important role in the evaluation and treatment of peripheral vascular diseases and, for at least the past two decades have expanded their efforts in cardiac rehabilitation. Some of the earliest writings by physical therapists describe tests available for the evaluation of the peripheral vascular system, as well as walking programs designed for the treatment of indolent ulcers and intermittent claudication.[1,2]

Today, the practice of physical therapy extends to all body systems and to nearly all disease entities. The cardiovascular system continues to require the expertise of physical therapists versed in this system and should be considered by any physical therapist who is screening particular signs or symptoms involving chest, neck, face, and the upper or lower extremities. This chapter describes disease entities that may give rise to such signs or symptoms. Information is provided on medical screening procedures and physical therapy evaluation techniques used to assess the cardiovascular system.

It is often difficult to differentiate the sources of local peripheral edema, jaw pain, or tingling in the fingers, any of which may have a cardiovascular origin. In the absence of a specific diagnosis, the physical therapist must decide when these complaints need to be referred to a physician for a differential diagnosis. The evaluation procedures described in this chapter will help the physical therapist provide vital information to the physician. By screening a patient's left shoulder pain and ruling out angina pectoris, the physical therapist can proceed to evaluate other potential sources of the complaint without imposing undue restrictions on the patient's activity. By recognizing angina the physical therapist can aid in the early and appropriate intervention for a life-threatening condition.

There is not always a clear-cut differentiation between cardiovascular causes of symptoms and musculoskeletal system dysfunction. Many complaints of pain in the upper or lower extremities are extremely confusing to the patient and the health professional, even after a thorough medical screen. The physical therapist's ability to provide pertinent information about these complaints can prove invaluable. In the event that cardiovascular disease is present, the physical therapist needs to recognize the implications this presents for treatment precautions. For example, heart disease may impose limits on the intensity and type of physical activity that are safe for the patient. Wound healing will be impaired in the patient with vascular compromise.

This chapter provides an overview of the anatomy and physiology of the heart and peripheral vasculature. The general symptoms and signs of cardiovascular diseases are described, and the screening procedures available to the physical therapist are presented. Objective tests used for the medical screening of these symptoms or signs are listed with parameters for normal or abnormal, such as blood pressure, pulse palpation, and electrocardiography (ECG). Specific common cardiovascular diseases are presented, including the pathophysiology, histology, and usual findings of diagnostic medical tests. Appendix 2-1 provides physical examination techniques for evaluation of cardiovascular diseases.

CARDIOVASCULAR ANATOMY AND HISTOLOGY

The cardiovascular system is a massive network of three types of blood vessels connected to a pump, the heart. Efferent flow of oxygenated blood is carried in arteries of progressively diminishing caliber. Veins convey blood back to the heart. The interface between these two types of vessels in many parts of the body is the third type of vessel, the capillary. Another network of vessels is the lymphatics, which carry a tissue fluid known as lymph away from peripheral circulation and toward the heart, ultimately draining into the venous system through the thoracic duct. The main transport function of the lymphatics is to remove fluid and large diameter molecules from the systemic circulation. The heart itself is somewhat pyramidal in shape and is encased in a double-layered sac known as the pericardium. It is located within the middle mediastinum and is divided into four chambers: the right and left atria and right and left ventricles. Three external surfaces can be identified: the sternocostal, or anterior; the diaphragmatic, or inferior; and the base, or posterior surfaces. In addition, the distal tip of the left ventricle defines the apex. Directed down, forward, and to the left, it is at the fifth left intercostal space, 3½ inches (9 cm) from the midline (Fig. 2-1).

Unoxygenated or venous blood returns to the heart through the inferior vena cava, passing into the right atrium. It then flows into the right ventricle, pulmonary artery, and pulmonary vascular bed, where carbon dioxide and oxygen are diffused. Freshly oxygenated blood returns to the heart through the pulmonary veins into the left atrium and left ventricle. Blood is ejected into the aorta for systemic distribution. The flow of blood out of each chamber is regulated by the presence of a heart valve. The tricuspid valve is located between the right atrium and right ventricle, the pulmonic valve between the right ventricle and pulmonary artery, the mitral valve between

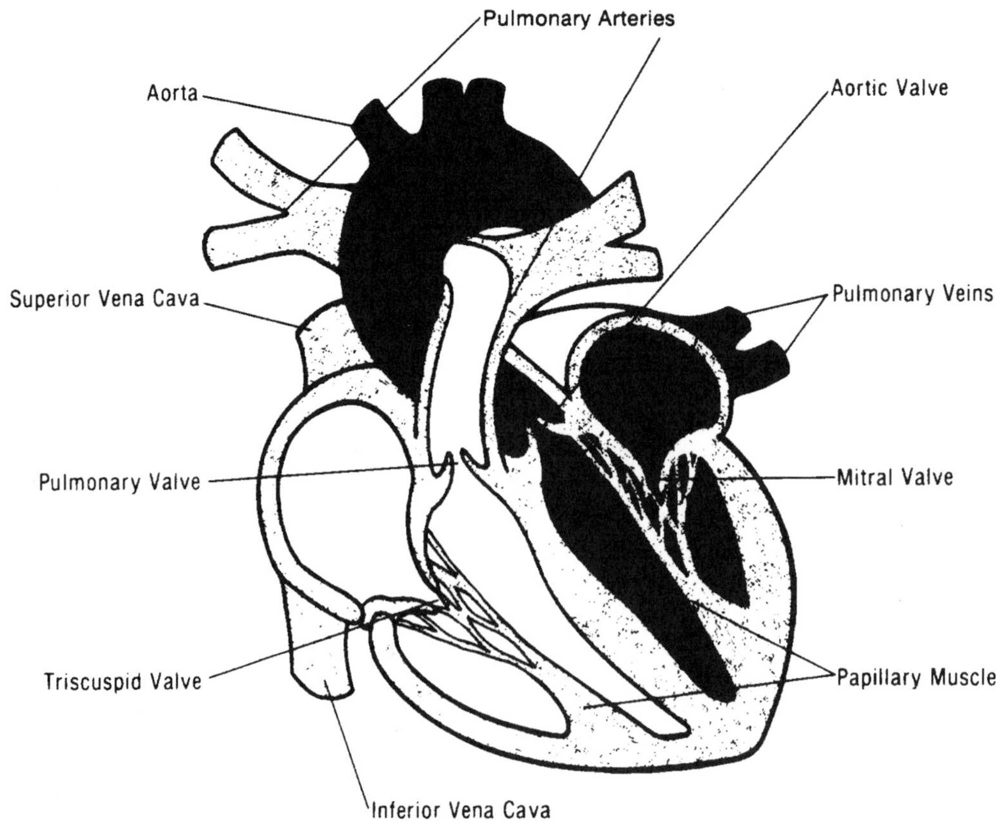

Fig. 2-1. Cross section of the heart and great vessels. (From Cohen and Michel,[3] with permission.)

the left atrium and left ventricle, and the aortic valve between the left ventricle and aorta (Fig. 2-1). The heart itself is composed of three layers of tissue. The thick cardiac muscle, the myocardium, is covered externally with serous pericardium, called the epicardium, and internally with a layer of endothelium, the endocardium.

The heartbeat originates in a specialized system of cardiac muscle cells that generate and conduct electrical impulses. Known as the conducting system of the heart, this system provides for the synchronized contraction of cardiac muscle and a cardiac output that meets the body's metabolic needs. Structurally it is composed of the sinus node, the atrioventricular (AV) node, the AV bundle with its right and left branches, and the subendocardial plexus of Purkinje fibers (Fig. 2-2). The heart is nourished by an arterial supply provided by the right and left main coronary arteries, which arise from the aorta directly above the aortic valve (Fig. 2-3). The number and configuration of branches that arise from these two vessels vary considerably from one individual to the next. In most cases, however, the right coronary artery travels anteriorly and inferiorly along the right side of the heart, perfusing the right atrium, the right ventricle, portions of the left ventricle, and the sinus and AV nodes. The left main coronary artery usually gives rise to the left anterior descending and circumflex branches and perfuses the entire left ventricle and most of the left atrium. Cardiac innervation is by both the sympathetic and parasympathetic fibers of the autonomic nervous system. Sympathetic fibers arise from the cervical and upper thoracic portions of the sympathetic trunks and the parasympathetic supply from the vagus nerves.

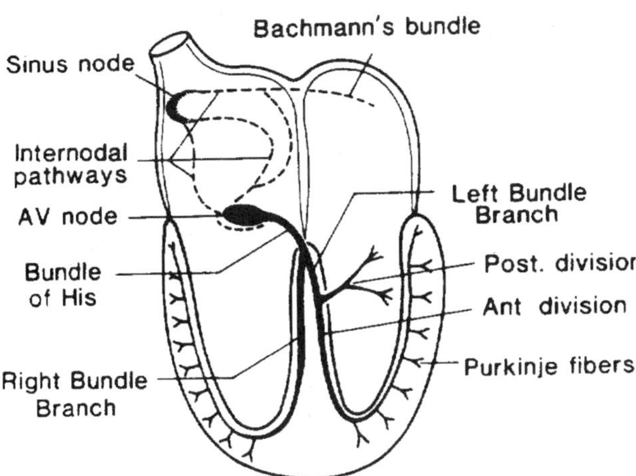

Fig. 2-2. Diagrammatic representation of the conducting system of the heart. (From Albarran-Sotelo et al.,[4] with permission.)

The flow of oxygenated blood to the peripheral tissues is carried by arteries. Regardless of their diameter, all arteries consist of three microscopic layers: the intima, media, and adventitia. From inside out, the intima is thin and forms the interface between the vessel and the circulating blood. It is composed of the endothelium, a basement membrane, and an elastin membrane. The media is formed by layers of smooth muscle cells and an elastic membrane. Finally, the adventitia of the artery appears with its collagenous support structure through which pass blood vessels, lymphatics, and nerves to the artery itself (Fig. 2-4). At the level of the arteriole, blood passes to the capillary, where it equilibrates with the interstitial fluid. Capillaries drain through venules to veins. While the same microscopic layers are present in veins, they contain little smooth muscle tissue in the media. Vein walls are, therefore, thin, and easily distended. In the veins of the extremities, a series of bicuspid valves are present, preventing the retrograde flow of venous blood.

Cardiovascular Physiology

The cardiovascular system transports substances absorbed from the gastrointestinal tract and oxygen from the lungs to the tissues and returns the products of metabolism to the kidneys and carbon dioxide to the lungs. It has a role in controlling body temperature and distributes hormones and other substances important to cell function. The functions of the cardiovascular system and the influences on it can best be appreciated by looking separately at the heart and the circulation.

The Heartbeat

The heartbeat consists of an orderly sequence of events involving contraction of the atria, known as atrial systole, followed by contraction of the ventricles, ventricular systole. This is followed by diastole, during which all four chambers are relaxed. The heartbeat originates in the specialized myocardial cells of the cardiac conduction system. Because of faster rates of discharge, the sinus node has the role of cardiac pacemaker. The electrical impulses it generates spread across the atrial myocardium, through

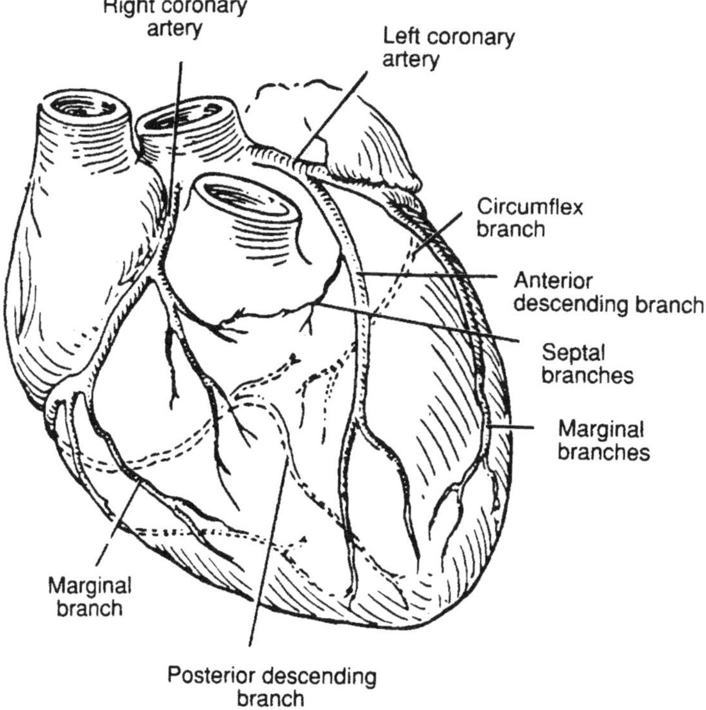

Fig. 2-3. Coronary arteries, showing the arterial supply to the surface of the heart. (From Ross,[5] with permission.)

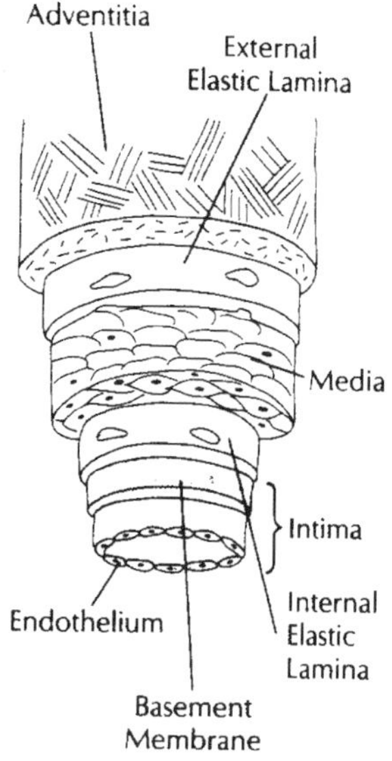

Fig. 2-4. Cellular architecture of the artery. (Modified from Stein et al.,[6] with permission.)

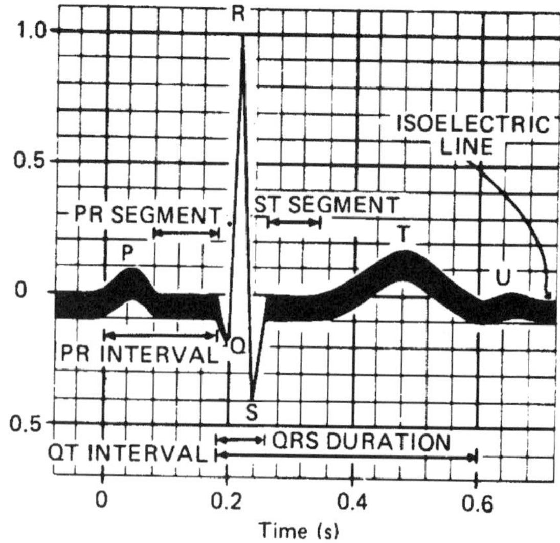

Fig. 2-5. PQRST pattern of the electrocardiogram. (From Ganong,[7] with permission.)

the AV node, and into the ventricles. The ventricles are depolarized in an "inside–outside" fashion, stimulating the endocardium, myocardium, and finally the epicardium. An inherent property of all excited muscle cells is the ability to produce an action potential that is transmitted along its membrane. The electrical event that occurs is a result of chemical changes resulting from ion fluxes across the muscle cell membrane. A transmembrane action potential is composed of rapid depolarization, plateau, and slow repolarization phases. When electrodes are placed on the skin, the action potential that is recorded extracellularly resembles the PQRST pattern of the ECG (Fig. 2-5). More correctly, it is the sum of all myocardial action potentials for any one heartbeat. When detected from certain body surface locations, the ECG is a record of the electrical behavior of the heart during the cardiac cycle. The P wave is generated at the time of atrial depolarization, the QRS by ventricular depolarization, and the ST segment and T wave by ventricular repolarization. The size and shape of any one PQRST complex vary with the placement of the electrodes, or leads, used to record it.

Mechanical Events of the Cardiac Cycle

Once activated, myocardial contraction begins shortly thereafter. Contraction of the atria, known as atrial systole, begins after inscription of the P wave on the ECG. Ventricular contraction or ventricular systole begins near the end of the R wave and ends just after the T wave. With all chambers relaxed in late diastole, the tricuspid and mitral valves that partition the atria and ventricles are open, and the pulmonary and aortic valves are closed. Blood is able to flow throughout the heart, filling the four chambers. While 70 percent of left ventricular filling occurs now, the remainder is accomplished during the next phase, atrial systole. With the onset of the next phase, ventricular systole, the tricuspid and mitral valves close. The ventricular muscle mass contracts very little, but intracavity pressures rise sharply. This period of ventricular systole is referred to as isovolumic contraction. It will last approximately 0.05 seconds, until pressure in the right ventricle exceeds pulmonary artery pressure (10 mmHg) and left ventricular pressure exceeds aortic pressure (80 mmHg), and the respective pulmonary and aortic valves open (Fig. 2-6). Ventricular ejection occurs with peak left ventricular pressure reaching 120 mmHg and peak right ventricular pressure, 25 mmHg. The amount of blood ejected by each ventricle per stroke is 70 to 90 ml, approximately 65 percent of total volume of blood present in the left ventricle at the time of systolic contraction. It is this value of 65 percent that is referred to as the left ventricular ejection fraction.

Contraction of the heart muscle forces blood out into the aorta in a pulsatile fashion. As this pressure wave travels along arterial walls, the walls expand. This expansion is palpable as the pulse. The rate at which this pressure wave travels is dependent on the characteristics of the vessel in which it is traveling and is faster than the velocity of blood flow. For example, there is a 0.1-second delay between peak left ventricular systolic ejection and palpation of the radial pulse at the wrist. Various characteristics of a pulse can be described. The most obvious—strength of pulse—is determined by the pulse pressure, and not the mean pressure. While the pulse is generated by the arterial pressure wave and is palpated over an artery, it can be transmitted to the great veins of the neck. Palpation of the jugular venous pulse can be important for analysis of heart function.

A series of vibratory sounds, known as heart sounds, are set up with each cardiac cycle. Two heart sounds produced by the normal heart are S1, the first heart sound, caused by closure of the tricuspid and mitral valves at the start of ventricular systole; and S2, the second heart sound, which arises when the aortic and pulmonary valves close. While both sounds are a mix of vibrations caused by different events of the cardiac cycle, two components of S2 can be discerned by the trained human ear. The first, known as A2, is due to closure of the aortic valve. The second, P2, stems from pulmonic valve closure. A third heart sound (S3) and a fourth heart sound (S4) can occur during diastole in both normal and abnormal states. Other sounds, not necessarily abnormal, which are generated in various parts of the vascular system by turbulent flow, include murmurs, bruits, clicks, rubs, and hums. Murmurs can be a cause for concern, as they may reflect disease in one or more heart valves. Murmurs are sounds made up of many frequencies. The characteristics of a particular murmur depend on the velocity of blood flow, the morphology of the valvular orifice, and the resonating properties of the surrounding structures. A valve can malfunction in two ways. Normal forward flow of blood can be hindered by a narrowed valve, a condition known as stenosis. A valve that fails to close adequately and that leaks blood back into the

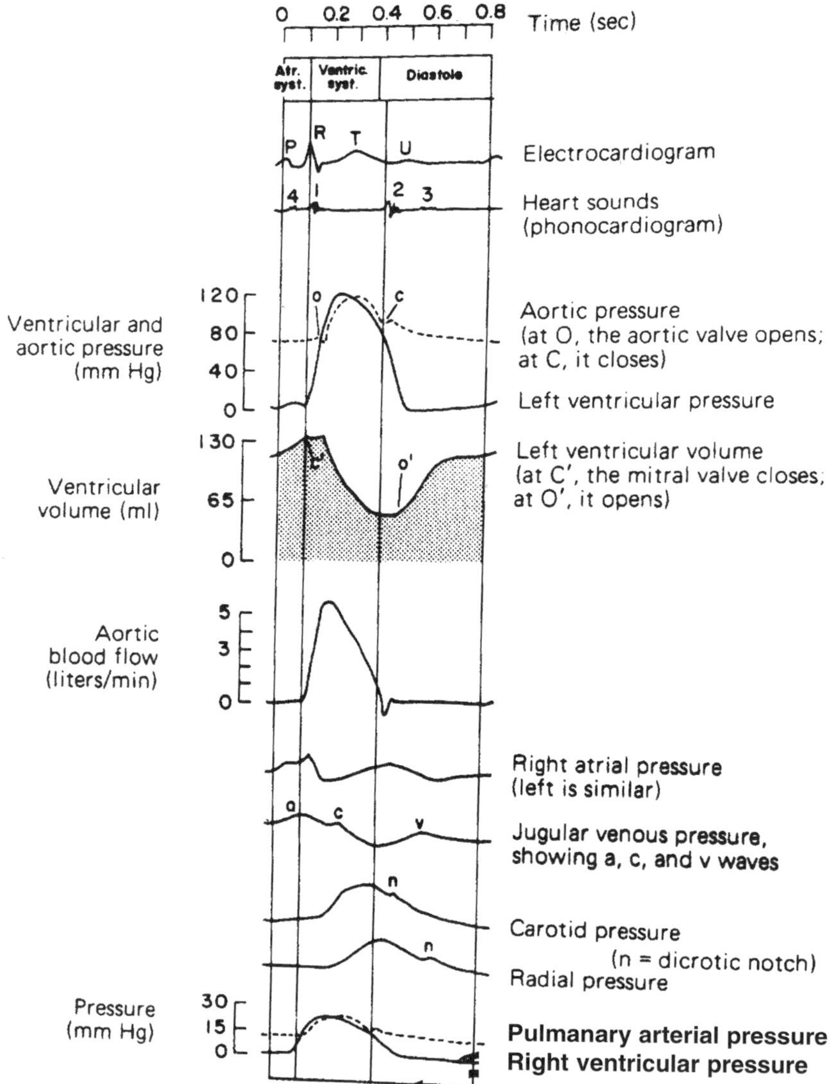

Fig. 2-6. Events of the cardiac cycle. (From Cohen and Michel[3] as adapted from Ganong,[8] with permission.)

chamber from which it just came is called incompetent or insufficient. This condition is referred to as regurgitation of the valve. Appropriate location of the stethoscope on the chest wall (Fig. 2-7) can determine which valve is producing the murmur. Whether the lesion is stenotic or insufficient can be decided by correlating the timing of the murmur (whether in diastole or systole) with knowledge of the mechanical events of the cardiac cycle. Blood normally flows through the aortic and pulmonary valves in systole. A murmur in systole will be caused by a stenotic lesion and a murmur in diastole by a regurgitant flow. Because the normal flow of blood through the mitral and tricuspid valves is in diastole, the reverse is true. A murmur arising from either of these valves in systole is caused by regurgitation, and stenosis of the valve will be heard in diastole.

Cardiac Output

The pumping function of the heart is regulated by a number of different mechanisms that match the output of the heart to tissue perfusion needs over a large range

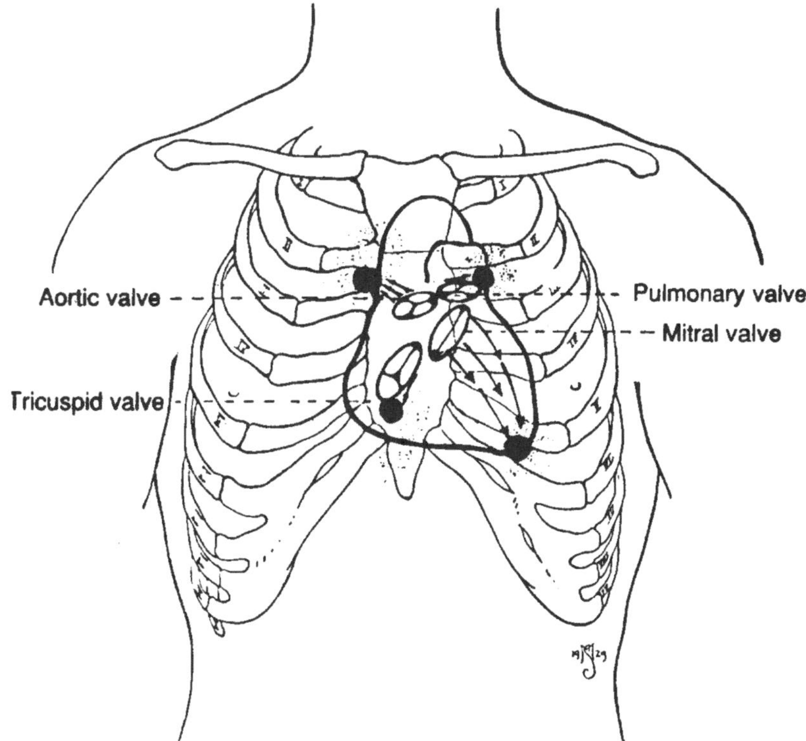

Fig. 2-7. Anatomic location of heart valves and of areas in which sounds are best heard. (From Delp and Manning,[9] with permission.)

of physiologic demands. Cardiac output is the amount of blood moved per minute by the heart from the great veins into the aorta. It is also referred to as minute volume, defined as the product of stroke volume and heart rate. Because the size of the individual determines the perfusion needs, cardiac output is frequently expressed as a function of body surface area. The cardiac index (CI) is the cardiac output (CO) in liters per minute (L/min) divided by the body surface area (BSA) in square meters (m^2).

$$CI = \frac{CO\ L/min}{BSA\ m^2}$$

Cardiac output can range from 20 to 30 percent below normal resting supine values, as with assumption of the upright position from a supine value, to 700 to 800 percent above resting levels with extreme effort. The two major clinical measurements of cardiac output use either the Fick principle or the indicator dilution technique; cold saline is the indicator and thermodilution the specific technique. This measurement is accomplished by injecting saline into the right atrium through one port of a Swan-Ganz catheter. Temperature change is registered at a thermistor in the pulmonary artery at the balloon tip of the catheter.

Regulatory mechanisms can work on either or both components of the cardiac output equation: heart rate or stroke volume. Heart rate is controlled primarily by autonomic nervous system input. Sympathetic stimulation causes an increase in heart rate, and parasympathetic stimulation decreases it. Stroke volume is also influenced by neural stimulation, with sympathetic afferents giving greater strength to muscle fiber contraction at any given length and parasympathetics having the opposite effect. The effect of the release of catecholamines by sympathetic stimulation on heart rate is referred to as chronotropic action. Their effect on the strength of myocardial contraction is known as inotropic action. An inherent property of the myocardial muscle mass, independent of innervation, to regulate stroke volume stems from the generation of tension within the fiber at any given cardiac muscle fiber length. Classic physiologic studies of this length–tension relationship for the isolated muscle strip plot sarcomere length against isometric tension. This force of contraction depends on preload, the initial load on the muscle before contraction, and afterload, the tension at which the load is lifted. In the individual patient, preload translates into the degree to which heart muscle is stretched before contraction and afterload, the resistance against which blood is expelled. When preload is thought of more generally as venous return and afterload as peripheral resistance or impedance, it becomes clear that these variables can be manipulated therapeutically to affect myocardial fiber shortening, stroke volume, and cardiac output. Other regulatory mechanisms of cardiac output that work more slowly, effecting change by determining extracellular volume and secondly blood volume, are the renin–angiotensin system and centrally mediated release of antidiuretic hormone, or vasopressin.

Blood Pressure

Whereas cardiac output is the amount of blood ejected from the heart throughout a complete cardiac cycle, actual tissue perfusion over a broad spectrum of physiologic demands is determined by the arterial (or blood) pressure. The highest pressure point of the pulse wave is the systolic pressure, and the lowest pressure, at the end of diastole, is the diastolic pressure. The difference between systolic and diastolic pressures is the pulse pressure. Mean pressure is the average pressure during the cardiac cycle. It is not an arithmetic average, but rather a geometric mean, that can be approximated with the following formula (Fig. 2-8):

$$\text{Mean pressure} = \text{diastolic pressure} + \tfrac{1}{3}\ \text{pulse pressure}$$

Multiple cardiovascular regulatory mechanisms for controlling blood pressure have evolved. These adjustments include both local and systemic mechanisms that (1) affect the diameter of arterioles and other resistance vessels, (2) increase or decrease blood storage in the venous system, and (3) vary the rate and stroke volume of the heart. The autonomic nervous system has a major regulatory role, involving sensory input from peripheral baroreceptors and from chemoreceptors located in the walls of the heart. In the major blood vessels, sensory input is relayed to a center of cardiovascular control in the medulla. This area, when stimulated, results in vasoconstriction or vasodilation of various vascular beds. Also contributing to pressure control at the individual organ or vascular bed are metabolic end products and other vasodilatory peptides that affect vascular smooth muscle tone, as well as the inherent response of resistance vessels to varying degrees of stretch.

Oxygen Consumption of the Heart

Unlike skeletal muscle, which requires glucose or glycogen for metabolism, cardiac muscle can take advantage of a number of energy sources, including esterified and nonesterified fatty acids, lactate, ketone bodies, and amino acids. All metabolic pathways are aerobic, however, requiring oxygen for adenosine triphosphate (ATP) regeneration. Oxygen consumption of the heart is determined by heart rate, intramyocardial wall tension, and contractility of the myocardium. Measurements of wall tension and contractility are not readily available clinically. An excellent correlation exists, however, between myocardial oxygen consumption and the rate pressure product or double product obtained by multiplying heart rate and systolic blood pressure measured at any given workload.

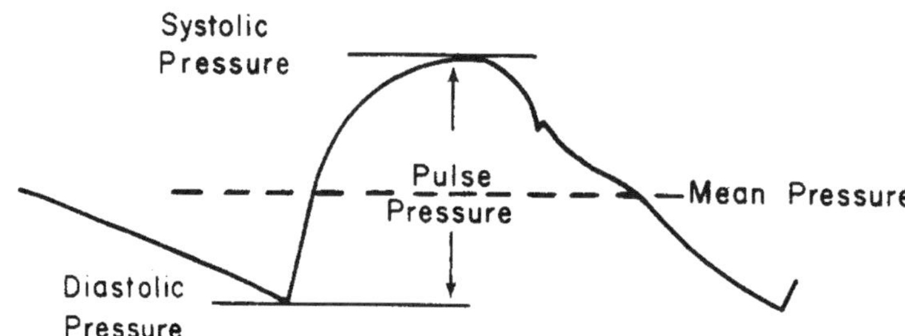

Fig. 2-8. Schematic arterial pressure pulse-labeled to show pressure values usually measured. (From Little,[10] with permission.)

SIGNS AND SYMPTOMS OF CARDIOVASCULAR DISEASE

Every organ in the human body relies on the anatomic integrity and physiologic effectiveness of the cardiovascular system for tissue nutrition. Impairments in this system can cause symptoms anywhere throughout the body. Some of these symptoms can be very clear-cut sequelae of cardiovascular disease, such as intermittent claudication. Many symptoms are confusing, such as fatigue, and are likely to be presented to a physical therapist. The physical therapist should be familiar with those symptoms that are likely to implicate the cardiovascular system: pain, irregular heartbeat (palpitations), lightheadedness, syncope, fatigue, dyspnea, and cough.

Pain

Pain that is cardiac in origin is referred to as *angina pectoris*. This condition is defined as an imbalance of myocardial oxygen supply and oxygen demand, arising when the available blood supply is inadequate to meet the metabolic requirement of cardiac muscle. Angina pectoris is a symptom of myocardial ischemia. Typical angina occurs substernally, with a referral pattern to the left shoulder and along the inside of the left arm in the usual ulnar pattern following the C8 and T1 distribution. Atypical angina may occur in the face, jaw, teeth, either or both shoulders, posterior thorax, and down either or both arms. Angina is usually described as a pressure and not necessarily as a pain. It may be accompanied by nausea, vomiting, epigastric distress with burping, or none of these. Because of these associated symptoms, it may easily be mistaken for indigestion. Often patients will remember sensations of numbness or tingling in their left hand associated with angina. These, too, are often misleading for patients who do not know they have coronary artery disease (CAD).

To aid in making a differential diagnosis for the source of thoracic pain, the following rules of thumb are presented. Angina is most likely relieved by rest and rarely lasts longer than 5 minutes at rest. Thoracic pain that worsens with inspiration, is sharp and improves with a change in position, is usually pericarditis, not angina. A sharp stabbing pain that occurs with a deep breath, described as a knife in a local area, is probably pleurisy. Myocarditis and endocarditis do not necessarily produce chest pain, but a chest tightness with breathlessness may easily be confused with angina. There is often low-grade fever and malaise, as well as arthralgias accompanying cardiac infections or inflammations. The pain associated with aortic aneurysm is usually a hot sensation, throbbing in nature, and increasing in intensity with increased physical activity. A dissecting aortic aneurysm presents as a pain, sudden in onset, a searing heat, often located in the patient's back, and accompanied by a rapid decrease in blood pressure. Pain that is burning, limited in area over the cutaneous distribution of a nerve, and accompanied by swollen local lymph nodes may indicate herpes zoster, especially if it is brought on by recent stress or in an immunocompromised patient. Skin vesicles eventually appear.

Angina can occur from etiologies other than coronary artery disease or coronary vasospasm. Aortic stenosis and outflow tract obstruction caused by hypertrophy of the septum known as hypertrophic cardiomyopathy (HCM) can result in inadequate blood flow into the coronary circulation during diastole. Chest pain on exertion accompanied by breathlessness can be a symptom of inadequate blood flow, rather than coronary vessel disease. Another clinical entity that sometimes causes chest pain attributable to blood flow dysfunction is mitral valve prolapse.

Typical angina is described in the following terms:

Onset: exertional, or under conditions of stress
Location: substernal with left shoulder and arm radiation
Quality: pressure, tightness that may not be perceived as pain
Intensity: ranging from pressure or tightness to severe crushing sensation
Duration: usually longer than 1 minute but less than 10 minutes
Relief: stopping exercise, sublingual nitroglycerin
Associated symptoms: breathlessness, diaphoresis; sometimes nausea and vomiting when severe

Atypical angina usually refers to angina that is nonexertional. It can occur as a pain, tightness, or tingling located in the jaw, in the neck, or in the back, radiating down either or both arms, or as something quite unique to the patient. Atypical angina can occur at rest and often awakens a person between 2 and 5 AM. It is thought that there is a relationship to the peak in catecholamine plasma levels, which occurs then.

Myocardial ischemia may be "silent," and not at all perceived as pain. Anginal equivalents can occur such as diaphoresis, dyspnea, or fatigue. If a patient has had angina in the past, the medical history should mention the specific anginal pattern with clear descriptors. In addition, the presence of CAD should be documented by tests and by an analysis of the risk factors for this disease.

Physical Therapy Evaluation of Myocardial Ischemia

High Suspicion of Myocardial Ischemia

1. *Chest pain brought on by exertion, cold air, drag on cigarette, and after a heavy meal:* This pain is often accompanied by dyspnea, diaphoresis, and nausea.
2. *Angina:* Stable angina has a regular, consistent, predictable onset, location, relief, and duration. Unstable angina is characterized by increasing frequency; onset is now earlier, more easily induced, and spreading or radiating in location; it requires more sublingu al nitroglycerin and takes longer to obtain relief.
3. *Variant angina:* Rest angina occurs during sleep and is unrelated to exertion, from vasospasm of coronary arteries. It may be associated with high anxiety.
4. *Prinzmetal angina:* Cardiac pain occurring almost always at rest. ECG shows pronounced ST segment elevation rather than depression.
5. *Non-CAD chest pain with exertion, accompanied by dyspnea, wide pulse (systolic vs. diastolic) pressure:* Other causes of myocardial ischemia such as aortic stenosis, hypertrophic cardiomyopathy, left ventricular hypertrophy.

Leg Pain

Leg pain is a very nonspecific symptom that can be very localized, quite general, and variable under different conditions. Causes of leg pain can be vascular, such as phlebitis, vasculitis, or ischemia, as in intermittent claudication or anterior compartment syndrome. Other causes of leg pain may be secondary to musculoskeletal disorders, as in arthritis. Leg pain may be neural in origin, as in sciatica or in neuropathy of diabetes mellitus, or may be due to soft tissue conditions, such as cellulitis. Muscle imbalance or weakness as occurs with shin splints can produce leg pain that may be confused with anterior compartment syndrome or pain associated with stress fractures. Descriptors of pain, location of discomfort, and associated findings may be the most critical aspects of the differential diagnosis. Localized edema of both ankles may be present with venous stasis ulcers. Skin discoloration (blue to black with gangrene, brown to purple with venous stasis) and presence of hair loss and trophic changes of skin will lead to the conclusion of arterial or venous insufficiency. Peripheral neuropathies and sympathetic neuropathies can produce trophic changes and pain as well. The physical therapist looks for long scars along the course of a vein as evidence of previous revascularization surgery, such as a saphenous vein for coronary artery bypass graft (CABG).

Pain with acute swelling in the anterior tibial compartment is associated with cramping, increases with walking or running, and stops with rest. It occurs secondary to increased capillary permeability or hematoma within tight connective tissue in the shin area. Calf pain with slow walking that develops into a cramp unless walking is discontinued is symptomatic of calf muscle ischemia caused by peripheral vascular disease. The former is usually found in young athletes and is known as anterior compartment syndrome.[11] A case study is provided by Cohen and Michel.[12] By contrast, the patient with intermittent claudication is usually older; often is found in association with type 2 diabetes mellitus; has a duller ache that may occur in the buttock, thigh, calf, or all of the above; and comes on with walking, intensifies if walking continues, and disappears with rest.

Other forms of leg pain relating to vascular insufficiency include gangrenous lesions yielding very intense, constant localized pain associated with blackened lesions in the skin, most often of the toes or heel. Venous stasis ulcers produce a raw, throbbing, constant, nauseating pain in an ulcerated area, usually surrounded by brownish discolored skin, and local edema. Pain over a localized distribution, associated with a red, hot area and swelling may be a symptom of thrombophlebitis. This occurs most commonly in patients who have been bedridden or immobilized for a long period.

Physical Therapy Evaluation of Leg Pain

Fingertip palpation of peripheral pulses is one of the most important procedures to employ. The femoral pulse is found in the groin, medial to the inguinal ligament. The popliteal pulse is behind the knee joint in the popliteal fossa. The tibial pulse is posterior to the medial malleolus, and the pedal pulse is found on the mid-dorsum of the foot. If a pulsatile mass is palpated anywhere in the body, such as in the abdomen or groin, it needs to be checked urgently, as it may be an aneurysm. Absent or diminished pulses and asymmetry of pulses on the two lower limbs should raise suspicion of peripheral vascular disease (PVD).

Another significant evaluation is that of reactivity of the arterial system. The reactive hyperemia test is the use of gravity to drain the limb of a significant volume of blood and the rapidity with which the arterial system can compensate for this blood redistribution. To perform this test, the patient is supine, and the lower limb being tested is elevated over the patient's head level, approximately 45 degrees of hip flexion. The leg is kept in this position for 1 to 3 minutes or until the color of the foot, ankle, and lower leg is quite blanched. With a stopwatch, the examiner times how long it takes for the skin to turn pink as soon as the limb is brought to the dangling position while the patient is sitting. Normally, this time is less than 1 second. Anything above 1.5 seconds represents some degree of arterial insufficiency. This test takes an eye sensitive to color change. Another similar test, perhaps a little more risky for the seriously impaired patient with arterial insufficiency, measures reactive hyperemia to cold water immersion. Instead of gravity, the use of cold water immersion will produce blanched or mottled skin, which can be rewarmed with rapid immersion in warm water, and the time to return to pink skin is taken as the test of arterial insufficiency. Again, normal reaction time is less than 1 second. In highly pigmented skin this test may be less sensitive.

To determine the pressure of the systolic pulse wave in a peripheral vessel, a sphygmomanometer cuff is inflated above the site of the suspected lesion. The Doppler probe is placed along the vessel being studied. As the pressure is slowly released, flow is first detected at the point of systolic pressure. When the sphygmomanometer is applied at serial points along the limb, a gradient in pressure between any two measurement sites will localize the segment in which arterial obstruction is significant. This test may be performed by a physical therapist or may be done in a vascular diagnostic laboratory. Skin temperature can be a useful measure, and a temperature map can help assess areas in which arterial supply is inadequate. Thermography provides the same measurement but is a much higher, more sensitive technology. It is also more expensive.

Physical Therapy Evaluation of Leg Pain

High Suspicion of Vascular Cause of Leg Pain

1. Gangrene anywhere on the peripheral body part indicates arterial insufficiency.
2. Nonhealing ulceration on the peripheral body part indicates a vascular problem—either arterial insufficiency or venous stasis.
3. Absent or diminished pulse.
4. Ischemic pain with activity of muscle involved in the activity is the result of arterial insufficiency. Intermittent claudication is the peripheral example, in which onset occurs with walking; pain is in the calf muscle, in the hamstring muscle group, or in the gluteal group. Testing for reactive hyperemia will result in delayed skin coloration. Doppler tests, especially under low-level exercise conditions, help pinpoint location and identify severity of stenoses.

Irregular Heartbeat

By definition, irregularities of heart rhythm (palpitations) are abnormal but may be quite benign or dangerous to the patient. Some patients may not perceive them at all, while others may find them quite bothersome. The physical therapist must distinguish between irregularities that are not hemodynamically compromising and those that need immediate medical attention. In general, atrial arrhythmias, or extra beats originating in the atria but not from the sinus node, are of the benign variety. However, a new onset may be significant hemodynamically, especially if the ventricular response rate goes above 160, at which rate diastolic filling time may be sufficiently reduced to undermine the cardiac output. There is also a much increased risk of clot formation with atrial arrhythmias leading to the potential risk of thrombus or embolus. Ventricular arrhythmias are more likely to lead to serious hemodynamic compromise. In addition, a primary conduction defect can lead to a rhythm disturbance, which can be quite serious. First-degree AV block appears as a prolongation of the PR interval and represents a slowing of conduction through the atria. This block does not challenge the patient hemodynamically. Second-degree AV block appears in two forms: Mobitz type I (or Wenckebach), and Mobitz type II. Both types occur when some impulses are conducted from atria to ventricles, while other impulses are blocked. Wenckebach AV block almost always occurs at the AV node and is often due to increased parasympathetic tone or to drug effect. It is usually transient and does not compromise the patient. Progressive prolongation of the PR interval indicates decreasing conduction velocity, until finally an impulse is completely blocked. Only a single impulse is blocked, and the cycle is repeated. Type II AV block occurs when the block is below the level of the AV node in the bundle of His, generally the result of an organic lesion. Thus, it is associated with a deterioration to third-degree or complete heart block. In type II second-degree AV block, the PR interval does not lengthen before a dropped beat. The block may be intermittent, or the conduction ratio may vary. If it is a constant conduction ratio, the palpable pulse is regular. Third-degree AV block indicates complete absence of conduction between atria and ventricles. P waves occur at their own rate and rhythm; QRS complexes appear at a different (slower) rate and rhythm without any relationship to each other. The block is usually below the AV node, thereby carrying a poor prognosis. In this case, the QRS rate is the ventricular escape rhythm, with its inherent firing rate of less than 40 per minute. There may be periods of asystole in this case. Figure 2-9 presents an overall view of the major arrhythmias.

Physical Therapy Evaluation of Irregular Heartbeat

Since not all patients have symptoms associated with their irregular heartbeat, the physical therapist's pulse palpation may demonstrate the first sign of this problem. Any pulse point will reflect the irregularity. The first step is to define the nature of the irregularity, then determine the amount of hemodynamic dysfunction caused by the arrhythmia. The vital signs should be taken. Heart rate must be counted for a full minute to determine the total number of fully perfused beats. The heart rhythm, taken peripherally, may be described as regular, regularly irregular, or irregularly irregular. When an irregular pulse is found, an apical auscultation simultaneously performed with a peripheral palpation will help elucidate the significance. The presence of the S1 or S2 (lubb-dupp) heart sound during a peripheral pause in pulse is noted. If there is no palpable pulsation, even when a normal heart sound is heard, there is no perfusion with the beat. The frequency and regularity of the pause in palpated pulse should be noted to help assess its severity. Blood pressure may be difficult to perform accurately during an irregular heartbeat, since the systolic reading depends on the normal Korotkoff sound, which will be absent during the pause of a premature contraction. The absence of a timely beat may be misread as the diastolic pressure rather than as a pause, since it may appear as cessation of sound.

Lightheadedness

Lightheadedness is a common experience. There are many causes, some simple and easily removed, such as hyperventilation, others complex and associated with severe compromise. For this reason, it is critical to ascertain whether there are any associated symptoms accompanying the experience of lightheadedness. The most frequent etiologies are ventricular ectopic activity, hypotension, hyperventilation, hypoglycemia, and cerebral ischemia.

A person who feels lightheaded may appear pale and may also be diaphoretic, but may in most respects be reasonably normal in appearance. If a patient loses consciousness, there is more cause for alarm (see under Syncope). Patients experiencing a transient ischemic attack (TIA) may also have slurred speech, loss of motor control on one side or a portion of their body, or incoordination of motion.

The medical history should help the physical therapist determine any previous history of any of the above. The physical therapist should be especially on the alert for mention of diabetes mellitis (hypoglycemic reaction to insulin); TIAs (cerebral ischemia); and any sign of arrhythmias, such as ventricular ectopic activity (VEA). If this symptom has occurred frequently, the chart may have a description of what provokes it. For example, orthostatic intolerance produces lightheadedness with postural change from recumbancy to the upright position. There may also be an indication of how long this symptom lasts, how frequently it appears, what relieves it, and whether it leads to loss of consciousness. Hyperventilation is often a result of anxiety and may become chronic. If chronic, lightheadedness may be a persistent experience, accompanied by tingling of the fingers, numbness, and an increase in respiratory rate. Sustained VEA will result in hypotension and may represent a serious dysfunction of the myocardium. However, many people experience transient VEA,

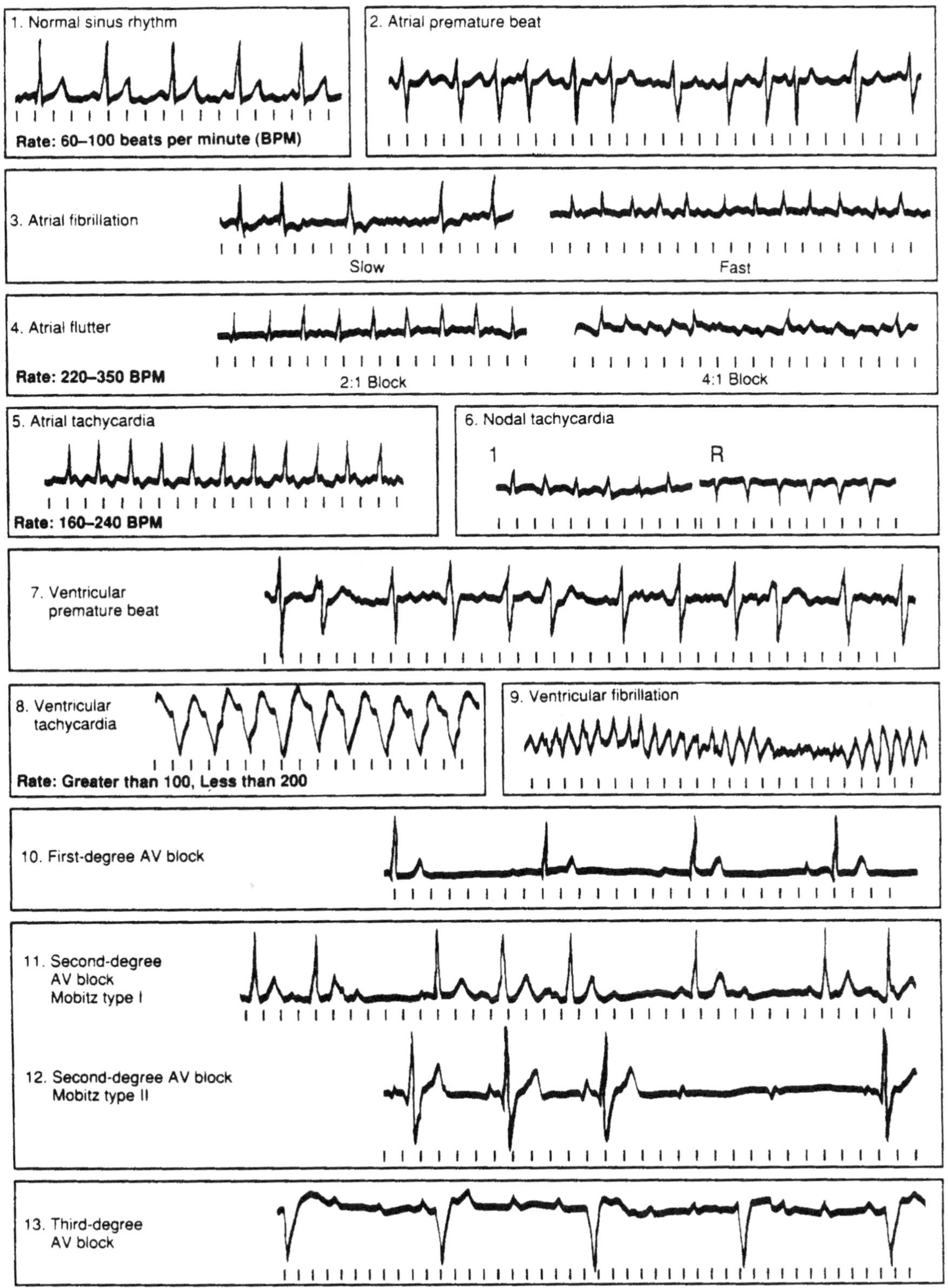

Fig. 2-9. Patterns of the major arrhythmias.

which is well tolerated. VEA can occur from caffeine ingestion, with lightheadedness resulting from lack of perfusion to the brain. Hypotension with change of position may be transient, may be associated with prolonged bed rest or recent surgery, hypovolemia, or may represent congestive heart failure and a seriously failing left ventricle. It is therefore important to look at the patient's chart for concurrent diagnoses, such as diabetes, sustained VEA, and TIAs. Certain drugs such as antihypertensives and antiarrhythmics can produce lightheadedness when the dose is being adjusted in some patients, as blood pressure may become more labile, or a cardiac rhythm may be stimulated by the altered dose. Examples of these types of such drugs are methyldopa and quinidine sulfate.

Syncope

Syncope, or loss of consciousness, is generally caused by cardiovascular problems. It is not always serious, however. It can range from nothing more than vasovagal syncope, with a spontaneous rapid recovery, to ventricular fibrillation or cardiac standstill, prompting immediate emergency intervention to prevent death.

A medical history for a patient who has experienced loss of consciousness in the past should include a description of the conditions that provoked this state, as well as the probable cause. Vasovagal syncope can be triggered by fear, pain, the sight of blood, hunger, and fatigue and is most frequently encountered in persons in a high anxiety state. Common premonitory signs or symptoms include pallor, yawning, sighing, hyperventilation, epigastric discomfort, nausea, and/or blurred vision. In the case of loss of consciousness caused by orthostatic hypotension, the blood pressure will fall precipitously when the patient moves from a supine to standing position and is preceded by lightheadedness when the person is upright. There is also a compensatory tachycardia, which would not be present during vasovagal syncope. Hypoglycemia in diabetes mellitus may result in loss of consciousness, especially during or after exercise. A seizure is typically characterized by muscle jerking, breath holding, and choking sounds, and the patient may lose consciousness. Grand mal seizures generally abate spontaneously after 3 to 4 minutes and are characterized by lip or tongue biting and by incontinence of the bowel and bladder. The seizures are followed by a state of mental confusion. Most other causes of loss of con-

Physical Therapy Evaluation of Lightheadedness

Rule out cardiac cause:

1. *Take the blood pressure:* If hypertensive or normotensive, hypotension is not the cause. In the case of orthostasis, hypotension occurs only in response to position change (i.e., from the supine to upright position), causing lightheadedness.
2. *Check heart rate:* If not less than 60 beats per minute (bpm), bradycardia is not the cause.
3. *Check respiratory rate:* If elevated, the probable cause is not cardiac but respiratory.
4. *Check the ECG for ventricular arrhythmia and for signs of ischemia:* Since both arrhythmia and ischemia result in some myocardial dysfunction, there may be hypotension with resulting lightheadedness. The presence of chest pain with or without ST segment change and with lightheadedness must be further worked up for myocardial ischemia.
5. *Check blood sugar level:* If low and accompanied by diaphoresis, pallor, and fatigue, the probable cause is hypoglycemia.
6. *Check motor coordination:* If patient is not incoordinated or hemiparetic, and speech is normal, the cause is probably not cerebral ischemia, although there certainly can be less straightforward presentations of cerebral ischemia.

High suspicion of cardiac cause:

1. *Skipped beats on pulse taking:* Check the ECG for VEA, paroxysmal atrial tachycardia (PAT), bradycardia, and heart block.
2. *Hypotension:* A low systolic reading suggests hemodynamic compromise. A low pulse pressure (narrow margin between systolic and diastolic reading) and not necessarily hypotension per se also suggests cardiac problem.
3. *Chest pain:* Chest pain may also be present with or without ST-segment depression on ECG.

sciousness are life threatening or could become so, such as ventricular ectopy (ventricular fibrillation or tachycardia), asystole, pulmonary embolus, aortic stenosis, and HCM. Carotid sinus hypersensitivity could produce loss of consciousness when a patient wearing a high collar turns the head, which causes spontaneous stimulation of the carotid sinus. Other types of syncope include micturition syncope, Stokes-Adams attacks (i.e., transient asystole or ventricular fibrillation in the presence of atrioventricular block), sinus arrest, hyperventilation syncope, and cough syncope. Exertional syncope has been found in patients with aortic stenosis, HCM, pulmonary hypertension, asystole, and ventricular tachycardia.

Physical Therapy Evaluation of Syncope

High suspicion of cardiac cause:

1. Check supine and standing blood pressure for orthostatic intolerance as a cause of loss of consciousness.
2. In cases of prolonged unresponsiveness, consider cardiac arrest. Check for pulse, respirations, pupils. Call a code and begin CPR.
3. Check for the presence of ventricular ectopic activity on the ECG.

Fatigue

Fatigue is defined as the loss or lack of energy with which to perform a necessary activity. Sources of fatigue at very low-level exertion may be neurologic, muscular, metabolic, psychiatric, cardiac, or pulmonary. A medical history is an important reference for sorting out the cause of fatigue in any given patient. However, fatigue is rarely the single presenting symptom reported on the patient's medical chart. Most tests are not specific for fatigue, but the combination of many test results may elucidate the cause of fatigue and whether it is pathologic.

If the patient's history indicates that fatigue is a major complaint, an interview should provide descriptors. Fatigue may be general whole-body fatigue, or it may be quite localized. It may be accompanied by other associated symptoms, such as pain in a muscle, chest pain, or dyspnea. Normal causes of fatigue, related to high levels of energy output, include local muscle glycogen depletion after very prolonged high-level effort, lactate accumulation in muscle and blood, poor motivation or loss of motivation, calcium ion depletion, and dehydration. In addition, some pathologic conditions that contribute to early fatigability include a low cardiac output state, such as CAD, aortic valve dysfunction, cardiomyopathy, and myocarditis. Anemia can cause extreme fatigue. Hypothyroidism results in lethargy and a general loss of energy. Hyperthyroidism may also lead to chronic exhaustion. Psychiatric disorders, especially depression, are usually associated with chronic fatigue. Conditions resulting in hypoxia also result in fatigue and other associated symptoms of increased respiratory rate, dyspnea, and lightheadedness. These conditions include respiratory failure, acute pulmonary embolus, and arte-

Physical Therapy Evaluation of Fatigue

High suspicion of cardiac cause:

1. Look for signs of falling blood pressure, which occurs in cardiac tamponade, congestive heart failure (CHF), and inotropic incompetence. In CHF, check for appearance of rales in both lung bases, using the diaphragm of the stethoscope, and check for a gallop rhythm using the bell of stethoscope over the apex with the patient in a left side-lying position (see Auscultation, under Physical Examination). In cardiac tamponade, look for dyspnea, weakness, malaise, chest pain, anorexia, and weight loss with diaphoresis.
2. Check for hypotension with tachycardia or with severe bradycardia.
3. Check the patient for pallor.
4. Check pulses and ECG for frequent VEA.
5. Look for results of exercise tolerance test (ETT), echocardiography, cardiac catheterization or magnetic resonance (MR) imaging to indicate the presence of CAD, aortic valve dysfunction, cardiomyopathy, cardiac catheterization, or myocarditis.

riovenous shunt of the heart or lungs. Finally, hyperglycemia such as may occur in a diabetic patient with an insulin deficiency will result in extreme fatigability. General metabolic derangements and systemic illnesses that create fatigue include some cancers, chronic renal failure, and chronic liver failure.

Dyspnea

Breathlessness, or dyspnea, is a common experience whenever we engage in fairly strenuous exercise. It is accompanied by a respiratory rate usually over 40 breaths per minute and can be extremely frightening if extreme. The fear of suffocation accounts for associated symptoms and behaviors. Breathlessness can be an acute problem, such as occurs in the choking victim, or can be chronic, under conditions of low-level exertion in severe chronic obstructive pulmonary disease (COPD), or at rest, in CHF. There may be several causes for dyspnea. The increase in metabolic demand for oxygen provides a chemical stimulus to increase respiration, which may lead to the patient's perception of breathlessness. It may actually be caused by the inappropriate length–tension relationship of the diaphragm muscle when the muscle length is too short, as in high exercise demand, or when the muscle length is too overstretched, as in COPD patients, to meet the tension requirement of a particular activity. In left ventricular congestive failure, caused by a failing pump, fluid is retained in the left atrium, which backs up in the pulmonary circulation. The fluid leaks out into the alveoli, blocking the exchange of gases and creating the demand for better oxygenation or better ventilation. The impossible demand, unable to be met by the inadequate supply, produces dyspnea.

The medical history will enlighten the physical therapist about the likely etiology of the breathlessness. What is the smoking history of the patient? The higher the pack-year exposure to smoking, the more damage to the tissue. Environmental exposure to damaging substances can also be a cause of breathlessness. Air pollutants may include chemical substances, fibrous particulate substances (e.g., asbestos), and dust from occupations working with substances (e.g., coal dust and flour dust), which can all contribute to long-term lung disease. The result is chronic breathlessness because of the loss of available lung tissue for gas exchange.

Cardiac causes of dyspnea include coronary insufficiency, mitral valve disease, myocardial dysfunction, and constrictive pericarditis. Breathlessness may occur under different conditions, and it may help to delineate which condition is pertinent to each patient. Dyspnea on exertion (DOE) is one condition common to both cardiac and pulmonary disease. Many patients have some elements of both diseases (attributable to many common etiologies, such as smoking). In DOE, breathlessness is brought on by activity. In severe DOE, activities are curtailed when they induce the unpleasant sensation of dyspnea. Thus begins the spiral of deconditioning, which produces a lower anaerobic threshold and an earlier onset of DOE. Thus, dyspnea induces more deconditioning, which exacerbates the symptom of breathlessness.

Another condition is paroxysmal noctural dyspnea (PND), in which a patient awakens from prolonged sleep with dyspnea. Its frequent occurrence implies CHF. Chronic pulmonary edema or cor pulmonale is worsened by a long period of recumbency and by consequent shifts in hydrostatic fluid. Orthopnea is the final condition, in which the supine position is not tolerated; propping several pillows below the head can relieve dyspnea.

Findings from the maximum stress test with gas analysis can illuminate the various etiologies of dyspnea. If deconditioning is the primary cause, expected findings will be early dyspnea, a low maximal oxygen consumption ($\dot{V}O_2$), and a low anaerobic threshold. If the patient has CHF, made worse by exercise, there will be a low, nonresponsive cardiac output, reflected in the systolic blood pressure by a flat or dropping measurement with increasing exercise. In addition, there will be early onset of anaerobic metabolism and a rapid rise in heart rate. The third heart sound may become audible during exercise. When the peripheral circulation is the limiting factor to a patient's exercise tolerance, dyspnea may occur early in the test because of earlier anaerobic metabolism in the local ischemic muscle bed. There will be a low maximal $\dot{V}O_2$, low anaerobic threshold, and, very likely, local muscle pain in an area of active contraction.[13]

Cough

Cough occurs as a protective reflex to expel foreign matter from the large airways, thus avoiding obstruction of the airways. In general, a cough should not be suppressed, but when it becomes chronic, ineffective, and irritating, cough

Physical Therapy Evaluation of Dyspnea

High suspicion of cardiac cause:

1. If the blood pressure (BP) is low, heart rate (HR) is high, rhythm of ECG shows premature atrial contractions (PACs), respiratory rate is high, oxygen saturation is normal, and temperature is normal, it is likely to relate to CHF.
2. Pulses paradoxus, inspiratory weakening of the pulse, along with a low blood pressure, fatigue, dyspnea, anorexia, weight loss, and malaise may indicate cardiac tamponade.
3. Auscultate for the diastolic murmur of mitral stenosis.
4. Pulmonary embolism will produce abrupt onset of dyspnea, which may be very severe, and should correlate with a drop in oxygen saturation by pulse oximetry.
5. Chronic pericarditis will produce tachycardia with dyspnea and may flare up acutely with sharp chest pain.
6. Check for cyanosis of nail beds and lips as an indication of tissue hypoxia.
7. Check whether the patient has secretions chronically, or suddenly, with acute onset of pulmonary edema.

suppression is sometimes a goal. The therapeutic goal, however, is most likely to enhance cough effectiveness.

Most causes of cough involve infectious, neoplastic, or allergic disorders of the lungs and tracheobronchial structures. Cardiovascular diagnoses that contribute to the symptom of cough include left ventricular failure with pulmonary edema, pulmonary venous hypertension, pulmonary infarction, and expanding aortic aneurysm that compresses the tracheobronchial tree. In some patients, a premature ventricular beat can cause a cough.

A medical history should describe whether myocardial damage or mitral stenosis in the past may account for CHF before this episode or new-onset CHF. If pulmonary edema has occurred, there is usually a description of the sputum produced, which is frothy and pink, and the cough will be bubbling, loose, and rattling. Cough caused by pulmonary venous hypertension secondary to mitral stenosis or chronic CHF tends to be dry, irritating, and nocturnal.

Physical Therapy Evaluation of Cough

High suspicion of cardiac cause:

1. Chest radiography showing cardiomegaly, a boot-shaped heart, and Kerley B lines points to a cardiac etiology.
2. Sputum that is pink and frothy and copious suggests a cardiac diagnosis.
3. An echocardiogram that shows myocardial wall hypokinesis, akinesis, dyskinesis, or mitral valve dysfunction and an ejection fraction of less than 40 percent implicates myocardial dysfunction.
4. Adventitious breath sounds, such as rales and rhonchi, may implicate either pulmonary or cardiac problems, or both, but, in the presence of a gallop rhythm heart sound, certainly suggest myocardial dysfunction.

HISTORY

One of the most important means to obtain information is the patient interview. Key questions about each symptom listed in Table 2-1 as well as questions about the patient's medical history and family history can be very instructive in ascertaining the likelihood that a given symptom is cardiovascular in origin. The interview can also indicate the significance or severity of symptoms.

Patient's Past and Current Medical History

Many signs and symptoms of the cardiovascular system stem from atherosclerotic disease. Questions about risk factors for CAD are therefore important. If a patient has used tobacco in any form or been exposed to secondary tobacco smoke, one should have a low threshold for considering signs and symptoms as cardiopulmonary in origin. Other cardiac risk factors, such as hypertension, diabetes, dyslipidemia, postmenopausal status in women, physical inactivity, being overweight, and having predisposing psychological factors can provide valuable insight into the probability that the patient has CAD or PVD. The physical therapist should ask about the patient's own knowledge of CAD and whether the patient has ever had a heart attack, angina, a problem with heart rhythm, or been told that he or she has high blood pressure.

Family Medical History

CAD and often PVD have a strong family history. Thus, a patient who is a reasonable historian should know whether parents and/or siblings experienced similar signs or symptoms or carried the diagnosis. Questions designed to uncloak this information can be very enlightening, since a positive response gives a much higher suspicion for cardiovascular disease.

Table 2-1. Key Questions for Cardiovascular Symptoms

Angina
Description of chest pain
Where is it?
When does it occur?
How long does it last?
What gives relief?
Sweating
Do you sweat with chest pain?
Do you ever sweat without exercise (cold sweat)?
If so, when?
Palpitations
When do these occur?
How do they affect you (e.g., scared, dizzy, weak)?
How do you get rid of them?
Breathlessness
What brings on breathlessness: activity, sleep, certain positions?
What gives relief (pursed-lips breathing, sitting upright, leaning forward with support, rest)?
Lightheadedness/loss of consciousness
Have you ever felt dizzy or blacked out?
If so, how often?
If so, what brings it on?
If so, how do you get relief?
Fatigue
How is your energy level in general?
How well do you sleep at night?
Cardiac risk factors
Have you ever been told that you have high blood pressure?
Do you now, or have you ever, smoked? Cigarettes? Other? How long, and how many?
Have you ever had your blood cholesterol checked? Do you know the level? Do you know what it should be?
Do you have diabetes?
What is your best body weight? Are you over, under, or OK now?
What activities do you do regularly?
Has anyone in your immediate family ever had a heart attack?
Has anyone had chest pain or cardiac surgery?
Have you ever had a heart attack, chest pain, or cardiac surgery?

PHYSICAL EXAMINATION

Observation

The observer's eye, when fully opened to postural, color, skin, or other changes that occur with cardiovascular disease, can be decisive in assessing the presence and extent of a disease process. The most obvious example is in PVD. Skin color changes and skin texture can define arterial or venous insufficiency. Arterial problems result in blue to black skin lesions in regions of smooth, hairless skin. Venous problems produce brown or purple areas of discoloration, often extending much farther than areas of arterial lesions, with roughened skin texture. Edema of both ankles occurs with venous stasis, which tends to be relatively painless.

In CHF, edema of both ankles can occur when right ventricular failure is involved. This edema is not associated with discoloration, is painless, and is usually associated with rapid weight gain (4 to 5 pounds over 2 to 3 days), jugular venous distention (JVD), and ascites. JVD is determined by placing the patient supine in a 30-degree head-up position and measuring the number of centimeters up from the right atrium that the distention of the jugular vein appears in the neck (Fig. 2-10). Normally there will be no jugular venous filling in 30 degrees of head-up position.

Left ventricular failure results in breathlessness, which can be quite acute. In the situation of acute pulmonary edema, the patient appears to be starved for air. The patient will be gasping, often leaning forward on both arms to fix the shoulder girdle, which facilitates the accessory muscles of breathing. This appearance is identical to that of the person with primary lung disease who is air hungry. A cough may be present that will be productive of frothy pink sputum. In chronic CHF, the cough may be productive of white bubbling sputum and accompanied by a wheeze.

In the case of a cardiac or pulmonary shunt, in which blood bypasses the pulmonary alveoli and arrives insufficently oxygenated in the periphery, chronic tissue hypoxemia is the result. Fingernail and toenail clubbing can be observed (Fig. 2-11).[15]

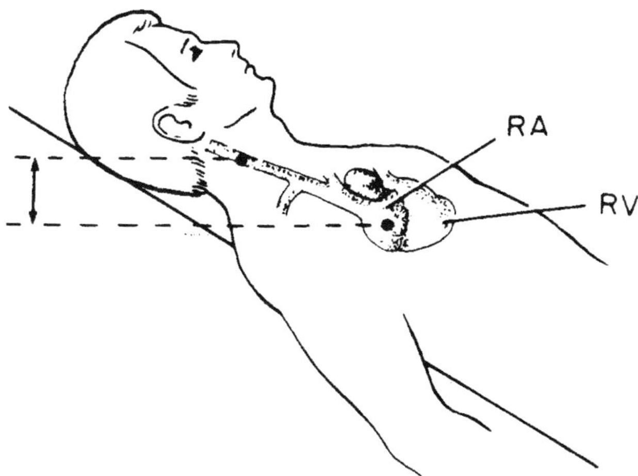

Fig. 2-10. Examination of jugular venous pulse and estimation of venous pressure. RA, right atrium; RV, right ventricle. (From Sokolow and McIlroy,[14] with permission.)

Patients with heart disease may experience angina in a variety of ways. They may appear anxious but otherwise show no obvious signs of cardiac embarrassment. When patients are pale, diaphoretic, cyanotic, or weak, there is usually hemodynamic compromise with a poor cardiac output. For the patient who has irregular heartbeats or palpitations, the physical appearance provides important clues about the hemodynamic significance of their arrhythmia. A compromised patient will appear pale, even ashen, may be diaphoretic, and may have cyanotic lips and nail beds.

Palpation

Palpation is a very useful technique for differentiating chest pain syndromes. Chest wall pain may be elicited by finger probing over trigger points, by applying pressure over joint structures (especially costochondral junctions), or by applying pressure with the heel of the hand at the sternocostal joints. Angina will not be elicited by palpation techniques.

Pulse counting is usually done by palpation. Usual sites for determining a patient's heart rate is the radial pulse or the brachial pulse. The carotid pulse may be used but at a site below the sensitive carotid pressure receptors, at the level of the thyroid cartilage. In some thin patients, an apical pulsation can be palpated by placing the hand over the cardiac apex position at the fifth intercostal space to feel for the point of maximal impulse sensation. This is a very effective point in children.

For the patient experiencing a cardiac arrhythmia, palpation by the physical therapist may provide the first evidence of the source of the problem. What the physical therapist feels should help a physician or someone trained in arrhythmia detection to recognize it and initiate appropriate treatment. A pulse pattern should be described as follows:

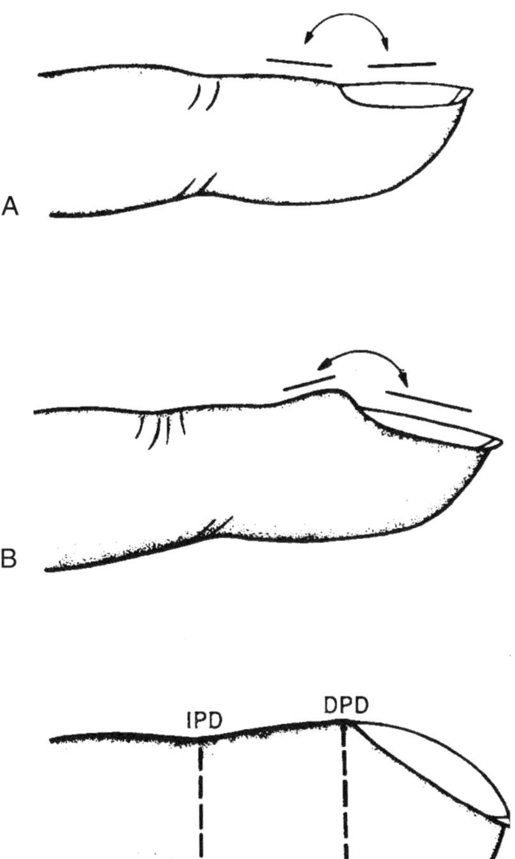

Fig. 2-11. (A) Normal digit configuration. **(B)** Mild digital clubbing with increased hyponychial angle. **(C)** Severe digital clubbing. Depth of finger at base (DPD) is greater than depth of interpharyngeal joint (IPD) with clubbing. (From Wilkins et al.,[15] with permission.)

Is the rate regular or irregular? (Count for a full minute if necessary.)
If the ECG is observed, are there P waves?
Are P-to-P wave and R-to-R intervals regular or irregular?
Is there a P wave before each ventricular complex?
Are the P waves and QRS complexes identical and normal in configuration?
What is the hemodynamic significance of the arrhythmia?

The systolic blood pressure should be taken and the patient's appearance noted. In hemodynamic compromise the blood pressure may be very low, at less than 80/40, or there may be a very high reading, over 200/110. The patient will look pale and agitated and may become cyanotic and show altered mental status.

The peripheral pulses are palpated primarily to determine the presence or absence of a pulse. Primary sites for palpation include the carotid, radial, brachial, femoral, popliteal, and tibial pulses. A carotid pulse will be absent or distant in patients who have carotid stenosis. This leads to symptoms of lightheadedness, loss of consciousness, and strokelike symptoms of slurred speech, sagging facial muscles on one side, and weakness on one side of the body. TIAs, by definition, are reversed, leaving no sequelae, but should be considered as serious warning signs of vascular disease.

Patients who lack a tibial pulse in one or both feet (dorsum) should have their popliteal pulses checked, as well as the femoral pulses, to determine if these too are absent. Thus, the presence of a palpable pulse should mean that blood supply is adequate; when the pulse disappears to palpation, there may be vascular insufficiency.

Palpation can also be useful in early detection of an aneurysm. When a throbbing mass is palpable along an artery, the presence of an aneurysm should be suspected, and immediate referral to a physician for a diagnostic evaluation is indicated. An abdominal aortic aneurysm can be palpated with a two-hand technique above the umbilicus with the patient supine. Pressing the fingers down on points spreading outward from the midline should enable the investigator to feel the pulsations in the aorta, normally at 2 inches apart. Once the spread is wider but the pulsation continues, an aneurysm is suspected (Fig. 2-12). Ausculating for a bruit over the vessel would then be warranted.

Lymphedema is an abnormal accumulation of lymph in the extremities that occurs with infections of the lymphatics, with trauma to lymph channels (e.g., in burns and radiation), with allergic reactions, and with tumors obstructing a channel. The form this edema takes is localized edema, which can lead to extensive fluid accumulation from the level of the obstruction to all distal parts. Body parts thus affected feel pulpy and appear quite bloated.

Local edema may result from any loss of fluid balance between the interstitial and vascular compartments in any segment of the body. Hydrostatic pressure, inside blood vessels, develops as a result of gravity, the force of systolic ejection, and total blood volume. When one or more of these forces prevails over the tissue tension and oncotic pressures, tending to push fluid inward into vessels, edema can result. It may remain local to an area of dependency, characterized by insufficient fluid supply. This fluid accumulation can be palpated but may be less obvious than central or lymphatic sources of edema. It will feel boggy but sometimes will resist pitting.

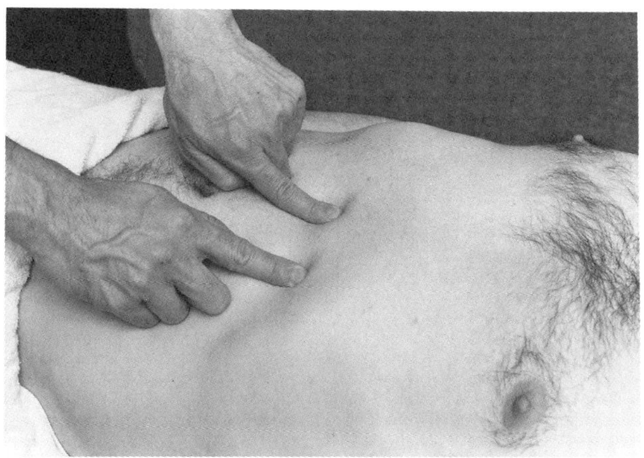

Fig. 2-12. Palpating for the lateralmost borders of the aortic pulse. The therapist should assess the entire length of the palpable portion of the aorta.

It is difficult to assess a patient's vascular status accurately by palpating skin temperatures. The only useful evaluation is to compare the temperature of bilateral extremities by palpation and to note any obvious difference. Skin temperature should be accurately measured with a skin thermometer or thermistor, which will enable the therapist to draw a temperature map of limbs. This map can help assess the areas in which arterial supply is inadequate, as the skin distal to a vascular lesion will be significantly cooler than the proximal skin. Localized distribution of hot, red skin, often accompanied by swelling, may be thrombophlebitis, or deep venous thrombosis (DVT). This condition occurs most commonly in patients who have been bedridden or immobilized for a long period and does not correlate with other vascular diseases.

Auscultation

In order to gain insight into the source of a symptom that may be cardiovascular, or pulmonary, both breath sounds and heart sounds should be auscultated. The patient who is experiencing chest pain may avoid taking a deep breath for fear of worsening the sensation. Muscular splinting may reduce air movement at the bases of both lungs. Patients who are extremely anxious may breathe shallowly or may hyperventilate. Typically, patients with central nervous system (CNS) depression breathe very shallowly. Inspiratory rales will be heard bilaterally in the presence of pulmonary edema. In patients who have chronic CHF, a wheeze may develop if their failure is worsening; rales (crackles) should be audible as well.

Heart sounds normally occur as four distinct sounds: two very prominent high-frequency sounds, the *lubb-dupp* or S1 and S2, and two low-pitched, less obvious sounds, heard most distinctly in pediatric populations because of the lack of subcutaneous tissue and in adult patients who have exaggerated S3 and S4 heart sounds resulting from disease states. Both the S3 and S4 heart sounds are diastolic filling sounds generated by the influx of blood from atria to ventricles during diastole. In patients with CAD who have ventricles with decreased contractility caused by a scar from a myocardial infarction or by ischemia, the decrease in ventricular compliance results in greater volume of blood entering and even greater sloshing of blood as it enters the chambers. These factors amplify the filling sounds. The S3 heart sound occurs shortly after S2, or after semilunar valve closure. When this sound is auscultated, it most likely indicates a large area of noncompliant ventricular muscle, and the entering blood is unable to be accommodated by a stretchy, elastic wall. Patients with an S3 heart sound are typically in heart failure and will require medical attention to compensate for their failure. The S4 heart sound occurs at the end of diastole, when the last bit of blood enters the ventricles from an atrial "kick" as both atria contract. An area of scar or poor wall motion in the ventricles will magnify the S4 heart sound. It does not indicate CHF per se. However, the presence of both an S3 and S4 heart sound is described as a gallop rhythm and represents decompensated CHF.

Auscultation of heart sounds requires skill, which can only be acquired with practice. However, this skill may be one of the most critical for the patient who has known CHF compensated by medication. This patient needs to perform exercise and may be pushed over the edge by exercise into decompensation.

To auscultate for S3 and S4 heart sounds, the patient is placed in the left lateral decubitus position to increase the volume of blood returning to the heart. The bell of the stethoscope is used on the xiphoid, lower left sternal border and listened to during inspiration. The bell of the stethoscope is placed on the apical space over the 5th intercostal space left of the sternal border. The physical therapist listens for S3, S4 on expiration. The sounds may be heard immediately after the "dupp" of "lubb-dupp" (S3) and immediately preceding the "lubb" for S4. The following is a useful mnemonic for each:

"Ken-	tuck-	key"
S1	S2	S3

"Ten-	nes-	see"
S4	S1	S2

Blood Pressure

A clinical measure of blood pressure is one of the most useful simple measures available for assessing cardiac status and patient response to treatment, position change, exercise, and anxiety. The systolic blood pressure represents the product of the cardiac output and the total peripheral resistance. As such, it is an index of myocardial contractility. Unfortunately, there is a high degree of error in the measurement as compared with that taken with an arterial line (anywhere from 5 to 20 mmHg difference), even by experienced clinicians. For therapists who are unaccustomed to auscultation techniques and to the sounds produced in the circulatory system known as Korotkoff sounds, this technique may be quite inaccurate.

When the systolic reading is high, there may be a high cardiac output (as during exercise), or a high degree of peripheral resistance, as in anxiety states or under conditions of stress, or both. Conversely, a low systolic reading implies low cardiac contractility, although this is not necessarily low. There may be a low cardiac output, a low degree of total peripheral resistance, or both. The patient who fails to show an "adaptive" blood pressure response to exercise and who has a flat or falling systolic reading with exercise probably has an inadequate cardiac output, may have a failing ventricle with loss of contractility, and may also have inappropriate peripheral vasodilation.

The product of the systolic blood pressure and the heart rate (rate pressure product or RPP) during exercise at any point is an index of myocardial work. Thus, a patient who has known cardiac disease and who performs exercise should always have both systolic blood pressure and heart rate monitored to determine the degree of work the heart is placed under. If the patient experiences angina with exercise, the RPP will always be the same at the threshold for angina, assuming no change in drug regimen or interim cardiovascular intervention. This stands to reason, since myocardial ischemia occurs when there is an imbalance between myocardial supply of oxygen and the demand for oxygen. The supply is determined by the caliber of coronary vasculature and consequent blood flow, and the demand is the work of the heart. Since the heart functions as a pump, it is intuitively easy to see why it pumps harder when it must work faster (increased heart rate) and when it must increase the power of its contraction (increased contractility, or systolic blood pressure).

Systolic readings during exercise may become very high at maximal levels, and the upper limits of safety are a matter of controversy and not at all standard. Younger subjects can easily tolerate high readings of 220 mmHg, whereas older people may not, even if they have no disease. There is no agreement about setting upper limits for specific age groups, and there must be a high degree of individualization. Common sense dictates that the person with an aortic aneurysm should have a low upper limit for systolic blood pressure, perhaps 170 mmHg. Many elderly subjects may be subject to aortic disease without clinical manifestations and should therefore be held to an upper limit of perhaps 190 mmHg. However, the patient with hypertension has accommodated to much higher pressures over time and should show excessively high systolic responses to exercise.

Diastolic blood pressure should not be higher than 90 mmHg but can drop to zero by auscultation in certain exercising subjects. For people with resting diastolic readings above 90 mmHg, significant hypertension is present that should be reported to the patient's doctor if it is an uncommon finding for this patient. Some patients, however, have labile pressures with a diastolic reading that may be as high as 105 from time to time. This is usually well tolerated and is often left untreated. The significance of the higher diastolic reading is that the myocardium at rest is still facing a high fluid pressure, which implies that there may be a loss of contractility or onset of failure.

The difference between the systolic and the diastolic blood pressure is called the pulse pressure. This difference should not narrow with exercise, or it is a grave sign of pending cardiac failure. Clearly, if the cardiac output is falling with a resultant drop in systolic pressure, and the amount of pressure in diastole is rising with fluid backup and loss of contractility, the pulse pressure is narrowing. This becomes an important indicator for eventual distress.

All patients who have known heart disease, and any who exhibit signs or symptoms of heart disease, should have their blood pressure measured. Blood pressure should be measured at rest and with the patient in supine, sitting, and standing positions, to determine orthostatic adjustment before exercise, and certainly during and after exercise.

ELECTROCARDIOGRAM

The ECG is the surface recording of the electrical activity of the heart. It tells nothing about the mechanical, contractile function of the heart or about its effectiveness as a pump. However, the ECG does shed light on two overall aspects of myocardial function: the excitability of cardiac tissue and the nutritional status of regions of the heart. When 12 leads are monitored, representing the standard measurement of electrical activity, the nutritional status of all the different aspects, from base to apex, from anterior to posterior, and from lateral to inferior, can be assessed. When ischemia is present, the sensitive segment on the ECG is the region representing ventricular repolarization, known as the ST segment. When injury and/or necrosis is present, the same segment will register a different change. Ischemia depresses the ST segment; injury elevates it. The particular lead(s) where these signs are found indicate(s) the location of injury, without specifying an anatomic distribution.

Hyperexcitable states of the myocardium include extra beats generated from irritable foci; hypoexcitability may be seen as conduction pathway delays or blocks. For this parameter, any lead will show the same information, although some may be easier to see than others. Thus, a rhythm-strip ECG is a single-lead tracing over a period of time in order to track the relative excitability of the tissue. On a single-lead rhythm strip, taken at rest, consecutive beats should be checked for regular intervals of P-QRS-T, (see Fig. 2-5), which do not vary from beat to beat. In heart block or sinus arrest, segments of this normal waveform may be prolonged, missing, or dissociated, thereby creating pauses in the palpated pulse. Premature beats can readily be found as those appearing early and therefore too close to the previous beat for the normal R-to-R interval. The configuration of these premature beats is critical. If they resemble the normal beat, but occur early, and have a P wave before the QRS complex, they are usually atrial, whereas if they have a wide, quite different configuration from the normal beat, and have no P wave before the QRS, they are ventricular. If there is more than one premature beat, they may all be the same in configuration, or there may be more than one type, or multiform. Uniform beats originate from a single ectopic focus; multiform beats originate from several ectopic foci.

The significance of an irregular heartbeat can be determined from a functional evaluation. The physical therapist can choose one or more pertinent activities for the patient to perform while being monitored with a rhythm-strip ECG. In addition, vital signs will help determine the hemodynamic status of the patient during the activity. Since activity increases myocardial work, this may induce an irregular heartbeat, especially in cases in which myocardial dysfunction or hypoxia is responsible for the arrhythmia. Some arrhythmias occur at rest or at low levels of activity and are abolished with higher energy requirements because of the overriding influence of the sinus node when exercise demands induce sympathetic stimulation to that node. Many arrhythmias will not be influenced by activity, but activity will be tolerated less well than rest. This is due to the inadequate hemodynamic response available to support activity requirements under conditions of myocardial arrhythmias.

Some additional problems with cardiac rhythm can arise. These include severe sinus bradycardia, which may result in serious hemodynamic compromise and require emergency measures but yield no irregularity of pulse. Severe sinus tachycardia may not be well tolerated by some patients because of severe anxiety associated with the sensation of flutter in their chests and because of inadequate diastolic filling time. Medical treatment may be necessary, although usually not on an urgent basis.

CARDIOVASCULAR PATHOPHYSIOLOGY

The seven most frequently encountered cardiovascular disease states seen in patient populations from an indus-

Observations that the physical therapist should make during activity on the patient who has a rhythm-strip ECG recording include the following items (see Fig 2-9):

1. Describe heartbeat in terms of rate and rhythm, whether premature or not.
2. Describe P waves, PR and QRS intervals, and morphology. If ventricular in configuration, what is the frequency of the premature beat? If it is less than 6 per minute, this is probably well tolerated. If it is greater than 6 per minute, check vital signs for evidence of hemodynamic intolerance.
3. Describe signs and symptoms of hemodynamic compromise.
4. Note what provoked the arrhythmia.
5. Note what caused any change in it.
6. Check the relationship of P waves to QRS complexes. If P waves appear at their own rhythm, unrelated to QRS complexes, the patient may have third-degree heart block, which will not be tolerated well for long. Some cases of atrial to ventricular dissociation are tolerated without any problem.
7. If P waves occasionally trigger QRS complexes in a normal sequence, but at other times are not followed by a QRS complex, the patient may have second-degree heart block, and that could deteriorate into third-degree heart block.
8. PVCs are more serious if they occur frequently, are multiform, and/or if they occur early (R on T), because they are more likely to deteriorate into ventricular tachycardia.
9. Ventricular tachycardia, seen as three or more PVCs, may deteriorate into ventricular fibrillation and become life-threatening or may not promote adequate peripheral perfusion, resulting in hemodynamic compromise.
10. Ventricular fibrillation calls for immediate electrical countershock as an emergency measure. Cardiopulmonary resuscitation (CPR) should be initiated and a code called.

trialized society are CAD, arrhythmias, heart failure, hypertension, valvular heart disease and endocarditis, pericardial disease, and aortic and vascular tree disease.

Coronary Artery Disease

Whether presenting as chronic angina pectoris, unstable angina, myocardial infraction (MI), sudden death, or congestive ischemic cardiomyopathy, the underlying pathologic lesion will be a unifying one in most cases (i.e., atherosclerosis of the coronary arteries). Atherosclerosis involves a progressive thickening and hardening of the medium-sized and large muscular arteries, usually the coronary, carotid, basilar, vertebral, aortic, and iliac vessels. Epidemiologic efforts have identified various risk factors that predispose to the development of atherosclerosis. These include a family history of CAD before the age of 60; male gender; women who are postmenopausal; a history of hypertension or diabetes mellitus, dyslipoproteinemia involving an elevation in the low-density lipoprotein (LDL) fraction and/or depression of the high-density lipoprotein (HDL) cholesterol fraction; recent tobacco abuse; obesity; physical inactivity; and psychological profile characterized by high levels of stress, hostility, and anger.

Current understanding of the mechanisms of atherogenesis recognizes a complex process involving several key cell types, including endothelial cells, platelets, macrophages, and smooth muscle cells. Vascular thickening is a consequence of plaque formation, which results from endothelial injury, platelet–endothelial interaction, and lipid accumulation. Initial change is thought to occur as early as age 3 years with the development of the fatty streak, a slightly raised lesion in which limited numbers of smooth muscle cells and lipid-containing macrophages invade the endothelium or inner lining of the blood vessel wall. In the genetically predisposed person or one with known risk factors, these lesions may mature, becoming fibrotic and more obstructive. Endothelial damage occurs with increasing shear stress from blood flow, hyperlipidemia, hypertension, immune injury, homocystine, or cigarette smoking. Endothelial lining cells release several growth factors that trigger platelet activation and aggregation as well as vascular smooth muscle contraction. If exposed to elevated levels of circulating lipids, fibrotic portions of atherosclerotic plaques develop with further accumulation of lipid-laden macrophages, migration of smooth muscle cells, and collagen synthesis. Further maturation of the lesion, elevated cholesterol concentration within the lipid fraction results in cholesterol crystal formation in the older, deeper layers.

Presumably the gradual narrowing of coronary flow can cause the chronic pattern of exertionally related angina pectoris. Rupture or fissure of a plaque causes a sudden change in lesion shape, triggering the cascade of events that leads to intraluminal thrombosis, resulting in unstable angina (Fig. 2-13). Whether a person goes on to suffer an MI will depend on the degree and duration of inadequate coronary blood flow. Sudden ischemic death can result, too, in this setting of prolonged coronary insufficiency, in which fatal ventricular arrhythmias are triggered.

Patients with atherosclerotic CAD can present with (1) a chronic pattern of effort- or stress-related chest pain known as angina pectoris; (2) chest pain that is new, increasing in intensity or frequency, occurring at lower workloads, or requiring more sublingual nitroglycerin for relief, called unstable angina; (3) chest pain and other constitutional symptoms associated with MI; or (4) death. Indeed, of the roughly 1.5 million people in the United States who suffer an MI annually, 540,000 (36 percent) will die—350,000 of those before medical attention can be obtained.[16] While patients typically present in middle or advanced age, coronary atherosclerosis progresses over decades. Autopsies of young adults killed in military combat or accidentally frequently demonstrate evidence of coronary atherosclerosis. Both sexes are susceptible, with incidence rates of disease for women increasing and surpassing those of men once into the postmenopausal years.

Several tests and studies are frequently done to evaluate patients suspected of having or known to have CAD. A resting ECG is normal up to 50 percent of the time in those with chronic stable angina. Evidence of previous injury may be seen in the form of Q waves in a particular distribution. The most common findings are nonspecific ST segment and T wave abnormalities. If the patient is unstable, transient depression or elevation of the ST segment often associated with T wave inversions is seen. Recording of an ECG during and after some type of stressful intervention, such as exercise, is valuable in assessing cardiovascular reserve and the possible degree of hemodynamic compromise. Exercise tolerance tests are often performed in this group of patients. A definitive diagnosis of CAD requires highlighting of the coro-

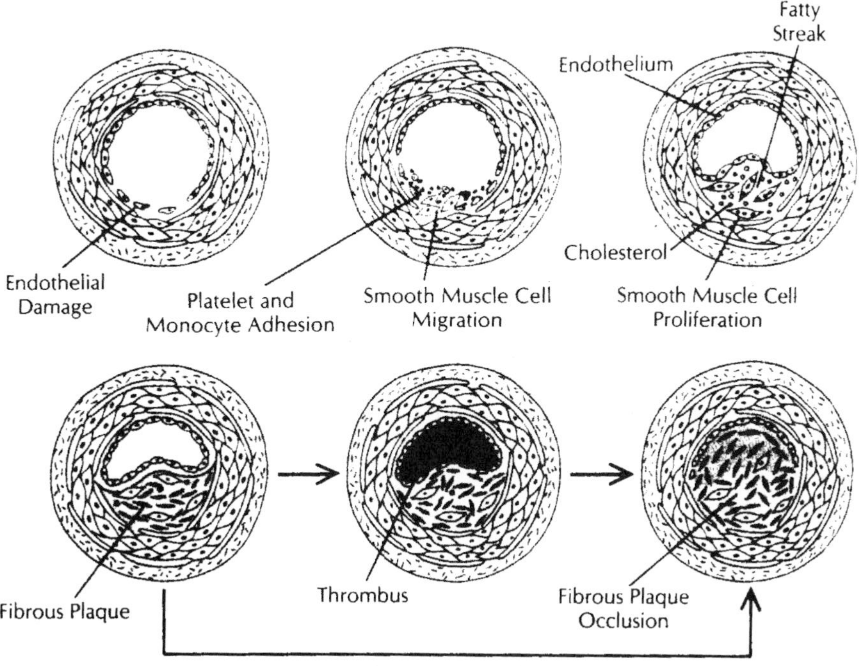

Fig. 2-13. Proposed cellular changes involved in plaque formation, thrombosis, and vascular occlusion. (Modified from Stein et al.,[6] with permission.)

nary blood vessels with radiocontrast in a procedure known as coronary angiography. This technique is part of cardiac catheterization, with left ventriculography also performed at this time. By injecting radiocontrast into the left ventricle, an estimation of cardiac performance and evidence of any prior injury can be obtained. Noninvasive evaluations of left ventricular performance can be obtained by cardiac ultrasound (echocardiography) and radionuclide angiography with a first-pass radionuclide angiogram and the gated blood pool study.

Exercise Tolerance Test

Patients with suspected CAD, whether the symptom of chest pain is present or not, will most likely be evaluated in a cardiology stress-testing laboratory. Although diagnosis is an important goal of the ETT, other very significant items of information can be derived. These include definition of a dose–response relationship between exertion and cardiovascular adaptation, establishment of an optimal prescription for exercise, identification of a patient's limitations to exercise, induction of arrhythmias, and assessment of efficacy of a recent addition to one's antianginal regimen or recent procedure. A variety of protocols exist using either a treadmill or a cycle ergometer. The advantages of using a standardized protocol are many. A patient's response can be compared with that of a larger pool of similar subjects. Also, a baseline can be established in the patient's dose response, which can be compared with a future ETT after an intervention, after a period of time has elapsed, or upon the appearance of a new sign or symptom. Exercise is carefully titrated in increasing doses. This is why a consistent protocol with known energy requirements must be used, so that the cardiac responses to each "dose" or exercise level may be identified. Cardiac responses monitored include heart rate, blood pressure, and ECG changes. The ECG provides information about the status of myocardial perfusion (ST segment) and the rhythm. Arrhythmias arise when the myocardium is hypoxic, with metabolic abnormalities, or because of inherent conduction problems. Blood pressure monitoring gives important information about the hemodynamic responsiveness of the heart under exercise conditions. Systolic readings may be abnormally high or low, may drop when they should be rising, or may be normal, all of which can help determine the significance of the chest pain. When a standard Bruce treadmill protocol is used, the normal systolic rise is 12 mmHg per stage. With cycle ergometry, the blood pressure rise should be higher than with treadmill testing because of the muscular activity in the arms contributing to stabilizing the torso.

In the case of chest pain, the ETT can be used to determine the symptom threshold, in terms of either the workload at which chest pain arises or the heart rate and/or blood pressure at which chest pain appears. The product of heart rate and systolic blood pressure at the point that angina occurs can be used clinically as the RPP at angina threshold. This index correlates highly with actual measurement of myocardial oxygen consumption, providing a handy clinical tool for the indirect measure of myocardial work. The equation that no longer balances supply with demand demonstrates an RPP at which angina occurs and supply is inadequate. This relationship is relatively fixed until one of several things happens: the disease progresses and the RPP is lower at a given angina threshold; a therapy such as β-blockade is instituted that affects heart rate and blood pressure even at angina threshold; or an exercise training program is successfully undertaken that can raise the RPP where angina is experienced or eliminates the experience of angina, even up to maximal exercise.

In using the ETT results to establish an exercise prescription, the anginal threshold heart rate is taken as the symptom-limited maximal heart rate, and not the true physiologic maximum. A percentage of this symptom-limited maximum heart rate is then used as a target heart rate for training. Frequently, 10 bpm less than symptomatic maximum is chosen for a target. American College of Sports Medicine guidelines[17] recommend 70 to 85 percent of the symptom-limited maximum heart rate level or use of the Karvonen equation:

$$\text{Target heart rate} = (HR_{max} - HR_{rest}) \times 0.7 + HR_{rest}$$

The ETT results may show that a patient who experiences chest pain has no ischemic ST segment change. The question arises as to whether the chest pain is actually not of cardiac origin or is a false-negative ECG finding. The test may demonstrate no chest pain but a positive ST segment change. Is this silent ischemia or a false-positive ECG finding? When a test is negative for both chest pain and ischemic ST segment change, is the patient actually free of hemodynamically significant CAD, or was the exercise level attained inadequate to produce diagnostic information? To clarify such situations, current practice is to perform a diagnostic ETT with myocardial imaging techniques using thallium in order to observe myocardial perfusion.

The physical therapist may be in a position to need such information about a patient for whom a standard stress test is unavailable or not possible. It is quite reasonable to perform a standardized exercise at initial low levels with gradually increasing increments of effort with appropriate patient monitoring without calling it a formal stress test. If an appropriate activity can be identified that can be performed under relatively controlled conditions (e.g., 6-minute walk test, one flight of stairs, or wheelchair propulsion over an identified distance), the method of performance must be documented to make it repeatable, and the same parameters must be monitored in order to develop the dose–response relationship.

Arrhythmias

Rhythm disturbances involve an abnormality in the generation and/or propagation of the heartbeat. This can occur as an isolated situation or may be related to other underlying problems of the cardiovascular system. Its presence may be unknown to the patient, may cause troublesome symptoms resulting in no blood pressure abnormalities, or may lead to sudden death. Separate from this general discussion of the pathophysiology of arrhythmias is the earlier discussion on recognition of specific arrhythmias.

Cardiac arrhythmias are thought to arise as a result of one of two possible mechanisms. The first involves a disturbance in automaticity, the inherent property of the conduction system to generate a heartbeat. If the rate of the normal cardiac pacemaker is too fast or too slow, this is referred to as sinus tachycardia or sinus bradycardia. Other parts of the conduction system (i.e., the AV nodal junction), as well as the atrial and ventricular myocardium, are capable of impulse generation. These can be single beats arising early, known as premature ventricular or atrial beats (also contractions, complexes, and depolarizations), or accelerated junctional beats. Sustained rhythms of more than three beats in duration include the atrial, supraventricular, and ventricular tachycardias.

The second mechanism for arrhythmia generation results from a disturbance in conductivity, the appropriate distribution of a normal heartbeat throughout the myocardium. The conduction abnormality can result from AV block. As such, it is classified as first-, second-, or third-degree block.

First-degree AV block: The site of conduction delay is nearly always in the AV node. Recognition is made by prolongation of the PR interval on the 12-lead ECG.

Second-degree AV block: This abnormality is divided into Mobitz type I, in which delay is within the AV node, and Mobitz type II, with delay occurring below the AV node in the His-Purkinje system.

Third-degree AV block: Also referred to as complete heart block in which conduction of the heartbeat from atria to ventricles is completely blocked, the actual site of the block is in the bundle-branch system.

Further disturbances in conduction can give rise to the phenomenon known as re-entry. In re-entry, an impulse that would normally reach a branch point and travel at equal rates of speed down both branches on toward the ventricle is slowed in one branch and blocked in the other. The impulse will be delayed in reaching its destination down one branch. Because the block experienced by the impulse in the other branch was unidirectional, the stage is set for the delayed impulse now to go backward up the unidirectionally blocked branch, re-entering the system as an ectopic or abnormal beat. This mechanism is seen with such cardiovascular diseases as CAD and cardiomyopathy. It too can give rise to isolated or sustained premature beats or rhythms.

Also seen in conduction disturbances is the phenomenon of bypass tract conduction or pre-excitation. In this condition, depolarization of the ventricular myocardium occurs earlier than expected because conduction is occurring by way of an anomalous pathway or bypass tract that conducts much more quickly than the normal conduction system. Wolff-Parkinson-White syndrome is an example of this phenomenon. It is characterized on the ECG by a short PR interval and frequently with a delta (δ) wave preceding each QRS complex, lending a widened, bizarre appearance. Clinically, these patients will present with palpitations or lightheadedness resulting from a variety of tachyarrhythmias that can develop.

The 12-lead ECG and rhythm strip are the most important tools for diagnosing these disorders. A Holter monitor is often ordered to diagnose rhythms or conduction abnormalities that may be transient and not present at the time an ECG is obtained; to quantify frequency of a problem; or to determine possible arrhythmic precipitants of a symptom complex. The Holter monitor continuously scans and records two chest leads over a 24-hour period.

A recently developed technique, known as signal-averaged ECG, is used to identify patients at risk of future malignant arrhythmias, as is the case in postinfarction patients or in patients with a cardiomyopathy. With this technique, low-amplitude electrical activity occurring in the late phase of the QRS complex is amplified and averaged in a computer-assisted process. These late potentials are the presumed substrate for re-entrant ventricular arrhythmias. If a patient has been discovered to have serious arrhythmias that will require drug therapy, or if a serious arrhythmia is suspected but cannot be documented, electrophysiologic studies (EPS) may be pursued. These invasive studies require the placement of one or more intracardiac catheters to record and stimulate portions of the heart that are electrically silent on the body surface ECG (e.g., sinus node, right or left atrium, His bundle, right bundle branch, left bundle branch, and specific sites within the right or left ventricle).

Heart Failure

Defined broadly, heart failure is the condition in which the heart is unable to supply all body tissues adequately with oxygenated blood. Heart failure can occur even though the heart muscle is normal, as in situations in which venous return to the heart is impaired (e.g., constrictive pericarditis or restrictive cardiomyopathy). Most cases result from the actual inability of the myocardium to contract sufficiently. This condition is generally produced by cumulative ischemic injury, as seen with ischemic cardiomyopathy. It can also result from chronic alcohol exposure, the peripartal state, Adriamycin toxicity, diabetes, sarcoidosis, Chagas disease, or amyloidosis. Frequently no etiology is found, and recent viral infection is suspected.

Patients with heart failure will present with congestive symptoms, the particular pattern of which can help in defining the failure as left sided, right sided, or biventricular. A distinction is made between chronic and acute heart failure. A chronic condition is present and unchanged for a minimum of 3 months, and an acute situation is manifested within minutes to hours, usually in association with myocardial ischemia or infarction. The acute presentation is often referred to as pulmonary edema.

Hemodynamically, abnormalities include decreased cardiac output and elevated ventricular filling pressures. Hypoperfusion, as a result of a drop in cardiac output, can lead to confusion, weakness, and cold and clammy extremities. Elevated left ventricular filling pressures, clinically measured as mean left atrial pressure or left ventricular end-diastolic pressure, cause pulmonary venous congestion, leading to exertional dyspnea, nonproductive and nocturnal cough, orthopnea, and paroxysmal nocturnal dyspnea. Elevated filling pressures of the right heart, measured by use of a central venous pressure (CVP) catheter, are associated with systemic venous congestion manifested by pedal edema, abdominal discomfort and/or distention, and anorexia.

A major component in the clinical presentation of these hemodynamic abnormalities is the compensatory attempts made by the body. While initially helpful, these efforts invariably become counterproductive. The sympathetic nervous system and the renin–angiotensin system are stimulated, leading to increased heart rate, increased filling pressure, and increased contractility. In addition, myocardial hypertrophy occurs. When carried to the extreme, increased arterial vascular tone results in increased peripheral resistance and afterload on the already failing left ventricle. Venoconstriction shifts blood volume into the central circulation, worsening congestive symptoms. Finally, filling pressures past an optimal point simply add to congestion.

Once heart failure becomes even moderate in extent, the patient will be easily fatigued with minimal effort, will often require multiple daily medication, and will have a host of cardiac management problems. Whether the CHF patient is being examined de novo, having the efficacy of a new drug assessed, or being seen for follow-up management, left ventricular function must be evaluated. The most accurate and thorough determination of left ventricular performance is invasively at cardiac catheterization when pressure, flow, and volume can be measured and dimensions calculated. Noninvasive measures can be done with echocardiography and radionuclide angiography. Increasingly, structured exercise protocols are being added to these assessments of left ventricular performance for better definition of the functional response to interventions and overall prognosis.

Hypertension

Arbitrarily defined as a blood pressure above 140/90 mmHg, hypertension affects 20 percent of adult Americans. Of those, 90 percent have no identifiable secondary cause of the hypertension and are said to suffer from essential or primary hypertension. The remaining 10 percent have treatable or reversible causes of hypertension, such as renal parenchymal disease, renovascular disease, primary aldosteronism, Cushing syndrome, pheochromocytoma, coarctation of the aorta, or hyperparathyroidism. Although largely asymptomatic, left untreated, hypertension will shorten life by 10 to 20 years, primarily because of acceleration of atherosclerosis, but also by leading to stroke, heart failure, peripheral vascular disease, renal insufficiency, and retinopathy.

Blood pressure is determined primarily by cardiac output and peripheral resistance. The multifaceted, regulatory networks that control cardiac output, fluid status within and outside the vascular bed, and vascular caliber and responsiveness all must respond to the increased pressure load of hypertension. Many observations have been made about hypertension, but the underlying cause has not yet been identified. Two main mechanistic theories prevail: (1) an increased level of cardiac function results from overstimulation by the sympathetic nervous system, and (2) primary retention of salt and water by the kidneys may lead to elevated blood pressure levels. Heredity obviously has a role to play in many instances of essential hypertension. Another contributing factor is the person's lifestyle including percentage body weight above ideal, dietary habits, level of habitual physical activity, tobacco use, and possible oral contraceptive use.

The diagnosis of hypertension can be made during the physical examination, requiring no more than a stethoscope and sphygmomanometer. Because most hypertension by far is classified as essential hypertension, the standard evaluation initially includes only a few simple laboratory tests of blood and urine to determine severity of cardiovascular disease, possible causes of hypertension, overall cardiovascular risk, and baseline values for judging therapeutic efficacy. These include hemoglobin and hematocrit values; complete urinalysis; serum potassium, calcium, creatinine, and uric acid; and plasma lipid profile (total cholesterol, LDL and HDL cholesterols, and triglycerides) and plasma glucose.

Valvular Heart Disease and Endocarditis

The four heart valves can develop abnormalities either obstructing the forward flow of blood (stenosis) or allowing blood to leak backward into the preceding chamber (regurgitation). Involvement of either the mitral or aortic valve is more common and more debilitating than right-sided lesions.

Mitral Stenosis

Mitral stenosis is almost always a result of rheumatic fever. There is always a delay of many years between the acute fever and the development of symptoms. Rheumatic fever distorts the valve apparatus in a number of ways, all of which result in fusion of the valves. A normal valve opening or orifice is 4 to 6 cm^2. A reduction to 2 cm^2 is considered mild and to 1 cm^2 critical. At this level of stenosis, a pressure gradient between left atrium and left ventricle develops. This increase in pressure is transmitted backward, in turn raising the pulmonary venous and capillary pressures. This results in exertional dyspnea. Further clinical compromise is dictated by the degree of increased pulmonary vascular resistance and lowered cardiac output.

Women have a higher incidence of mitral stenosis. Typically, the patient with mitral stenosis will present with dyspnea, largely the result of reduced compliance of the lungs. Other complications of this lesion include infective endocarditis, hemoptysis, chest pain of unclear etiology, and thromboembolism. Often atrial fibrillation will develop. Once patients become moderately symptomatic, medical management becomes more difficult, and invasive procedures are entertained. In certain situations, mitral valvuloplasty is a consideration. Operative approaches that are available for rheumatic mitral stenosis include closed mitral commissurotomy (reopening of the valve leaflets by splitting along the fused commissures), open commissurotomy with the aid of cardiopulmonary bypass, and mitral valve replacement.

Mitral Regurgitation

Abnormalities of any portion of the mitral valve apparatus can result in incompetence. Leaflet involvement is seen most commonly in chronic rheumatic heart disease. The mitral annulus, a portion of the fibroskeleton of the heart that is the attachment point of the leaflet base, can become dilated or calcified, resulting in regurgitation, especially in the elderly. Abnormalities of the chordae tendineae, either congenital or a consequence of infective endocarditis, trauma, rheumatic fever, or myxomatous degeneration, can result in problems, often acutely and without warning. Finally, the papillary muscle, which completes the connection between leaflet and chordae to the ventricular wall, can rupture, usually as a result of ischemia. Pathophysiologically, the left atrium receives a significant portion of the blood flow in systole, which would normally have been ejected into the aorta. There is also overloading and eventual dilatation of the left ventricle as the left atrium chronically discharges its excessive blood volume into it during diastole.[18] Whether the patient presents with fatigue and exhaustion from a low-output state or with pulmonary edema and right-sided failure depends on the chronicity of the lesion.

Because of the multiple etiologies resulting in mitral regurgitation, the natural history of the disease is quite variable and appears to be dependent on both the regurgitant volumes as well as on the underlying etiology. Acute pulmonary edema, hemoptysis, and systemic embolization are less likely to occur than in mitral stenosis. If symptoms do develop, the presenting picture is that of CHF. Medical management is focused on afterload reduction. Once surgery is decided on, options include annuloplasty (repair or support of the existing valve structure) or valve replacement.

The mitral valve prolapse syndrome involves a common cardiac valvular abnormality that can include mitral regurgitation. For most people with this diagnosis, it remains an echocardiographic finding with no resultant symptoms, functional implications, or effect on future outcomes. In a few cases, symptoms can include palpitations, chest discomfort, and, when mitral regurgitation is severe, symptoms of heart failure. Etiology of the chest discomfort is postulated to involve increased papillary muscle tension and left ventricular wall motion abnormalities. The clinical course can be complicated by arrhythmias, endocarditis, progressive mitral regurgitation requiring valve replacement, and cerebral embolization.

Aortic Stenosis

Valvular aortic stenosis is usually either congenital or degenerative in origin. In most cases, nodular calcium deposits on the valve cusps prevent normal opening during systole. With obstruction to left ventricular output, a pressure gradient develops between the left ventricle and the aorta. Output is maintained by hypertrophy of the left ventricle. Patients with aortic stenosis can remain symptom free until late in the course of the disease, when the heart can no longer meet the oxygen demands of the massively hypertrophied left ventricle.

The natural history of patients with aortic stenosis is characterized by a long latent period. Despite increasing obstruction of the aortic valve and myocardial hypertrophy, the patient is asymptomatic. Typically, symptoms develop in the sixth decade of life and include angina, syncope, and dyspnea. By the time symptoms appear, the prognosis is poor, and only with invasive intervention is there any hope of interrupting the projected 2- to 5-year survival. Angina experienced by the patient with aortic stenosis is attributed to the increased oxygen demands of the hypertrophic myocardium as well as diminished oxygen supply caused by compression of the coronary vessels. CAD can co-exist and can also contribute to symptoms.

The ECG will demonstrate left ventricular hypertrophy in most patients, seen as a marked increase in voltage of the QRS complex. Chest radiography commonly demonstrates post-stenotic dilatation of the ascending aorta. If the aortic stenosis is severe, calcification of the valve is almost always present in the adult patient. The most sensitive and specific noninvasive test is the echocardiogram. With its various modes of inquiry, it can define abnormal valvular shape and restricted leaflet motion, measure blood flow through the valve, measure the pressure gradient across the valve, and calculate valve area. When surgery is contemplated, cardiac catheterization is usually performed to assess pressure gradients and valve area, using catheter measurements, as well as to evaluate for coronary atherosclerosis. Aortic valve replacement is the definitive procedure for critical aortic stenosis. Valvuloplasty of the aortic valve is generally reserved for patients considered too frail to withstand surgery.

Aortic Regurgitation

Aortic regurgitation can result either from valve leaflet abnormalities (e.g., rheumatic fever or infective endocarditis) or from abnormalities of the aorta (e.g., Marfan syndrome, syphilis, or rheumatoid arthritis). In a patient with chronic regurgitation of blood, the left ventricle compensates by dilating. Symptoms arise when the heart fails to achieve an effective forward cardiac output. When acute, the left ventricle is unable to compensate by dilating; left ventricular failure quickly occurs as the ventricle is unable to meet the burden of acute, severe volume overload.

Chronic aortic regurgitation is characterized by a latency period during which the left ventricle is slowly dilating; the patient is asymptomatic until late in the course of the disease, once left ventricular dysfunction has developed. These symptoms include exertional dyspnea, orthopnea, and paroxysmal nocturnal dyspnea. The left ventricle tolerates acute, severe regurgitation poorly; the patient with acute regurgitation usually presents with sudden cardiovascular collapse (i.e., weakness, severe dyspnea, and hypotension).

Electrocardiographic findings of aortic regurgitation are relatively subtle. The chest radiographic findings are dependent on the duration and severity of regurgitation as well as left ventricular function. In chronic aortic regurgitation, marked enlargement of the cardiac silhouette and dilation of the ascending aorta are common findings. The echocardiogram demonstrates abnormal valve function, the effects of regurgitation on surrounding structures, changes in left ventricular size and function, and turbulent regurgitant flow across the aortic valve in diastole. Severe aortic regurgitation is an indication for surgical replacement of the valve.

Infective Endocarditis

Heart valve leaflets are derived from endocardium. When they become infected, the condition is referred to as endocarditis. A large variety of bacteria can infect the heart valves, as can yeast and fungi. In general, normal valves in a healthy person do not become infected. An abnormal, damaged, or prosthetic valve is much more vulnerable to infection. The likelihood of infections is increased by other systemic illnesses, burns, placement of inert material (e.g., a catheter line or pacemaker wire near or through the valves), and intravenous drug abuse. Once infected, vegetations develop on the leaflets. These vegetations can embolize to other parts of the body; rupture the surrounding structures, leading to valvular lesions; produce a persistent bacteremia; or develop into an immunologic disorder.

Patients with endocarditis can present with symptoms of only a few days' duration, yet be critically ill. This condition is referred to as acute bacterial endocarditis. Conversely, chronic illness with symptoms of fatigue, weight loss, low-grade fever, and arthralgia is the picture of subacute bacterial endocarditis. The diagnosis is made when multiple blood cultures demonstrate the offending organism. Echocardiography can demonstrate valvular and myocardial function and the presence of valvular vegetations. Patients are treated with organism-specific intravenous antibiotics for extended periods.

Pericardial Disease

The double-layered tissue lining the heart can become inflamed and accumulate fluid, known as an effusion, between the two layers. The usual presentation is that of chest pain, a pericardial friction rub, and typical ECG abnormalities. The numerous causes of this inflammation include viral infection, bacterial infection, uremia, trauma, postpericardiotomy syndrome, neoplasia, and postinfarction syndrome. Effusions usually resolve spontaneously, but some can become chronic. In the event of scarring of either the parietal or visceral pericardium, constrictive pericarditis develops, interfering with cardiac filling. The patient presents with exertional dyspnea, abdominal swelling, fatigability, and edema. Cardiac tamponade arises when the accumulation of fluid around the heart is hemodynamically compromising. Typically urgent in nature, cardiac tamponade often requires hemodynamic support and periocardiocentesis.

Aortic and Vascular Tree Diseases

The aorta can be afflicted by any of four entities. Aneurysms or widening of the aorta can arise. If all three layers of this large artery are involved, it is a true aneurysm. If the intima and media are disrupted and it is only the adventitial layer with a perivascular clot expanding outward, it is referred to as a false aneurysm. Most aneurysms are caused by atherosclerosis, but trauma, infections, or genetically weakened media, known as cystic medial necrosis, can have the same result. Dissection of the aorta can occur in which the intima is disrupted. Blood enters between the vessel layers, separating them further. A weakened medial layer predisposes to this predicament, as seen with cystic medial necrosis, Marfan syndrome, chronic hypertension, pregnancy, coarctation of the aorta, or a bicuspid aortic valve. A third entity is occlusive disease of the aorta caused by atherosclerosis. As in the coronary vascular bed, there is plaque formation, rupture, hemorrhage, and thrombus formation. Fourth, aortitis, or inflammation of the aorta, can also occur. Syphilis is the best known etiology, although other infectious and noninfectious agents have been identified.

Aneurysms of the aorta in the abdominal region are generally asymptomatic, picked up incidentally on a routine physical examination. Aneurysms can cause a sense of fullness or a continuous, gnawing pain in the low back. Expansion of the aneurysm produces sudden, severe pain in the same low back or lower abdominal region. Actual rupture links excruciating pain with hypotension and shock. A physical examination is limited in that it can reveal an enlarged, pulsatile mass at best. Diagnoses and definition of the aneurysm are accomplished with a variety of procedures, which may include plain films of the chest and abdomen, ultrasound, computed tomography scanning, and angiography. Because aneurysms will continue to expand and lead to rupture if left alone, elective surgery is recommended once aneurysms reach a certain diameter. Whether elective or emergent, surgery involves resection of the aneurysm and insertion of a prosthetic vascular graft.

In an older patient population the effects of atherosclerosis involving the vascular system are seen more distally. Patients typically present with intermittent claudication. As the blood supply to the lower extremity is further impaired, pain can be present at rest, and ulcers or gangrene of the toes and distal foot develop. The more distal vasculature can also be acutely occluded or interrupted by embolism, thrombosis, or injury.

The symptoms, findings on physical examination, and testing procedures are discussed earlier in this chapter. Older patients may have symptoms for many years; efforts are aimed at modifying risk factors, such as cessation of smoking, weight loss, and exercise training. If pain becomes intolerable even without exertion, tissue appears threatened by insufficient blood supply, or testing suggests critical occlusive disease, patients may undergo percutaneous angioplasty by means of fluoroscopically guided catheters or surgery for either vascular repair or bypass graft placement.

SUMMARY

This chapter discusses the anatomy, physiology, and pathophysiology of the cardiovascular system as it applies to patients seen by health care providers in daily practice. The clinical entities identified are discussed according to the symptoms presented to the physical therapist. By building on this information with the appropriate physical evaluation and diagnostic testing, the therapist can develop a practical approach to data collection, understanding, and management of the patient with cardiovascular disease.

PATIENT CASE STUDY 1

History

The patient was a 42-year-old social worker who came to the clinic with a diagnosis of mechanical low back pain syndrome. Her chief complaint was a constant dull ache in the central lower thoracic and upper lumbar regions. Sitting and standing for more than a couple of minutes would increase the intensity of the aching. Assuming a supine or side-lying position for 20 to 30 minutes would decrease the intensity of the ache to its usual level of discomfort. The aching was least intense early in the morning but increased progressively through the remainder of the day. Although the ache made falling asleep difficult, once asleep, the patient was not awakened by pain. The symptoms began 18 months before the physical therapy evaluation. The patient described the aching as beginning 4 to 5 days after she had cleaned her closet. She underwent physical therapy for 6 weeks, receiving ultrasound, hot packs, transcutaneous electrical nerve stimulation (TENS), and electrical stimulation. The patient received no relief of symptoms. She also described an intermittent deep throbbing pain in the same general area. The onset of this symptom was associated with increased exertion, such as climbing stairs or walking uphill. She could obtain relief by stopping and sitting or by leaning forward with her upper body supported by a car, railing, or tree. She noted shortness of breath when the throbbing sensation was present. These symptoms began insidiously 12 months before the evaluation. She had not seen a physician specifically for these symptoms.

The patient also described an intermittent sharp pain in the right lumbosacral junction region. This symptom was associated with a few repetitions of bending or lifting. Stopping the activity usually eliminated the pain within minutes. This symptom dated back to the L4–L5, L5–S1 lumbar fusion operation she had undergone in 1983.

The patient's medical history included a lumbar decompression surgery L4–L5, L5–S1 in 1980 and subsequent decompression and lumbar fusion of L4–L5, L5–S1 in 1983. Her surgical history also included a hysterectomy. Outside of being treated for colitis in 1983, the patient stated that her general medical history was negative. She also denied any history of smoking. The only medication she was taking was cyclobenzaprine (Flexeril). The only significant family medical history item she offered was that her father had died from a cerebrovascular accident.

Physical Examination

In a standing position, the patient presented with a decreased low lumbar lordosis and a markedly increased lordosis in the mid-lumbar region. A slightly increased mid-thoracic kyphosis was also noted. Slight increase in muscle tone was noted in the left and right paraspinals from T10 to L3. Trunk active ROM in standing demonstrated provocation of the sharp right lumbosacral junction pain with one repetition of backward bending. There was a marked increase in the mid-lumbar spine lordosis, as if she were hinging at that region during the movement. A sharp stretching sensation was provoked in the right middle and lower lumbar spine region extending to the right iliac crest with side bending to the left and forward bending. She experienced immediate relief from this discomfort when returning to the upright posture.

The neurologic examination was negative; peripheral pulses were symmetric and perceived to be normal. Muscle length testing demonstrated moderate tightness of hamstrings and hip flexors, as well as weakness in the abdominals and hip extensors. There was no palpatory tenderness at the interspinous spaces of the thoracic or lumbar spine, but central pressures (passive accessory vertebral motion testing) at T4, T8, and T12 provoked significant local tenderness, accompanied by segmental hypomobility. Central pressures at L3 increased the intensity of the patient's chief complaint, deep aching. Right unilateral pressure at the L5–S1 segment provoked sharp pain at the lumbosacral junction. Passive intervertebral physiologic motion testing of the spine demonstrated hypermobility at the L3–L4 and L2–L3 segments in backward and forward bending. With the patient positioned supine, abdominal palpation was carried out. Significant tenderness was provoked with palpation along the linea alba, approximately 2 to 3 inches above the umbilicus. Palpating the lateral extent of the aorta, the arterial pulse indicated a localized, enlarged, pulsatile mass, approximately 3 inches above the umbilicus. After maintaining slight to moderate pressure over this tender site for 20 to 30 seconds, the patient noted the deep throbbing pain in the lower thoracic and upper lumbar region. This was the same sensation she experienced when walking up flights of stairs or uphill. The throbbing sensation receded quickly when the palpatory pressure was released. At this point, the patient was again questioned regarding her past medical history, especially noting any cardiovascular system involvement. She denied any significant history initially but then remembered going to the emergency department because of severe palpitations 5 months before this clinical visit. She stated that her pulse rate had been 200 bpm, but nothing was found medically; by the next day, the symptoms had passed and had not occurred since. She was again asked about family medical history related to cardiovascular system conditions. This time she offered that three of her grandparents had died of MI and that her brother had been diagnosed as having a mitral valve prolapse condition.

Assessment and Outcome

The patient had come to Minneapolis from another state to see the physician who had done the lumbar fusion surgery. Possible surgery to the L3–L4 segment was to be considered for the thoracolumbar junction symptoms (aching). The patient was referred to the physical therapist for consultation regarding the appropriateness of physical therapy treatment for her current complaints. She was scheduled to have a discogram at the L3–L4 and L2–L3 segments the day after the physical therapy consultation. She was then to see the physician.

On the basis of the clinical examination, it was apparent that the sharp pain in the right lumbosacral junction and the dull ache at the thoracolumbar junction region were related to dysfunction of the musculoskeletal system. Provocation and alleviation of these symptoms were related to specific movements or postures. Also, both symptoms were provoked during the initial evaluation with passive segmental testing (central pressures at L3 and right unilateral pressures at L5–S1). However, the third complaint, deep throbbing pain, immediately raised suspicion. A throbbing sensation is not a description generally used by patients who present with mechanical dysfunction conditions. Throbbing or pulsating sensations are often associated with involvement of components of the cardiovascular system. A symptomatic aortic aneurysm could cause this type of pain complaint anywhere in the thoracic spine (usually midline), the chest, or abdominal regions. Because of the anatomic location of the aorta, numerous other structures may be impinged on by the aneurysm, causing a multitude of seemingly unrelated symptoms. These structures include spinal nerves, the esophagus, and the bronchi. The fact that the throbbing pain was brought on by physical exertion, such as stair and hill climbing, and was then relieved by cessation of the activity also suggests possible cardiovascular system involvement. Even though the throbbing pain and the dull ache were located in the same body region, the behavior of the symptoms was very different. The dull ache was provoked by sitting or standing for more than a few minutes, while physical exertion was what provoked the throbbing sensation. Physical examination findings also suggested two different lesions responsible for the different symptoms at the thoracolumbar junction. Passive intervertebral segmental testing provoked the aching at the L3 level, and abdominal palpation provoked the throbbing pain in the same area. The fact that the patient had a significant family medical history for cardiovascular system pathology also added weight to the concern regarding the origin of the throbbing complaints.

At completion of the initial evaluation, the patient was asked to remain in the clinic while the referring physician was contacted. The above information was communicated with emphasis on the factors that raised concern regarding the origin of the throbbing pain at the thoracolumbar junction. The discogram was put on hold and tests were run to check for the presence of an aortic aneurysm. A large aneurysm was found, and the patient returned home for medical consultation. She was also referred to a physical therapist at home for treatment of the dysfunction related to the complaints associated with the L5–S1 and L3–L4 segments.

Abdominal palpation played an important role in the decision to contact the physician regarding this patient's status. The abdomen is an important area to be assessed by the physical therapist. Multiple musculoskeletal system structures are located in the abdominal cavity (e.g., anterior lumbar spine, psoas major, and abdominal muscles) that, when dysfunctional, could affect the patient's symptoms and response to treatment. A number of other structures, including the visceri, and any aortic enlargement may affect the clinical picture as well. Screening this region may prevent a delay in the patient receiving important medical treatment (see Ch. 4 for a detailed description of abdominal anatomy and how to screen this region; Chs. 5 and 6 also present relevant information).

PATIENT CASE STUDY 2

History

The patient was a 66-year-old retired man who came to the clinic with a diagnosis of right sacroiliac joint pain. His chief complaint was intermittent aching in the right buttock and right calf. Walking was the only activity that provoked his symptoms. He would be pain free when ambulation was initiated, but consistently after walking 10 to 15 minutes the aching in the right buttock and calf would begin. If the patient continued to walk, the intensity of the pain increased tremendously; if he sat down, he would be pain free within minutes. The patient also described the sensation of restless legs periodically after he had been in bed for a short period. Walking short distances would relieve this discomfort. The patient's chief complaint and symptom behavior pattern were consistent from early morning to bedtime.

These symptoms began insidiously 16 months before the initial evaluation. During the past 16 months, the patient had received two 4-week sessions of physical therapy consisting of lower-extremity stretching and strengthening exercises, ultrasound to the right buttock and sacroiliac joint, hot packs to the lumbar and buttock regions, and prone press-up exercises. Outside of feeling a little looser, the patient's symptoms did not change. He received cortisone injections to the right sacroiliac joint and to trigger points in the gluteus medius, with only slight, temporary decrease in the intensity of the symptoms.

The patient's medical history included lumbar decompression surgery for a herniated nucleus pulposis at L5–S1 in 1963. He stated that the only residual effect was low lumbar stiffness. He had also suffered a heart attack in 1981 and received a pacemaker. The patient has smoked one pack of cigarettes daily for the past 50 years. He denied any bowel or bladder dysfunction. Special tests over the past 16 months included radiographs that he recounted as indicating loss of disc space height at L5–S1 and possible right lateral stenosis at L5–S1.

Physical Examination

In the standing position, slight atrophy of the right gluteals, thigh, and calf was noted. A reduced lumbar lordotic curve and increased midthoracic kyphosis were present. There was no provocation of symptoms with active movement of the trunk in standing or with overpressure, including the quadrant positions. Backward bending and right-side bending ROM were significantly reduced in the low lumbar spine. Right hip internal rotation and the combined motion of hip flexion and adduction were moderately reduced compared with the left hip. Neurologic evaluation and sacroiliac joint and hip provocation tests were negative. Muscle length tests demonstrated bilateral lower-extremity tightness of the hip flexors, external rotators, and adductors, with the right side being tighter than the left. Manual muscle testing showed weakness of the right hip extensors and abductors. Muscle palpation produced numerous tender areas with increased muscle tone of the right gluteals and hip external rotators. There was no palpatory tenderness over the posterior sacroiliac joint ligaments or at the interspinous spaces of the lumbar and thoracic spine. Joint mobility testing demonstrated hypomobility at the right hip joint, right sacral base, L5, and thoracolumbar junction. There were no palpable differences between the lower-extremity pulses.

Because of an inability to provoke the patient's symptoms, the patient was instructed to walk until the symptoms were severe, just before the second physical therapy visit. Although symptoms were not aggravated by stressing the thoracic and lumbar spine, sacroiliac and hip joints, and corresponding soft tissue structures, there was greater difficulty in palpating the right lower-extremity pulses compared with the left. This had not been the case during the initial evaluation, when the patient was asymptomatic.

Assessment and Outcome

The referring physician was contacted after the second physical therapy visit. He was informed of the several factors suggesting a vascular occlusive disease as a possible source of the patient's symptoms: intermittent claudication, weaker right lower-extremity pulses after ambulation, and a history of smoking and heart attack. Of equal concern was the inability to provoke symptoms with palpation and active and passive testing. Because of the presence of significant right hip, sacral, and lumbar dysfunction, as well as muscle imbalances that might be related to the symptoms, it was agreed that physical therapy was to continue for 2 or 3 weeks including the initiation of a lower extremity conditioning exercise on a stationary bicycle. Depending on the patient's response to treatment, a decision would then be made regarding any additional medical tests to be carried out. The patient was seen twice a week, receiving joint mobilization for the right hip, right sacral base, and hypomobile segments of the lumbar and thoracic spine. In addition, soft tissue mobilization and muscle-stretching exercises and strengthening exercises were carried out for the involved areas. Objectively the patient improved; backward bending and right-side bending ROM improved significantly, as did right hip joint mobility. Despite these improvements, the patient's tolerance for walking only slightly improved as the behavior of the right buttock and calf symptoms changed little. The patient was sent back to the physician for additional tests, which indicated significant occlusion of the right iliac artery. Subsequent treatment of the occlusion completely eliminated the patient's symptoms.

This patient presented with many of the important findings discussed in Chapter 1 (i.e., the possible presence of pathology, including insidious onset of symptoms, an inability to provoke symptoms by stressing the structures of the musculoskeletal system, and the lack of subjective improvement despite significant objective improvement). In addition, numerous symptoms and signs suggested a vascular condition, including intermittent claudication symptoms, the complaint of restless legs, a long history of smoking, a previous heart attack, and decreased pulses after long enough ambulating to provoke symptoms. Sufficient dysfunction was present in the lower quarter, however, to raise suspicion of a mechanical origin of the symptoms of musculoskeletal dysfunction as well. At times the significance of musculoskeletal system dysfunction related to the patient's complaints presents a difficult clinical situation. Careful and frequent reassessment of symptoms and signs after treatment help the clinician decide whether the patient should be assessed medically to rule out the presence of pathology. Communication with the physician regarding clinical findings that have raised suspicion in the therapist's mind is then essential to ensure the proper course of treatment for the patient. In this patient's case, months of symptoms and unnecessary treatments might have been avoided had a more complete and concise evaluation been made initially. Fortunately for this patient, his condition was treated successfully. For other pathologies, such as cancer, a few months can make a difference in the prognosis for recovery.

REFERENCES

1. Wise CS: Physical medicine in disease of peripheral circulation. JAPTA 30:499, 1950
2. Stillwell DM: Bisgaard treatment for static edema and its sequelae in the lower extremity. Arch Phys Med Rehabil 37:693, 1956
3. Cohen M, Michel TH: Overview of the cardiac system. p. 15. In: Cardiopulmonary Symptoms in Physical Therapy Practice. Churchill Livingstone, New York, 1988
4. Albarran-Sotelo R, Atkins JM, Bloom RS: Arrhythmias. p. 48. In American Heart Association: Textbook of Cardiac Life Support. American Heart Association National Center, Dallas, 1987
5. Ross G (ed): Essentials of Human Physiology. Year Book Medical Publishers, Chicago, 1978
6. Stein B, Israel D, Cohen M, Fuster V: Ischemia and infarction III: pathogenesis of coronary occlusion. Hosp Pract 23:87, 1988
7. Ganong WF: The heartbeat and electrical activity of the heart. p. 445. In Review of Medical Physiology. 13th Ed. Appleston & Lange, E. Norwalk, CT, 1987
8. Ganong W: Review of Medical Physiology. 8th Ed. Lange Medical Publications, Los Altos, CA, 1977
9. Delp M, Manning R: Major Physical Diagnosis. 8th Ed. WB Saunders, Philadelphia, 1979
10. Little RC: Physiology of the Heart and Circulation. 4th Ed. p. 238. Year Book Medical Publishers, Chicago, 1978
11. Mubarak SJ, Hargens AR: Compartment Syndromes and Volkmann's Contractures. Saunders' Monographs in Clinical Orthopedics. Vol. 3. WB Saunders, Philadelphia, 1981
12. Cohen M, Michel TH: Case profiles. p 252. In: Cardiopulmonary Symptoms in Physical Therapy Practice. Churchill Livingstone, New York, 1988
13. Kanarek DJ, Hand RW: The response of cardiac and pulmonary disease to exercise testing. Clin Chest Med 5:181, 1984
14. Sokolow M, McIlroy M: Clinical Cardiology. Lange Medical Publications, Los Altos, CA, 1981
15. Wilkins RL, Sheldon RL, Jones-Krider S: Clinical Assessment in Respiratory Care. 2nd Ed. CV Mosby, St. Louis, 1990
16. American Heart Association: Textbook of Advanced Cardiac Life Support. p. 2. American Heart Association National Center, Dallas, 1987
17. American College of Sports Medicine: Guidelines for Exercise Testing and Prescription. p. 67. Lea & Febiger, Philadelphia, 1986
18. Braunwald E: Valvular heart disease. p. 1123. In Braunwald E (ed): Heart Disease: A Textbook of Cardiovascular Medicine. 1st Ed. WB Saunders, Philadelphia, 1980

SUGGESTED READINGS

Chatterjee K, Cheitlin M, Karliner J et al: Cardiology. Mosby-Year Book, St. Louis, 1991

Cohen M, Michel TH: Cardiopulmonary Symptoms in Physical Therapy Practice. Churchill Livingstone, New York, 1988

Degowin R: Degowin and Degowin's Diagnostic Examination. 6th Ed. McGraw-Hill, Summit, PA, 1993

Eagle KA, Haber E, DeSanctis RW, Austen WG (eds): The Practice of Cardiology. 2nd Ed. Little, Brown, Boston, 1989

Froelicher V: Exercise and the Heart. 3rd Ed. McGraw-Hill, Summit, PA, 1993

Hillegass EA, Sadowsky HS: Essentials of Cardiopulmonary Physical Therapy. WB Saunders, Philadelphia, 1994

Hurst JW (ed): Cardiovascular Diagnosis—The Initial Examination. Mosby-Year Book, St. Louis, 1993

Spittell JA: Contemporary Issues in Peripheral Vascular Disease. FA. Davis, Philadelphia, 1992

Tilkian SM, Conover MD, Tilkian AG: Clinical Implication of Laboratory Tests. 4th Ed. CV Mosby, St. Louis, 1987

Waugh R, Ramo B, Wagner G, Gilbert M: Cardiac Arrythmias: A Practical Guide for the Clinician. 2nd Ed. FA Davis, Philadelphia, 1994

Appendix 2-1

Physical Examination in Cardiovascular Diseases

Technique	Findings	Entity
Observation	Cyanosis of nailbeds, lips	Hypoxia
	Clubbing of fingernails	Tissue hypoxemia (shunt)
	Jugular venous distension (JVD)	Right ventricular CHF
	Cardiac apical pulsations	Normal 20% of the time; left ventricular CHF, 80%
	Discolorations of skin	Peripheral arterial and venous disease
	Ulcerations, trophic changes of skin	PVD and DM
	Peripheral edema	CHF, venous stasis, lymph edema
Palpation	Point of maximal impulse	
	LV bulge	LV aneurysm
	Lateral and downward	Cardiac dilatation as in aortic regurgitation, Right pneumothorax
	Hyperdynamic apical impulse (thrust)	Heightened myocardial tone: mitral/aortic regurgitation, exertion, emotion, thyrotoxicosis, LVH
	Sustained and enlarged LV impulse	CHF
	Chest pain	Trigger points, costochondral tenderness, r/o angina
	Deep abdominal midline pulsations—finger span wider than 2 inches	Abdominal aortic aneurysm
	Peripheral pulses—rate rhythm, symmetry, strength	
	<60	Bradycardia
	>100	Tachycardia
	Irregularly irregular	Atrial fibrillation
	Regularly irregular (skipped beats)	PVCs, heart block, check EKG
	Weak, thready distal pulse	Hypotension
	Asymmetric peripheral pulses	Arterial occlusive disease
	Temperature of skin	
	Red and hot	Could be thrombus, infection, inflammation
	Cold and clammy	Could be hypotension, arterial occlusive disease, autonomic dysfunction, Raynaud's phenomenon
Auscultation	Ventricular gallop (S3)	Rapid filling normal in young people; mitral regurgitation, thyrotoxicosis, CHF
	Atrial gallop (S4)	Altered compliance of ventricle; CHF, HTN, atrial stenosis, pulmonary HTN, previous MI
	Summation gallop (S1, S2, S3, S4)	Anemia, hyperthyroidism, CHF
	Murmurs	Valvular disorders, arterial aneurysm, thyrotoxicosis
	Bruits (arterial)	AV fistula, occlusive disease
	Blood pressure	
	>140 SBP	Hypertension, anxiety, pain, exercise
	<90 SBP	Hypotension, hypovolemia, orthostatic intolerance, shock, low EF
	>100 DBP	Hypertension, CHF
	<0 DBP	Exercise vasodilation, shock
	Wide pulse pressure SBP↑ DBP↓	Outflow obstruction

Continues

Technique	Findings	Entity
	Narrow pulse pressure, SBP↑ DBP↓	CHF
	Breath sounds	
	Crackles, symmetrical and bibasilar	CHF
	Friction rub over ribs	Pericarditis
Percussion	Dullness at lung bases	CHF, atelectasis
Exercise	EKG	
	ST↓	Ischemic myocardium
	ST↑	Aneurysm or acute injury to the heart
	T wave inversion	Ischemic myocardium
	PVCs, VT-salvos	Ischemic or irritable ventricle
	VF	Cardiac arrest
	SBP	
	Rises	Normal to maximum
	Excessive rise	Hypertensive
	Flat or falling	Nonadaptive, could mean failing heart
	Dyspnea	
	Early, at low workloads	CHF or lung disease or deconditioning
	At rest	CHF, ischemic heart, lung disease
	Chest pain	Ischemic heart; correlates with ST↓ on ECG
	Fatigue	Normal at 60–70% maximum
	Early	Poor endurance, deconditioning, outflow tract obstruction (aortic stenosis or hypertrophic cardiomyopathy), peripheral circulatory deficits, inefficient heart as in atrial fibrillation

3 SCREENING FOR PULMONARY SYSTEM DISEASE

David Arnall, Ph.D., P.T.
Michael Ryan, M.D., F.A.C.P.

The physical therapist is a valued member of the health care team, providing care for patients with lung disease in both outpatient and inpatient settings.[1–3] As the need for physical therapy services increases subsequent to the aging of the American public, the accurate assessment of ventilatory muscle strength and pulmonary function will become increasingly important. Since diagnosis-related groupings (DRGs) frequently determine the length of hospital admissions, the role of physical therapy services in the after-discharge care of the patient will become more important in the home health and outpatient settings. Physical therapists interested primarily in orthopaedics or sports medicine cannot reasonably expect to treat a patient adequately without knowing about baseline measurements of both ventilatory and respiratory functions.[4–7] With so many patients, young and old, having respiratory disease, physical therapists need the assessment and treatment tools necessary to address respiratory problems, as well as orthopaedic conditions.

To help prepare the therapist for screening and assessing the pulmonary system, this chapter presents an overview of pulmonary anatomy. The assessment and interpretation of breath and vocal sounds by auscultating the chest wall with a stethoscope are also presented in great detail. Pertinent evaluation information obtained through chart review, history taking, and physical examination is also discussed. The disease entities presented in this chapter are those that physical therapists are most likely to encounter in the clinical setting.

PULMONARY ANATOMY

Anatomy and physiology are the foundations upon which evaluation and treatment are built. Before auscultating the patient's chest wall, it is imperative that the physical therapist clearly understand the external chest wall markings that overlie the lung and the relationship the external landmarks have to internal pulmonary anatomy. The anatomy reviewed briefly in the following paragraphs will help the clinician understand that the placement of the stethoscope has meaning with reference to the underlying lobes and bronchopulmonary segments.

The left and right lungs are grossly comprised of regional lobes demarcated by the presence of fissures that penetrate deep into the lung fields frankly dividing the lung into upper, middle, and lower lobes on the right and upper and lower lobes on the left lung. The left lung does not have a middle lobe (Figs. 3-1 and 3-2).

The lobes of the right lung are separated from each other by two large pulmonary fissures: (1) the horizontal or transverse fissure and (2) the oblique fissure. The horizontal or transverse fissure divides the right upper lobe from the right middle lobe (Fig. 3-1). The oblique fissure divides the right middle lobe from the right lower lobe (Fig. 3-1). The upper and lower lobes of the left lung are separated by the oblique fissure (Fig. 3-1).

The major lobes of the left and right lungs are further comprised of bronchopulmonary segments that are not immediately seen in the cadaver because there are no anatomic fissures that divide the major lobes into the

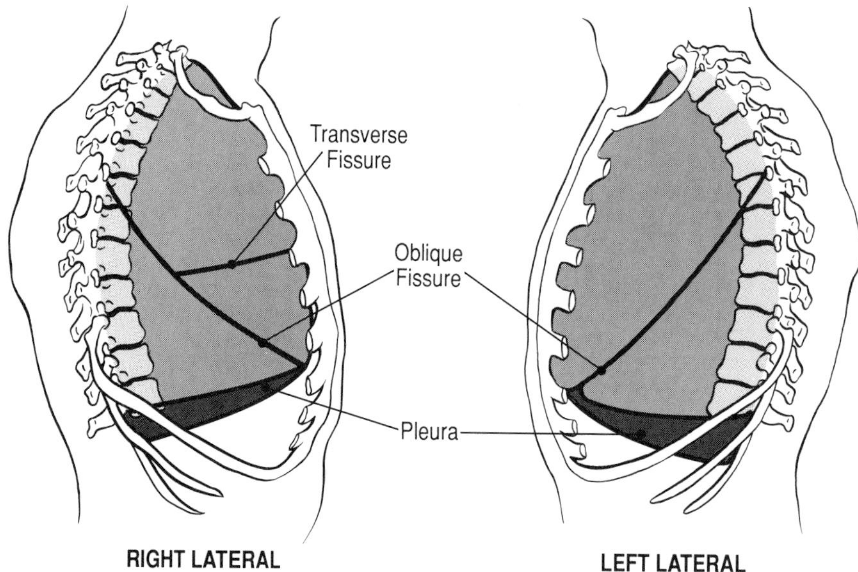

Fig. 3-1. Lateral views of the lobes, fissures, and pleura of the lungs in relationship to elements of the bony thorax.

smaller bronchopulmonary segments. Rather, the bronchopulmonary segmental divisions of the lobes and their corresponding names are determined by the names of the segmental bronchi that serve these areas of the lung. The various bronchopulmonary segments of each major lobe are listed in Table 3-1.

When the physical therapist learns the external surface anatomic landmarks that overlie specific bronchopulmonary segments, auscultation of the patient's lung fields becomes meaningful. Figures 3-3 and 3-4 outline pictorially the thoracic cage bony structure and the surface markings overlying the bronchopulmonary seg-

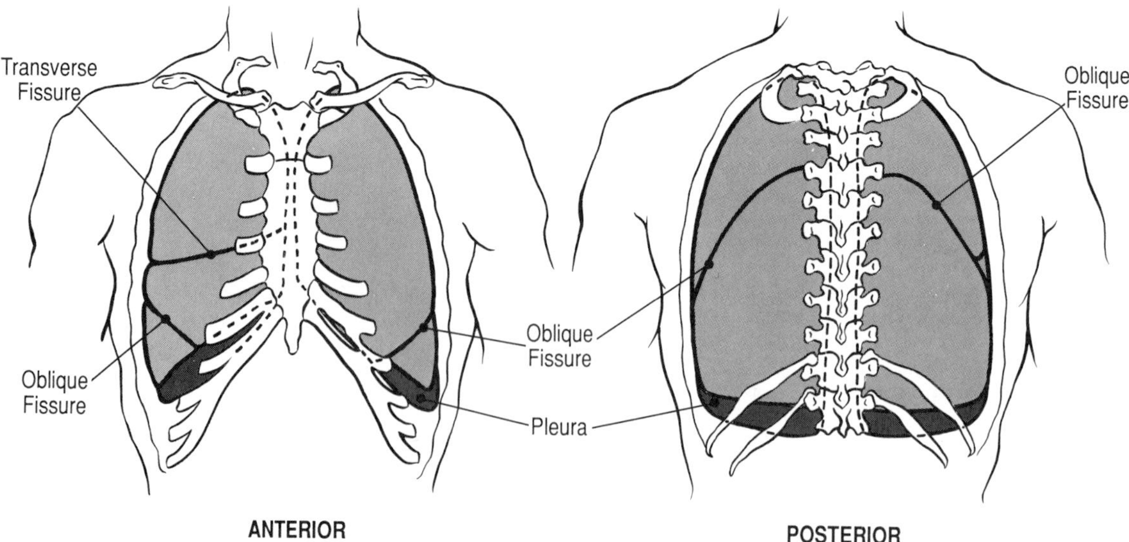

Fig. 3-2. Anterior and posterior views of the lobes, fissures, and pleura of the lungs in relationship to elements of the bony thorax.

Table 3-1. The Bronchopulmonary Segments of Each Lobe of the Right and Left Lung

Right Lung
Upper lobe
Apical segment
Anterior segment
Posterior segment
Middle lobe
Medial segment
Lateral segment
Lower lobe
Anterior basilar segment
Superior segment
Medial basilar segment
Posterior basilar segment
Lateral basilar segment
Left Lung
Upper lobe
Apicoposterior segment
Anterior segment
Superior lingular segment[a]
Inferior lingular segment[a]
Lower lobe
Anterior basilar segment
Superior segment
Posterior basilar segment
Lateral basilar segment

[a]The lingular segments are part of the upper lobes of the left lung but are anatomically analogous to the medial and lateral segments of the right middle lobe.

ments. From these drawings, it is easy to determine which major lobe and often which bronchopulmonary segment is being auscultated.

The following discussion describes placement of the stethoscope on the chest wall to listen to specific regions of the lung.

The Right Lung

The Upper Lobe

The right upper lobe is comprised of three bronchopulmonary segments—apical, posterior, and anterior.

The Apical Segment

The apical segment is not often auscultated because it is not as frequently involved in disease pathologies as other bronchopulmonary segments. The apical segment of the right upper lobe can be auscultated by placing the diaphragm of the stethoscope over the upper trapezius muscle just above and behind the clavicle. This segment can be auscultated at this point because the tip of the apical segment peaks out over the clavicle. In the adult, the vesicular breath sound or the bronchovesicular breath sound is the normal breath sound heard through the stethoscope. When the vesicular breath sound is heard, the inspiratory to expiratory (I:E) ratio is usually 1:¼, meaning that normally the expiratory phase is only one-fourth the duration of the inspiratory phase. It is also common while listening to the vesicular breath sound not to hear the expiratory phase at all. Therefore, in a normal vesicular breath sound, the expiratory phase will be abbreviated or completely absent compared with the inspiratory phase.

If the bronchovesicular breath sound is heard, the clinician will usually hear the vesicular portion during the inspiratory phase of the respiratory cycle, while the more tubular, high-pitched bronchial portion of the sound is heard during exhalation. The I:E ratio is usually close to 1:1, meaning that inspiration is heard as long as expiration. In children and teenagers, the normal breath sound is usually the bronchovesicular breath sound. The differences in the breath sounds in teenagers and children compared with adults is probably due to maturational factors.

The Posterior Segment

The posterior segment of the right upper lobe can be auscultated if the diaphragm of the stethoscope is placed over the lower trapezius just below the spine of the scapula. The medial border for this lobe is the thoracovertebral border of the spine (some anatomists call this region the paraspinous gutter), while the lateral border is located approximately between the third and sixth ribs along the mid-axillary line. The inferior border of this bronchopulmonary segment is along the sixth rib as it approaches the spinous process of T5. The inferior border of the posterior segment of the right upper lobe is also demarcated by the oblique fissure. The superior border is just anterior to and at the same level as the spine of the scapula, which lies immediately to the right of the dorsal spinous process of T3. The vesicular breath sound is most commonly the normal breath sound that is heard in this segment in the adult. The I:E ratio for this breath sound is normally 1:0 or 1:¼.

However, it is also normal to hear the bronchovesicular breath sound, with the softer, breathy vesicular sound being heard in the inspiratory phase and the harsher, more tubular, hollow, and high-pitched bronchial sound being heard during expiration. The I:E ratio is usually 1:1 for the bronchovesicular breath sound. Teenagers and children

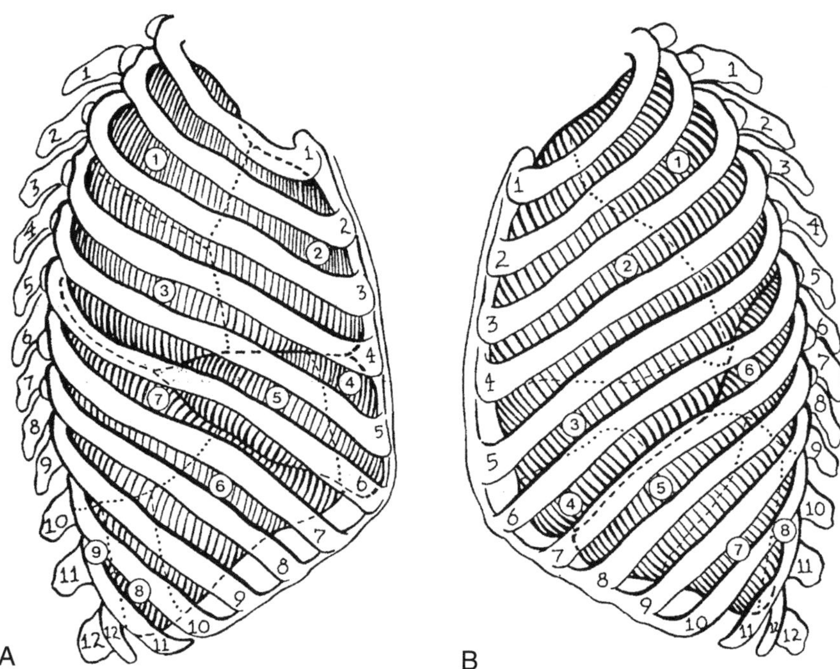

Fig. 3-3. Bronchopulmonary segments of the lungs in relationship to elements of the bony thorax. **(A) Right lung.** *Right upper lobe:* 1, apical segment; 2, anterior segment; 3, posterior segment. *Middle lobe:* 4, medial segment; 5, lateral segment. *Right lower lobe:* 6, anterior basilar segment; 7, superior segment; 8, lateral basilar segment; 9, posterior basilar segment;*, medial basilar segment not shown. **(B) Left lung.** *Left upper lobe:* 1, apicoposterior segment; 2, anterior segment; 3, superior lingula; 4, inferior lingula. *Left lower lobe:* 5, anterior basilar segment; 6, superior segment; 7, lateral basilar segment; 8, posterior basilar segment.

will very often demonstrate the bronchovesicular breath sound in this bronchopulmonary segment.

The Anterior Segment

The anterior segment of the right upper lobe can be easily auscultated because the surface area for auscultation is extensive. The anterior segment can be auscultated at its inferior border above or on the level of the fourth rib, lateral to the sternocostal margin at its medial border, just below the clavicle at its superior border, with the lateral border extending to just posterior to the mid-axillary line. The normal breath sound is a vesicular breath sound in the adult. The I:E ratio for this breath sound is usually 1:0 or 1:¼. In some adults a bronchovesicular breath sound can be heard immediately over the sternocostal border and immediately below the clavicle. In children below the age of 12 to 14 years, the bronchovesicular breath sound predominates throughout the lung field of the anterior segment.

The Middle Lobe

The right middle lobe consists of two bronchopulmonary segments—the medial and lateral segments. The medial bronchopulmonary segment is medial and anterior to the lateral segment. Unless the clinician is experienced, it can be difficult to know which segment is being auscultated. These two relatively small segments can be auscultated over the wedge-shaped area shown in Figures 3-3 and 3-4. This area is between the fourth and the sixth ribs anteriorly and encompasses the nipple of the right chest wall. (The nipple is a good landmark only in young males, young females before pubescence, and adult males who do not have substantial upper body fat reserves that mimic breast tissue. In other sex and age groups the nipple will frequently have too much inferior displacement, making it an unreliable external thoracic wall landmark.) Moving laterally and posteriorly along the fifth rib, the wedge-shaped area narrows and terminates just posterior to the mid-axillary line. If the stethoscope is

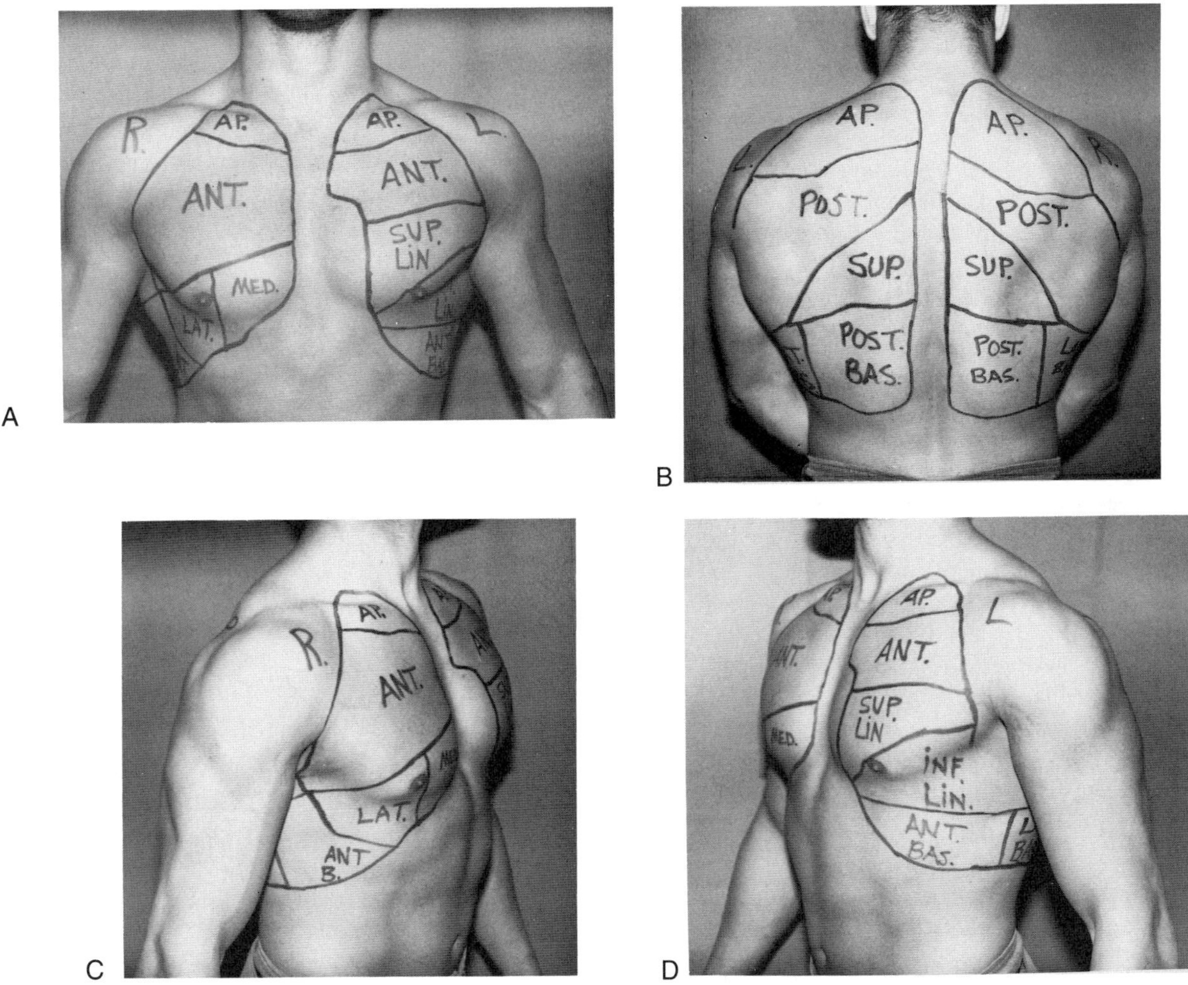

Fig. 3-4. Bronchopulmonary segments of the lungs in relationship to surface anatomy. **(A)** Anterior view. **(B)** Posterior view. **(C)** Right lateral view. **(D)** Left lateral view. AP, apical segment; ANT, anterior segment; MED, medial segment; LAT, lateral segment; SUP LIN, superior lingula, left lung; INF LIN, inferior lingula, left lung; ANT BAS, anterior basilar, left lung; POST, posterior segment; SUP, superior segment; POST BAS, posterior basilar.

placed on the anterior surface of the chest wall between the fourth and sixth ribs on or medial to the nipple and lateral to the sternum (Fig. 3-3), the chances are fairly good that the medial segment is being auscultated. If the stethoscope is placed lateral to this area, the lateral segment is probably being auscultated (Fig. 3-3). The normal breath sound heard in the healthy adult is always the vesicular breath sound for both the medial and lateral segments of the right middle lobe. As mentioned before, in children and young teens, the bronchovesicular breath sound is a normal variant.

Often the most posterolateral area of the right middle lobe can be identified by following the sixth rib along its posterior and oblique upward direction toward the mid-axillary line. When coming to the point on the chest that marks the junction of the transverse and oblique fissures (slightly posterior to the mid-axillary line) and crossing over that point, one will often hear a change in the breath sounds going from a higher pitched to a lower pitched vesicular breath sound. The subtle change in pitch is an indication that one has crossed over from the middle lobe to the lower lobe in the vicinity of the superior segment of the lower lobes.

The Lower Lobe

The lower lobe of the right lung consists of five segments—anterior basilar, lateral basilar, posterior basilar, superior, and medial basilar segments.

The Anterior Basilar Segment

The anterior basilar segment of the right lower lobe can be auscultated by placing the diaphragm of the stethoscope on the anterior chest wall on its superior border at the sixth rib and as far down as its inferior border at the tenth rib 2 to 3 inches above the costal margin. The stethoscope can be moved laterally within this lobe as far as the mid-axillary line. The medial border for this segment is along the mid-clavicular line. The normal breath sound that is heard in the basilar segments is always the vesicular breath sound in the adult with an I:E ratio of 1:0 or 1:¼. The bronchovesicular breath sound may still be heard in children and in young teens.

The Lateral Basilar Segment

The lateral basilar segment of the right lower lobe is lateral to the anterior basilar segment. It occupies an area below the eighth rib on the lateral surface of the chest wall and 2 to 3 inches posterior to the mid-axillary line. In the adult, the normal breath sound that is heard in this basilar segment is always the vesicular breath sound, with an I:E ratio of 1:0 or 1:¼. The bronchovesicular breath sound may still be heard in children and in young teens.

The Posterior Basilar Segment

The posterior basilar segment of the right lower lobe is auscultated by placing the stethoscope on the posterior surface of the thoracic wall between the vertebral column as its medial border and the lateral basilar segment as its lateral border. The superior border of this segment is located below the dorsal spinous process of T9 vertebra, with the inferior border located at the dorsal spinous process of T11 vertebra. The normal breath sound in the healthy adult is always the vesicular breath sound, with an I:E ratio of 1:0 or 1:¼. The bronchovesicular breath sound will often be heard in children under the age of 12 to 14 years.

The Superior Segment

The superior segment of the right lower lobe is located on the posterior wall of the thorax below the oblique fissure that runs generally along the sixth rib. The inferior border of the superior segment curves posteriorly from the mid-axillary line to the dorsal spinous process of the ninth thoracic vertebra. The medial border for this segment is the vertebral column between the dorsal spinous processes of T5 through T9, with the lateral border being the oblique fissure that angles obliquely downward along the sixth rib. The normal breath sound that is always heard in this segment of the lung in healthy adults is the vesicular breath sound, with an I:E ratio of 1:0 or 1:¼. The bronchovesicular breath sound will often be heard in children under the age of 12 to 14 years.

The Medial Basilar Segment

The medial basilar segment of the right lower lobe, also known as the cardiac bronchopulmonary segment, cannot be auscultated because it is located medial to the anterior basilar segment juxtapositioned to the heart. It has no thoracic surface area exposure from which to be auscultated.

The Left Lung

The Upper Lobe

The left upper lobe is divided into four segments: apicoposterior, anterior, superior lingula, and inferior lingula segments.

The Apicoposterior Segment

The apicoposterior segment of the left upper lobe is positioned in the thoracic cage similarly to that of the right apical and posterior bronchopulmonary segments. The landmarks for auscultation are very similar. The normal breath sounds heard in these segments may be vesicular to bronchovesicular, depending on the body size, percent body fat, and age of the patient. The vesicular breath sound, as mentioned before, is a breathy, muffled, whispy, low-pitched sound that usually has an I:E ratio of 1:0 or 1:¼. If the bronchovesicular breath sound is heard, the vesicular portion of the breath sound is often heard during the inspiratory cycle, while the bronchial portion is frequently heard during exhalation. The I:E ratio for the bronchovesicular breath sound is usually 1:1.

The Anterior Segment

The anterior segment of the left upper lobe has virtually the same location as the anterior segment of the right lung. The normal breath sound that is typically heard in a healthy adult will be the vesicular breath sound, although the bronchovesicular breath sound is a common variant when auscultating near the sternoclavicular, sternocostal, and clavicular borders. In young teens and children the bronchovesicular breath sound is heard as the normal breath sound.

The Superior and Inferior Lingula

These two segments occupy roughly the same space as the medial and lateral segments of the right middle lobe. As mentioned previously, the left lung does not have a middle lobe. However, the analogous structures in the left lung are the superior and inferior lingula. In the adult, the normal breath sound that is heard in these segments is always the vesicular breath sound. The bronchovesicular breath sound can often be heard in young teens and children.

The Lower Lobe

The lower lobe of the left lung is composed of four segments: anterior basilar, superior, posterior basilar, and lateral basilar segments.

The Anterior Basilar Segment

The anterior basilar segment of the left lung has an anatomic distribution similar to that of the analogous segment on the right side. The normal breath sound that is always heard in the adult is the vesicular breath sound. The bronchovesicular breath sound can often be heard in young teens and children.

The Superior Segment

The superior segment of the left lower lobe is positioned in the thoracic cage in an area analogous to the same segment on the right side. The normal breath sound heard in this segment is always the vesicular breath sound in the adult. The bronchovesicular breath sound can often be heard in young teens and children.

The Posterior Basilar Segment

The posterior basilar segment of the left lower lobe is located at its superior border just below the spinous process of T9 along the vertebral column extending inferiorly to about the dorsal spinous process of T11. It extends laterally out to a point on the posterolateral thoracic wall roughly analogous to a line dropped vertically between the surgical neck of the scapula and the glenoid fossa of the scapula. The vertebral column is its medial border and the lateral basilar segment its lateral border. The normal breath sound heard in the healthy adult is always the vesicular breath sound. The bronchovesicular breath sound is often heard in the young teen and in children.

The Lateral Basilar Segment

The lateral basilar segment of the left lower lobe is located analogously to the right lateral basilar segment. The normal breath sound that is heard in healthy adults is always the vesicular breath sound. The bronchovesicular breath sound may be heard in young teens and in children.

PHYSICAL ASSESSMENT OF PULMONARY STATUS: AUSCULTATION

The Stethoscope As An Evaluation Tool

The physical therapist should understand how to perform a chest assessment using a stethoscope. This is a basic tool in the pulmonary evaluation and is of immense help in understanding the patient's condition. The following is a brief overview of how to auscultate or listen to the chest using a stethoscope. Practice under the tutelage of an experienced auscultator is invaluable. However, it is hoped that the rudimentary information presented here will stimulate the reader to become a knowledgeable auscultator.

The stethoscope is a diagnostic tool that has been used for well over 150 years to determine the condition of certain organs. Laennec, a French physician, was an early proponent for using the stethoscope to ausculate or listen to the lungs. Laennec's stethoscope was a simple tube considerably different from the stethoscopes today. The modern stethoscope is divided into three major components (Fig. 3-5):

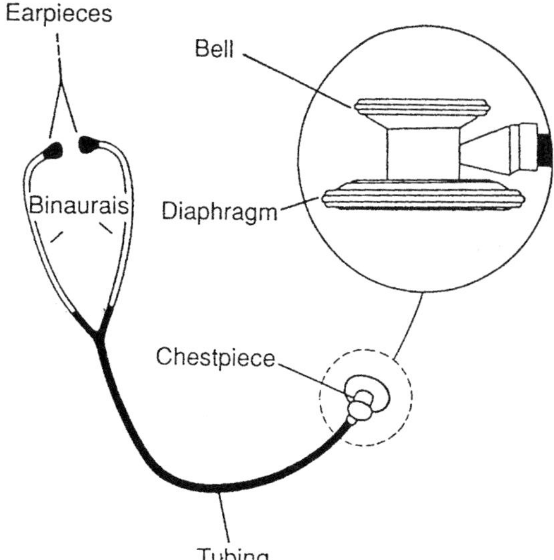

Fig. 3-5. Components of the stethoscope.

1. The head (or chestpiece);
   a. The bell
   b. The diaphragm
2. Tubing
3. Ear pieces

Head

The modern stethoscope is most often duosonic. This means that there is a bell on one side and a diaphragm on the other side. Stethoscopes are, however, still made that are unisonic (i.e., they have a diaphragm only).

The bell transmits low-frequency tones at the expense of the high-frequency tones. It is therefore very useful for listening to rhonchi or wheezes in the central airways of the lung or for a heart murmur such as the murmur that frequently appears in patients with mitral valve stenosis. The diaphragm facilitates tone transmission of high-frequency tones at the expense of low-frequency tones. Therefore the diaphragm is useful for hearing bronchial breath sounds and bronchovesicular breath sounds. While the bell and the diaphragm have these sound transmission characteristics, in actuality most practitioners simply use the diaphragm to assess sounds emanating from the thoracic wall.

Tubing

The tubing is usually thick walled and flexible, with the inner bore diameter the size of the metal earpiece tubing. Double tubing (i.e., a tube running from each earpiece) is superior to a single-tube stethoscope construction, because double-tube stethoscopes transmit sound better than single-tube stethoscopes. The length of the tubing connecting the head and the earpieces should be between 12 and 16 inches long. The shorter the tubing the better the transmission of the sound waves. The length of the stethoscope tubing has to be long enough for the clinician to use comfortably during a chest examination.

Earpieces

Earpieces should be chosen so that they fit into the ears comfortably and exclude as much extraneous room noise as possible. Many physical therapists, nurses, respiratory therapists, and physicians choose soft rubber earpieces instead of the hard plastic earpieces that frequently come with the stethoscopes. The soft rubber earpieces not only conform more easily to the ear channel but also block some of the room noise more efficiently than do the plastic ones.

What Can You Hear With the Stethoscope?

Vocal and Breath Sounds

While listening with the stethoscope placed on the chest wall, the sounds produced by the passage of air in and out of the lung during respiration will be heard. These sounds are created by the turbulence and vibration of air passing in and out of the lung through the various generations of the bronchopulmonary tree. Some of the sounds that a clinician will encounter are normal breath sounds heard in patients with healthy lungs. These sounds will be made by air passing in and out of clear, unobstructed bronchial passages. Sounds known as adventitious sounds are abnormal and are typically created by having air pass through bronchial passages obstructed by mucus. The ease with which these sounds or vibrations are transmitted depends on the elasticity (or compliance) of the tissue, the mass (or volume) of the transmitting medium, and the density of the transmitting medium. For example, the alveoli or air sacs surrounding all of the bronchial structures dampen sound transmission. In a healthy lung this has the effect of damping the higher frequency sounds in favor of the lower frequency sounds. Therefore, what is heard over the lateral and posteroinferior chest walls is a muffled and breathy sound. In areas of the chest wall in which there is a small number of alveoli, such as near the trachea and over the costosternal border, the sounds are of higher frequency and tend to be tubular, harsh, and somewhat metallic in quality, much like hearing air blowing through a tube.

Transmission of Vocal or Voice Sounds

During a standard chest assessment, the clinician listens to the chest wall with a stethoscope, while the patient utters a word such as "ninety-nine" or a long vowel sound such as the letter "E" or "A". The quality of the spoken or whispered word whether clearly understood or so muffled as to be unintelligable through the stethoscope should be noted. Two types of vocal or voice sounds can be heard: normal vocal sounds and abnormal vocal sounds.

Normal Vocal Sounds. As air passes over the vocal cords, vibrations are produced in the larynx, and sound is created. The sound waves are transmitted through the respiratory tract and through the chest in all directions to the thoracic wall. The vocal sounds are loudest near the trachea and the major bronchi because there is less lung tissue to muffle the transmission. Words spoken while auscultating in the area of the trachea or costal sternal borders will be "fuzzy" but intelligible. Vocal sounds heard during auscultation in the more distant areas of the lung field (e.g., the posterior basilar segments) are less intense and much more muffled. Indeed, in a normal lung, the syllables of the words cannot be understood at all. The clinician hears what sounds somewhat like talking with a mouth full of food. No one can understand what has been mumbled, only that something has been said.

Abnormal Vocal Sounds. There are several common abnormal vocal sounds in patients with consolidation disorders (e.g., pneumonia, atelectasis). Consolidation is a process in which the lung becomes less compliant (flexible and extensible) because of the presence of larger than normal amounts of fluid collecting in the interstitial spaces and in the bronchial passages. Bronchophony, whispered pectoriloquy, and egophony are examples heard over an area of consolidation in the lung.

Bronchophony. Bronchophony is an abnormal vocal sound in which the transmission of the spoken word is increased in both intensity and clarity. During the examination, the clinician will ask the patient to utter a specific word or a letter such as "ninety-nine" or "EEEEEE." If the patient has a bronchophony, the clinician will be able to hear through the stethoscope the word or the enunciated long vowel sound. The clarity of the word or vowel phonation is related both to how well developed the consolidation is and to the size of the consolidated area. To some degree, it is clear enough to understand the exact words or vowel sound. The presence of bronchophony is a sign that sound is being transmitted through fluid-filled spaces (i.e., there is fluid in the airways or in the interstitial spaces that makes the lung more solid and enhances sound transmission).

At this juncture it is wise to insert a cautionary note. When practicing auscultation of the lung fields with the stethoscope, it is important to remember that the bronchopulmonary segments have normal or typical sounds that are associated with the surrounding anatomy and the location of the bronchopulmonary segment. For instance, the apical segments of the upper lobes are juxtaposed to the trachea, the clavicle, and the sternum and may transmit voice sounds more clearly than other more distal bronchopulmonary segments. There simply is not a great deal of parenchymal and alveolar tissue in the upper lobes to muffle the sound waves that are transmitted from the larynx to the chest wall. Additionally, there is a great deal of cartilagenous and bony anatomy as well as the substantial cartilagenous ring structure of the upper airways, all of which permit sound waves to be effectively transmitted to the thoracic wall. It may appear to the beginning auscultator listening to the thoracic wall around the trachea, the costosternal borders, or the thoracovertebral borders that the patient may have a bronchophony, when this is not the case, simply because the sounds are so easily transmitted in the upper lobes next to the trachea and mainstem bronchi. However, in all other lung fields, the vocal sounds will be unintelligible in a clear lung. If the phonated word or vowel sounds can be heard in these areas (the anterior bronchopulmonary segment of the upper lobes, right middle lobe, left lingula, bilateral basilar segments), it can be strongly suspected that the area is consolidated. Bronchophony is always an abnormal vocal sound and is diagnostic for lung disease.

Additionally, the beginning auscultator has to learn to isolate extraneous background noise from the sounds emanating across the thoracic wall. Background noise may come from the stethoscope's diaphragm rubbing against body hair, from the contact of the stethoscope tubing against the patient, from the crepitus of the auscultator's finger joints, or from noises in the room. All of these distractions make listening to thoracic sounds somewhat difficult. The auscultator must learn to ignore extraneous sounds and hear only those coming from the patient—a skill that comes to all who persist.

Whispered Pectoriloquy. During whispering, the vocal cords do not oscillate because there is no turbulent air flow through the trachea, glottis, and larynx. In a normal lung, the whispered voice is not heard at all or, at best, only faintly and indistinctly. No syllables can be distinguished throughout the entire chest, except perhaps very faintly around the sternum and the trachea in the upper lobe areas of the lung, where the bony anatomy transmits the sound.

To test for a whispered pectoriloquy, the patient is asked to whisper the number series "1, 2, 3, 4." If a whispered sound can be heard that is definitely and clearly recognizable, then the patient has a whispered pectoriloquy. The patient must very quietly whisper (no phonated words) if this test for consolidation is to be of value. Whispered pectoriloquy is never a normal sound and always indicates consolidation of the lung field in the area being auscultated. It is important for the auscultator to remember to isolate the sound from the chest wall from all other extraneous sounds. The beginning auscultator can easily mistake the whispered sound heard extraneously from the patient's lips for a whispered pectoriloquy heard across the chest wall. It is sometimes tempting to hear what we have consciously asked the patient to whisper when, in fact, the whispered words are only heard by our ears and not through the stethoscope.

Egophony. The word *egophony* comes from the Greek "voice of the goat." Egophony refers to the nasal or bleating quality of speech transmitted through consolidated lung tissue. The uttered word will frequently sound much like when children playfully talk with their noses pinched, having a very nasal, whinning, or bleating character. Egophony is a modified form of bronchophony in which there is not only an increase in the clarity of the spoken voice but also a change in the character of the sound. When the patient phonates the long vowel sound of "EEEEE," the auscultator hears the long vowel sound "AAAAA." With egophony, when sound waves pass through the consolidated lung tissue, the sound is transmuted, producing the phenomenon known as an E-to-A egophony. The precise mechanism for this abnormal vocal sound is not clearly understood but is no doubt related to the way sound waves are transmitted through a fluid-filled or obstructed lung field. Egophony is always an abnormal sound and indicates consolidation of the lung in the area that is being auscultated.

Transmission of Breath Sounds

Normal Breath Sounds. There are four basic types of normal breath sounds: tracheal, bronchial, vesicular, and bronchovesicular sounds. Each of these has a normal regional location in the lung. For example, in most patients, the bronchial breath sound is normally only heard over the manubrium, but is occasionally heard at the costosternal margins of some individuals. The four breath sounds are completely normal when heard through the stethoscope in their appropriate anatomic region of the lung. However, when the tracheal, bronchial, and bronchovesicular breath sounds are heard outside of their normal regional distribution, they are considered to be abnormal and signs of disease pathology.

Tracheal Breath Sounds. Tracheal breath sounds are only heard over the trachea below the larynx. Since this breath sound is located only over the trachea, and not in the lung fields, the tracheal breath sound is usually not auscultated. However, it is important to know what a tracheal breath sounds like because the bronchial breath sound has many of the same qualities.

The tracheal breath sound is heard through the stethoscope as a high-pitched, loud, tubular, hollow, raspy, metallic sound. It has been likened to wind rushing through a hollow tube. On auscultation, both the inspiratory and expiratory phases of the ventilatory cycle are clearly heard. The I:E ratio is almost always equal in length; occasionally the expiratory phase is slightly longer (i.e., I:E ratio = 1:1 or 1:1½). There is a pause between the expiratory and inspiratory phases. The expiratory phase is usually coarser or louder than the inspiratory phase. It can be represented diagramatically as follows:

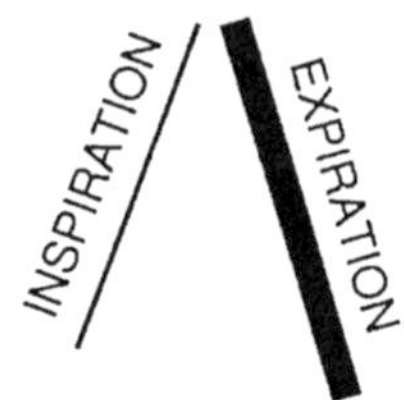

Bronchial Breath Sounds. Bronchial breath sounds are normally heard over the upper lobes of the lungs close to the sternum along the anterior midline of the thorax at the jugular notch of the manubrium as well as directly over the manubrium. They are sometimes also heard along the costosternal margins of the sternum. On auscultation, they are tubular and metallic in quality, high pitched, and resonant. Like the tracheal breath sound, the bronchial breath sound is much like hearing air being blown through a hollow tube.

Bronchial breath sounds differ from tracheal breath sounds in that the bronchial breath sound is not as loud because there is more soft tissue muffling the sound transmitted to the sternal chest wall from the trachea and the mainstem bronchi than on the neck anterior to the trachea.

When a bronchial breath sound is heard on or next to the sternum it is considered a normal breath sound. Bronchial breath sounds have a louder and longer expiratory phase (I:E ratio = 1:1¼ to 1:1½). There is usually a characteristic pause between inspiration and expiration, but on occasion this pause may be absent especially during hyperventilation. A normal bronchial breath sound can be represented diagramatically as follows:

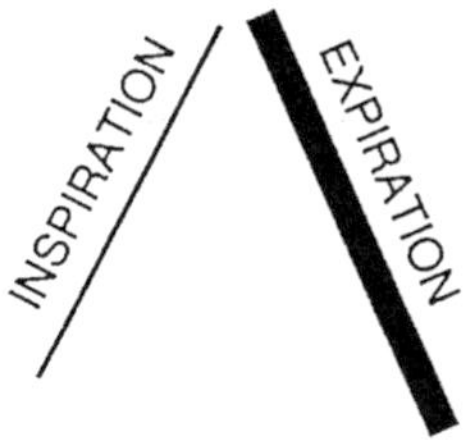

However, if the bronchial breath sound is heard in any other area of the lung, such as the anterior bronchopulmonary segment of the upper lobes, the lingula, the right middle lobes, or the bilateral lower lobes, it is considered an abnormal sound of serious import. It is then an indication of enhanced sound transmission due to fluid filling the lungs, of atelectasis, or of a compressed consolidated lung.

Vesicular Breath Sounds. Vesicular breath sounds are normally heard over the entire anterior, lateral, and posterior chest walls, excluding the areas described under Bronchial Breath Sounds (Fig. 3-6).

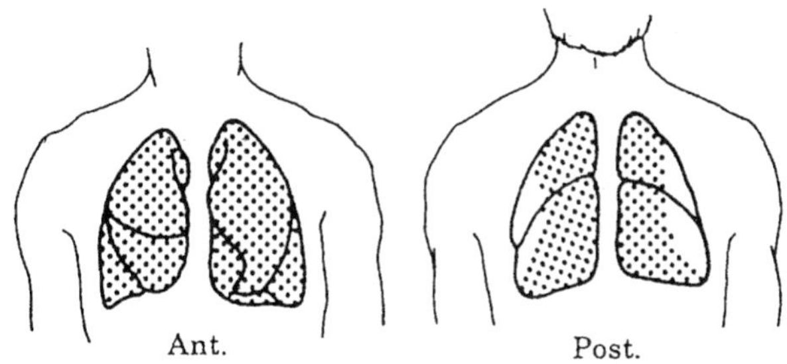

Fig. 3-6. Dots signify where vesicular breath sounds are normally heard. Anterior (ANT) and posterior (POST) views of the trunk.

Vesicular breath sounds are muffled and low pitched compared with bronchial and tracheal breath sounds. It has often been said that vesicular breath sounds are like wind rustling through the leaves of a tree. Vesicular breath sounds are so muffled compared with the other breath sounds that they sound like respirations in the next room through a house wall.

Inspiration will be low pitched and more audible than expiration, with inspiration being three times longer than expiration (I:E ratio = 3:1). Therefore, expiration will be much shorter and much more faint. There is usually no pause between the longer inspiratory and shorter expiratory phases. Often the expiration phase is completely absent (I:E ratio = 1:0). The length relationship of inspiration to expiration is diagramatically represented as follows:

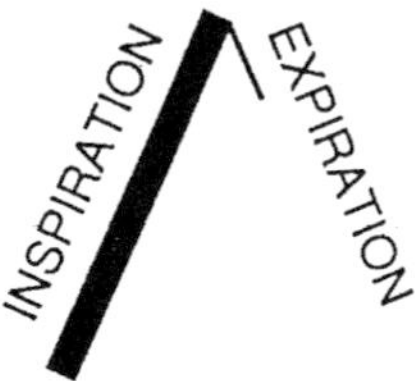

Unlike the bronchial breath sound, which is considered to be an abnormal breath sound when it is heard in an atypical area of the lung, the vesicular breath sound is not considered abnormal solely on the basis of geographic location. Rather, the vesicular breath sound may be viewed as abnormal when it is diminished in normal intensity or is distantly heard in its wide lung field distribution. This occurs when the lung tissue is no longer being adequately ventilated, producing a faint or a distant breath sound. Distant vesicular breath sounds are commonly heard in patients who are in the early stages of pnuemonia, in patients who are experiencing the onset of atelectasis, and in patients with chronic obstructive pulmonary disease (COPD). An abnormal vesicular breath sound (depressed vesicular breath sound) may have a pause between the inspiratory and expiratory phases, or its I:E ratio may no longer be 1:0 but more like 1:½, giving it characteristics more like a bronchial breath sound.

Bronchovesicular Breath Sounds. As the name implies, the bronchovesicular breath sound is a combination of vesicular and bronchial breath sounds. It is unique because the vesicular characteristic appears usually on inspiration while the bronchial characteristic appears during the expiratory phase. The pitch will change between respiratory phases to reflect the dual character of this breath sound (i.e., a soft muffled sound for the vesicular breath sound and a high-pitched, tubular sound for the bronchial breath sound). There is a pause between inspiration and expiration that sets this breath sound uniquely apart from the vesicular breath sound. Expiration is usually as long as inspiration, with an I:E ratio of 1:1. These sounds are normally heard on the anterior chest wall over the sternum at the angle of Louis and along the lower costosternal borders of the sternum, as well as the interscapular region between T3 and T6 (Fig. 3-7). The bronchovesicular breath sound is the predominant and normal breath sound in children under age 13 years. It is represented diagrammatically as follows:

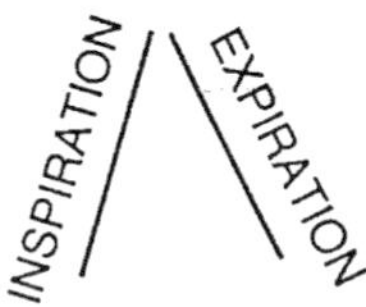

However, when the bronchovesicular breath sound is heard in an area of the lung that normally has vesicular breath sounds, it is considered abnormal. Bronchovesicular breath sounds designate partial consolidation in the lungs typically seen with the build up of secretions, atelectasis, or a combination of both.

Diminished Breath Sounds. These are often called decreased breath sounds. They designate an interference

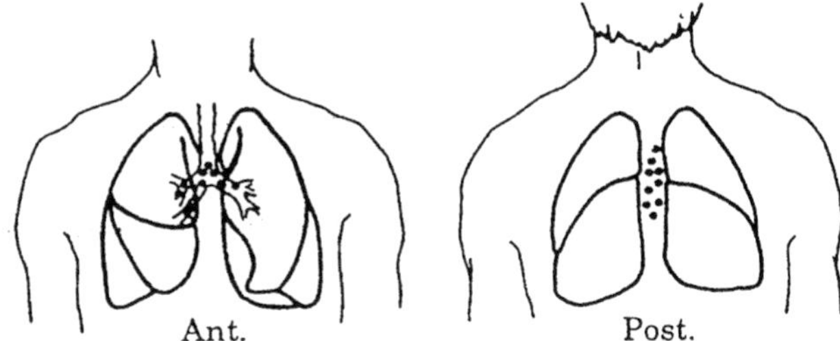

Fig. 3-7. Dots signify where bronchovesicular breath sounds are normally heard. Anterior (ANT) and posterior (POST) views of the trunk.

with the conduction of breath sounds and will therefore be decreased or absent. Diminished breath sounds indicate decreased air entry to a particular region of the lung.

The causes of diminished breath sounds are as follows:

1. Fluid in the pleural space
   a. Hemothorax (blood)
   b. Inflammatory pleural effusion
2. Air in the pleural space: pneumothorax
3. Thickening pleura caused by fibrosis: effusion, empyema
4. COPD, caused by decreased air velocity and sound conduction as a result of overinflation of the lung
5. Bronchial obstruction: mucous-plugged lumen
6. Hypoventilation of the lung caused by pleurisy or splinting secondary to a thoracic incision

In all but the first case, decreased breath sounds are a result of an interposed liquid medium as well as a definite decrease in ventilation of the underlying lung.

Adventitious Sounds

Adventitious sounds are not heard normally over any anatomic region of the chest. Adventitious sounds are not like the breath sounds previously discussed. Adventitious sounds are superimposed on top of the breath sound. They indicate air passing through obstructed regions of the lung. The most common adventitious sounds are rales, rhonchi, and stridor.

Rales.

Rale is a French word meaning "rattle." This term was in common use during late eighteenth century and early nineteenth century Europe and indicated impending death. Its usage today is no longer associated with the impending death of the patient. It is now a word that suggests distal airway mucous plugging and the obstruction and collapse of the acinus—the basic functional unit of the lung responsible for gas exchange and comprising the following structures: respiratory bronchioles, alveolar ducts, alveolar sacs, and the alveoli. Since rales is a word of European origin, its meaning in modern American English over the past several decades has become obscured. Clinicians have sought a more descriptive word that accurately describes the quality of this adventitious sound. The recent change in medical nomenclature for rales is *crackles*. In truth, both terms are still used and appear with frequency in medical charts. The terms in this section are presented side by side in an effort to ease the transition to the new term.

Rales or crackles are popping sounds that are heard through the stethoscope during the inspiratory phase of ventilation. They sound like popcorn popping or like the crackles or popping of burning wood. Because the crackles can be heard separately and clearly one from another, they are sometimes called discontinuous sounds. Rales or crackles result from the passage of air through mucous secretions in the distal regions of the bronchopulmonary tree, that is, the last four to five generations of the lung. The crackle or popping sound occurs during inspiration as a result of re-inflation of the lung's airways and possibly the sudden re-opening of collapsed alveoli. Crackles may also reflect air passing through secretions and the subsequent movement of the obstructive mucous plugs as a result of the negative inspiratory pressures generated during labored breathing. Occasionally crackles can be heard in the beginning third of expiration in patients with severe COPD. The exact reason for this is difficult to explain, since crackles are adventitious sounds produced by the opening of formerly closed terminal airways—an inspiratory phenomenon. One possible explanation for this may be the severity of the patient's COPD. If the patient's lung damage is great enough, airflow characteristics may be changed such that there is not a sharp and distinct change in air movement; hence, while exhalation may be starting, the airflow of inspiration is not completely finished (i.e., the transition between the end of inspiration and the beginning of exhalation is not discrete).

The sound of a rale will vary according to the size of the space involved and the character of the secretions that are responsible for the collapse. Rales or crackles may be wet or dry depending on the amount of moisture in the lung. Also, rales can be classified as fine, medium, or course in character.

Fine Rales (Fine Crackles). Fine crackles are heard when secretions have collected in the deep, terminal areas of the tracheobronchial tree. Through the stethoscope, fine crackles are frequently not well separated out, and individual popping is less distinct. Fine crackles sound like the slurping of the last portions of a milk shake through a straw or like the rapid close-ordered popping of a string of firecrackers. These sounds indicate inflammation and congestion involving the alveoli. They can be heard at any stage during inspiration but are commonly heard at the beginning. Diagrammatically, they can be portrayed as follows:

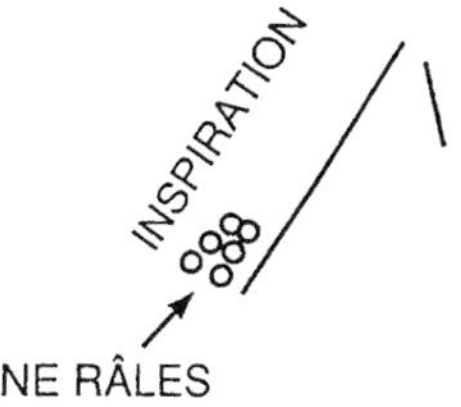

Medium Rales (Medium Crackles). Medium rales sound heavier or louder than do fine rales. They can be heard at any stage of inspiration but are commonly heard halfway through the inspiratory phase. They tend to be the result of air passing through mucus in the acinus and tend to reflect a more tenacious secretion in the distal airway. Diagrammatically they can appear as follows:

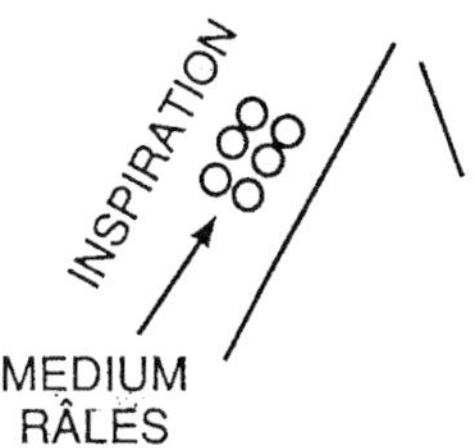

Course Rales (Course Crackles). Course rales are a sign of heavy involvement of the distal airway in that the secretions are very wet and tenacious. They can frequently appear early but may be heard throughout the entire inspiratory phase and are a serious sign of pulmonary involvement. Diagrammatically they can can appear as follows:

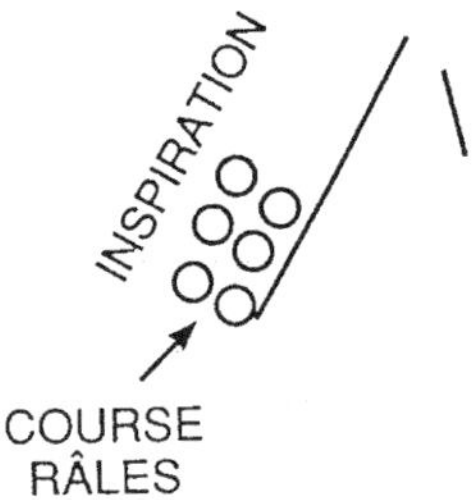

Rhonchi

Rhonchi, like rales, have been given a new name that more accurately describes the sound. The newer term cohabitating in the medical records with the older term of rhonchi is *wheeze*.

Rhonchi or wheezes are continuous in their sound, unlike rales, which are discrete, discontinuous and singularly crackly. Rhonchi or wheezes are continuous "snoring" or rumbling-type sounds that can be heard throughout inspiration and expiration. Rhonchi or wheezes are sounds produced by the passage of air through the trachea, bronchi, and bronchioles, which have been narrowed or nearly closed by disease and mucous plugging. Rhonchi or wheezes represent obstructive events occurring in the central airways. They can be cleared by coughing and suctioning, whereas rales are not cleared in this manner.

Some clinicians make a distinction between a high-pitched wheeze and a low-pitched wheeze. A high-pitched wheeze, sometimes called a *sibilant* wheeze, sounds remarkably like the distant calls of migrating whales. On the other hand, the low-pitched wheeze, often called *sonorous* is a low-pitched growling or snoring type of sound.

Stridor

Stridor is a particularly loud musical sound most prominent during inspiration. It can be heard at a distance from the patient without the use of a stethoscope. Stridor is produced when the patient is experiencing laryngeal or tracheal obstruction. Stridor is the sound heard in children with croupe. It is that high-pitched raspy, throaty, wheezy, or crowing sound that is so indicative of the child's respiratory distress.

Although stridor is usually heard during inspiration, it can be heard during inspiration *and* expiration as the airway becomes increasingly obstructed. The larynx or the trachea can be increasingly obstructed by the growth of laryngeal tumors, by a worsening tracheal stenosis, or when some object has been inhaled or aspirated into the upper airway of the lung. When particularly severe, stridor is associated with gasping respiration and the use of accessory respiratory muscles in an attempt to increase airflow. Stridor should be viewed as potentially indicating a life-threatening illness especially if there is inflammation involved. In these conditions, such as in croupe, severe tracheitis, or when a toy has been inhaled into the upper respiratory tract, the patient can become so hypoxemic as to need emergency services to restore a patent airway.

Pleural Friction Rub

The visceral and parietal pleural surfaces of the lung glide over each other without difficulty because they are smooth and glistening. The thin fluid layer between these pleural coverings acts to lubricate the surfaces and allows them to slip past each other noiselessly and effortlessly during the respiratory phases of breathing. However, when these surfaces become inflamed they can become rough and self-adherent, creating a pleural friction rub.

A pleural friction rub is a continuous sound that is usually heard at the middle to end of the inspiratory phase and perhaps at the beginning of the expiratory phase. Pleural friction rubs have a characteristic squeaking, grating, creaking, or clicking sound. A tell-tale sign of the presence of a pleural friction rub is the cessation of breathing at the point the patient feels pain during the respiratory cycle—a phenomenon called splinting. The patient will splint or momentarily hold his breath because of the pain caused by the roughened and inflamed pleural surfaces sticking together. The adherence of the pleural surfaces will then release quickly and the patient will continue the rest of the inspiratory cycle. During exhalation, the patient may again experience a momentary splinting episode at the same point where the pleural pain was felt during inspiration. This cyclic adherance and release of the pleurae is diagnostic of a pleural friction rub. Rubs are most commonly heard over the posterolateral and anterolateral chest wall and on the posterior chest wall. Pleural friction rubs are often caused by pneumonias, blunt trauma to the thoracic wall, tumors, bacterial infections of the pleurae, and thoracic surgery.

Helpful Hints for the New Auscultator

New auscultators should practice in a quiet room. In the hospital intensive care unit, the background noise can be so loud as to make it almost impossible for the new auscultator to hear any sound emanating from the thoracic cavity. It is useful to practice on healthy individuals first, in a quiet place, to learn the normal breath sounds and where they are located. It would be wise to practice on many people and to evaluate the different regions of the lung methodically. In review, the tracheal breath sound is normally heard only over the trachea. The bronchial breath sound is normally heard only over the manubrium of the sternum and occasionally along the sternocostal border. A bronchial breath sound heard anywhere else is considered abnormal and portends the presence of lung disease. The vesicular breath sound is normally heard over the remaining portions of the chest wall. The clinician has to remember that certain sounds are normal when found in the right place in the lung. However, that same sound heard in a region of the lung field where it is not normally heard is a sign of pathology. The clinician must become very familiar with the lung sounds heard in their normal anatomical location. This will be essential when a real pathology is present and altered lung sounds are heard.

For proper evaluation of the gradations of sounds, the clinician should move the stethoscope in an orderly pattern from side to side, that is, move from the right basilar segments to the left basilar segments or from the anterior segment of the right upper lobe to the left anterior segment of the left upper lobe. Essentially, the auscultator listens to one full inspiratory and expiratory cycle on the right and then repeat this on the left. In so doing, one can compare right side to left side and can detect differences in amplitude and pitch between the right and left lung fields.

The new auscultator may at first have a problem filtering out local extraneous noise: noises transmitted through the stethoscope that originate from either the patient or the clinician. Extraneous local noises might include the following:

1. Sounds in the therapist's phalangeal joints are easily mistaken for chest sounds; they are transmitted to the ears while the stethoscope is handled and as the diaphragm is firmly pressed on the patient's chest.
2. The sound of thick chest hair scratching across the diaphragm of the stethoscope is often mistaken as fine rales. Once the source of this local noise is identified, the auscultator can learn to ignore the sound or can try dampening the area with some water to make the hair lay close to the chest wall.
3. Local extraneous noise may come from clothing rubbing on the stethoscope.
4. The crepitant noise from arthritic joints can interfere with listening to the chest wall.
5. Speech as well as bowel sounds can also provide considerable interference with the sounds of a patient's lungs, especially the patient who is on bed rest.

Practice makes perfect, and this adage applies to anyone learning chest auscultation. The idea is to start out slow and listen to normal, healthy lungs first. Some tapes and book publications discuss in great detail how to listen to the chest when conducting a pulmonary assessment.

ASSESSMENT OF THE PULMONARY PATIENT

Chart Review

The physical therapist should have a thorough understanding of the patient's past medical history. Knowledge of the patient's medical background can help in forming a meaningful rehabilitation plan and in making realistic goals to meet the needs of the patient. The discussion offers a practical approach to pulmonary assessment based on common simple techniques applicable in both outpatient and inpatient settings (see Table 3-2).

Table 3-2. Pulmonary Evaluation Techniques

Outpatient	Inpatient
History (including medications)	History (including medications)
Physical examination	Physical examination
Spirometry (FVC, FEV_1, PEFR, $\dot{V}_E$)	Spirometry (FVC, FEV_1, PEFR, V_T)
Maximum inspiratory or expiratory force	Maximum inspiratory or expiratory force; PEEP
Compliance (dynamic)	Compliance (static and dynamic)
	Arterial blood gases
Oximetry	Cardiac monitor, oximeter
ECG, chest radiography	Ventilation-perfusion calculated
Functional capacity (VO_{2max})	shunt or V_D/V_T

Medical History

If the medical chart is accessible, the medical history should be thoroughly reviewed for information pertinent to the patient's current medical problems. Does the patient's current hospital visit represent a repeat admission for the same problem, or is this an admission completely unrelated to the acute or chronic respiratory problems? For example:

1. Is an emphysemic patient being admitted for removal of plates and screws from an open reduction internal fixation (ORIF) performed several months or years ago? If this is the case, the patient's emphysema is a secondary problem and will have to be managed while the patient is in physical therapy for gait training and muscle strengthening. It may well be necessary to address the respiratory problem first before working with the patient's musculoskeletal system.
2. Is the patient being readmitted because of a recurrent infection in a total hip prosthesis? The infection may well be accompanied by a secondary pneumonia resulting from the patient's inactivity or bedrest. Once the infection is under control, the therapist may well be asked to see this patient for muscle strengthening, range of motion (ROM), exercises and increasing out-of-bed activities such as gait or bicycle exercises. However, the lung condition will be the major acute obstacle for the patient needing to increase physical activity.

It is clear that as Americans age, more patients will have multiple system impairments. It may well become the exception, rather than the rule, for a therapist to treat a patient for a single problem.

Psychosocial History

The physical therapist should know the patient's psychosocial history. This information should readily be available in the medical chart. However, if it does not or if the chart is not available for review, the psychosocial history may be obtained from the patient, the family, or the relatives. Psychosocial information may be extremely helpful to the therapist in understanding the patient's attitudes toward members of the rehabilitation team, motivations or lack of motivations for recovery, and interactions with family members. The complexities of a patient's emotions and feelings is best understood with this type of knowledge. All too often, the success or failure of a patient's rehabilitation program rests on the level of trust, support and love the patient feels in the family. The behavior of a patient reflects the nuances of familial interaction.

Some of the information gleaned by the therapist may include the age of the patient and the patient's marital status. Marital status can be an important piece of background information to be used to enhance the patient's desire to participate in the rehabilitation process. It may also explain why the patient is not participating in the program. For example, the patient may become despondent as discharge from the hospital grows nearer because there is no one to "go home to". Such patients may feel as if there is no reason to live anymore. They may have no incentive to participate actively in their own rehabilitation and may well refuse to take responsibility for their own recovery.

Radiographic Results

It is important to read the radiographic reports. These reports are useful in determining what part of the lung field is involved in the disease process. The radiographic report will indicate whether the patient has a panlobar (diffuse) problem or a discrete lobar involvement. In many instances, the radiologist will have access to old films and will state in the report how the most recent radiograph compares with older ones. These comments indicate whether the patient is improving, has remained the same, or is deteriorating. Radiographic reports also indicate whether the disease process is acute or chronic. All of this information helps the therapist plan reasonable rehabilitation goals.

Medication History

It is important for the physical therapist to have a good understanding of the pulmonary medications that patients are taking. Generally, respiratory medications fall into four classes: sympathomimetics, methylxanthines, mucolytics, and corticosteroids.

Sympathomimetics

The sympathomimetics are widely prescribed because of their usefulness as β_1- or β_2-adrenergic agonists (i.e., they mimic the actions and have the same side effects observed when patients are given either epinephrine and norepinephrine). Some medications possess the ability to stimulate one β-adrenergic receptor more than another. If sympathomimetic medications are selective in the type of β-adrenergic receptor they stimulate, they are called β-selective sympathomimetics. Those medications that stimulate both the β_1- and β_2-receptors are called nonselective β-adrenergic medications.

Medications that have an affinity for binding to β_1-receptors are medications that will strongly stimulate cardiac function (e.g., stimulate heart rate and stroke volume). Because these medications have a dramatic impact on the heart, the β_1-drugs are said to have inotropic and chronotropic effects. β_1-selective drugs as well as nonselective β-adrenergic drugs have fallen into disfavor because they are potentially harmful to some patients who are susceptible to developing tachyarrhythmias and suffer from hypertension. Patients with cardiac disease should not be given medications with β_1-selective or nonselective β-adrenergic properties. On the other hand, β_2-selective adrenergic medications are very desirable because their effects are largely restricted to the lungs (i.e., bronchodilatory). These drugs become vitally important when it is necessary to bronchodilate a patient who has an accompanying heart condition that would be made worse if a nonselective β-adrenergic drug was administered. Hence, most pulmonary medications prescribed today are largely β_2-selective. Some of the important members of this group in common use are terbutaline sulfate (Brethine), metaproterenol (Alupent), albuterol sulfate (Ventolin), isoetharine hydrochloride (Bronkosol), pirbuterol (Maxair), and bitolterol mesylate (Tornalate). See Table 3-3 for potential side effects that warrant immediate contact with a physician.

Methylxanthines

Methylxanthines represent a very small class of pulmonary bronchodilatory medications. The mechanism of action is not well understood but is believed to be related to the inhibitory effects these drugs exert on the destructive enzyme phosphodiesterase. Phosphodiesterase destroys cyclic 3′,5′-adenosine monophosphate (cAMP), a nucleotide that activates a large number of chemical pathways. When methylxanthines are taken, the intracellular levels of cAMP rise dramatically and bronchodilation results. By association, if the half-life of cAMP can be prolonged by inhibiting the enzyme that destroys it, then the bronchodilatory effects brought about by the activation of cAMP are also prolonged. The medications in this group are theophylline (Theo-Dur), oxtriphylline (Brondecon), aminophylline, theophylline Na^+ glycinate (Asbron G), and dyphylline. There are other methylxanthines (caffeine and theobromine), but they are not used very often for medical treatment. See Table 3-4 for potential side effects that if noted would warrant physician contact.

Table 3-3. Sympathomimetics

Side effects that warrant immediate physician contact
Chest pain
Hallucinations
Breathing difficulties
Irregular heartbeat
Severe dizziness
Severe headache
Marked increased blood pressure
Nervousness
Severe weakness

Table 3-4. Methylxanthines

Events that warrant immediate physician contact
Onset of fever or flu as the chance of side effects increases
Side effects that warrant physician contact
Melena
Diarrhea
Dizziness
Headache
Irritability
Confusion
Skin rash
Insomnia
Stomach pain/vomiting
Unusual fatigue
Irregular heartbeat

Mucolytics

Mucolytic medications are used to thin secretions in the tracheobronchial tree so that the mucociliary elevator

Table 3-5. Mucolytics

Side effects that warrant physician contact
Mood/mental changes
Sore throat and fever
Chest tightness
Unusual bleeding
Irregular heartbeat
Unusual fatigue
Headache
Increased sweating
Trembling

can clear them from the lung more easily. There are a variety of mechanisms that these medications activate to achieve this effect (e.g., thinning of bronchial secretions by cleaving mucin's disulfide bonds [N-acetylcysteine] and thinning secretions by cleaving some components found in the mucous secretions [rhDNase]). These medications help thin the secretions so that the patient can clear them from the lungs by deep breathing and coughing or undergoing postural drainage and percussion. See Table 3-5 for potential side effects that if noted warrant physician contact.

Corticosteroids

Corticosteroids are employed widely in pulmonary medicine to control the injurious effects of inflammatory processes in the lung. Inflammatory processes are responsible for the increased production of mucus in the lungs as well as fibrotic destruction of the tracheobronchial tree. Steroids in small doses effectively block all of the mediators of inflammation and inhibit fibrosis and scarring of the pulmonary system.

Medications in this group are popular, when given in the appropriate doses, because they do not cross over into the systemic circulation. These medications are delivered most often by a metered-dose inhaler. Because the effects of these medications are largely restricted to the tracheobronchial tree after inhalation, they do not have the detrimental effects on connective tissue that are commonly associated with larger doses of corticosteroids typically administered by enteral (oral) or parenteral (injection) routes. Common members of this medication group are triamcinolone acetonide (Azmacort), beclomethasone dipropionate (Beclovent), and flunisolide (Aerobid). See Table 3-6 for potential side effects that if noted warrant physician contact.

Table 3-6. Corticosteroids

Side effects that warrant physician contact
White, curdlike patches in the mouth
Edema of the face
Skin rash
Tachycardia
Mouth, throat, lung infections

The Pulmonary Function Test

The chart should be reviewed to see whether pulmonary function studies have been completed. These tests measure the patient's lung volumes and capacities. They are very useful because they are a measure of the patient's ability to ventilate and exchange two critical gases—oxygen and carbon dioxide—in and out of the lung.

Pulmonary function tests are particularly useful in the diagnosis of COPD such as asthma, emphysema, chronic bronchitis, and bronchiectasis. In suspected COPD, the patient will have a classic reduced ability to exhale air forcibly from the lungs. Therefore, critical volume measurements of the patient's ability to expire air forcibly from the lungs will be reduced; that is, forced expiratory volume in 1 second (FEV_1), forced expiratory volume in 3 seconds (FEV_3), peak expiratory flow rate (PEFR), mid-expiratory flow rate ($FEF_{25\%-75\%}$), and forced vital capacity (FVC) will all be smaller than in patients with normal lung function.

Pulmonary function tests are also useful but less diagnostic in patients suspected of having restrictive lung disease. Restrictive lung diseases such as adult respiratory distress syndrome (ARDS), infant respiratory distress syndrome (IRDS), coccidioidomycosis (Valley Fever), sarcoidosis, and any number of pulmonary fibrosis syndromes all make the lung less flexible or compliant. The lung affected with a restrictive disease is a stiffer lung. Expansion and contraction of the bronchopulmonary tree are much more difficult, and the volume of air that can be brought in and out of the lungs is reduced. Also, a number of medical conditions restrict normal expansion and contraction of the lung, such as a flail chest, a thoracic cage affected by ankylosing spondylitis, rib fractures, as well as blunt chest trauma, in which case patients refuse to deep breathe because they are splinting against the pain that deep inspiration might cause. These conditions affect the normal mechanics of breathing. Patients with these medical problems will have pulmonary function tests that display a normal tidal volume but smaller than normal FEV_1 and FVC values. The FEV_1 to FVC ratio ($FEV_1\%$) will be very close to 1.00 because the FEV_1 and FVC are equally affected by the restrictive pathology. The patient usually has an FEV_1 close to the FVC because of the difficulty of expanding the chest wall during inspiration.

If the patient has had a pulmonary function study, the report will describe the results in terms of obstructive or restrictive lung disease. These reports coupled with the information on the radiographic report, as well as the blood gas report, are very helpful in determining the patient's pulmonary disease state.

It is also helpful to find out whether serial pulmonary function tests (PFTs) are available. These tests will show whether the patient's pulmonary status has changed over the past few months or years.

Blood Gases

The therapist should read the blood gas reports. They will show whether the patient has adequate gas diffusion. Blood gas reports have a wealth of information describing the acid–base balance of the patient. Some of the information the therapist should have is the partial pressure of oxygen (PaO_2), partial pressure of carbon dioxide ($PaCO_2$), pH, and bicarbonate ion concentration in the blood.

Normal blood gas readings are described as partial pressures of a specific gas (oxygen and carbon dioxide) and are given the units of millimeters of mercury pressure (mmHg). Normal values for oxygen are between 90 and 100 mmHg and for carbon dioxide, 35 and 45 mmHg. If the patient has a partial pressure of oxygen (PaO_2) less than 80 mmHg, severe central nervous system effects will be noted because the central nervous system does not function well when the patient is hypoxic. If the $PaCO_2$ rises above 60 mmHg, the patient will likely be in respiratory distress because of the retention of carbon dioxide, a condition known as hypercapnia.

The normal pH of the blood is between 7.35 and 7.45. For a number of reasons the pH of the blood can be altered. If the pH falls below 7.35, the patient is said to be acidotic. Acidosis is usually caused by failure to ventilate the lungs adequately. The exchange of oxygen and carbon dioxide across the alveolar–capillary interface is reduced, and the blood begins to collect everincreasing amounts of carbon dioxide because of continued cellular metabolism. As carbon dioxide collects in the blood, the pH of the blood rapidly falls, pushing the patient further into acidosis. The reasons for acidosis are legion. Millions of patients each year experience respiratory acidosis because of COPD, drug overdose, or airways obstruction.

Chronic Obstructive Pulmonary Disease

Patients who smoke constitute the largest class of individuals who experience chronic acidosis. People with emphysema and chronic bronchitis experience increasing difficulty in exchanging oxygen and carbon dioxide over the years of their smoking lifetime. This is directly attributable to the constituents of the burning tobacco that stimulate an inflammatory reaction in lung tissue, causing fibrosis and scarring of the gas-exchange surfaces of the lung. The alveolar–capillary interface where oxygen and carbon dioxide are normally exchanged is so eroded by fibrosis as to impede the movement of oxygen and carbon dioxide across this delicate interface. The smoker becomes increasingly short of breath because of poor gas-exchange mechanics. These patients will have slightly lower PaO_2 values and very much higher $PaCO_2$ values on the blood gas report. Patients with COPD will often be seen with PaO_2 values in the range of 80 to 90 mmHg and $PaCO_2$ values in the range of 50 to 60 mmHg. As the destruction of the gas-exchange surfaces continues as a result of continued tobacco abuse, the patient will experience increasingly severe respiratory difficulties. Death by respiratory failure can eventually be the end result if the smoking behavior is not stopped.

Drug Overdose

Drug overdose patients will be acidotic as a result of severe central nervous system and respiratory center depression. The poor blood gas values in these patients are a direct result of the failure of the respiratory system to stimulate adequate ventilation of the lungs. The poor respiratory mechanics must be corrected immediately to avoid irreparable damage to the central nervous system.

Airways Obstruction

Airways obstruction is another common reason that patients may experience acute blood–gas derangements. Objects or mucous secretions may be obstructing the upper airways of the tracheobronchial tree, resulting in inadequate ventilation.

The Laboratory Reports

The therapist should read the laboratory reports for bacteriology, for sputum cultures, for hematology, and for urine analysis. Some common blood laboratory values are

Platelets: 200,000–400,000/mm^3
Red blood cells: 5,000,000–6,000,000/ml
White blood cells: 4,500–10,800/ml
Hemaglobin
- Females: 13–14 g/dl
- Males: 15–16 g/dl

Hematocrit
- Females: 34%–46%
- Males: 40%–52%

Work History

What is the work history of the patient? Is the patient retired or is it likely that the patient will return to work? How happy was the patient with the job before the present illness? How anxious is the patient to return to the workplace? Is the patient involved in a worker's compensation dispute subsequent to an injury on the job? Is a lawsuit pending in the courts during the course of rehabilitation? The answers to many of these questions may influence the patient's desire to participate actively in rehabilitation.

Discharge Planning

Will the patient return home immediately after discharge, or will there be the need for a short stay at an extended care facility? Is there the likelihood of home discharge and the need of some health services in the home? Will treatment be continued on an outpatient basis? The excitement of getting out of the hospital is sometimes dampened by the need to go to an extended care facility. The patient's zeal for rehabilitation can be affected by what type of discharge is expected. The therapist can help the patient to see the benefits of an extended care facility. The time spent in helping patients cope with discharge can go a long way in helping them work hard for rehabilitation, making the therapist's job much easier. Depression concerning the illness frequently encumbers that patient's speedy progress in rehabilitation, but when it is complicated by depression about discharge to an extended care facility, the therapist can find it very difficult to motivate the patient to work hard to recovery.

History

The therapist should interview the patient or the patient's family for the relevant history concerning the illness for which the patient is being admitted. The following questions should be included:

1. What is the patient's smoking history? How long has the patient been a smoker? How much did the patient smoke per day?
2. What is or was the patient's occupation? Did the patient's job present an occupational risk to pulmonary health? If yes, to what extent was that health hazard responsible for the present hospital admission?
3. Can the patient document a history of shortness of breath secondary to smoking, or does the patient think the shortness of breath started just before admission to the hospital?

The next step is to determine the patient's responses to activity. How is the patient able to tolerate mild to moderate activity? The following questions should be considered.

1. Can the patient get out of bed and walk unattended or is he restricted to bed rest?
2. Does the patient require oxygen supplementation during exercise? Is oxygen necessary even at rest? What are the blood oxygen saturation values for the patient at rest, during ROM exercises, and during ambulation? Oxygen saturation is determined by an oximeter and is useful in estimating the oxygen-carrying capacity of the patient.
3. Does the patient tolerate positional changes? Can the patient lie flat in the bed during sleep or must he sit up in bed during sleep hours? Many patients in respiratory distress cannot tolerate the supine or prone flat positions. These patients will often feel less shortness of breath when in the sitting position. While in the sitting position, the abdominal contents are being pulled on by gravity and pulled away from the diaphragm, permitting maximal downward excursion of the diaphragm. This position allows for a deeper inspiratory effort and therefore reduces the sensation of shortness of breath.

Physical Examination

The examination begins with manually evaluation of the chest wall. This aspect of the evaluation looks at the anatomic and mechanical movement of the thoracic wall. The following information should be included in the evaluation notes:

1. Can the patient take a deep breath, or does the patient complain of being unable to take a deep breath? What is the cause of the patient's complaint of shortness of breath? Frequently patients with pneumonia or other diseases such as asthma, bronchitis, or emphysema will complain of shortness of breath. They will try to ventilate the entire lung by taking in deep breaths, but the complaint of shortness of breath

persists. This problem is due to either fluid filling in the acinus (the basic respiratory unit of the lung, consisting of the respiratory bronchioles, the alveolar duct, the alveolar sac, and the alveoli) or obstruction of the conducting airways (trachea, mainstem bronchi, lobar bronchi, segmental bronchi, small bronchi) and the peripheral airways. Very often the patient who complains of shortness of breath will have evidence of this in the movement of the chest wall. The therapist should place the palmar surfaces of the hands firmly on the lateral chest wall. The patient should be asked to take a deep breath while the therapist determines the amount of chest wall excursion. Using this simple test, the therapist can often feel the loss of chest wall excursion on the side that is affected with disease. The therapist should note whether there is equal bilateral expansion of the chest wall. If there is less excursion on the right or the left, that outcome should be noted. Additionally, the overall amount of rib flaring should be noted. This can be done by placing a tape measure around the thoracic cage an three points—the axilla, the level of the nipples, and the bottom of the thoracic cage—and recording the chest wall circumference both at rest and during maximal inspiration.

2. Is there pain on deep breathing? Pain frequently accompanies pulmonary problems. Patients with pneumonia frequently experience pain in the region of the atelectasis and fluid infiltration of the lung. This pain is usually encountered on inspiration and can be so severe at times as to limit the depth of the inspiratory effort. The splinting and shallow breathing that results from chest wall pain only complicates the patient's recovery. Deep breathing and coughing are effective treatments for clearing secretions from the lung. Many times the therapist's greatest task in treating patients experiencing chest wall pain is to get them to produce an effective deep cough and to breathe deeply.
3. Is there any use of the accessory respiratory muscles? Patients in respiratory distress will recruit the accessory muscles of respiration (e.g., the sternocleidomastoids, the paraspinal muscles, and the shoulder girdle muscles). The neck, back, and shoulders should be observed during inspiration to see whether the patient is activating the accessory muscles. Cavitation of the thoracic wall—a depression of the thoracic wall between the ribs during inspiration—is a sign that the patient is experiencing respirtory distress. Cavitation is seen especially in children who are diagnosed with IRDS. In these infants, every inspiratory muscle is called into action in order to mount enough driving pressure to open up the collapsed or collapsing lung. The negative driving pressure exerted by the infant during the inspiratory manuever is so great as to cause the interthoracic spaces to be drawn inward below the surface level of the ribs, giving the appearance that there are indentations or cavitations between the ribs.
4. Does the patient suddenly halt inspiration and splint or exhibit a chest wall "catch"? This can be indicative of the presence of a pleural friction rub. Also, if there are rib fractures, there usually is crepitus and muscle splinting present because of movement of the bony ends of the fractured ribs that cause chest wall pain.
5. What is the rate and depth of respiration?

Productive or Nonproductive Cough

1. Can the patient elicit a good round double cough? Patients must be able to take in a deep breath and produce a deep double cough in order to clear the secretions from their lungs. Deep coughing mobilizes the secretions, while a shallow in-the-throat cough does little but inflame the throat.
2. What is the quantity, color, and general consistency of the mucus that is brought up from the lungs? Green mucus is a sign that infection is present. Frothy and pink or red mucus indicates that blood is most likely also being coughed up.

Breathing Patterns

1. Is there any paradoxical breathing? Paradoxical breathing is a pattern seen frequently in high paraplegics and in quadriplegics. Normally, the abdomen and the chest concomitantly rise during inspiration because, as the chest wall expands and rises, the contracting diaphragm pushes down against the abdominal contents, forcing the abdomen to rise as well. In patients who have lost innervation to the intercostal musculature (especially the external intercostals), the chest will not rise as much and may actually appear to fall during inspiration while the abdomen rises. Quadriplegic patients who only have a neurologically intact diaphragm via the phrenic nerve (C3–C4–C5) and who have lost all thoracic innervation will exhibit this type of paradoxical breathing.

2. Is expiration longer than inspiration? Patients who have COPD will very often breathe with pursed lips. Breathing through pursed lips in effect creates a back pressure in the lungs to prevent the small bronchi and the terminal bronchioles from collapsing during mid to end expiration. The back pressure that these patients deliver to their lungs is much like the positive end-expiratory pressure (PEEP) given to ventilator-bound patients to prevent collapse of the acinus. In both cases—in the COPD patient and the ventilator patient—PEEP is designed to keep the terminal airways open as long as possible in order to ensure a longer oxygen–carbon dioxide exchange period.
3. Can the patient speak while breathing or are breaths interspersed between words in a labored, gasping type of speech?
4. Is there any vocal fremitus? Vocal fremitus decribes the vibratory or buzzy sensation the therapist will feel if the hands are placed on the patient's chest as the patient speaks. Usually the therapist will place the palmar or the hyothenar regions of the hands on the thoracic wall while evaluating the patient for the presence of vocal fremitus. As the patient speaks, the rattling of the chest wall will be evident and is due to the passage of air and sound through secretions in the major airways. Vocal fremitus is often observed in patients with COPD and pneumonia.
5. What is the rate of breathing?

Finger Percussion

Finger percussion is useful in determining which areas of the thoracic wall should be auscultated. The technique involves placing the middle finger—the "anvil"—of the nondominant hand on the chest wall and sharply and quickly tapping it over the distal interphalangeal joint (DIP), using the middle finger of the dominant hand as the "hammer." When the hammer firmly raps the anvil, a resonant note is heard. For those who do not have the power to create a nice resonant note with the hammer finger, sometimes using a reflex hammer instead of the hammer finger produces a loud enough note to be easily heard.

The therapist will listen for variations over the chest wall in the transmitted sound, much like the technique used when auscultating the chest wall with a stethoscope. A side-to-side movement should be employed to compare the sounds heard over the right lung field with the sounds heard over the left lung field.

Normally the percussion note should be the same on both sides when moving over the thoracic wall. However, in areas of consolidation, there will be a reduced resonance or a dullness to the sound produced during finger percussion.

Auscultation

The therapist should first listen for normal breath sounds (bronchial and vesicular) in the areas of the lung field in which they normally appear. The therapist should also listen for adventitious sounds over the entire lung field such as rales, rhonchi, stridor (inspiratory stridor), pleural friction rub, as well as the voice sounds such as bronchophony, egophony, and whispered pectoriloquy.

When auscultating the lung fields, start by listening to the anterior chest wall. Listen to one side and then the other side in the same segment of the lungs. Listening to the same segment of one lung permits a comparison between the sound that was heard and the sound that will be generated on the opposite lung. This side-to-side movement of the stethoscope enables the therapist to evaluate the amplitude of both lung fields and to determine whether or not abnormal breath sounds or adventitious sounds are present. After evaluating the anterior chest wall, the therapist moves to the lateral chest wall and the posterior chest wall in a similar side-to-side evaluation method.

FUNCTIONAL RESPIRATORY CAPACITY ASSESSMENT

The basic assessment techniques mentioned in Table 3-2 contrast the normal pulmonary state discussed in the preceding portion of this chapter with the abnormal, given the specific disease state. The emphasis in the disease state is on basic outpatient assessment techniques unless the patient's situation, as in the intensive care unit in coma, renders the basic technique inadequate. In such circumstances, additional special techniques are suggested elsewhere.[8]

Some basic tests that are or should be readily available to physical therapists for completing their assessment include simple spirometry, used to obtain an FVC and an FEV_1; a manometer to measure maximum inspiratory pressure or force; ear or fingertip oximetry; the ECG; and the chest x-ray.

As with cardiac rehabilitation, the therapist needs an estimate of the individual's functional respiratory capacity. Several regression equations have been developed to measure the patient's respiratory capacity. One such equation is given below[9]:

$$VE_{max}\ (L/min) = 37.5 \times FEV_1$$

This particular measurement of functional capacity has the additional advantage of proving useful in predicting maximum oxygen uptake, as follows[9]:

$$VO_{2max}\ (ml/min) = 216.8 + 22.3\ (VE_{max})$$

A third equation has value because it also measures the patient's ventilatory muscle strength for baseline as well as for trending purposes:

$$VE_{max} = 21.34 \times FEV_1\ (L) + 6.28 \times PIFR\ (L/sec)$$

The test and equation results should provide adequate information for the therapist not only to evaluate the patient accurately, but also to provide an exercise prescription for that patient. These equations and assessment techniques will be effective in all types of respiratory disease.

Summary—Signs and Symptoms

The pulmonary system is a highly specialized organ with a singular task: to oxygenate the blood and to rid the body of carbon dioxide. All of the objective tests mentioned in this chapter help to determine if there are any pathologies present. There are a variety of signs and subjective symptoms the patient may demonstrate or divulge during the physical assessment examination. Some of the signs of respiratory distress that the therapist should be aware of are shortness of breath, dyspnea, cyanosis, rapid and shallow breathing, blood-streaked mucin, perulent mucin (sign of infection), cavitations of the chest wall during inspiration, recruitment of accessory muscles for breathing, paradoxical breathing patterns, unequal excursion of the chest wall during inspiration, shifting of the trachea away from its midline position in the neck (sign of pneumothorax), pursed lip breathing (common in COPD patients), the presence of adventitious breath sounds and vocal sounds on auscultation, and the inability to maintain continuous speech (sign of shortness of breath).

The signs indicating respiratory distress may be caused by the loss of lung tissue compliance (distensibility), the loss of gas diffusion capacity and exchange surface area (obstructive lung disease), the loss of the flexibility of the thoracic cage itself (restrictive lung disease), and loss of normal neuronal control over respiratory musculature (spinal cord injury). The patient may complain of symptoms such as hypoxia, shortness of breath, dyspnea, fatigue, malaise, bronchoconstriction (asthma), palpitations, tachycardia, and chest pain (sign of infection, atelectasis, pneumothorax). Some of the signs and symptoms require rapid medical assistance. Chest pain and shortness of breath may indicate the presence of a pneumonia, a pneumothorax, or a pulmonary embolism. Shortness of breath, dyspnea, cyanosis, or pursed lip breathing may indicate the patient is experiencing an asthma attack, especially if accompanied by bronchoconstriction. Shortness of breath and hypoxemia may also indicate the beginning pulmonary deterioration in a Guillain-Barré syndrome patient, the worsening of a pneumonia, or the presence of a pulmonary embolism. See Table 3-7 for a summary of symptoms and signs suggesting involvement of the pulmonary system.

In a private practice setting, any of these signs and symptoms require the therapist to refer the patient on for additional medical testing. The presence of pulmonary symptomatology demands additional tests that are not part of the armamentarium of the physical therapist. A thorough chest assessment involving auscultation, mediate (finger) percussion, measurement of chest excursion, determination of pulmonary function, assessment of skin color, observation of breathing patterns, and evaluation of the subjective history and symptoms offered by the patient is essential to determine the presence or absence of pulmonary disorders. In states where direct access is

Table 3-7. Signs and Symptoms of Pulmonary Distress

Review of systems checklist for pulmonary system
Dyspnea
Cyanosis
Palpitations
Tachypnea
Fatigue
Malaise
Chest pain
Cough: onset or change in typical pattern
Sputum: green, red, pink and frothy
Observations suggesting pulmonary system distress
Wheezing
Stridor
Paradoxical breathing patterns
Trachea positioned off-midline
Cavitations of chest wall during inspiration
Unequal excursions of chest wall during inspiration

part of the Physical Therapy Practice Act, the therapist would be wise to incorporate chest assessment techniques as part of the patient's medical evaluation to ensure that no pulmonary problems, which complicate the practice of physical therapy and compromise the patient's health, are present.

DISEASES OF THE PULMONARY SYSTEM

We will now consider four general categories of pulmonary disease with which the physical therapist will need to be familiar. The four categories of respiratory disease are as follows (Table 3-8): (1) Obstructive pulmonary disease, which is the most common disease entity and includes obstructive sleep apnea, asthma, chronic bronchitis, emphysema, bronchiectasis, and cystic fibrosis; (2) restrictive pulmonary disease, which includes obesity (the most common limitation to chest expansion), ventilatory muscle dysfunction (i.e., denervation of the muscles of respiration—the ventilatory pump), cervical cord injury, and diaphragmatic paralysis (this category also includes common disease entities that can compress or infiltrate the alveoli, including pneumonia, interstitial lung disease, lung tumors, and diseases of the pleural space); (3) pulmonary vascular diseases, such as pulmonary heart disease, pulmonary thrombosis, and embolism and heart failure; and (4) errors in ventilatory regulation, such as central hypoventilation (sleep apnea) and central hyperventilation.

OBSTRUCTIVE PULMONARY DISEASE

Obstructive pulmonary disease is defined by increased residual volume and obstruction to air flow during both inspiration and expiration.

Certain historical information must be obtained in order to concentrate the therapist's treatment approach effectively. Of primary importance is a history of (1) those irritants that worsen the individual's symptoms, such as smoking, exposure to pollen, fumes, or other particles that seem to cause acute respiratory difficulty and repeated lung infections; and (2) possible influence of that individual's job, such as coal mining, uranium mining, working around cotton gins or silage. It seems self-evident that if the individual cannot avoid the irritant that is aggravating, if not causing, his lung disease (such as smoking), the efforts of the therapist are unlikely to be effective.

The interview should document the presence of cough, particularly if it is persistent (greater than 3 months per year on a daily basis) and whether it is accompanied by wheezing, as with asthma, or by sputum production. If the individual is producing more than 3 to 4 tablespoons of mucopurulent or purulent secretion each day, such production suggests that postural drainage and percussion (frappage) may be of benefit. The therapist should note sputum appearance, whether clear, mucoid, purulent, or bloody. The presence of blood in the sputum should alert both the individual and the therapist to the possibility of another more serious illness than bronchitis, even though chronic bronchitis is probably the most common cause of hemoptysis.

The patient's functional capacity should be estimated. Questions that may serve to give that information include the distance the individual can walk continuously at any rate on the level and whether shortness of breath (dyspnea) is present at rest or only with activity. Shortness of breath present during the night such that the individual must arise in order to obtain relief suggests paroxysmal nocturnal dyspnea and orthopnea, these two symptoms relating more to left ventricular heart failure than to lung disease per se. An estimate of the individual's nutritional status, if only to ask about weight loss, is well worthwhile.

Table 3-8. Types of Lung Disease

Clinical Type	Distinguishing Features
Obstructive: emphysema, asthma, bronchitis, bronchiectasis, obstructive sleep apnea	Obstruction to inspiratory and expiratory airflow (↓FEV_1/FVC); increased residual volume
Restrictive: obesity, interstitial lung disease (ARDS), ventilatory muscle weakness, lung volume loss	Decrease in all lung volumes; no obstruction to airflow
Pulmonary vascular disease: pulmonary artery embolism, pulmonary heart disease, chronic heart failure	Normal lung volume; decreased functional alveolocapillary membrane area for O_2–CO_2 exchange
Ventilatory regulation: hypoventilation (central sleep apnea); hyperventilation	Slowed or accelerated respiratory rate; normal A-a O_2 difference

Inspection should include an estimate of mucous membrane cyanosis, specifically of tongue and buccal membranes, bearing in mind that an individual must have at least 4 g of desaturated hemoglobin per 100 ml of blood to make cyanosis visible; notation of membrane pallor, which suggests significant anemia, is important. Respiratory rate and manner should be noted since a prolonged expiratory phase particularly in the presence of chronic cough and pursed lip breathing is good confirmatory evidence that the individual suffers from significant obstructive pulmonary disease. The patient's ability or inability to speak fairly long sentences before taking a breath is also a valuable clue to the severity of obstructive lung trouble.

The patient's seated position as if supporting the torso on extended arms is a further clue to the presence of significant obstructive pulmonary disease. Another sign of obstructive disease is the chest appearing to be in continuous full inspiratory pause (i.e., a barrel-shaped chest). Clubbing of the terminal phalanges is associated with chronic lung, heart, and liver disease (Fig. 3-8).

The severity of the clubbing is probably related best to duration of the disease state as well as severity. The presence of ochre-brown stains between the index and second finger of either right or left hand characterizes the smoking of at least two packs of cigarettes per day.

Such evaluation of outpatient status must be expanded or varied with regard to the hospitalized patient, particularly one in the intensive or intermediate care unit.[8] Some information can be obtained from other personnel or from the individual's relatives. Under these circumstances, the therapist must rely on observations as noted above.

In addition, one should note ventilator settings, if such are in use. Observation should include whether the individual is on spontaneous, assisted, or mandatory ventilation; tidal volume (V_T), respiratory rate; and fraction of inspired oxygen (FIO_2). Furthermore, one should note whether PEEP or continuous positive airway pressure (CPAP) is being used. In general, PEEP will not be commonly used for an individual with COPD, but is used very effectively for other disease categories discussed later.

If the hospitalized patient is breathing spontaneously, the therapist should evaluate for thoracoabdominal dyssynchrony, defined as a loss of the synchronized outward movement of the lower chest and upper abdomen during diaphragmatic contraction.[10] The chest will appear retracted as the epigastrium expands and vice versa. This finding is of particular importance as an early indicator of ventilatory muscle fatigue, the cause of which must be corrected if physical therapy is to be of benefit. To return to those techniques that are useful for both inpatient and outpatient evaluation: palpation and percussion of the patient's chest with obstructive pulmonary disease frequently will reveal that the chest wall does not move when the individual takes a deep breath and that percussion of the lung bases will elicit no evidence of diaphragmatic motion, that is, level of dullness between complete expiration and full inspiration. Percussion will also frequently indicate a hyper-resonance of the chest, expected in an individual who has a significant amount of air trapping in emphysematous lung disease. The resonance felt by the percussed finger is a more sensitive indicator than the audible or auscultated note for detecting subtler changes of tissue density within the chest.

Palpation with the examining hand over the precordial area may reveal a right ventricular heave just left of

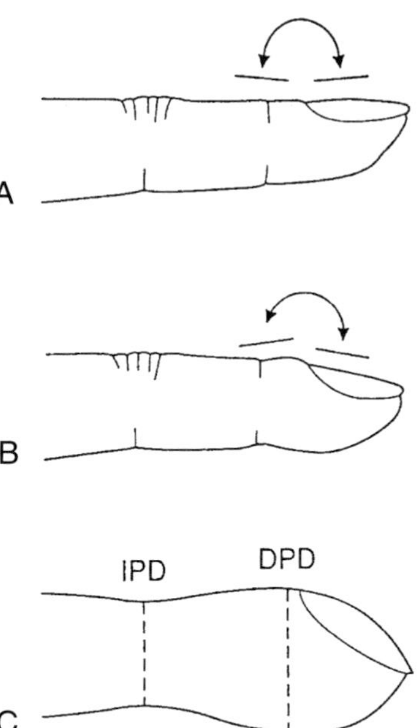

Fig. 3-8. Clubbing of the digits. **(A)** Normal digit configuration. **(B)** Mild digital clubbing with increased hyponychial angle. **(C)** Severe digital clubbing; depth of finger at base of nail (DPD) is greater than depth of interphalangeal joint (IPD). DPD, distal phalangeal depth; IPD, interphalangeal depth. (From Wilkins et al.,[13] with permission.)

the sternum or just beneath the xiphoid process. This finding is a reasonably good indicator of right ventricular hypertrophy or strain from pulmonary hypertension. Occasionally when one palpates the radial artery pulse or the apical cardiac impulse in the presence of COPD with pulmonary hypertension, the therapist will find that during inspiration the radial pulse, systolic pressure, or apical impulse will noticeably diminish ("paradoxical pulse").

Auscultation of the chest in chronic obstructive pulmonary disease of any type is limited not only by the fact that the best stethoscope hears no deeper than about 3 to 5 cm into the chest, but also by the decreased breath sounds related to air flow obstruction. In general, one will find that the vesicular breath sounds are diminished during inspiration and the first portion of the expiratory phase and that adventitious sounds, such as rhonchi, will frequently be very prominent during the expiratory phase, especially during a forced expiration maneuver. A bronchospastic component occurs not only in the asthmatic, but also frequently in the chronic obstructive lung disease patient such that expiratory wheezing will be present. Inspiratory wheezing, on the other hand, usually suggests that there are multiple bronchiolar plugs. The presence of inspiratory rhonchi, particularly in an individual with severe asthma, is worrisome, since such a finding is associated with recurrence of the asthma attack, the development of *status asthmaticus* (cessation of respiration), and death. Such a finding is also sometimes difficult to separate from pneumonia, but in general the inspiratory rhonchi will be present throughout the lungs rather than in an isolated lobe or lobes. The finding of coarse rhonchi and rales in an isolated area of lung, which clears with a deep breath or cough, objectively denotes an atelectasis of that segment of lung and suggests that more vigorous pulmonary therapy and evaluation for obstructing tissue are needed.

A useful measurement of ventilatory muscle strength is maximum inspiratory pressure (P_{imax}), also known as maximum inspiratory force (MIF), or negative inspiratory force (NIF), which should be at a minimum −20 cm of water to produce adequate resting vital capacity. Maximum expiratory pressure (P_{emax}) can also be used.[7] A generated pressure of −40 to −60 cm of water is necessary to sustain activities of daily living, including walking. Such measurement should always be obtained in the outpatient setting and a similar measurement can be acquired in the inpatient setting if the patient is responsive to command.[6–8]

The muscular power needed to provide a vital capacity (VC) of approximately 15 ml/kg (the capacity necessary for an adequate cough and respiratory reserve) is produced by a negative inspiratory force greater than −20 cm of water or more negative than −20 cm of water pressure in 20 seconds.[7] It should be noted that the normal NIF is in excess of a −80 cm of water, with a range from −60 to −90.[6] In addition, other readily measured clinical evaluations of respiratory capacity include minute ventilation, which should be between 6 and 10 L/min in an adult and is frequently used in correlation with the FVC.[6]

Oximetry with either ear or finger probe gives an adequate measurement of respiratory function, that is, oxygen exchange across the alveolar–capillary membrane both at rest and with activity but does not reflect CO_2 exchange. Because of their simplicity and reproducibility, the maximum inspiratory pressure or maximum negative inspiratory force and oximetry should be repeated as a guide to the success or lack of success of therapeutic maneuvers.

Under the general category of obstructive pulmonary disease exists a subcategory of upper airway obstructive disease that overlaps with two other categories discussed later. This disease is obstructive sleep apnea.[11]

This entity is considered separately within the category of obstructive pulmonary disease for a number of reasons: (1) This disease process, unlike most obstructive pulmonary diseases, will respond readily to ventilatory muscle strengthening and weight loss. (2) It is not a problem of intrathoracic airway obstruction, but rather oropharyngeal upper airway obstruction secondary to decreased muscle tone. (3) The disease overlaps with restrictive pulmonary disease because it is almost always seen in persons who are morbidly obese; it overlaps with central respiratory diseases because of the apparent insensitivity of the brain stem respiratory centers to hypoxemia and/or hypercapnia.

The characteristic history obtained concerning these individuals is that of overweight state, daytime somnolence, morning headache, nocturnal snoring, and episodes of apnea lasting more than 10 seconds and occurring more than five times in any given hour of sleep.

Inspection finds an overweight, thick and short-necked individual, usually with red face and a somewhat "froggy" voice, an increased respiratory rate when awake, and an irritable affect.[12] Palpation, percussion, and auscultation will rarely reveal anything of major importance other than poor thoracic expansion and decreased breath sounds. The FVC and maximum minute volume (MMV) will generally indicate the classic decrease in lung volume measurements associated with restrictive defects. Oximetry during the patient's sleep will usually indicate significant hypoxemia, that is, to less than 88 percent oxyhemoglobin saturation. Hypercapnia may also occur. Observation of the individual's sleep pattern will demonstrate more than five episodes per hour of ventilatory muscle activity, but no air movement at nose and mouth. The apneic episodes last more than 10 seconds each. Frequently such episodes will cease with a loud snort or cough and be interspersed with loud snoring.[11] This disease process offers the physical therapist an excellent opportunity to attain real success with ventilatory muscle strengthening in association with a weight loss program. Additionally, continuous positive airway pressure will be necessary during the night for a period of weeks and months.

Restrictive Pulmonary Disease

Restrictive pulmonary disease is characterized by a decrease in all lung volumes. In contrast to the preceding respiratory disease state, the flow rates (FR), such as forced expiratory flow rate (FEFR) are normal or increased.[8]

The diseases in this general category include (1) abnormalities of the thoracic cage, either congenital or acquired (multiple rib fractures); (2) respiratory muscle dysfunction as with muscle weakness of any kind, including medication effect or myasthenia gravis; (3) diseases that invade the lung tissue, including interstitial lung disease and pneumonia; and (4) diseases occupying the pleural space or lung parenchyma, including tumors, pleural effusions, and pneumothorax.

This category of disease is less common than the preceding obstructive category but offers the physical therapist, assuming primarily patient muscle and structural dysfunction, a good opportunity to improve the patient's respiratory status. The basic concept that must be kept in mind with regard to restrictive pulmonary diseases is that the ventilatory muscles must generate a pressure great enough to overcome the recoil of the lung tissue. A measure of the ventilatory muscle strength required to increase the lung volume against the resistance of the lung tissue is called compliance.[6] A rough measure of dynamic compliance can be obtained by measuring the vital capacity of an individual at the peak of the maximum inspiratory pressure (NIF) of which the patient is capable. The ratio of vital capacity in milliliters of air to the maximum inspiratory pressure (NIF) in negative centimeters of water gives a direct measurement of compliance including the ventilatory muscle function. Vital capacity/maximum inspiratory pressure:

$$\text{VC} = \text{Compliance (dynamic) } [C_{DYN}]$$

This equation demonstrates that the more inspiratory pressure required to attain a given volume or a lesser lung volume obtained with a given maximum inspiratory pressure causes a decreased compliance. To obtain eupnea the work of the ventilatory muscles must increase.

Abnormalities of the Thoracic Cage

The most common disease state having to do with abnormalities of the thoracic cage is obesity. This morbid state restricts the expansion of the chest wall and restricts diaphragmatic function. Individuals with this particular type of ventilatory disease have been given the diagnostic term obesity-hypoventilation syndrome. The history of these individuals will frequently document that they have been overweight for many years and have become progressively sedentary. Information from a family member may well indicate symptoms discussed in the preceding section concerning obstructive sleep apnea. Objective information frequently includes an elevated blood pressure (even with an oversized sphygmomanometer) and an elevated red blood count (secondary erythrocytosis) because of the hypoventilatory state and resultant hypoxemia. The chest circumference will not expand during inspiration to a significant degree when measured with a tape at the nipple line. If the individual is examined sitting upright, percussion will demonstrate inadequate descent of the diaphragm over the posterior portion of thoracic cage during inspiration. Auscultation will simply reflect decreased breath sounds and occasional basilar rhonchi.

Ventilatory Muscle Dysfunction

Ventilatory muscle dysfunction[7] includes generalized muscle weakness as from myasthenia gravis, Guillain-Barré syndrome, muscular dystrophy, metabolic disease states such as severe potassium deficiency or phosphate deficiency, and specific antibiotic effects, particularly the commonly used aminoglycoside. One should also include cervical spinal cord damage with or without diaphragmatic paralysis in this category.

A common theme of this group of disease states is that diffuse neuromuscular weakness does not necessarily interrupt adequate ventilation and respiration unless the diaphragmatic function is also severely damaged.

The physical therapist's evaluation or assessment done accurately is of great help in this particular category. As always, history is critical in evaluation. Since these patients will almost always be hospitalized and frequently will be in the intensive care unit, the history may have to be obtained from the chart and other from individuals rather than from the patient. Of particular importance will be a history of (1) infectious disease, not only for the obvious possibility of developing and perhaps correcting Guillain-Barré syndrome, but for sepsis with attendant aminoglycoside antibiotic use; and (2) metabolic disease states such as hypokalemia or hyperkalemia, caused by alcohol and diuretic use or acute renal failure, respectively. A history of cervical spine damage with the attendant possibility of intercostal muscle paralysis or diaphragmatic paralysis, including chest trauma with nonfunctional intercostal muscle and chest wall motion, will clarify the physical therapist's approach.

The objective findings in this particular disease state must include observation of intercostal muscles and diaphragm contraction, especially the diaphragm. Palpation and inspection will demonstrate whether or not the normal expansion of the lower rib cage and epigastric area occurs during inspiration. The therapist must be alert to the presence of the paradoxical inward motion of the lower thorax as such thoracoabdominal dyssynchrony would indicate that the diaphragmatic function is failing either from paralysis of the nerves innervating the diaphragm or from muscle weakness of any cause. Auscultation will generally indicate little or no air movement in the bases of the lungs. Decreased breath sounds in general correlate with the patient's inability to clear secretions from lung bases. The decreased ventilation in association with ventilation–perfusion mismatch at the same lung bases weakens general muscle function, including the diaphragm. Negative inspiratory or positive expiratory force will be decreased, as will the FVC and the FEV_1.

Should the physical therapist find diaphragmatic failure, he must as a member of the team caring for this individual notify other members so that corrective action can be taken. From the therapist's point of view the presence of true diaphragmatic failure requires the nonventilated patient to be repositioned supine in such a manner that any diaphragmatic function present can be enhanced by moving the dome of the diaphragm cephalad upward with the passive motion of the abdominal viscera, thus giving the diaphragm more efficient contractile effect. Such positioning will be particularly effective in those quadriplegic patients who may have little intercostal muscle function, but an intact diaphragm.

Bedside observations that the physical therapist should make include FVC and a maximum inspiratory pressure or similar to measure the lung volume produced and obtain baseline ventilatory muscle strength. Oximetry is also useful because of the previously mentioned problem with ventilation–perfusion mismatching in the lung bases. Auscultation is frequently useful for finding poorly cleared secretions in the form of rhonchi. Such findings should alert the therapist to two things: that the ventilatory efforts are as yet inadequate and that there is an impending atelectasis and/or pneumonia.

Diseases that Invade the Lung Tissue or Occupy the Pleural Space or Lung Parenchyma

Another category of restrictive diseases includes those that restrict lung volume, including intrapulmonary diseases of such diffuse types as pneumonia, interstitial pneumonitis, and adult respiratory distress syndrome or intrathoracic space-occupying lesions, most commonly pneumothorax or pleural effusions.

Once again the history is basic to understanding the disease process with which the therapist must work; it includes history of pneumonia, congestive heart failure, multiple injury, and so on. This information will determine to a large degree what progress the therapist might expect to make. For example, very little will be accomplished by the therapist until a large pneumothorax or pleural effusion is evacuated or a lung tumor, particularly endobronchial lesions and mass-effect lesions, can be either removed or relieved.

An example of this category of restrictive lung disease that is perhaps not so common, but is devastating in its effects on the patient and carries a high morbidity and mortality rate, is the adult respiratory distress syndrome.[12] This disease, with its profound hypoxemia due to severe alveolar–capillary membrane block, as well as ventilation–perfusion abnormalities and worsening compliance, poses one of the most severe problems requiring the efforts of all members of the team, including the physical therapist, to obtain the best possible result.

The objective findings of this category are those of the given disease process: the space-occupying lesion frequently will produce dullness to percussion and absent breath sounds, particularly with pleural effusions, whereas a large pneumonia, particularly a multilobed variety, will produce dullness but increased breath sounds, including E-to-A voice transmission change. Interstitial diseases including adult respiratory distress syndrome will produce the typical "velcro" rales to auscultation, while the breath sounds are usually enhanced, not absent, and percussion usually indicates resonance. However, if a pneumothorax intervenes, as it frequently does during the therapy of adult respiratory distress syndrome, the resonance remains the same or increases, whereas breath sounds will diminish and there will be abrupt worsening in the patient's respiratory status.

Pulmonary Vascular Disease

The third general category of pulmonary pathophysiologies states with which the physical therapist must deal is pulmonary vascular disease, which diminishes the available alveolar–capillary membrane for oxygen and CO_2 exchange. This general category can be considered as the lung disease with changes in ventilation–perfusion secondary to other disease states. As the name implies, pulmonary vascular disease is usually accompanied by normal lung volume measurements, but the restriction in pulmonary function is in the arterial and capillary flow to segments or regions of lung tissue. Decreased perfusion allows a major ventilation–perfusion mismatch with subsequent hypoxemia of the pulmonary venous blood. Usually a decrease in the carbon dioxide level of the blood occurs because of hyperventilation. "Dead space" ventilation increases above normal (normal is approximately 1 ml per pound of ideal body weight[6]). Since the hypoxemia increases the pulmonary vasoconstriction, a vicious cycle develops, increasing ventilation–perfusion mismatch. Characteristically the abnormalities noted above increase in severity with any exercise.

The other disease states most commonly associated with this particular situation include pulmonary heart disease secondary to any pathophysiology within the lung vascular bed, including vascular changes attending severe obstructive pulmonary disease or primary disease entities as lupus erythematosus, rheumatoid vasculitis, sarcoidosis, and interstitial lung disease of any type. Diseases primarily affecting the vascular bed include deep vein thrombosis with subsequent pulmonary embolism and pulmonary arteriolar obstruction. Left heart failure can over a period of time cause a significant pulmonary vascular disease state, primarily by back pressure from an elevated left ventricular end-diastolic pressure. This allows a transudation of serum into the interstitial portion of the lung, decreasing the diffusion of oxygen from alveolar surface to capillary bed.

The history is of critical importance in this disease category. It will generally clarify the underlying or primary disease state, such as rheumatoid arthritis, sarcoidosis, lupus erythematosus, and so forth, and gives some index of their severity and current treatment. Acute symptoms are also of great importance in that dyspnea on exertion is an outstanding feature, as is a chronic nonproductive cough. Occasionally family members will note the development of cyanosis when the patient walks even a short distance. The individual rarely recognizes any fever, nor is one usually documented; however, profuse nightsweats are common within this general category. A history of abrupt pleurisy is often obtained not infrequently from those individuals with rheumatoid arthritis and lupus erythematosus, but commonly (in about 20 to 30 percent of cases) abrupt pleuritic chest pain can be dated to the minute by an individual who has suffered a pulmonary embolism and infarction. Subsequent hemoptysis is characteristic.

If the examiner suspects pulmonary thromboembolism, a history of swollen painful legs particularly with walking or pelvic heaviness or pain from those who have recently travelled a long distance, should be sought. Such history should prompt examination of the lower extremities for increased girth, swelling, tenderness, and redness along the great veins of the lower extremity.

The physical findings in regard to this category include the physical manifestations of the underlying disease state. Such obvious things as the malar rash of lupus erythematosus or the joint destruction of rheumatoid arthritis can be observed. One notes nonspecific cyanosis that occurs at rest, but particularly with exercise. Respiratory rate will generally be increased above normal. The individual with pleurisy is easily recognized by a guarded set of the trunk. Palpation may demonstrate a right ventricular heave or lift, and, if pulmonary hypertension has become chronic and significant, *pulsus paradoxum* (vida supra) will frequently be palpable. The patient will generally demonstrate a resonant chest, whereas auscultation may frequently show the same "velcro" rales that we associate with any interstitial disease state. On occasion the examiner will occasionally hear an evanescent pleural friction rub attending a pleuritic disease state, including pulmonary embolism and infarction.

Of particular interest in individuals with superimposed right heart failure secondary to hypertension and pulmonary vascular disease is the finding of fingernail and toenail bed clubbing or the finding of pretibial edema, suggesting decompensation of the right ventricle. These two findings will generally indicate a poor prognosis. A great deal of care must be taken with these individuals for any kind of rehabilitative therapy. The development of ischemic heart disease or of superventricular dysrhythmias such as multiple atrial tachycardia or atrial fibrillation is very frequent in these individuals.

Pulmonary function measurements will generally show a combination of obstructive and restrictive defects in those individuals with interstitial lung disease. There will frequently be a decrease in compliance. As with other categories the maximum exercise ventilation will be diminished. Such decrease in maximum ventilation should be correlated with oxygen consumption and measured in any of these categories in order to estimate the functional capacity at which physical therapy, for instance, by bike or treadmill walking, can be started.

Ventilatory Regulation Disorders

The fourth and final general category of pulmonary pathophysiology to consider is that of a disordered ventilatory regulation.[7,8] The characterization of this category is defined by the limits of hypoventilation or hyperventilation. This category is generally a secondary disease state found in patients with other types of pulmonary disease already considered. These individuals seem to have a disordered central brain stem response to either elevated carbon dioxide or lowered oxygen concentration or both. If the brain stem is not the center of the disordered response, then the peripheral chemoreceptors, for instance, in the carotid bodies, are at fault.

General disease states that are included in this section are those of a central sleep apnea, usually related to previous damage to the brain stem by various insults, including blood vessel occlusion, injury, neoplasia (either benign or malignant), or infection including viral. Central sleep apnea is on occasion idiopathic. A peculiar disease state is that of "Ondine's curse." Such individuals are noted to breathe normally when they are awake, but when asleep do not respire. Peripherally insensitive states to oxygen and/or carbon dioxide changes in the bloodstream include hypothyroidism in which an individual lacking adequate thyroid hormone simply is insensitive to oxygen and carbon dioxide fluctuations. These individuals also have significant myxedematous acretion within the lung tissue. A common cause of death in hypothyroid patient is hypothermia in coma, but also pneumonia to which they cannot respond. Probably the most common state of hypoventilation noted and usually suspected by history is that associated with the intake of narcotic and sedative medications. This is particularly true in those with underlying chronic lung disease of any kind. While history is important in these individuals, frequently necessary information will be lacking. Observation will indicate a hypoventilatory state with a slow or absent respiratory rate, despite a drop in oxygen saturation. If the individual is awake, he or she will be subject to confusion and hallucinatory disorientation.

To define this particular pattern of disease state, one can measure the alveolar–arterial oxygen gradient, which should be normal in central or chemical hypoventilation assuming normal lungs.[8] As a corollary to the normalcy of the A-a oxygen gradient, other lung volume measurements will generally be normal, although in the case of hypothyroidism a restrictive pattern sometimes will be noted.

In the case of hyperventilation as a subcategory under disorders of ventilatory regulation, one should note that hyperventilation or the "hyperventilation syndrome" is certainly the most common of these states and seems to be in large part a stress reaction to either psychological or physical stimuli. This particular central hyperventilation pattern should not, however, be accepted as the diagnosis initially, but rather should be a diagnosis of exclusion. Once again and there should be a demonstrably normal A-a oxygen gradient.

A number of medications or drugs will cause hyperventilation on the basis of either central or peripheral stimulation, although most of these act centrally. Most notable are such drugs as the amphetamines and cocaine and for therapeutic reasons most importantly progesterone, used in the treatment of central sleep apnea and the obesity-hypoventilation syndrome. The hyperventilatory response to acidosis of any kind, whether lactic acidosis or a diabeta ketoacidosis, is an obvious example of chemical hyperventilation.

A careful history will describe the basis for the presence of these disease states. Objectively an individual who has an increased respiratory rate above 18 breaths per minute at rest, for example in the presence of Kussmaul breathing (deep rapid respirations) with either lactic acidosis or diabetic ketoacidosis, is particularly impressive. The appearance is that of a "driven" respiratory pattern. A peculiar fruity or acetone odor to the breath is a reasonably good tip indication of either ketoacidosis or early salicylate excess. Physical findings are rather minimal, although with diabetic ketoacidosis one will frequently note evidence of dehydration with dry mucous membranes, cracked lips, decreased skin turgor, and so forth. Lowered blood pressure is frequently present as well. The lungs will show no particular evidence of decreased chest expansion or dullness to percussion, unless some other process is present. Auscultation will generally detect clear breath sounds unless such entities as aspiration have supervened. Generally speaking, lung functions will be normal, including the A-a oxygen gradient.

SUMMARY

The assessment of the patient with chronic lung disease of any type requires a knowledge of the normal in order to detect and work with the abnormal. This chapter has presented a system for assessing such individuals in order to develop a reasonable program for treatment. This chapter stresses basic techniques, including history taking and physical examination, as the basis for both the above intents. These techniques have passed the test of time, are applicable in many situations, and are based largely on capabilities available to all therapists.

The second portion of the chapter presents the abnormal clinical states in a format of four disease categories that are practical disease categories roughly separated by basic physiologic measurements. They include chronic obstructive pulmonary disease, restrictive pulmonary disease, vascular diseases of the lung, and disorders of ventilatory regulation. The ability of the therapist to use the basic techniques noted above, to separate the individual's disease state into one of the four categories, largely determines the therapist's most effective approach and therefore makes the best therapeutic approach. The therapist's assessment of the individual with pulmonary disease is the foundation for therapy without which progress can be made in the proper care and follow-up of these patients.

REFERENCES

1. Hogkin JD: Home care and pulmonary rehabilitation. p. 216. In Kacmarek RM, Stroller JK (eds): Current Respiratory Care. Mosby, St. Louis, 1988
2. Petty TL: Pulmonary rehabilitation: why, who, when, what, how? J Respir Dis 2:200, 1990
3. American College of Sports Medicine: Guidelines for Exercise Testing and Prescription. 3rd Ed. Lea & Febiger, Philadelphia, 1986
4. Skinner JS: Exercise Testing and Exercise Prescription for Special Cases. Lea & Febiger, Philadelphia, 1987
5. Altose MA: The Physiological Basis of Pulmonary Function Testing: Clinical Symposia 31:2. Ciba Pharmaceutical, Summit, NJ, 1979
6. Shapiro BA, Harrison RA, Kacmarek RM, Cane RD: Clinical Application of Respiratory Care. 3rd Ed. Yearbook Medical Publishers, Chicago, 1985
7. Bates DV: Respiratory Function and Disease. 3rd Ed. WB Saunders, Philadelphia, 1989
8. Luce JM, Tyler ML, Pierson DJ: Intensive Respiratory Care. WB Saunders, Philadelphia, 1984
9. Carter R, Linsenbardt S, Blevins W et al: Exercise gas exchange in patients with moderately severe to severe chronic obstructive pulmonary disease. J Cardiopulmonary Rehabil 9:243, 1989

10. Carter R, Nicotra B: Recognition and management of respiratory muscle fatigue and chronic obstructive pulmonary disease (COPD). IM 9:171, 1988
11. Smith PL, Schwartz AR: Sleep disordered breathing in adults. Contemp Intern Med June, 1990
12. Petty TL: Acute respiratory distress syndrome (ARDS). Dis Monogr XXXVI:9, 1990
13. Wilkins RL, Sheldon RL, Krider SJ: Clinical Assessment in Respiratory Care. 2nd Ed. CV Mosby, St. Louis, 1990

SUGGESTED READINGS

Cherniak RM, Cherniak L: Respiration in Health and Disease. 3rd Ed. WB Saunders, Philadelphia, 1983

Enright PL, Hyatt RE: Office Spirometry—A Practical Guide to the Selection and Use of Spirometers. Lea & Febiger, Philadelphia, 1987

Frownfelter DL: Chest Physical Therapy and Pulmonary Rehabilitation. 2nd Ed. Year Book Medical, Chicago, 1987

Irwin S, Tecklin JS: Cardiopulmonary Physical Therapy. 2nd Ed. CV Mosby, St. Louis, 1990

Lane EE, Walker JF: Clinical Arterial Blood Gas Analysis. CV Mosby, St. Louis, 1987

Morgan WKC, Seaton A: Occupational Lung Diseases. 2nd Ed. Keith C. Morgan and WB Saunders, Philadelphia, 1984

Murray JF: The Normal Lung—The Basis for Diagnosis and Treatment of Pulmonary Disease. 2nd Ed. WB Saunders, Philadelphia, 1986

4 Screening for Gastrointestinal System Disease

Michael B. Koopmeiners, M.D.

The gastrointestinal (GI) system is responsible for providing the body with the essential nutrients for survival. The extraction of these essential nutrients from ingested food—digestion—begins in the mouth with the mechanical breakdown of food. As the bolus of food moves to the esophagus and progresses through the intestinal tract, chemical processes complete the digestive process. Undigestable food particles are stored in the sigmoid colon until they are eliminated through the rectum. The liver and pancreas are also part of the GI system. These organs produce digestive enzymes and hormones to facilitate the breakdown of food particles.

Pathology of the GI system can lead to low back pain, leg pain, and thoracic spine complaints; less obviously, it can lead to shoulder pain. The physical therapist can identify markers of GI pathology. Once alerted to the possibility of visceral pathology, the physical therapist can facilitate appropriate consultation and referral. Once it is established that the presenting complaints are secondary to biomechanical dysfunction rather than to visceral pathology, appropriate patient care can be initiated.

This chapter reviews the normal anatomy and physiology of the structures of the GI system. Figure 4-1 presents an anatomic overview of the GI system. It is not my intent to highlight all possible diseases of the GI system—only those conditions most likely to be encountered by the physical therapist are discussed. These conditions may mimic musculoskeletal system dysfunction or may have an impact on the type of physical therapy modality used.

ANATOMY AND PHYSIOLOGY OF THE GASTROINTESTINAL SYSTEM

The mouth provides an entrance to the GI system, as well as initiating digestion by the mechanical breakdown of ingested food material. The normal swallowing mechanisms, facilitated by cranial nerves IX, X and XII, move the food bolus from the mouth to the esophagus. The esophagus is a hollow muscular tube that connects the mouth to the stomach. It runs in the chest cavity, lying in the midline in front of the vertebral column. High in the chest cavity, the esophagus runs behind the trachea; lower down, it runs behind the heart, with the descending aorta on its left. It attaches to the stomach just below the diaghram. The lower esophageal sphincter is a one-way valve that prevents stomach contents from regurgitating into the lower esophagus.

The upper esophagus is striated muscle under voluntary control. The lower esophagus and lower esophageal sphincter are smooth muscle under involuntary control mediated by the vagus, or 10th cranial nerve. The involuntary activity of the esophagus and of the intestinal tract is primary peristalsis, rhythmic progressive pulsatile contractions of the hollow viscus tube. The lower esophageal sphincter relaxes as a peristaltic wave approaches so that food can enter the stomach.

Blood supply of the upper esophagus comes from the branches of the thoracic artery. Lower esophageal blood supply comes from the branches of the left gastric artery and inferior phrenic arteries. A plexus of veins drains the esophagus, forming multiple anastomosis with the portal venous system of the stomach. The esophagus has two

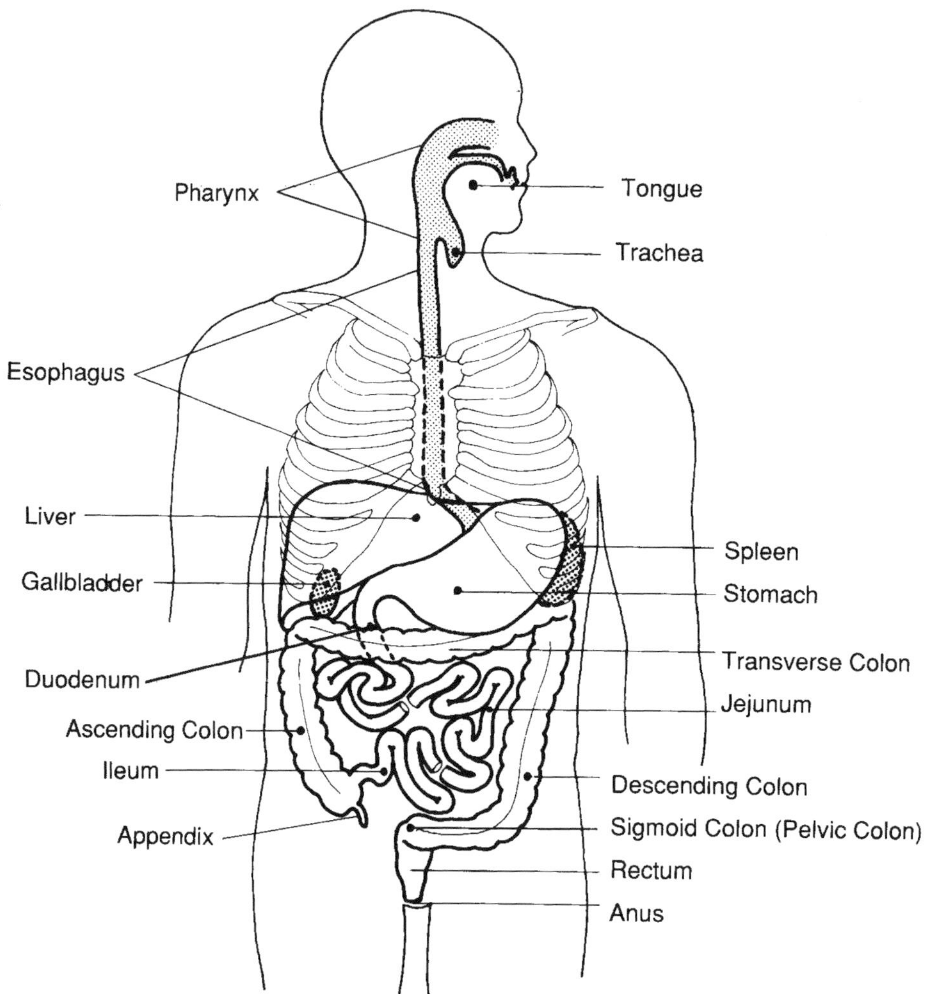

Fig. 4-1. Anatomic view of the gastrointestinal system.

main functions—transport of food and mechanical dispersion of food—the first step of digestion.

The stomach is a dilatation of intestinal tract separated from the esophagus by the lower esophageal sphincter and from the first part of the small intestine by the pyloric valve. It is located in the mid-epigastric area of the abdomen immediately behind the transverse colon. It partially covers the pancreas, which is located retroperitoneal, deep in the abdominal cavity (Figs. 4-2 and 4-3). Arterial blood supply comes from the celiac trunk off the aorta and from several branches off the splenic artery. The gastric veins enter the portal venous system. With obstructive liver pathology, such as cirrhosis, this venous system becomes engorged because of increased pressure necessary to "push" blood through the liver. This condition subsequently leads to esophageal varicose veins. The nerve supply is from the vagus nerve. A pacemaker in the proximal stomach initiates peristalsis for the upper intestinal tract.

Three mechanical functions of the stomach are identified: storage, mixing, and grinding. Outflow regulation of processed food particles to the small intestine is another important function. The rate of movement of the stomach contents to the small intestine must be balanced with the rate of pancreatic and biliary secretions, to permit efficient extraction of nutrients.

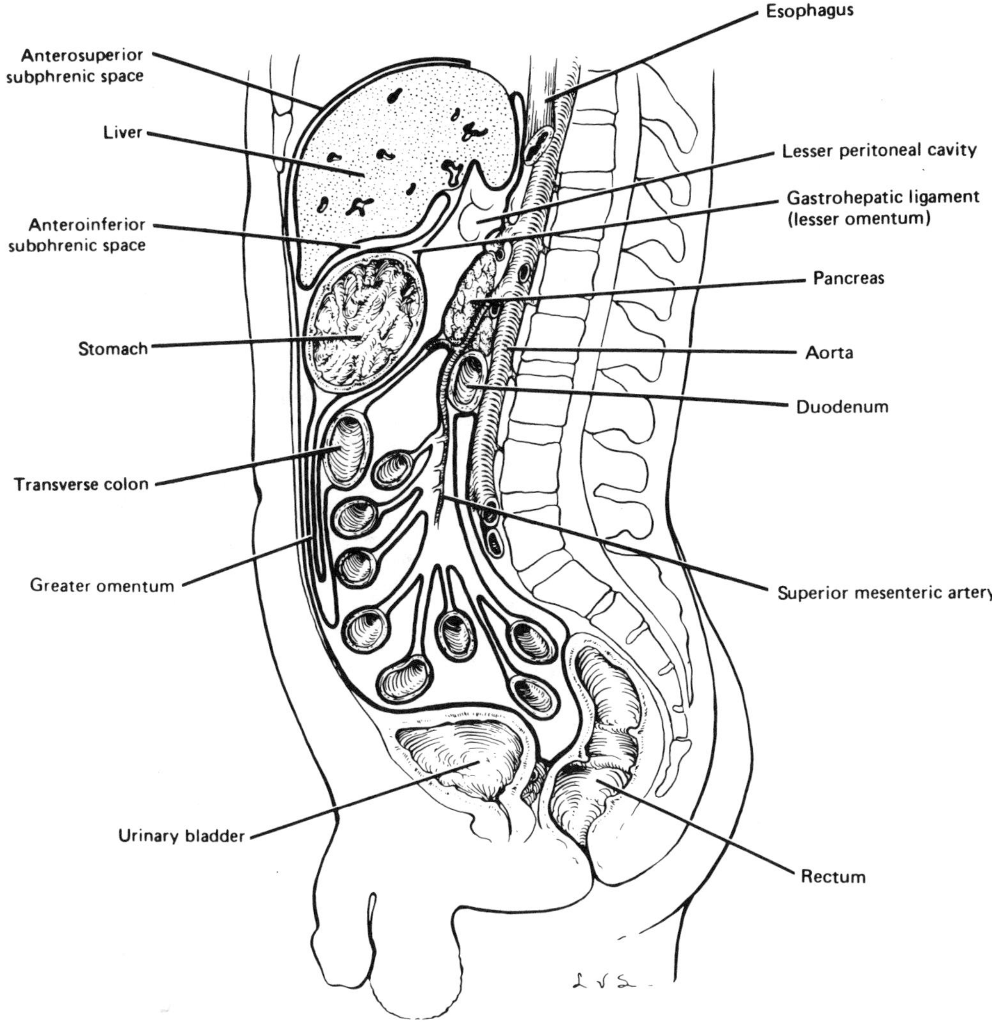

Fig. 4-2. A sagittal view of the trunk, demonstrating the proximity of the pancreas and duodenum to the thoracic spine. (From Way LW: Current Surgical Diagnosis and Treatment, 6th Ed. Lange, East Norwalk, CT, 1983, with permission.)

The stomach also has exocrine and endocrine functions. Exocrine functions (local secretion of chemicals) include secretion of acid, intrinsic factor, pepsin, mucus, and bicarbonate. All these ingredients are important for digestion. Although these secretions are normally very balanced, a mismatch of these secretions can lead to peptic ulcer disease.

Endocrine function is the secretion of hormones, which are chemicals produced in one part of the body that have an action in another part of the body. Specifically, the stomach produces various hormones that stimulate the pancreas, liver, and gallbladder to release their digestive enzymes into the duodenum.

The small intestine begins at the pyloric valve and ends with its connection to the large intestine in the right lower abdominal quadrant. It has three distinct parts: duodenum, jejunum, and ileum. The duodenum is the first 25 cm of the small intestine and lies in the right upper quadrant just below the liver. It is almost entirely retroperitoneal (Fig. 4-2), surrounding the pancreas and lying on top of the ileopsoas muscle and moving across the vertebral column at approximately the level of L3.

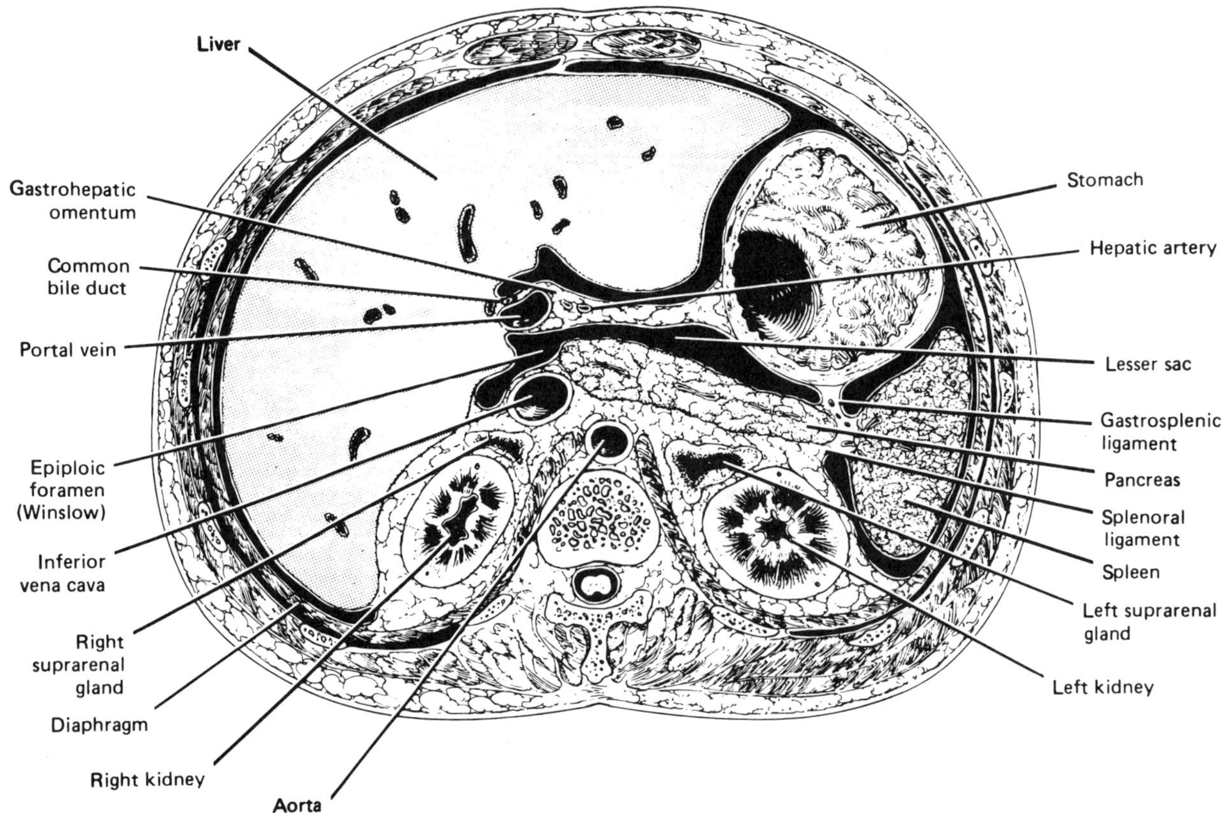

Fig. 4-3. A transverse plane view of the abdomen through T12 demonstrating the proximity of the pancreas to the spine. (From Lindner HH: Clinical Anatomy. Appleton and Lange, East Norwalk, CT, 1989, with permission.)

The duodenum receives the slurry from the stomach through the pyloric valve, as well as the fluids from the pancreas and liver through the common bile duct. This is the area of the small intestine that is most susceptible to ulcers. The blood supply is from the inferior mesenteric artery and gastric artery and is drained by the portal veins. The vagus nerve through the celiac ganglion provides the nerve supply to the duodenum and to the rest of the small intestine. Pain in the small intestine is produced by distention or violent cramps. The function of the duodenum is to neutralize the acid in the food slurry delivered from the stomach, as well as mix the food slurry with the pancreatic and biliary secretions.

The jejunum makes up the bulk of the small intestine. This undulating hollow viscus tube in the abdominal cavity stretches for 2.4 m. It is attached by the omentum to the posterior aspect of the abdominal cavity over the vertebral column. The omentum is the conduit through which the blood supply, nerve supply, and lymphatic supply attach to the small intestine. The superior mesenteric artery and portal vein and the vagus splanchnic nerve provide the small intestine with the necessary blood and nervous functions. The jejunum is mainly concerned with absorption of nutrients, water, and electrolytes. It has a significant capacity for absorption, since its surface area is greater than that of a double tennis court.

The ileum is the terminal 40 cm of the intestinal tract. It is located in the right lower abdominal quadrant and attaches to the colon through the ileocecal valve. The ileum provides the same functions as the jejunum, but it has a unique function of absorbing bile acids and intrinsic factor, recycling these chemicals in the body. Inability to reabsorb intrinsic factor causes a major disability in the form of vitamin B_{12} deficiency, which leads to pernicious anemia.

The large intestine (colon) stretches 1.5 m, beginning in the right lower abdominal quadrant, traverses the periphery of the abdominal cavity, and ends with attachment to the rectum in the posterior pelvis. The cecum located at the beginning of the colon is the blind-ended pouch to which the appendix is attached. The appendix and cecum are frequently retroperitoneal in the right iliac fossa, lying on top of the ileopsoas muscle. The ascending colon, on the right side of the abdominal cavity, is a retroperitoneal structure that lies on top of the quadratus lumborum, ileopsoas, and iliacus muscles. The transverse colon in the upper abdominal cavity runs over the stomach and the spleen, at the level of the umbilicus. The colon then turns caudally toward the rectum, becoming the descending colon, which, again, is retroperitoneal, lying on the psoas and quadratus lumborus muscles. The last part of the colon, or sigmoid colon, begins at the pelvic brim, crosses the sacrum, and curves and lies in the midline at the third sacral segment. The rectum lies in the mid-pelvis behind the prostate and bladder in males and behind the vagina in females.

The blood supply is from the superior mesenteric and inferior mesenteric artery. The portal vein drains the intestinal tract and goes through the liver before ultimately returning the blood to the central circulation via the inferior vena cava. The nerve supply is through the vagus nerve; the mid-colon contains an intrinsic pacemaker that controls the peristalsis activity of the mid- and lower colon. The function of the colon is to absorb water and electrolytes. The distal colon stores waste products in the form of feces. The rectosigmoid colon and anal canal have the function of expulsion of feces.

The liver is located in the right upper abdominal quadrant under the diaphragm, with its lower margins normally at the lower edge of the right rib cage. The gallbladder is located beneath the liver in the midclavicular line. A tight capsule surrounds the liver; stretching of this capsule causes the pain associated with liver pathology. The liver has two blood supplies: the hepatic artery makes up 10 percent of the blood flow and provides the necessary oxygen for the cells of the liver; and the portal vein makes up 90 percent of the blood flow coming into the liver. The portal vein carries recently absorbed nutrients from the stomach and intestine, as well as hormones secreted by the pancreas and GI tract, to the liver for processing.

The liver plays a major role in regulating the serum levels of solutes, such as fat, protein, and carbohydrate, needed by the muscles, brain, heart, and other organs to function adequately. Bile is produced in the liver and is instrumental in the absorption of lipids and lipid-soluble substances. The liver also has a role in drug metabolism, in the normal rate of production of red blood cells, and in vitamin K production, which is necessary for normal blood clotting.

Besides the plexus of arteries, veins, and lymphatics in the liver, there is another plexus of hollow collecting tubes, called the biliary tree. The biliary tree collects bile, the digestive enzyme produced in the liver, and transports it through the hepatic duct to the stomach. Branching off this hepatic duct and located beneath the liver is the gallbladder (Fig. 4-1). The gallbladder is a storage sac that holds the bile until a bolus of food presents itself to the stomach. Hormone stimulation causes the gallbladder to contract and expel its contents into the hepatic duct, which ultimately empties into the duodenum. In addition to storing bile, the gallbladder concentrates bile by preferentially absorbing water. When it goes awry, this process contributes to the formation of gallstones.

The pancreas is another gland that is extremely important to normal functioning of the GI tract. It is located retroperitoneally, lying on top of the vertebral column, and extends to the left upper abdominal quadrant (Fig. 4-3). It is surrounded anteriorly by the stomach, the duodenum on the right, the spleen on the left, and posteriorly by the vertebral column (at the T10 level), kidney, aorta, and inferior vena cava. The pancreas secretes bicarbonate and digestive enzymes, the production of which is stimulated by eating. Bicarbonate is a major defense against gastric acid in the duodenum. Large acid production or too rapid delivery of the gastric acid to the duodenum will overwhelm the bicarbonate production of the pancreas and contribute to the formation of duodenal ulcers.

The pancreas has important endocrine functions. It secretes insulin and glugacon, as well as multiple other hormones necessary for normal regulation of glucose levels and several other substances in the bloodstream. The blood supply is extremely generous. The several major arteries going to the pancreas have generous anastomosis, but the nerve supply to the pancreas is relatively poor. As a result, the pain of cancer infiltration is minimal, making early detection of cancer of the pancreas extremely difficult. The initial presentation frequently will be thoracolumbar junction back pain.

Although the spleen is not part of the GI tract, it is located in the left upper abdominal quadrant below the rib cage, surrounded by various organs of the GI system. It lies against the paraspinous muscles on the left side. The function of the spleen is to filter out foreign substances as well as old degenerating blood cells from the bloodstream.

The GI system is responsible for maintaining adequate levels of all the essential nutrients in the bloodstream to facilitate the normal activity of the organism. It does this through complicated mechanical and biochemical processes. Many of the organs that make up the GI system are located in close proximity to various "organs" of the musculoskeletal system. This association is not obviously appreciated at times, since the significant part of those relationships is hidden in the posterior (retroperitoneal) aspect of the abdominal cavity. The importance of additional knowledge concerning the GI tract to the physical therapist becomes obvious when these relationships are appreciated.

DISEASES OF THE GASTROINTESTINAL SYSTEM

Visceral pathology of the GI system can present with symptoms easily confused with conditions of mechanical dysfunction. For example, right shoulder pain is a frequent complaint with liver or gallbladder pathology, and back pain can be associated with peptic ulcer or metastatic colon cancer. An awareness of GI conditions and the associated signs and symptoms that can present as mechanical dysfunction will enhance the physical therapist's skills to identify these conditions and direct the patient to seek consultation with a medical colleague.

Infectious Diseases of the Mouth and Throat

The most frequent category of diseases that affect the mouth and throat are infectious diseases. The presenting complaint for an infection of the throat may be neck pain associated with a reactive lymph node. If a swollen mass is found during the examination of the neck, the physical therapist should ask about sore throat, sore teeth, mouth sores, and so forth. If the swollen gland persists for 4 weeks, medical follow-up is warranted.

Esophageal Spasm

Esophageal spasm is a combination of esophageal colic and dysphagia of unknown cause. The spasm is exacerbated by hot or cold fluids, carbonated beverages, and exposure to stress. The resulting dysphagia involves both liquids and solids. The pain is colicky or crampy in nature, located substernally, radiating to the back, neck, jaw, or arms. The intensity is extremely variable, from minimal to severe symptoms. It may last for a few minutes to several hours. This condition may be confused with angina. A physical therapist may confuse this condition with disorders of the mid- and upper thoracic spine, left shoulder, and the anterior rib cage.

Acid Peptic Disorders of the Stomach and Duodenum

A common pathology of the stomach and first part of the duodenum that the physical therapist will come across frequently is that of acid peptic disorders. This is a group of disorders with very similar pathologic processes, including reflex esophagitis, gastritis, gastric ulcer, duodenitis, and duodenal ulcer. The common pathologic process is that of damage to the mucosa. Simple irritation of the mucosa will lead to conditions such as gastritis, while an actual erosion through the mucosa is an ulcer, either gastric or duodenal, depending on its location. One or more organs can be involved simultaneously.

The precise mechanism of these conditions is unclear. It is not simply a condition of too much acid but an imbalance of the acid, pepsin, bicarbonate, and mucous production of the intestinal tract. An infection by *Heleobacterium pylori* has been strongly implicated as leading to chronic recurrent peptic ulcer disease. The incidence of acid peptic disease is 35 percent in males and 25 percent in females. However, only 5 to 10 percent of the individuals are symptomatic. Seventy-five percent of affected individuals will have recurrent disease. Heavy smoking, heavy alcohol use, and use of nonsteroidal anti-inflammatory drugs (NSAIDs) increase the likelihood of this disease.

Acid peptic disorders present with a pain in the epigastric or right upper abdominal quadrant area of the stomach. The pain may radiate to the back; this is especially true of posterior penetrating ulcers. It is frequently described as a gnawing episodic pain, worse at night or when the stomach is empty and usually improves with food intake. Some weight loss, nausea, vomiting, and anorexia may be associated with this condition. Black tarry stools (melena) and vomiting of blood (hematoemesis) signify bleeding, which is the major cause of death in these patients. Other major complications include perforation leading to acute abdominal pain and necessitating surgery, as well as gastric outlet obstruction.

Physical therapists should think of these conditions whenever they have patients with lower thoracic spine complaints and lower anterior rib cage and upper abdominal complaints. With the significant use of NSAIDs in the patient population seeking care from physical therapists, these conditions must also be monitored for in clients being treated for conditions other than thoracic spine/upper abdominal complaints. If a patient gives a history suggestive of acute bleeding (melena or hematoemesis) an immediate referral to a physician is indicated.

Liver and Gallbladder Disorders

Hepatitis, inflammation of the liver, and cholecystitis, inflammation of the gallbladder, are conditions that can present with right upper abdominal quadrant pain, but also quite frequently present with right shoulder pain. The liver has multiple functions to perform. One is the production of bile acids, which are secreted and collected in the biliary duct system, coalescing into the hepatic duct and ultimately draining into the duodenum. The gallbladder is a small sac attached to the hepatic duct that stores the bile acids that are continually produced by the liver until they are needed, such as occurs after a meal. The gallbladder also concentrates the bile acids during the storage process by removing water. In so doing, precipitates will sometimes form in the bile acids, which will act as nideses for the formation of gallstones.

Gallstones

Gallstones vary in size from sand consistency up to stones several inches in diameter. The precise cause of the formation of these stones is unclear. Once formed, these stones can then irritate the lining of the gallbladder and/or occlude the outflow tract of the gallbladder, leading to inflammation and/or infection of the gallbladder. Ten to 20 percent of Americans have gallstones. The incidence increases with age. Obese females over 40 years of age have a significantly greater incidence of cholecystitis. Gallstones are frequently asymptomatic. Symptoms develop with occlusion of the outflow tract or inflammation of the gallbladder secondary to the gallstones. Pain is located in the right upper abdominal quadrant and may radiate to the back. Pain may also be referred to the scapula, right shoulder, or neck area. Pain is frequently abrupt in onset with a gradual defervescence of symptoms. Nausea, vomiting, and fever will occur with this condition—if not at the onset, certainly within hours of the onset. These patients will have tenderness, and occasionally a mass can be palpated in the right upper abdominal quadrant.

Cholecystitis and Hepatitis

While cholecystitis can occasionally confuse the physical therapist working with patients with right shoulder and right mid-back pain, hepatitis can do the same. Hepatitis is inflammation of the liver caused by several agents, such as the infectious agents of hepatitis A, B, and C or a chemical agent of which alcohol is the most common. This disease may be entirely subclinical and unsuspected in an individual appearing relatively healthy, or it may be rapidly progressive and fatal. For the viral agents, the onset of symptoms is usually 2 to 8 weeks after exposure. Patients will be fatigued, anorexic, and nauseated, with occasional fever and emesis. Musculoskeletal complaints besides the right shoulder and right mid-back pain could include headache, myalgias, and arthralgias. Dark urine and light-colored stools are frequent observations made by patients with hepatitis. These patients will have tenderness in the right upper abdominal quadrant, and the liver itself will occasionally be palpable and tender.

Viral hepatitis is an infectious disease and is potentially transmissible to the therapist. Type A is transmitted by the fecal-oral route. This is an important consideration when working with patients who are incontinent or disabled. Type B and type C are transmitted by percutaneous, oral-oral, perinatal, or venereal means. Needle sticks are a significant route of hepatitis B infection among hospital personnel. Alcoholic hepatitis will present in an extremely similar manner but will also have associated with it the stigmata of chronic or acute alcohol use (gynecomastia, jaundice, muscle wasting, abdominal bloating, etc.) (see Ch. 12).

Pancreatitis

Besides causing hepatitis, heavy alcohol use is a leading cause of pancreatitis, an inflammation of the pancreas. Pancreatitis can also be caused by gallstones or blunt abdominal trauma. In 20 percent of cases, no clear etiology is identified. Acute pancreatitis occurs in 20 of 100,000 patients. While this condition resolves spontaneously in many patients, chronic pancreatitis develops in 15 percent.

Pain is the dominant presenting complaint in patients with pancreatitis. There is a constant waxing and waning pain in the mid-epigastric and left upper abdominal quadrant area. One-half of patients will have pain radiating to the upper lumbar and lower thoracic area. The pain may also radiate retrosternally, to the right upper abdominal quadrant and left scapular and supraspinous area. These patients are very uncomfortable. Eating, alcohol intake, and vomiting will lead to exacerbation of the pain. On physical examination, they are frequently very tender in the mid-epigastric area and can also be tender in the lower thoracic, upper lumbar spine area.

Colon Disorders

Colon Cancer

Colon cancer has several characteristics that make it extremely important for the physical therapist to be aware of this condition. It is the most frequently diagnosed cancer in the United States. It is more prevalent in developed countries; the United States has one of the highest incidences in the world. Five to 6 percent of the population will develop colon cancer. The clinical importance lies in the frequency; also, early detection leads to substantial improvement in outcome. The physical therapist will encounter this disease either by local spread of the disease leading to local pathology that mimics complaints of mechanical dysfunction or by metastatic presentation of this lesion leading to complaints anywhere in the body, but more frequently in the thoracic spine and rib cage.

Risk factors for colon cancer are (1) age over 40 years; (2) prior history of inflammatory bowel disease, such as Crohn's disease or ulcerative colitis; (3) prior cancer of another organ; and (4) benign polyps of the colon. Screening the stool for blood and routine flexible sigmoidoscopy are advocated for any patient over 40 years of age. It is important to bear in mind, however, that these are screening tests and are not definitive diagnostic procedures.

Patients with colon cancer may complain of gradually progressive constipation and/or a reduction in the stool caliber. New blood mixed in with the stools or old blood may also be a presenting complaint. Frequent nonspecific symptoms that are true of any cancer condition will also occur, such as weakness, malaise, anorexia, and weight loss. This cancer frequently metastasizes to the liver, lung, and bone. It is not uncommon for the diagnosis to be made by recognizing a metastatic lesion as opposed to the primary lesion in the colon. The physical therapist will find it extremely important to screen for this disease, especially in patients over 40 years of age.

Diverticulitis

Another relatively common colon disease process is that of diverticulitis. This local inflammation in the wall of the apex of the small outpouching of the colon is caused by trapped feces. It can occur anywhere in the colon but frequently presents in the descending or sigmoid colon in the left lower quadrant of the abdominal area. This, again, usually occurs in patients over 40 years of age and has no particular predilection for either sex. Constant left lower quadrant abdominal pain radiating to the low back, pelvis, or left leg are the complaints associated with this disease. Fever, if present, is usually low grade. Usually there is a change in the stooling pattern, becoming loose and watery or hard. Rarely is bleeding noted in this disease.

Enlargement of the Spleen

Enlargement of the spleen frequently presents with vague left upper abdominal quadrant pain, left flank pain, and mid-back pain. Two main causes of spleen enlargement are infectious mononucleosis and cancer. Both conditions occur in young individuals: mono, almost solely in individuals between 15 and 25 years of age; cancer, such as acute leukemia, and lymphomas, occurs in younger individuals more frequently, but can occur in any age. The most significant complication of spleen envolvement is splenic rupture, which can lead to massive bleeding and occasional death. The therapist must be very aware of this fact when doing soft tissue work in the left upper abdominal quadrant on patients with suspected splenic enlargement. Additional symptoms besides pain that should make the therapist suspicious of pathology other than biomechanical are fatigue, malaise, weight loss, and lymph node enlargement.

One other condition may be encountered by therapists, especially if their patient population includes a high percentage of blacks. Sickle cell disease, occurring almost exclusively in blacks, will most likely be diagnosed before seeing the therapist and can lead to chronic spleen enlargement.

Abdominal Hernia

An abdominal hernia is the protrusion of abdominal contents through an opening in the muscle walls that surround the abdominal cavity. Two common areas in which hernias occur are the inguinal area and the diaphragm. An enlargement of the normal opening for the esophagus in the diaphragm allows part of the stomach to protrude into the chest cavity. This common condition is called a hiatal hernia and leads to symptoms similar to those of esophageal spasm. Increased intra-abdominal pressure will frequently aggravate the symptoms of a hiatal hernia. Corsets used for pelvic or lumbar spine stabilization may be poorly tolerated by these patients.

Hernias in the lower abdominal area are direct or indirect femoral hernias or inguinal hernias. The differences, although important to surgeons, are not necessary for the physical therapist to appreciate—only to realize the multiple terms used for hernia. The inguinal canal is the normal opening in the three layers of abdominal wall musculature that allows the spermatic cord and related vascular and nervous structures to traverse from the testicle in the scrotum to their intra-abdominal connections.

A small enlargement of the canal may permit a small protrusion and lead to subtle lower abdominal, hip, and anterior thigh pain. A larger opening and protrusion of intestine, while leading to similar pain complaints, will be less subtle to diagnose because of the presence of an obvious mass. The wide range of defects can make hernias difficult to exclude as a diagnosis even for the astute surgeon. This condition should be thought of in patients presenting with lower abdominal wall complaints, as well as hip and anterior thigh complaints. Hernias will produce pain with contraction of the abdominal musculature. This may be intermittent; on one occasion, there may be trapping and pinching of abdominal contents in the hernia sac, and at other times, if no abdominal contents are present in the hernia sac, no complaints may be elicited from similar activity. If the onset of symptoms is sudden, the diagnosis is made easier. Frequently the onset is subtle, with gradually worsening symptoms over time as the opening enlarges with repeat minor injury.

Strangulation is the most serious complication of hernias. This occurs when the blood supply to the abdominal contents in the hernia sac is compromised by the pressure that builds in the canal. Ischemia causing pain is the clinical result of strangulation; left untreated, it can lead to bowel necrosis and bowel death. This not so subtle condition will be noted by a tender inguinal mass, progressively worsening pain, nausea, vomiting, and fever. If suspected, immediate physician referral is indicated.

Summary

Gastrointestinal pathology has multiple areas of symptomatic overlap, with conditions frequently cared for by physical therapists. Complaints can be as diverse as shoulder strap pain and local cervical pain, secondary to metastatic lesions from colon cancers, or low back pain from pancreatitis or hip pain from a hernia. The alert therapist along with collaborating medical care providers can ensure patients of high-quality appropriate medical care.

ABDOMINAL EVALUATION

A history of complaints that may be secondary to visceral pathology should prompt screening for GI pathology. The presenting complaints that should make a therapist suspicious of nonbiomechanical problems were reviewed above and are summarized in Figure 4-4.

Each question is tied to one or more of the pathologies discussed above. Negative answers to all the questions may be enough reassurance that visceral pathology is unlikely. If the patient reports several of the symptoms, a screening evaluation of the abdomen would be the next step to take. Positive responses to all the questions, especially if there is an exaggerated quality to the answers, should raise the possibility of psychological problems (see Ch. 12).

Review of Systems: Gastrointestinal System

Item	Yes	No	Comments
1. Hemoptysis	_____	_____	____________________
2. Nausea	_____	_____	____________________
3. Vomiting	_____	_____	____________________
4. Melena	_____	_____	____________________
5. Hematochezia	_____	_____	____________________
6. Fatty food intolerance	_____	_____	____________________
7. Change in stool color	_____	_____	____________________
8. Constipation	_____	_____	____________________
9. Diarrhea	_____	_____	____________________
10. Change in urine color	_____	_____	____________________
11. Jaundice	_____	_____	____________________
12. Drug use	_____	_____	____________________
13. Sexual activity	_____	_____	____________________
14. Previous history of hepatitis	_____	_____	____________________
15. Previous history of hernia	_____	_____	____________________

Fig. 4-4. Checklist for screening the gastrointestinal system.

Physical Therapy Evaluation of the Abdomen

A screening evaluation of the abdomen begins with inspection. Figure 4-1 shows the location of intra-abdominal contents in relationship to external landmarks. Figure 4-5 presents the common terminology for various abdominal regions. During inspection, the physical therapist looks for asymmetries in shape and size such as in the lower abdominal quadrant or the right upper abdominal quadrant possibly signifying hernia or gallbladder disease, respectively. Noting abdominal scars may remind the patient of surgery not mentioned during the subjective examination.

Auscultation/Percussion

Auscultation to screen for bruits and bowel sounds is the next part of an evaluation. Particular attention should be paid to the mid-epigastric, right, and left lower abdominal quadrants and to the femoral areas when listening for bruits since these are locations for aneurysms and obstructions of the blood vessels (see Ch. 2). Normal bowel sounds can be as infrequent as every minute. Absence of bowel sounds should increase the therapists suspicion of intra-abdominal pathology. Percussion, seemingly simple but time consuming to master, is useful in evaluating liver and spleen size. Normal liver percusses to 4 to 5 inches in the mid-clavicular line (Fig. 4-6 and 4-7). A dullness in the quality of the noise in response to the percussion will signify a solid organ underneath the fingers; this is opposed to a more hollow-sounding resonance when hollow organs or cavities are percussed. This would help differentiate the location of the liver versus just percussing over lung tissue or the abdominal contents caudal to the liver. The spleen, found in the left upper abdominal quadrant, should be percussed over the rib cage at the caudal end of the anterior axillary line (Fig. 4-8). If the spleen is of normal size a hollowness should be noted during the percussion. If the spleen is sufficiently enlarged, a dullness may be noted during the procedure. To protect these

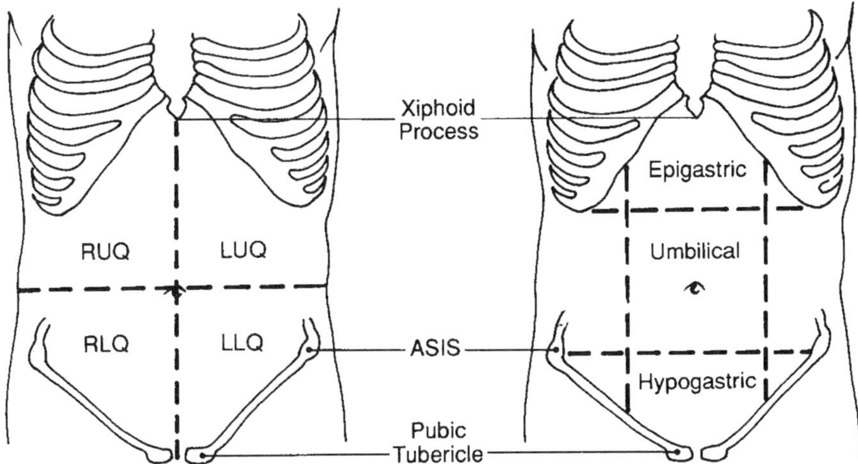

Fig. 4-5. Terminology used to delineate the regions of the abdomen. RUQ, right upper (abdominal) quadrant; LUQ, left upper (abdominal) quadrant; RLQ, right lower (abdominal) quadrant; LLQ, left lower (abdominal) quadrant.

structures, location of the liver and spleen should be noted before soft tissue mobilization techniques are performed in the upper abdominal areas. Percussion is one method to help delineate the boundaries of these two solid organs.

Palpation

Palpation in all four abdominal quadrants is the last part of the evaluation. Gastrointestinal system structures located in the right upper quadrant include the liver, gallbladder, and components of the small and large intestine. A portion of the stomach, the tail of the pancreas, components of the small and large intestine, and the spleen all lie in the left upper quadrant. The right and left kidneys also lie far posterior in the respective upper quadrant. Components of the large intestine, including the appendix, fill the right lower quadrant, while other components of the large intestine are located in the left lower quadrant. Masses associated with colon cancer or diverticulitis can be found anywhere in the abdomen but are more common in the left lower quadrant. Hernias will present as tender masses in the femoral triangle or groin area and can occur in both

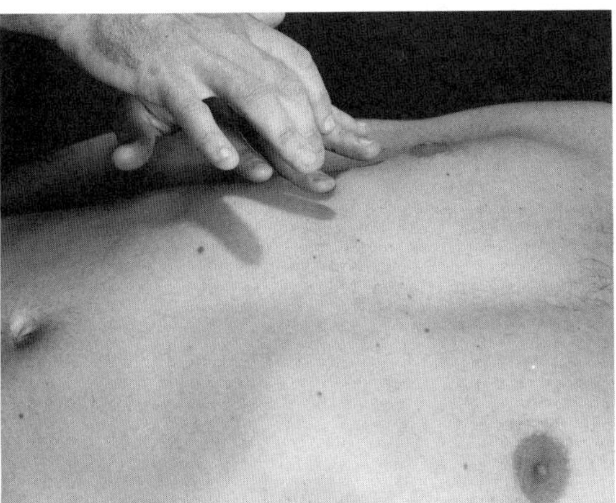

Fig. 4-6. Percussing for the cephalad edge of the liver in the midclavicular line.

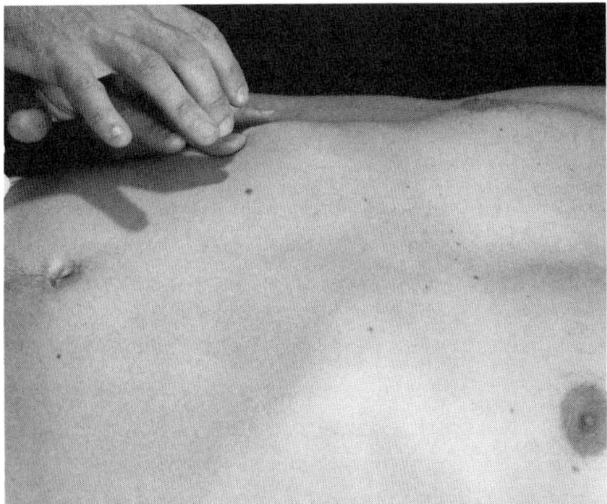

Fig. 4-7. Percussing for the caudal border of the liver in the midclavicular line.

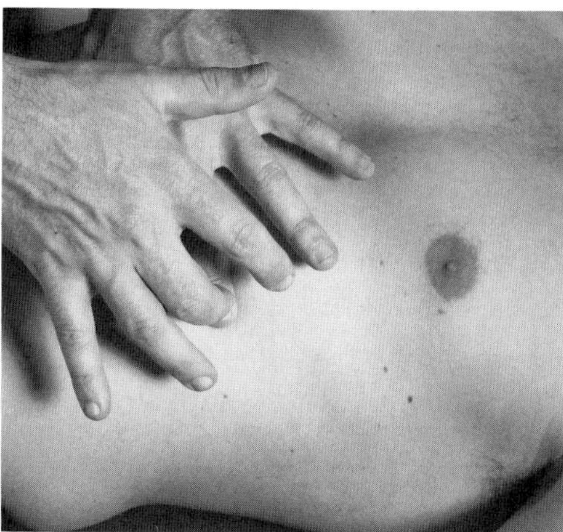

Fig. 4-8. Percussing for the spleen in the anterior axillary line.

men and women. Midline masses that are pulsatile may signify the presence of an aneurysm and should be referred for immediate consultation if noted. Generally speaking, the therapist should have difficulty palpating the specific abdominal visceral organs if they are not diseased because of the hollow soft nature of their structure. Exceptions may be solid organs, such as the liver, which may extend caudal to the rib cage, or fecal material, which may be palpable in the descending colon in the left lower quadrant.

The descending colon could be confused with the psoas musculature in this situation. To differentiate one structure from the other, the therapist must be aware that the psoas courses caudally and laterally and the descending colon courses caudally and medially. If palpating the psoas, the therapist will note a tissue texture change with a gentle hip flexion movement. A tissue texture change would not occur with hip flexion if the therapist is palpating over the colon.

Besides assessing for abdominal masses, tenderness and muscle guarding are other physical findings that may be elicited by palpation. A subset of tenderness that should raise concern is rebound tenderness. Rebound tenderness is when the pain experienced by the patient is worse with quick release of the palpatory pressure, as opposed to when the initial pressure was applied. If this sign is present, immediate referral to a physician should be made to rule out peritoneal irritation secondary to serious pathology, including abdominal bleeding. Abdominal muscle guarding or rigidity may occur in response to underlying visceral pathology. If noted, this self-protective reflex response should be correlated with other examination findings to help differentiate muscle guarding secondary to a local muscle injury, or to an injury to a deeper musculoskeletal system structure, from visceral pathology.

If the therapist finds a tender or painful area in the abdomen, the patient, in the supine position, can be asked to lift the head and neck off the table. As the abdominal muscles tighten, the therapist again applies pressure to the painful area; if the pain is still present, the lesion probably lies in the superficial myofascial wall of the abdomen, as opposed to a deeper visceral structure. If, instead, tenderness and pain disappear when the abdominals tighten but return when palpated with the abdominals relaxed, a deep visceral structure could be the source of the discomfort. Correlation of these findings with other examination findings should again help the therapist determine the involvement of musculoskeletal system structures versus elements of the GI system.

Diagnosis

A definitive diagnosis is not the goal for a physical therapy screening evaluation of the abdominal area. The evaluation can give clues that visceral pathology may be present. When suspicion is aroused in the astute physical therapist, physician consultation is warranted to ensure nonvisceral causes of the patient's presenting complaints.

SUMMARY

Patients presenting to the physical therapist may have visceral pathology as the primary cause of their presenting complaint. Therapists need to be aware of this possibility and should have a plan to address it. To help with this, the anatomy and physiology of the GI system are reviewed; common conditions are outlined to increase the awareness of visceral pathologies that present, such as mechanical dysfunction conditions; and an evaluation process of directed questioning and physical evaluation is presented as a suggested approach to patients in whom visceral pathology is suspected. By incorporating these suggestions into their practice, physical therapists will enhance the care given to patients who use their talents. For additional information regarding the GI system, the reader is directed to the Suggested Readings.

PATIENT CASE STUDY 1

History

The patient was a 32-year-old unemployed laborer who came to the clinic with a diagnosis of grade I spondylolisthesis at L5–S1. He presented with a long history of episodic low back pain, with the episodes usually precipitated by a lifting injury. He had been seen by a physical therapist previously and was referred to the clinic for consultation and subsequent treatment. When questioned, he described his chief complaint as severe deep aching pain in the central mid-thoracic spine region. He acknowledged central low lumbar spine pain but nothing that compared with the intensity of the thoracic pain. The thoracic pain was intermittent but daily; when severe, the aching seemed to wrap around the rib cage bilaterally. The patient was unable to relate a movement or posture to provocation, aggravation, or alleviation of symptoms. He stated that the pain just seemed to come and go for no reason. He reported that these symptoms began 2 weeks ago, after the physical therapist had tried a new joint mobilization technique on his back. When questioned further, the patient revealed that the pain began in the evening, a few hours after the physical therapy visit. He had no previous history of thoracic pain.

The patient's general medical and surgical history were negative, and he was not taking any medication. He had no history of smoking, recent weight loss, fever, or chills.

Objective Examination

In standing, the patient presented with an increased mid-thoracic kyphotic curve and an increased low lumbar spine lordosis. Abnormal muscle tone was not detected in the thoracic spine. The thoracic symptoms were not provoked with active movements of the trunk, but backward bending was moderately restricted in the mid-thoracic spine. The thoracic symptoms were also not provoked with central and unilateral pressures for the thoracic spine, but stiffness was noted in T5–T10. The corresponding portion of the rib cage was also stiff.

Assessment and Outcomes

The thoracic symptoms failed to be provoked with palpation, active and passive tests, and vertical trunk compression and distraction. Because of the suspicious behavior of the symptoms (i.e., unrelated to movement or change in posture), the patient was further questioned. When asked about abdominal symptoms, the patient stated that he had been experiencing heartburn after meals but was not sure whether there was a correlation between the heartburn and thoracic symptoms. The heartburn episodes had only been present for the past 1 to 2 weeks. When questioned about medications, the patient again stated that he was not taking any. He had taken Motrin for a couple of months but had not taken any for 2 to 3 weeks.

After the initial visit, the referring physician was contacted regarding the thoracic symptoms that had begun since the last patient visit to the physician. The suspicious pattern of symptoms and signs was discussed with the physician: the presence of abdominal symptoms (heartburn) and mid-thoracic pain (a common pain referral area for GI structures), an inability to provoke the symptoms during the examination, and a history of taking Motrin. (NSAIDs can cause GI ulcers but mask the ulcer symptoms while being taken.) The physician placed the patient on Tagamet and a bland diet. The thoracic symptoms were gone within 2 days and, according to the patient in a phone conversation, had not reappeared during the following 3-month period. The examination demonstrated numerous findings associated with the lumbar complaints. The mechanical musculoskeletal system dysfunctions related to these symptoms were subsequently treated.

PATIENT CASE STUDY 2

History

The patient was a 51-year-old unemployed nurse and physical therapy aide who came to the clinic with a diagnosis of mechanical low back pain syndrome. Initially her chief complaint was constant central low lumbar aching (Fig. 4-9). This aching was increased by sitting for more than 30 minutes, standing in one place more than 15 minutes, and assuming a forward flexed posture for more than a few seconds. The symptoms were lessened by assuming a recumbent position and, when weight bearing, by constantly changing her posture. She also experienced intermittent sharp pain in the same location. The sharp pain primarily occurred with sit-to-stand movements after sitting for more than 30 to 45 minutes. She could fall asleep without difficulty but woke one to two times a night due to her low back pain. These symptoms began approximately 2 years prior to this evaluation and were precipitated by catching a patient who was falling. She experienced a significant increase in the low lumbar aching 7 months prior to the evaluation, following a long car trip.

The patient denied any other symptoms including numbness or pins and needles. She also denied any symptoms or signs suggesting bladder dysfunction. Surgical history included tonsillectomy, appendectomy, and hysterectomy, and she was being treated for migraine headaches. The medication she was taking included Midrin and Tylenol No. 3 (Tylenol with codeine). A computed tomography (CT) scan had revealed a bulging disc at L4–L5.

Objective Examination

In standing, the patient presented with a slightly decreased low lumbar lordosis. Increased paraspinal muscle tone was noted in the low lumbar spine. Her chief complaint of aching was increased with one repetition of active trunk forward and backward bending and left side bending and rotation. Right hip flexion to 95 degrees also increased the aching sensation. Central and right unilateral pressures (passive accessory vertebral motion testing) at L4 also intensified the aching sensation. Significant hypomobility was noted at the L5–S1 segment, left sacroiliac joint, and thoracolumbar junction. The neurologic examination was negative.

Assessment and Outcome

The patient was seen for eight treatment sessions with a goal to increase pain-free range of motion (ROM) so that she could tolerate an aggressive exercise training program designed to prepare her for work as a physical therapy aide. She made excellent progress with the initial treatment and subsequent exercise program. She was no longer experiencing any sharp pain, and the central low lumbar ache was now intermittent. Her sitting and standing tolerance was much improved, and the low back pain no longer interrupted her sleep.

Approximately 1 month after the initiation of the exercise program, the patient began complaining of severe left lateral lumbar pain that spread out along the left iliac crest and into the left lower abdominal region. She returned to the original physical therapist for re-evaluation at that time. The patient described the symptom as an ache, but stated that she had never experienced the pain in these locations before (Fig. 4-9). The left mid- and lower lumbar pain was constant and increased if she sat for more than 30 minutes and with forward bending movements, especially those combined with left rotation. The aggravation or alleviation of the iliac crest and lower abdominal pain did not seem to be influenced by movement or assumption of various postures. The iliac crest and abdominal pain would come and go throughout the day and was severe enough to wake her at night. These new symptoms began 2 weeks prior to the re-evaluation, the day after Thanksgiving. She could not relate the onset of the symptoms to a particular traumatic incident or accident. When specifically questioned, in addition to these new symptoms, she revealed a recent onset of significant bowel dysfunction. The frequency of bowel movements had decreased, and she described a great deal of difficulty initiating a bowel movement. She denied ever having these problems previously.

During the objective re-assessment the left lumbar pain was increased with all active trunk movements in standing, but especially with forward and right-side bending. Left unilateral pressures (passive accessory vertebral motion testing) on L4 and, to a lesser degree, on L3 significantly increased the left mid- and lower lumbar aching. The iliac crest and left lower abdominal ache were not provoked during the objective examination, which included clearing tests for the thoracic, lumbar, sacroiliac joint, and hip joint regions. However, significant information was obtained with palpation of the abdomen.

With the patient in a supine position, severe muscle guarding was noted over the left mid- and lower abdominal regions. Generally, the lower abdominal area felt bloated compared to when it was assessed during the initial evaluation a number of weeks previously. Sharp local

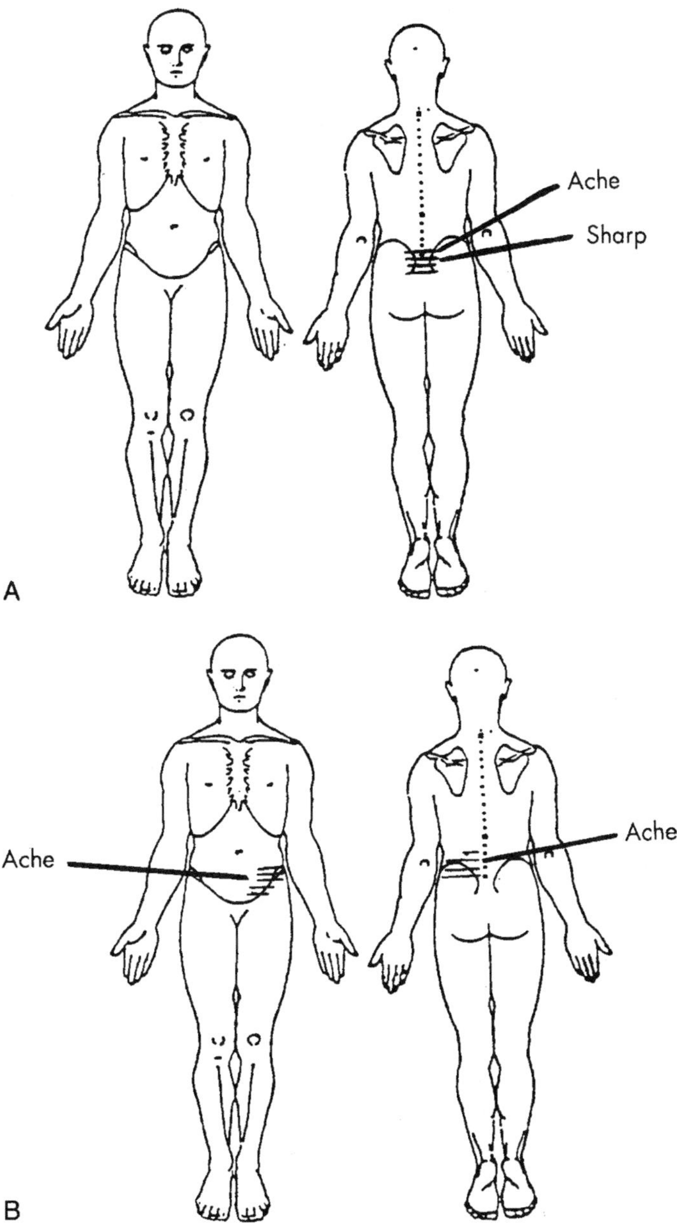

Fig. 4-9. (A) Chief complaint at the initial evaluation—constant central low lumbar aching and intermittent sharp central low lumbar pain. **(B)** Chief complaint at the re-evaluation—constant mid- and lower left lumbar aching and intermittent left iliac crest and lower abdominal aching.

tenderness was provoked with palpation at points in the mid- and left lower abdominal areas. The tenderness was not present over the same points when the abdominal muscle wall was contracted (she was asked to curl up to tighten the abdominal wall).

Conclusion

At the time of the re-evaluation visit, the patient received treatment for the mechanical dysfunction that was felt to be related to the mid- and lower lumbar region pain. She was also instructed to see her family physician regarding the iliac crest and abdominal symptoms. The family physician was called by the physical therapist to discuss why the patient was referred; the following information was communicated: insidious onset of symptoms in a new location (especially the iliac crest and abdominal pain), the nonmechanical behavior of these symptoms (the iliac crest and abdominal symptoms did not seem to vary with movement or postural changes), the recent changes in bowel function, the inability to provoke the iliac crest and abdominal symptoms during the objective examination, the significant mid- and lower abdominal muscle guarding and local tenderness, and the bloated nature of the abdominal region.

The patient returned to the physical therapy clinic 4 days later stating that she had been diagnosed by her family practice physician as having irritable bowel syndrome, a motility disorder of the small intestine and large bowel. She had been placed on a high fiber diet and began taking Metamucil. The iliac crest and abdominal pain quickly receded and had not been present 38 hours prior to her return to physical therapy. She also stated that she was not having difficulty with bowel movements any longer. Upon re-evaluation, palpation of the abdomen did not reveal the distention that was present previously; the abnormal muscle tone was not present, nor was local tenderness with palpation. The patient was once again treated for the mechanical dysfunction related to the left mid- and lower lumbar symptoms and subsequently returned to the group exercise class.

When the patient had returned for re-evaluation of the new symptoms, she was under the impression that this was a flare-up of her usual low back pain problem, despite the fact that the symptoms, especially the iliac crest and abdominal pain, were in a new location. Although she was aware of the changes in bowel movement pattern, she never considered contacting her physician regarding her symptoms because of the overriding nature of the increased low back pain. It was not until the specific location and behavior of the symptoms were discussed with the patient that she began to consider the possibility that these symptoms were not necessarily related to what she had originally been seen for. When initially asked about the presence of bowel dysfunction, she denied problems being present, but when given a specific list of bowel dysfunctions, she quickly noted the change in frequency of her bowel movements, as well as the difficulty in initiating them. Therapists should always include a list of specific examples of bowel dysfunction if a patient gives a negative initial response to the question, "Is bowel dysfunction present?" In this patient's case it was apparent after re-evaluation and response to treatment that the left mid- and lower lumbar symptoms were a result of local dysfunction, while the iliac crest and abdominal symptoms appeared to be related to a condition of the GI system. While irritable bowel syndrome was not discussed in this chapter, the use of the screening checklist (Fig. 4-4) would alert the therapist to the possible presence of this condition. Fortunately, both conditions responded quickly to the appropriate treatment, and the patient was able to resume the aggressive exercise program that had been initiated previously.

SUGGESTED READINGS

Isselbacher KJ, Braunwald E, Wilson JD et al (ed): Harrison's Principles of Internal Medicine. 13th Ed. McGraw-Hill, New York, 1994

Greenberger N: Gastrointestinal Disorder. A Pathophysiologic Approach. 3rd Ed. Year Book Medical Publishers, Chicago, 1986

Kelley WN (ed): Essentials of Internal Medicine. JB Lippincott, Philadelphia, 1994

Rubenstein E (ed): Scientific American Medicine. Scientific American, New York, 1990

Sleisenger M: Gastrointestinal Disease. Pathophysiology Diagnosis Management. 4th Ed. WB Saunders, Philadelphia, 1989

5 SCREENING FOR MALE UROGENITAL SYSTEM DISEASE

Dudley M. McLinn, M.D.
William G. Boissonnault, M.S., P.T.

The structures making up the male urogenital system include the kidneys, ureters, bladder, prostate gland, urethra, testicles, and epididymis. These structures are well known to cause both abdominal and low back pain. In addition, pre-existing conditions of the urogenital system, such as cancer or infections, may be associated with the development of disease processes and symptoms in other areas of the body. It is, therefore, essential that the physical therapist have the clinical tools to screen patients for the presence of disease of the urogenital system. The purposes of this chapter are to provide

1. A general review of the anatomy and function of the male urogenital system
2. An overview of the general symptoms and signs suggestive of urogenital system disease a physical therapist might expect to detect during the examination process
3. A more detailed analysis of the disease processes most likely to present primarily as pain syndromes and of prediagnosed conditions that could have an impact on the prognosis of physical therapy care

ANATOMY AND PHYSIOLOGY

The anatomic relationship of the urogenital system and of the abdomen, back, and peritoneum is shown in Figures 5-1 to 5-4. The kidneys and ureters exist bilaterally in the peritoneal cavity, separated from the gastrointestinal tract by the peritoneum. Normal kidneys can be difficult to palpate because of their anatomic location. Diseased kidneys could produce such symptoms as ileus or nausea because of the close proximity of the kidneys to structures of the gastrointestinal system. If pain is a presenting symptom, conditions of the kidneys and ureters (proximal portion) typically are manifested as back pain as opposed to abdominal pain due to their retroperitoneal location. The ureters connect to the bladder, which is extraperitoneal, existing inferior to the peritoneal cavity. As the bladder fills, its borders extend cranially to where the structure may be palpable superior to the pubic symphysis. The prostate and seminal vesicles are located caudad to the bladder and are connected to the urethra. The prostate and seminal vesicles lie close to the bladder and rectum and, if pathologically enlarged (particularly the prostate), may encroach on these two structures, impairing function (Fig. 5-5). The prostate is a chestnut-sized solid organ that can be easily palpated through the rectum. The testicles and epididymis lie in the scrotal sac and are connected to the vas deferens, which exits the scrotum through the inguinal canal. The vas deferens then empties into the urethra at its junction with the prostate gland. The vas deferens is also closely associated with the seminal vesicles at this junction. The testes are oval shaped and vary in size, with the left testicle commonly larger than the right. They are smooth and elastic in texture. The epididymis is posterior to, and distinguishable from, the testicles.

Neurologic control of the urogenital system originates in the brain stem and culminates in the sacral micturition center through the autonomic nervous system.

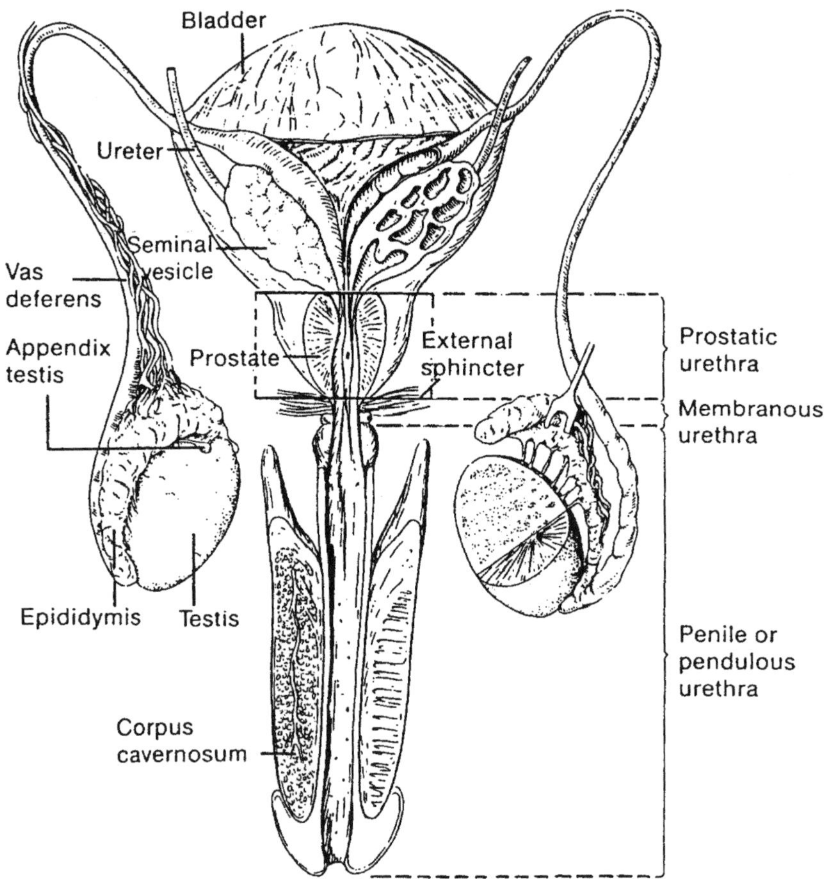

Fig. 5-1. Anatomic structures of the male urogenital system. (From Skögeland,[2] with permission.)

Table 5-1 designates the spinal segmental innervation levels for the structures of the urogenital system. This neurologic arrangement serves to stimulate or inhibit micturition through the two components of the autonomic nervous system. The cholinergic fibers stimulate micturition, whereas the sympathetic fibers inhibit micturition.

A primary function of the urogenital system is to act as a filter and drainage system for the body. An important function of the kidney is to regulate the body's extracellular fluid composition by filtering metabolic byproducts in the blood, thereby maintaining the fluid and electrolyte balance. The kidney can regulate the body's extracellular fluid by altering the composition of plasma as it courses through the vascular network of the kidney. The altered plasma influences the interstitial fluid of the body and the intracellular fluid composition as it circulates. The blood enters the kidney through a branch of the aorta, the renal artery (see Fig. 5-3). Ultimately the plasma brought into the kidney by the renal arteries filters through glomerular capillaries into the renal tubules.[1] As the filtrate passes through the renal tubules,

Table 5-1. Structures of the Male Urogenital System

Structure	Segmental Innervation	Possible Areas of Pain Referral
Kidney	T10–L1	Lumbar spine (ipsilateral) flank Upper abdominal
Ureter	T11–L2, S2–S4	Groin Upper/lower abdominal Suprapubic, scrotum Medial, proximal thigh Thoracolumbar
Urinary bladder	T11–L2, S2–S4	Sacral apex Suprapubic Thoracolumbar
Prostate gland	T11–L1, S2–S4	Sacral, low lumbar Testes Thoracolumbar
Testes	T10–T11	Lower abdominal Sacral

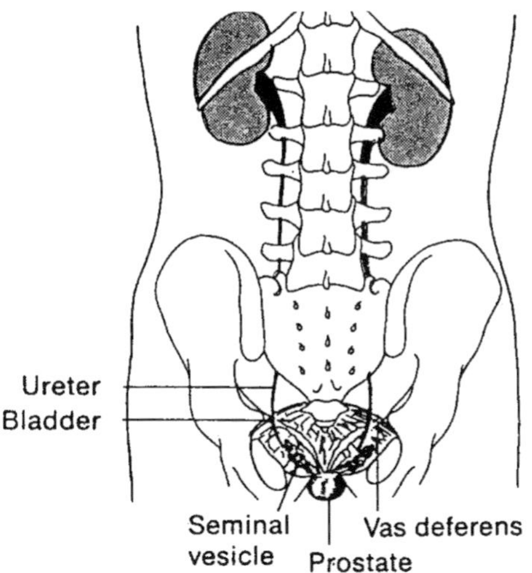

Fig. 5-2. Anatomic relationship of urogenital system structures and elements of the bony skeleton. (From Skögeland,[2] with permission.)

its volume is reduced and its composition altered. The volume is reduced by the absorption of water and certain solutes, such as sodium, calcium, potassium, and phosphate, which are used by the body. The composition is further altered by the secretion of the solutes magnesium, hydrogen, and ammonia into the remaining filtrate. The resulting filtrate eventually forms the urine that enters the renal pelvis and exits the body through the urine drainage system made up of the ureters, bladder, and urethra.[2] The kidney also produces hormones, including angiotensin II, prostaglandins, and kinins, which are important mediators regarding the regulation of blood pressure. The release of angiotensin increases extracellular fluid volume and elevates the blood pressure by enhancing sodium reabsorption within the kidney.[1] Through the production of the hormone erythropoietin, the kidney also helps regulates the synthesis of red blood cells. Therefore, if the kidneys are malfunctioning regarding hormone production, the patient may

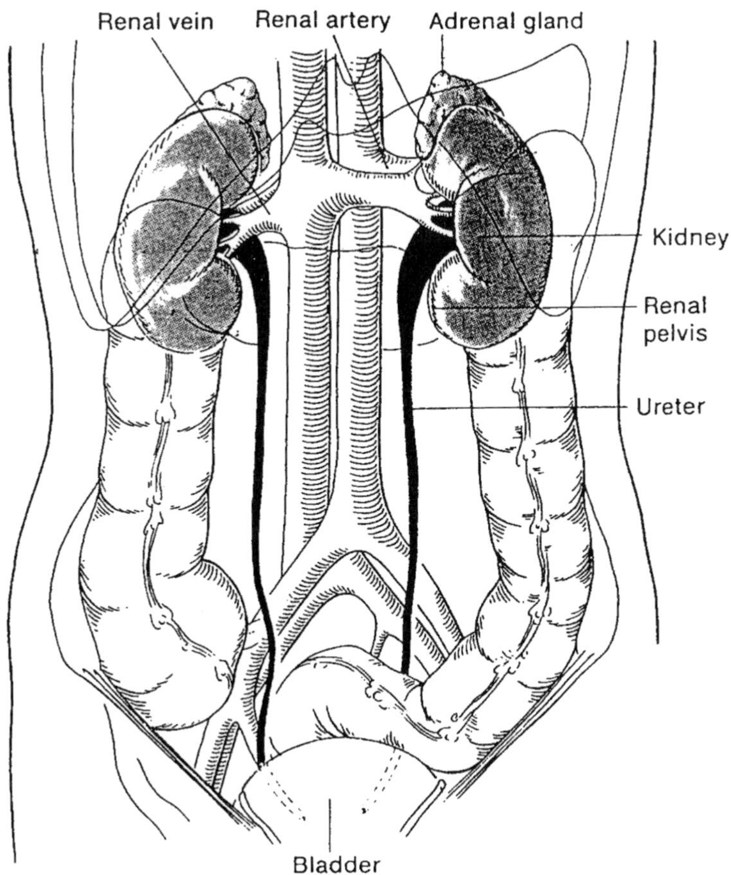

Fig. 5-3. Anatomic relationship of the kidneys and ureters and elements of the cardiovascular and gastrointestinal systems. (From Skögeland,[2] with permission.)

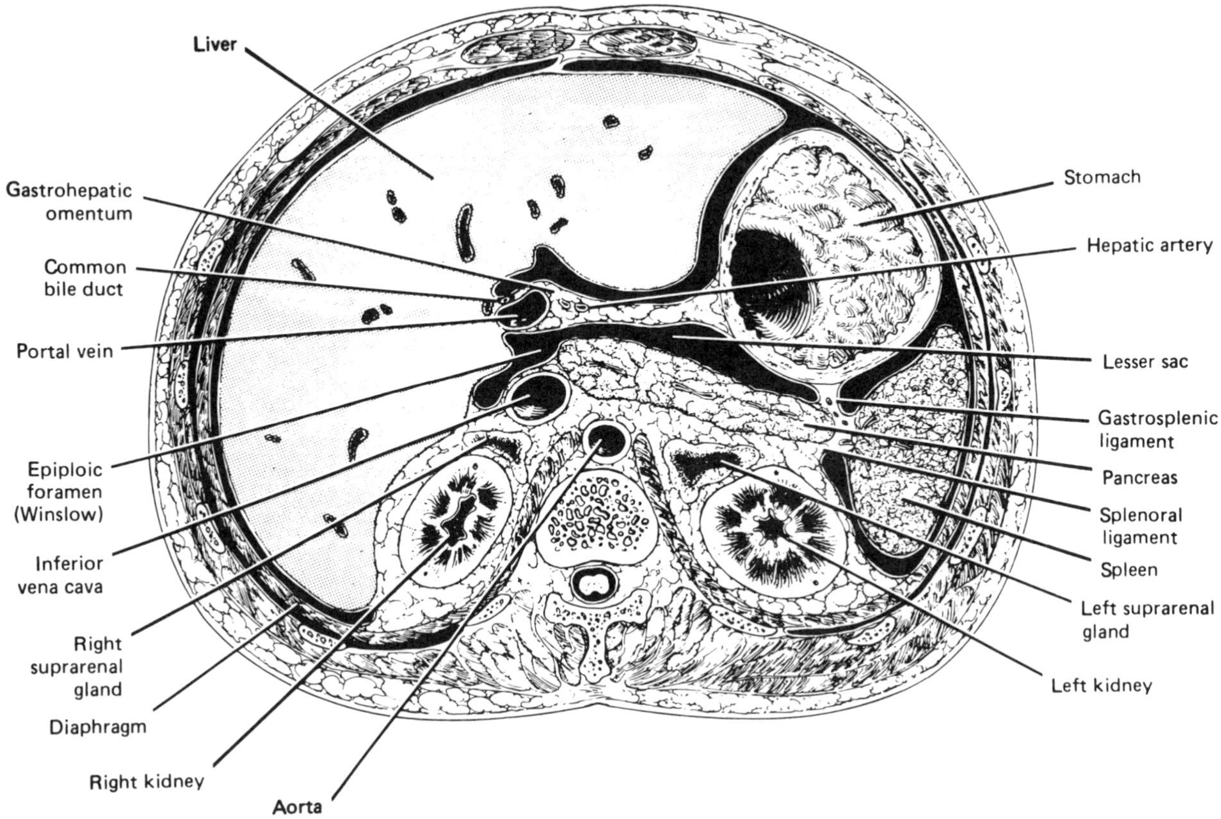

Fig. 5-4. Anatomic relationship of the kidneys to the spine. (From Linder,[14] with permission.)

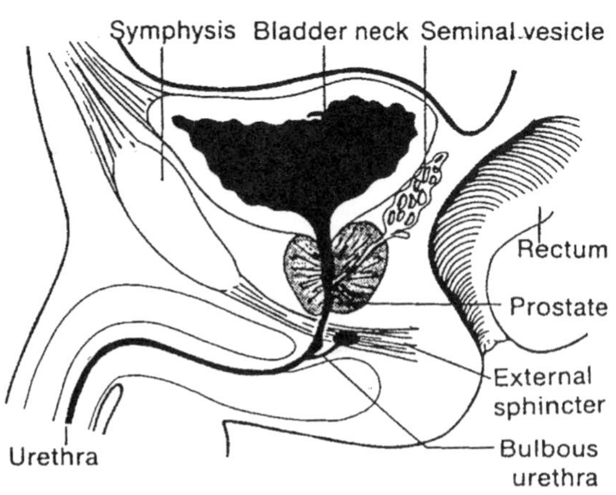

Fig. 5-5. Anatomic relationship of the prostate gland and the bladder, urethra, and rectum. (From Skögeland,[2] with permission.)

present with such conditions as hypertension and anemia. If the urine drainage system (the ureters, bladder, and urethra) is impaired, problems related to bladder distention and renal failure could develop.

The remaining structures of the male urogenital system include the testicles, epididymis, vas deferens, seminal vesicle, and prostate. The structures are involved in the important functions related to spermatogenesis, ejaculation, and male hormone production. Spermatozoa are formed within the testes and drain into the epididymis. Spermatozoa then pass into the vas deferens, which is continuous with the epididymis. Upon ejaculation, semen, including the spermatozoa, enters the urethra within the body of the prostate.[2] The testes also play an important role in male hormone production. The principal hormone produced within the testes, which is subsequently secreted, is testosterone. Luteinizing hormone (LH), released by the anterior lobe of the hypophysis (pituitary gland), stimulates the production of testosterone. Testosterone helps maintain the male secondary sex characteristics, including hair distribution, body configuration, and genital size, by acting as a prehormone for a number of sex steroids, such as androgens and estrogens.[3] Testosterone also exerts an important growth-promoting affect. Malfunction of these structures of the urogenital system could lead to sexual dysfunction (e.g., infertility, pain with ejaculation, and impotency).

Knowledge of the anatomy and physiology of the urogenital system can facilitate the therapist's understanding of the symptoms and signs of pathologic conditions that present in the clinical setting. This information should assist the therapist in formulating questions to be added to the history and should help in the interpretation of information volunteered by the patient regarding the function of this organ system. In addition, knowledge of anatomy will help the therapist differentiate these structures from musculoskeletal system structures during the objective examination and subsequent treatment. The remainder of this chapter focuses on the clinical presentation of diseases of the male urogenital system.

SIGNS AND SYMPTOMS OF DISEASE

History

The physical therapist must rely on the history for most of the information regarding screening this system for medical disease. Few physical therapy objective tests or measures provide data related to the function of the urogenital system as opposed to systems such as the cardiovascular or pulmonary. Therefore, questions regarding pain complaints, bladder function, and sexual function are crucial in screening patients for disease of the urogenital system. The medical tests commonly used to assess the health of the urogenital system include urinalysis, diagnostic ultrasound, radiology, and semen analysis.

The location, description, and behavior of symptoms are all important factors to be considered during the history. The PQRST method is commonly used by physicians to organize the history-taking process:

P Factors that provoke or palliate the pain.
Q Quality of pain, that is, sharp, dull, burning, wavelike (colicky), or stabbing
R Region and radiation of the pain
S Severity of the pain (usually graded mild, moderate, or severe)
T Timing as it relates to other events in daily living such as eating or sleeping (includes documenting whether the symptoms are constant or intermittent)

Urogenital system disease can result in abdominal, back, flank, or buttock pain. These symptoms may be described as a dull ache, burning sensation, or wavelike or colicky pain, depending on which structure is involved and the type of disease present. Organizationally, abdominal pain is best separated into regions. Right and left upper quadrant abdominal pain can reflect ipsilateral renal and proximal ureter abnormalities. Right and left lower quadrant abdominal pain can reflect ipsilateral distal ureteral, testicular, and epididymis disease. Bladder disease may result in right, left, or midline lower abdominal pain. Each of the urogenital system structures has the potential to refer pain to the remainder of the trunk, groin, or buttock regions, and the retroperitoneal location of the kidneys and proximal ureters may account for back pain complaints. Table 5-1 shows the possible areas of pain referral from these various structures. Figure 5-6 illustrates the specific pain pattern for the kidneys and ureters. Pain complaints noted in any of these areas should direct the therapist to ask questions regarding the behavior (provocation or palliation) of these symptoms related to urogenital system function in addition to the usual questions relating behavior of symptoms to assumption of specific postures and carrying out specific movements. On the basis of these pain complaints, questions regarding urinary or sexual dysfunction should also be asked.

Besides pain, additional information regarding the function of the urogenital system can easily be collected by the physical therapist. It is necessary to screen patients with the above-described complaints for disorders of voiding. Changes in frequency of urination from a patient's normal pattern can be suggestive of disease. Therefore, questions related to noted increase or decrease of the number of times a day a patient urinates are important.

Increased frequency at night, or nocturia, often reflects a bladder outlet obstruction disorder such as prostatism. Urinary urgency, sometimes to the point of incontinence, is often associated with infection, primarily of the bladder, urethra, and prostate. Complaint of

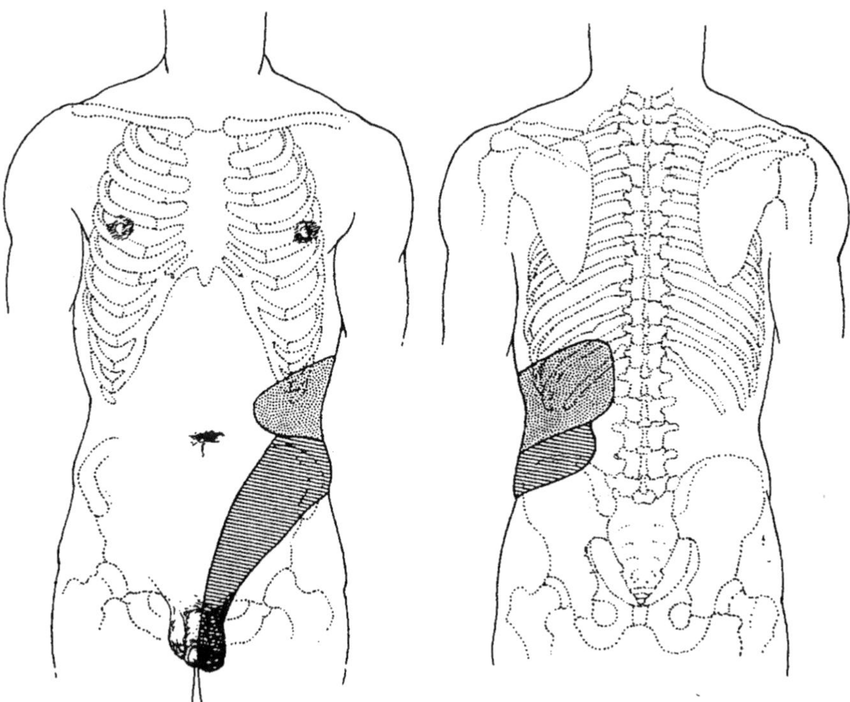

Fig. 5-6. Pain referral patterns for the kidneys (dotted areas) and ureters (horizontal lines). (From Smith,[13] with permission.)

pain and burning while voiding is known as dysuria and often reflects a urinary tract infection or outlet obstruction. Hematuria is always abnormal and a sign associated with serious pathology; any patient who notes blood in the urine should be referred immediately to a physician.[4]

Questions related to sexual function can also provide important information regarding the health of the urogenital system. These questions should address such issues as impotence, pain with ejaculation, premature ejaculation, and inability to maintain an erection.[4] Physical therapists may find it awkward at times to ask patients about sexual dysfunction, but if these questions are not specifically asked, the patient might not volunteer this information because of embarrassment or because he is unaware of the importance and relevance of these data. Figure 5-7 presents a checklist of items related to the urogenital system that should be included in the history if the patient describes pain in the areas previously discussed or has a significant medical history of involvement of this organ system, such as cancer or repeated infection.

Objective Examination

Few physical therapy objective examination techniques provide specific information regarding the status of the urogenital system. Physical therapists evaluate the abdomen by observation, palpation, and possibly percussion. Clinical findings may require the use of soft tissue mobilization techniques, to increase the extensibility of restricted tissue (e.g., scars) and to decrease the resting tone of muscles (e.g., abdominals, iliopsoas, and respiratory diaphragm). Physical therapists must be aware of the nonmusculoskeletal system structures within this region, that they may also be affecting with the assessment technique and soft tissue mobilization techniques. Of the urogenital system structures described, only the bladder (if distended) and the kidney may be palpable externally. When the therapist detects increased muscle tone or fullness in the suprapubic region associated with tenderness or provocation of symptoms, the therapist must differentiate between the abdominal muscle wall and pubic symphysis as the structures involved versus a

Review of systems checklist: Male urogenital system

Item	Yes	No	Comments
1. Dysuria	____	____	____
2. Hematuria	____	____	____
3. Incontinence	____	____	____
4. Frequency of urination	____	____	____
5. Urinary urgency	____	____	____
6. Decreased force of urinary flow	____	____	____
7. Impotence	____	____	____
8. Pain with ejaculation	____	____	____
9. Difficulties with maintaining an erection	____	____	____
10. Urethral discharge	____	____	____
11. History of urinary infection	____	____	____
12. History of venereal disease	____	____	____

Fig. 5-7. Checklist for review of the male urogenital system. (From Boissonnault and Bass,[12] with permission.)

deeper visceral structure (including the bladder). One of the special tests a therapist can use is to have the patient perform a partial curl-up (if cervical and upper thoracic spine flexion is not contraindicated) and to palpate the same area. If the area is no longer tender and then is tender again when the superficial muscle wall is more relaxed with the patient fully supine, a structure deep to the abdominal muscle wall should be suspected to be involved.

The therapist must be cognizant of the location of the kidney when assessing and mobilizing the lower thoracic and upper lumbar spine areas, including the 11th and 12th ribs. Pressure on the kidney could also possibly occur with soft tissue mobilization techniques for the quadratus lumborum, lumbar paraspinals, and the psoas muscle groups (see Fig. 5-2 for anatomic location of the kidneys). Using a hand/fist to percuss over the costovertebral angle is a technique utilized for provocation of symptoms related to kidney disease (Fig. 5-8). Marked exacerbation of symptoms with this technique warrants

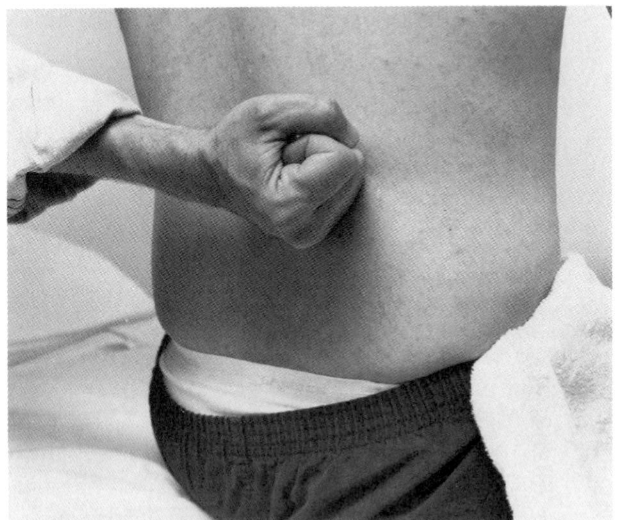

Fig. 5-8. Percussing over the costovertebral angle.

increased concern on the therapist's part regarding origin of the symptoms. Finally, related to palpation, the testes and penis should be considered. It is inappropriate for physical therapists to palpate these structures during an examination process, but the therapist should ask the patient whether he has noted any abnormal masses in the scrotum or change in size of the testicles upon self-examination. If the patient is unclear as to what is normal or abnormal, a description by the therapist of what is normal would be indicated. The description provided should include oval-shaped, firm, smooth, and elastic in texture, but also noting that the right and left testicle might not be the same size.

A correlation of the findings from the history and physical examination may provide the therapist with enough information to suspect involvement of the urogenital system. These specific findings should be communicated to the physician to decide whether the patient should see the doctor at that time for a detailed medical examination.

UROGENITAL SYSTEM DISEASE

Physical therapists should be knowledgeable of certain medical conditions of the male urogenital system. Infections, tumors, and impotence are the most common disease entities likely to confront physical therapists when treating patients with abdominal, lumbar spine, pelvic, and/or groin pain. This section discusses the etiology and symptoms and signs of these pathologic conditions. A brief overview of the medical testing procedures used to diagnose the conditions and of the common medical treatment approaches for these conditions is presented. Also addressed is chronic renal failure. The emphasis is on the secondary changes commonly associated with the disease, as well as their impact on physical therapy management.

Infections

Urinary tract infections are the second most common infection, after upper respiratory infections. Infections of the solid organs (i.e., kidney, prostate, testicles, and epididymis) will generally be associated with fever, chills, and malaise, with fever being the hallmark symptom.[2] Renal pain is often experienced in the ipsilateral lumbar region caudad to the rib cage. Table 5-1 and Figure 5-6 show additional possible areas of pain perception in the presence of kidney infection. Patients often describe the pain as being a dull constant ache.[4] Pyelonephritis, the most common renal disease, generally follows an untreated bladder infection. This disease should be strongly considered in immunocompromised patients, (e.g., a diabetic or cancer patient on chemotherapy) or in a patient with recent instrumentation (including cystoscopy or catheterization). Other factors predisposing to the onset of pyelonephritis include the presence of metabolic disease (e.g., diabetes mellitus), long-term immobilization, and medications (e.g., analgesics and corticosteroids).[2] A perinephric abscess, an abscess surrounding the kidney, lies in close proximity to the psoas muscle. Therefore, ipsilateral hip flexion may cause local pain secondary to psoas contraction. Pyelonephritis is not common in men but should be considered when a patient complains of unilateral lumbar pain associated with the presence of fever.

Prostatic pain is often experienced as a dull, diffuse, perineal pain. Pain referral patterns besides the perineal pain associated with prostate conditions are presented in Table 5-1. The intensity of the pain may vary with functions, such as bowel movements, urination, and intercourse. Certain perirectal conditions such as rectal fissures and hemorrhoids can mimic this disease, but a medical examination can quickly out rule these entities. Infections of the prostate behave much like bladder infections in that there may be a sense of urgency to void and increased frequency of urination. The increased frequency may be most noticeable to the patient at night, as he may be waking two to three times a night to urinate compared with the usual pattern of sleeping through the night. In addition, fever and chills may be present as well as dysuria, urge to defecate, and urethral discharge.[2,4]

Infections of the testicles (orchitis) and epididymis (epididymitis) are associated with rapid local swelling and scrotal tenderness. The patient may also present with fever and malaise. Testicular pain is usually experienced as a local dull ache, but pain can be referred to the lower abdominal or sacral regions. Patients with suspected involvement of the testicles should be seen immediately by a physician to rule out the presence of torsion of the testicle. This condition can compromise the local blood supply, requiring immediate medical attention and surgical release. Pain from epididymitis can be difficult to differentiate from testicular pain. Epididymitis causes pain secondary to swelling of the organ and is tender to touch. These infectious processes may be preceded by urethritis or prostatitis.

Infections of the hollow organs of the urogenital system (i.e., the ureters, bladder, and urethra) are associated with pain and other urinary tract symptoms, such as increased urinary frequency and urethral discharge. The hallmark symptom of infection of the solid organs, fever, is often absent.[2] Ureteral pain is often experienced as wavelike (colic) discomfort that can spread from the flank to the ipsilateral lower quadrant of the abdomen and into the ipsilateral testicle[4] (see Fig. 5-6). In the presence of a kidney stone, movement of the pain reflects movement of the stone as it traverses the ureter and bladder. Infection of the ureters can be secondary to multiple organisms, including *Gonorrhoeae*, *Chlamydia*, *Trachamatis*, *Trichomonas vaginalis*, Herpes simplex, *Candida albicans*, and such bacteria as *Escherichia coli*. Effective treatment includes treatment of the patient's sexual partner, to prevent recurrence.

As with pyelonephritis, bladder infections (cystitis) are not common in men. When present, however, the pain is usually constant and can be located in the suprapubic, sacral, or thoracolumbar regions. The pain may be associated with a sense of urgency to void. Although the pain may be constant, the intensity may vary, being wavelike (colicky), with urination intensifying the symptoms and possibly producing radiation of pain to the penis. Besides dysuria and urgency, other symptoms related to voiding may be increased frequency, including nocturia. Urethral pain associated with infection is often a burning sensation associated with urination. The patient may volunteer that he had urethral discharge.

In summary, although relatively uncommon in men, physical therapists should be familiar with the symptoms associated with urogenital system infections. Medical referral should be accomplished when these symptoms are present. The physician will make the diagnosis on the basis of urinalysis, urine culture, and other tests such as intravenous pyelogram and ultrasound of the kidneys, depending on the situation. The treatment is generally antibiotics, depending on the bacterial pathogen. In the case of infections of the solid genitourinary organs, it is often necessary to institute intravenous treatment initially. In immunocompromised patients, immediate consultation should be sought.

Cancer

Tumors of the male urogenital system can be either benign or malignant. Figure 5-9 indicates possible locations of the primary urogenital system tumors. Initially, most malignant tumors are clinically silent, but general symptoms, such as fatigue and malaise, may be present. Only after the mass has reached a certain size will the symptoms and signs of urogenital system involvement become apparent.[2] Of the body neoplasms, there is a high incidence of cancer of the prostate, bladder, and kidney. Neoplasms of the ureter, urethra, penis, epididymis, and seminal vesicles are rare.[4] As with tumors elsewhere in the body, the prognosis for treatment is enhanced by early detection. The physical therapist may be in a position to initiate referral to a physician for diagnosis on the basis of clinical findings.

Kidneys

Cancer of the kidneys can be divided into renal parenchymal and renal pelvis neoplasms. The most common renal tumor is renal cell carcinoma.[5] This disease rarely occurs before the age of 30, with increased incidence noted between the ages of 45 and 75. Peak incidence occurs during the sixth decade, affecting men two to three times more frequently than women.[5] The lungs, liver, and bony elements of the musculoskeletal system are the most common sites of metastasis.[4] The tumor may initially be asymptomatic, with sudden onset of painless hematuria precipitating concern on the patient's part. Pain, though, is the most commonly described symptom. Usually a dull ache is noted in the body regions described in Table 5-1 and Figure 5-6. Complaints of malaise, weakness, weight loss, and fever may also be a part of the patient's clinical picture.[4] A correlation between tobacco use and a higher incidence of renal cell carcinoma has been noted.[5] Enlargement of the kidney may make the structure palpable during the objective examination. Medical diagnosis is made by tests, including sonography, angiography, and computed tomography (CT) scanning. Treatment consists of nephrectomy, lymph node dissection, and postoperative radiation.

The renal pelvis (interior of the kidney) may also be a site of cancer development. This disease is also rare before the age of 30, with peak incidence during the sixth decade. Males are affected two times as frequently as women.[5] Carcinomas and papillomas present with a similar clinical picture. Hematuria of unknown cause is the primary finding of clinical concern, since enlargement of the kidney does not occur.[4] Pain, colicky in nature, though, may also be present. Other symptoms may include urinary frequency, malaise, weight loss, or fever. A medical diagnosis is made by intravenous or ret-

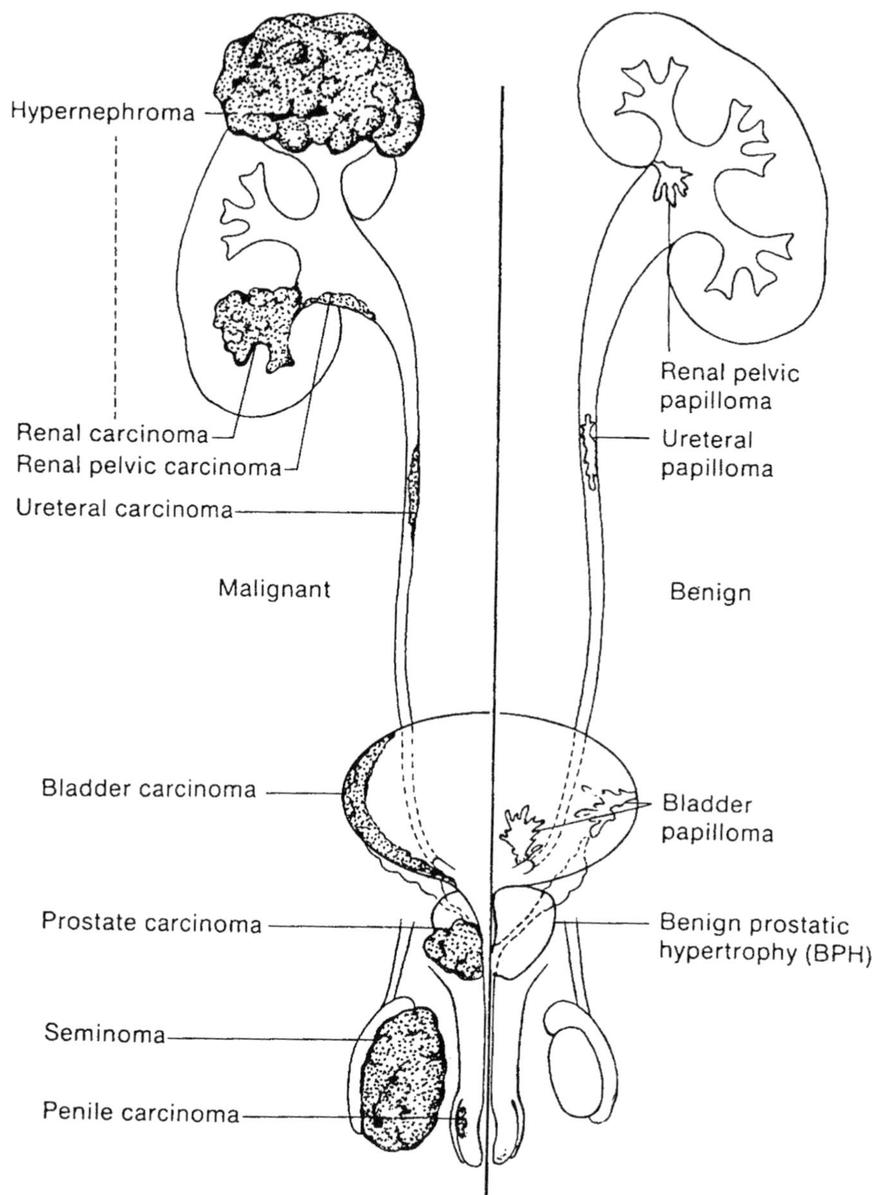

Fig. 5-9. Anatomic locations of malignant and benign lesions of the male urogenital system. (From Skögeland,[2] with permission.)

rograde pyelography, which permits visualization of the ureter and renal pelvis. Treatment would consist of nephroureterectomy, lymph node dissection, and postoperative radiation. Metastasis from this lesion may occur in the ureters and the bladder.

Bladder

Bladder cancer is the fifth most common cause of cancer death in men. Overall, bladder cancer is the second most common cancer of the urogenital system. The incidence is much higher in men than in women (ratio 3–6:1) and affects whites more often than blacks (ratio 4:1).[5] The incidence of bladder cancer is also higher in people in certain occupations (e.g., those exposed to chemicals, dyes, leather products, and rubber) and among cigarette smokers.[4] Cigarette smokers have an incidence of bladder cancer two to five times greater than that of the nonsmoking population.[5] Generally a poor prognosis is associated with bladder carcinoma, as most of the tumors are malignant. Metastasis can occur to the lungs, bony elements of the musculoskeletal system, and the liver. Presenting symptoms may include hematuria, dysuria, nocturia, and urinary urgency.[4] Diagnosis is made by tests including cystogram, cystoscopy, and biopsy. Treatment includes surgical resection of the tumor and postoperative radiation.

Prostate

After lung and gastrointestinal tract cancer, carcinoma of the prostate gland is the third leading cause of cancer death in men.[2,6,7] Prostate cancer is the second most common cancer in males.[5] The incidence of prostatic carcinoma and adenoma progressively increases after the age of 50 years.[7] Often no symptoms are noted in the early stages of this disease. The first symptom could be a dull, vague, diffuse ache localized to the central low lumbar spine or upper sacral regions. Early metastasis to the lumbar spine and pelvis (bony elements) is not uncommon. Besides these two sites, the femurs (proximal portion), thoracic spine, ribs, and sternum are sites of metastasis.[6] The most common visceral structures involved with metastasis are the lung, liver, and adrenal glands. These pathologic lesions resulting in local pain may be the initial symptoms noted by the patient. Only after the tumor is of sufficient size to compromise the urethra will urinary dysfunction be noted by the patient. The early stages of urinary dysfunction may include a sense of urinary urgency and possibly hematuria. In the more advanced stages of this disease, increased frequency of urination, particularly nocturia, slowing of the urine stream, and difficulty in starting the urine stream may also be present. In the early stages of cancer, palpatory abnormalities of the prostate are the primary diagnostic findings. Needle biopsy of the mass would then follow. Treatment may include prostatectomy, radiation treatment, chemotherapy, or hormone therapy.

Testes

Testicular tumors are relatively rare but, when present, are associated with a poor prognosis unless diagnosed early. Significant delay in diagnosis can occur if back pain is a presenting factor.[8] In some cases back pain may be the only symptom and the reason why the patient is seeing a physical therapist. The tumors tend to be very malignant, with peak incidence occurring between the ages of 20 and 40.[2] Testicular tumors are generally marked by painless but slow, progressive swelling of a testicle. Other symptoms may include abdominal pain, nausea, vomiting, and weight loss.[4] The patient may experience back pain as the disease spreads via the lymphatic system. The retroperitoneal lymphatics can be involved in the cephalic spread of the primary malignant disease from numerous structures, including the testes (Fig. 5-10). As the disease continues to spread, the supraclavicular node (left) may be involved, with the patient possibly experiencing local pain and the therapist observing/palpating a local mass. Owing to the endocrine function of the testicles, a tumor may result in gynecomastia (breast enlargement) and/or impotence.[2] Self-examination may reveal a unilateral, smooth, enlarged testicle or a testicular mass. Further diagnostic testing may include ultrasound, CT scan, and biopsy. Treatment consists of radical orchiectomy. Prompt surgical removal of the tumor may be life saving, with early detection paramount for a better prognosis. Therefore, men, especially between the ages of 20 to 40 years, should be encouraged to perform self-examination. Besides a tumor, scrotal enlargement may be caused by a hydrocele (benign fluid collection) or a spermatocele. An evaluation by the physician would help differentiate these entities from a neoplasm.

Chronic Renal Failure

Renal failure is defined as the deterioration of renal function associated with the accumulation of nitrogenous wastes not attributable to extrarenal factors.[9] Chronic renal failure is marked by irreversible loss of kidney function, resulting in a wide range of complications that affect numerous body systems. Patients prediagnosed as having chronic renal failure may be referred for physical therapy for conditions related or unrelated to renal disease. Regardless of why the patient has been referred, the therapist should understand the impact that the disease and associated secondary changes may have on the prognosis and outcome of the therapy sessions.

Chronic renal failure is marked by progressive loss of nephrons. The causes are numerous, with glomerulonephritis, interstitial renal disease, and polycystic kidney disease the most common.[10] Since the kidney functions to regulate the body's extracellular fluid composition, thereby influencing intracellular fluid composition, chronic kidney disease can have a wide-ranging effect on multiple body systems. These secondary manifestations of chronic renal failure can often be mistaken for primary conditions.

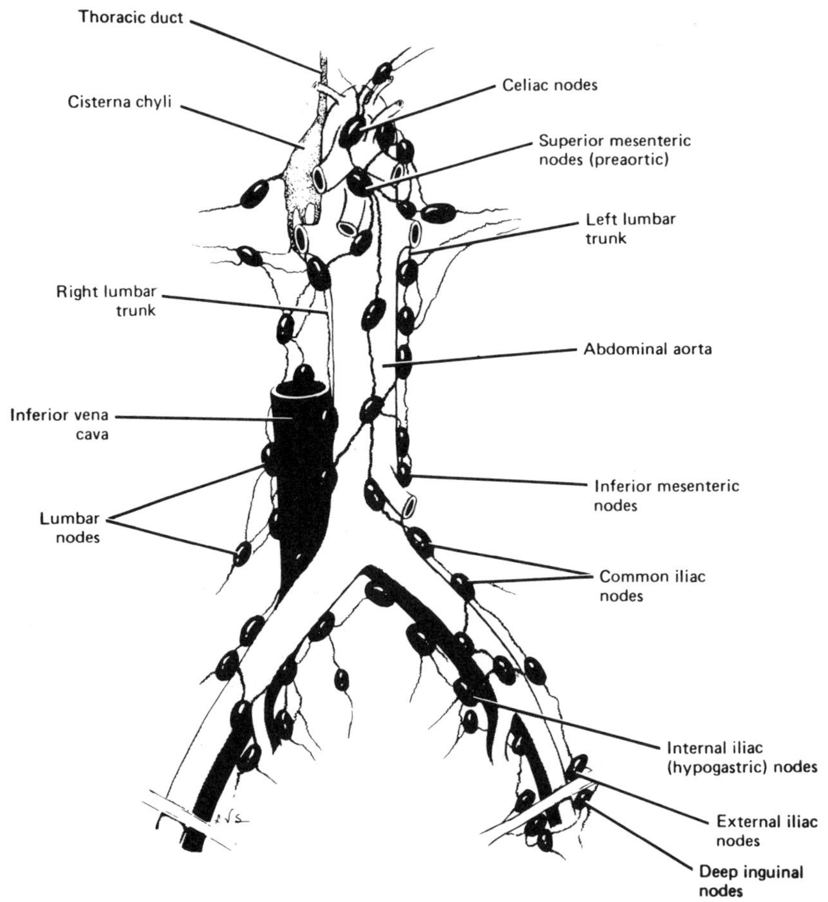

Fig. 5-10. Portions of the retroperitoneal lymphatic chain. (From Linder,[14] with permission.)

A number of symptoms and signs associated with chronic renal failure may interfere with physical therapy or may result in a confusing clinical picture. Common gastrointestinal system complaints associated with chronic renal failure include nausea and vomiting. Insomnia, inability to concentrate, and lack of alertness may also be present.[9] All these symptoms may interfere with the patient's ability to participate in a rehabilitation program, including tolerating exercises in the clinic as well as following through with a home exercise program. Neurologic changes may result in increased deep tendon reflexes,[9] intermittent paresthesias and hypesthesias of the hands and feet, cramping of limb musculature, and absence of sweating.[10] Proximal muscle weakness may also be present, making it difficult for patients to rise up from a chair or bed.[10] Differentiating these neurologic changes from those that occur from spinal or peripheral nerve entrapment may be difficult. Generally neurologic changes secondary to a systemic disorder will not follow the pattern of specific dermatomal or myotomal involvement. They will also not follow the pattern of a specific peripheral neuropathy. The therapist must be cautious, though, as a common clinical error may be to attribute a patient's complaints of numbness, weakness, or pins-and-needles sensations to the presence of chronic renal failure. Detailed investigation of the behavior of the symptoms may demonstrate changes in intensity or provocation of symptoms related to movements or assumption of specific postures. Similar findings may occur as active and passive range-of-motion (ROM) testing, and special tests are implemented in the objective examination. These findings may lead the therapist to suspect that all or a part of the patient's complaints are not related to the kidney pathology but rather to nerve involvement secondary to mechanical dysfunction. (See Patient Case History 2, Ch. 7, for an example.)

Other changes associated with chronic renal failure may have an impact on physical therapy management as well, including osteodystrophy. Elevated levels of parathyroid hormone secondary to the renal pathology can lead to increased bone resorption. The decreased bone density may lead to microtrauma of the bone resulting in local pain complaints. The most commonly involved bony elements include the vertebral column and femurs.[10] These patients will be more susceptible to fractures as well as other skeletal deformities. The therapist should be cautious when passively assessing spinal mobility, especially the thoracic spine, when using techniques such as central and unilateral pressures as described by Maitland[11] with the patient in a prone position. With the thorax stabilized anteriorly by the table and then stressed in a posterior to anterior direction by the therapist's pressure, the structurally weakened rib cage could be injured. Obtaining information regarding spinal segmental mobility and provocation of symptoms is an important goal of the objective examination. With patients coming to the clinic prediagnosed as having chronic renal failure, alternative patient positions and methods of passive interverterbral testing should be considered to protect the patient.

Finally, cardiovascular complications accompanying the chronic renal failure must be considered. Hypertension is commonly associated with chronic renal failure. Control of high blood pressure is important, to prevent the acceleration of nephrosclerosis and decrease the likelihood that other cardiovascular system disorders will develop.[10] Communication between the physician and physical therapist is important for setting the appropriate aerobic exercise workloads, using pulse rate and blood pressure measures, when appropriate, to monitor the patient and for determining the ideal days for rehabilitation in relationship to the days the patient undergoes dialysis. Finally, pericarditis can occur in up to one half of undialyzed patients.[10] This condition may develop while the patient is being treated by the physical therapist. (See Ch. 2 for a description of symptoms and signs associated with pericarditis.)

Impotence

In our fast-paced world, impotency is becoming a much more common problem. Many men will be reluctant to volunteer the fact that they are impotent, but will be relieved to discuss it if they are suffering from the problem. It is best to be sympathetic and not judgmental and suggest that they discuss it with their primary physician or with a urologist. In most cases, the problem is primarily psychological. Organic problems must be ruled out, however. Impotency can be secondary to a neurogenic problem such as polio, multiple sclerosis, tabes dorsalis, spinal trauma, or diabetic neuropathy. It can also be secondary to vascular conditions such as arteriosclerosis or thrombosis. Lastly, it may be secondary to endocrine conditions such as hypogonadism and hypopituitarism. It is also commonly associated with such drugs as sedatives, antidepressants, antihypertensives, as well as estrogens, which are often given in the presence of prostate cancer. Alcohol excess can also be associated with the presence of impotency. A careful screening of the patient's past and current medical history could be extremely helpful in directing the patient to the appropriate physician for a diagnostic examination.

SUMMARY

This chapter discusses the male urogenital system as it relates to the practice of physical therapy. The therapist must understand the basic anatomy of the urogenital system as it relates to other organ systems of the body, including the musculoskeletal system. It is important to remember that the signs and symptoms of disease, especially early stage disease of the urogenital system, are often nonspecific and general in nature. Since physical therapists are called on most frequently to help resolve pain or dysfunction, it is also helpful to remember that the original diagnosis may be mistaken, and a careful examination on the physical therapist's part may be extremely important in directing the patient to the appropriate physician and subsequent medical treatment. Two patient case histories follow.

PATIENT CASE STUDY 1*

History

The patient was a 58-year-old commuter van driver for a hospital who was referred to the clinic with a diagnosis of mechanical low back pain syndrome and cervical strain

* (From Boissonnault and Bass,[12] with permission.)

secondary to a motor vehicle accident. His van had been struck on the passenger side by a car as he pulled out of a parking lot 3 weeks before the evaluation. His chief complaints were left posterolateral cervical spine and left shoulder pain and central low lumbar spine pain. The patient described the left shoulder pain as a constant dull aching that was aggravated by driving for more than 1 hour. Limiting the driving time was his only method of controlling the symptoms. He also experienced intermittent sharp left cervicothoracic junction pain, which interfered with driving. This symptom was solely aggravated by left rotation of the cervical spine. He experienced significant stiffness in the cervical spine and slight aching early in the morning. A hot shower significantly reduced the stiffness, while the aching intensity varied with the amount of driving he did later that day. The cervical spine and left shoulder pain did not interfere with sleeping. The patient had never experienced cervical or shoulder symptoms before the motor vehicle accident.

The low back pain was described as a constant, low-intensity ache occasionally aggravated by repetitive lifting. He was able to obtain slight relief of the aching by assuming a supine or side-lying position for short periods. Driving did not seem to aggravate the lumbar symptoms. The patient stated that the low back pain was most intense early in the morning. He noted he was waking consistently around 3:00 AM with severe low back pain. Getting out of bed and walking for 15 to 20 minutes decreased the ache sufficiently so that sleep was possible again. He has experienced numerous episodes of low back pain over the past 5 to 6 years. None of the episodes was preceded by a traumatic incident or accident, but this most recent episode, which began 3 to 4 months before the evaluation, was the first marked by severe night pain. When questioned further, the patient revealed that the motor vehicle accident had not changed his low back condition.

The patient's medical history included surgical repair of a right lower abdominal hernia and an appendectomy. He was taking medication for high blood pressure, and ibuprofen had been prescribed since the motor vehicle accident. He denied any visual, auditory, or cognitive changes since the accident. The patient denied bowel dysfunction but had noted increased frequency of urination, including waking two to three times a night to urinate, and difficulty in starting the urine stream. He had not seen a physician specifically for the urogenital problems and had forgotten to tell the physician he saw following the motor vehicle accident. Radiographs were taken of the cervical spine after the accident, revealing degenerative disc disease at C5–C6.

Objective Examination

The objective examination revealed significant muscle guarding throughout the left posterolateral aspect of the cervical spine. There was also slight muscle guarding noted in the paraspinals, L4–L5. A moderately increased cervicothoracic junction kyphosis and decreased low lumbar lordosis was observed. Sharp left lower cervical spine pain and an increase in the left shoulder ache was noted with one repetition of cervical spine left rotation. Left rotation ROM was decreased by approximately 90 percent. Cervical left side bending and backward bending were moderately reduced, with the patient describing a "blocked" sensation in the left lower cervical region at end range. A slight to moderate loss of active backward bending and left and right side bending of the lumbar spine was also observed. The low lumbar symptoms were not provoked with any active movements of the trunk, nor with overpressures. The sharp left cervical pain was provoked with left unilateral pressures on C6. Segmental joint mobility testing also revealed hypomobility at C5, C7, and T1. In the lumbar spine, segmental hypomobility was noted at the L5–S1 segment, but, as with the active movements and overpressure in standing, there was no provocation of lumbar symptoms with segmental vertebral provocation or mobility tests.

Assessment and Outcome

The referring physician was contacted after the initial evaluation to discuss the discrepancy between the cervical and lumbar findings. There appeared to be a clear correlation between the motor vehicle accident and the cervical symptoms. The accident had precipitated the cervical and shoulder pain, whereas the lumbar complaints had been present before the accident and had not been changed by the accident. The primary reasons for referring the patient back to the physician were insidious onset of low back pain, low back pain being the most intense in the early morning (night pain), and dysuria marked by increased frequency, nocturia, and difficulty in starting the urine stream. It should be noted that when the patient was asked originally if he was experiencing any bowel or bladder dysfunction, he answered no. Further questioning regarding specific examples of bladder dysfunction, such as frequency, waking at night to urinate, and difficulty in starting the urine stream, revealed the important medical information. Clinicians should not assume that the patient understands such terms as bowel and bladder dysfunction. Further medical tests revealed that the patient had prostate cancer.

This case study demonstrates the importance of a thorough investigation of the behavior of all symptoms, including symptom variation over a 24-hour period. The report of severe low back night pain was the initial significant warning or suspicious clue picked up during the evaluation. This finding dictated that a very thorough review of organ system questioning be carried out that ultimately revealed the urinary system complaints.

Also demonstrated during this case is the importance of investigating the chronologic history of all symptoms. It was clear that while the traumatic incident was responsible for the upper-quarter complaints, the accident had nothing to do with the lumbar complaints. The last important factor differentiating the two primary symptomatic regions was being able to reproduce the upper-quarter symptoms with an active movement and passively stressing a cervical vertebral segment, while not being able to reproduce the lumbar symptoms with any of the objective tests.

PATIENT CASE STUDY 2

History

The patient was a 31-year-old bartender who was referred to physical therapy with a diagnosis of mechanical low back pain syndrome. He presented with the chief complaint of constant stiffness and soreness in the central low lumbar and upper sacral region. These symptoms began approximately 4 weeks prior to the evaluation and were attributed to starting a second full-time bartending job. Previous episodes of low back pain were mild and short lived, not requiring medical attention. The current symptoms were aggravated by driving for more than 1 hour and spending more than a couple of hours on his feet. The symptom intensity was decreased by changing positions and taking Nuprin.

The patient also noted intermittent sharp, shooting pain extending from the right flank area into the groin. Intermittent pressure was also noted in this area, but extended further into the right testicle. These symptoms began insidiously approximately 1 month prior to the evaluation and would appear and then resolve irrespective of patient posture or activities. On occasion the sharp pain would wake him from sleep. He had not told the physician of these symptoms, since they had not been present for a couple of days.

The patient's medical history included treatment for psoriasis, and Nuprin was the only medication he was taking. Review of systems questioning revealed intermittent problems of urinary frequency, urgency, and difficulty in starting the urine stream.

Physical Examination

Postural examination revealed a slightly reduced low lumbar lordosis and an absence of a lateral shift. The patient's chief complaint was increased with one repetition of backward bending and central pressures on L5. Backward bending was moderately reduced at L5–S1, as was right side bending, and a left-on-right sacral torsion was noted.

Percussion at and just caudal to the right costovertebral angle caused a slight local sharp sensation, similar to the intermittent pain described by the patient. Mild increased muscle tone was noted in the right upper and mid-abdominal areas compared with the left.

Neurologic examination was negative, and muscle length and strength tests revealed tight buttocks and hamstrings on the left and right sides. A slight weakness of the lower abdominals was also noted.

Assessment and Outcome

The referring physician was contacted regarding the patient's right flank and groin symptoms. Of concern were the urinary difficulties, the inconsistent nature of the symptoms appearing and disappearing regardless of position or activity, provocation only with percussion, and lack of mechanical dysfunction findings to account for these symptoms. These findings contrasted with those associated with the patient's chief complaint. The low lumbar symptoms worsened consistently with a certain amount of driving and a certain amount of time on his feet. These symptoms were increased during the physical examination and felt to be related to the patient's complaints. The referring physician (a neurosurgeon) recommended the patient see his primary care physician.

The patient was examined by the physician, including physical examination, urinalysis, and intravenous pyelogram. The physician called the therapist, stating the tests were negative and was unable to explain the patient's complaints. He recommended that the complaints be monitored by the patient and therapist and that the therapist call in 2 to 3 weeks to report on the patient's status.

There will be cases in which the report from the physician will state that tests are negative and the clinical examination findings inconclusive or negative. The fear of this scenario occurring should not dissuade therapists from referring patients to a physician. In fact, if every patient referred to a physician is diagnosed with disease, the therapist is probably not referring enough patients.

REFERENCES

1. Berne RM, Levy MN (eds): Physiology. 2nd Ed. CV Mosby, St. Louis, 1988
2. Skögeland J: Urology. 2nd Ed. Thieme Medical, New York, 1989
3. DeGroot LJ (ed): Endocrinology. 2nd Ed. Vol. 3. WB Saunders, Philadelphia, 1989
4. Tanagho EA, McAninch JW (eds): General Urology. 13th Ed. Appleton & Lange, E. Norwalk, CT, 1992
5. Schrier RW, Gottschalk CW (eds): Diseases of the Kidney. 4th Ed. Vol. 1. Little, Brown, Boston, 1988
6. Catalona WJ: Prostate Cancer. Harcourt Brace Jovanovich, Orlando, 1984
7. Rous SN: The Prostate Book. WW Norton, New York, 1988
8. Cantwell BM, Mannix KA, Harris AL: Back pain—a presentation of metastatic testicular germ cell tumours. Lancet 1:262, 1987
9. Walsh PC, Retik AB, Stamey TA, Vaughan ED (eds): Campbell's Urology. 6th Ed. Vol. 3. WB Saunders, Philadelphia, 1992
10. Stein JH (ed): Internal Medicine. 2nd Ed. Little, Brown, Boston, 1987
11. Maitland GD: Vertebral Manipulation. 5th Ed. Buttersworth, London, 1986
12. Boissonnault B, Bass C: Pathological origins of trunk and neck pain: part 1—pelvic and abdominal disorders. J Orthop Sports Phys Ther 12:192, 1990
13. Smith DR: General Urology. 11th Ed. p. 28. Lange Medical Publications, Los Altos, CA, 1984
14. Linder HH: Clinical Anatomy. Appleton and Lange, East Norwalk, CT, 1989

SUGGESTED READING

Isselbacher KJ, Braunwald E, Wilson JD et al (eds): Harrison's Principles of Internal Medicine. 13th Ed. McGraw-Hill, New York, 1994

Krane RJ, Siroky MB, Fitzpatrick JM (eds): Clinical Urology. JB Lippincott, Philadelphia, 1994

Tisher CC, Brenner BM (eds): Renal Pathology With Clinical and Functional Correlations. 2nd Ed. Vols. 1, 2. JB Lippincott, Philadelphia, 1994

Walsh PC, Retik AB, Stamey TA, Vaughan ED (eds): Campbell's Urology. 6th Ed. WB Saunders, Philadelphia, 1992

6 Screening for Female Urogenital System Disease

Patricia M. King, M.A., P.T.
Frank W. Ling, M.D.
Craig A. Myers, P.T., M.D.

The female urogenital system includes anatomic structures of the female reproductive tract and the urinary system. The former consists of the uterus, fallopian tubes, ovaries, vagina, external genitalia, and perineum, while the latter includes the kidney, ureters, bladder, and urethra. The anatomy of the upper urinary tract and conditions that affect the kidney and ureters are discussed in Chapter 5. Because of their common embryologic origins, as well as their anatomic juxtaposition, lower urinary tract disorders are discussed in conjunction with those of the female genital tract.

Abdominal, pelvic, and back pain are common symptoms associated with urogenital diseases and frequently encountered by primary care practitioners of obstetrics/gynecology or family medicine. Symptoms in these areas also frequently arise from musculoskeletal dysfunctions of the trunk, spine, and pelvic girdle and are potential points of interface between the physical therapist and physicians. It is essential for the physical therapist to be aware of obstetric and gynecologic concepts that might affect encounters with patients to the degree that the therapist can screen for urogenital disease and make appropriate medical referrals.

This chapter focuses on (1) normal anatomy and physiology of the female reproductive tract, including the normal physiology of pregnancy; (2) the relationship of normal physiology to signs and symptoms frequently seen in a physical therapy evaluation; (3) specific diseases of the female reproductive tract that may be seen by the physical therapist, including common clinical signs and symptoms associated with each; and (4) a summary of historical keys and physical examination findings that will assist the therapist in identifying the patient who may require gynecologic evaluation.

NORMAL ANATOMY AND PHYSIOLOGY

The bony pelvis, which consists of the sacrum, coccyx, and the two innominate bones, houses the female reproductive tract and urinary system. The innominate is composed of the ilium, ischium, and pubis, which are fused in the adult patient. Mobile articulations remain throughout adult female life at the pubic symphysis and the sacroiliac joints. The articular surfaces of the female sacrum are irregularly shaped, with considerable variation from individual to individual. The female sacrum is usually wider and has a shorter articular surface with the ilium than does the male sacrum.[1,2]

The irregular design of the sacrum and its articular surfaces creates sacroiliac articulations that present with the mobility necessary to accommodate the changes in pelvic position associated with pregnancy, labor, and delivery. Weight-bearing of the trunk is provided by the ischium when the patient is sitting, while the lower limbs share in the support of the trunk when the patient is standing, with weight-bearing forces transferred through the sacroiliac articulations. Figures 6-1 and 6-2 depict these structures.[2] The muscles of the pelvic wall or pelvic diaphragm are illustrated in Figures 6-3 to 6-5.[2]

The primary musculature supporting the pelvic floor is the levator ani, which has three components: the iliococcygeus, the pubococcygeus, and the puborectalis muscles. The fascial sheath surrounding these muscles is derived from the transversalis fascia. The pelvic floor muscles provide support for the pelvic viscera and must also withstand the force of gravity as well as intra-abdominal pressure increases that occur with straining, lifting, and elimination. Despite their significant functional role, the pelvic floor muscles are often poorly developed in women,[3] particularly those with sedentary lifestyles and those who have gone through pregnancy and childbirth without attention to physical conditioning.

The musculature of the perineum is shown in Figures 6-6 and 6-7. The primary neurologic supply for this area is demonstrated in Figure 6-8. The pudendal nerve, supplied by the 2nd, 3rd, and 4th sacral nerve roots, is the primary motor and sensory nerve to the perineum. The pelvic viscera is supported anteriorly by the abdominal musculature, which derives innervation from spinal nerve root levels T7–L1. Considering these levels of innervation and the referred pain phenomena, it can be concluded that symptoms of urogenital dysfunction can easily be confused with or masked by symptoms of musculoskeletal dysfunction in the trunk, pelvic girdle, and spine.

The internal genital organs are pictured in Figures 6-9 and 6-10. The organs of the female reproductive tract include the ovaries, the fallopian tubes, the uterus and cervix, and the vagina. The bladder, distal aspects of the ureter, and the urethra lie in close proximity to these internal genital organs. Also in close anatomic proximity are loops of small intestine, the ileocecal junction on the right and the sigmoid colon and rectum on the left.

The ovaries are normally 1 × 2 × 3 cm and lie against the lateral pelvic sidewall. These are the female gonads, the organs of the female reproductive tract that produce hormones, primarily estrogen and progesterone. The fallopian tubes are attached medially to the uterus and open distally at their fimbriated end, which is open to the abdominal cavity. This relationship between the uterus and abdominal cavity can be significant in the spread of infection and endometriosis, both of which are addressed later in this chapter (Fig. 6-11). The fallopian tube is normally approximately 10 cm in length. Its location in the pelvis varies, as it is fairly free to move about within the pelvis. The uterus is the organ in which a normal pregnancy implants and develops. It is also the origin of menstrual flow. It is situated between the rectum posteriorly and the bladder anteriorly (Fig. 6-9). The uppermost portion is termed the fundus. The junction between the uterus and the vagina is the cervix, the portion of the uterus visible upon vaginal inspection. The vagina (birth canal) is the fibromuscular tube that connects the internal genital organs with the labia. It is in close contact posteriorly with the rectum, as it is with the bladder anteriorly. Poor pelvic muscle support may

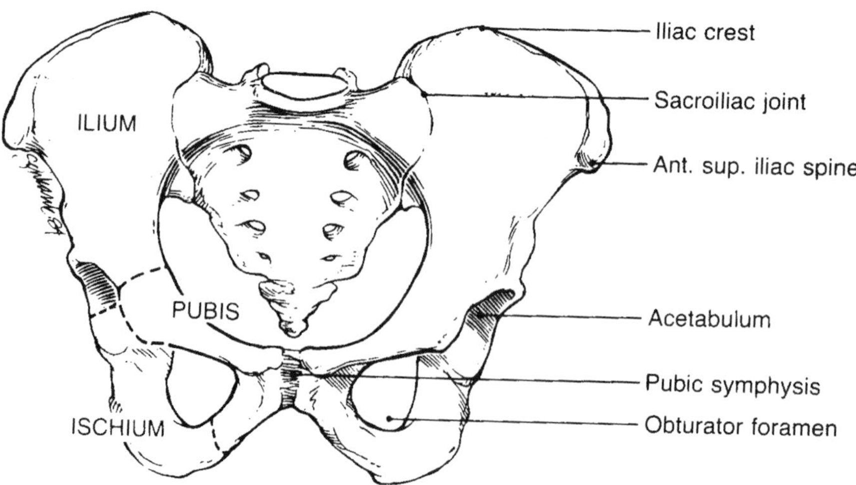

Fig. 6-1. Osseous anatomy of the pelvic girdle. (From Gould,[2] with permission.)

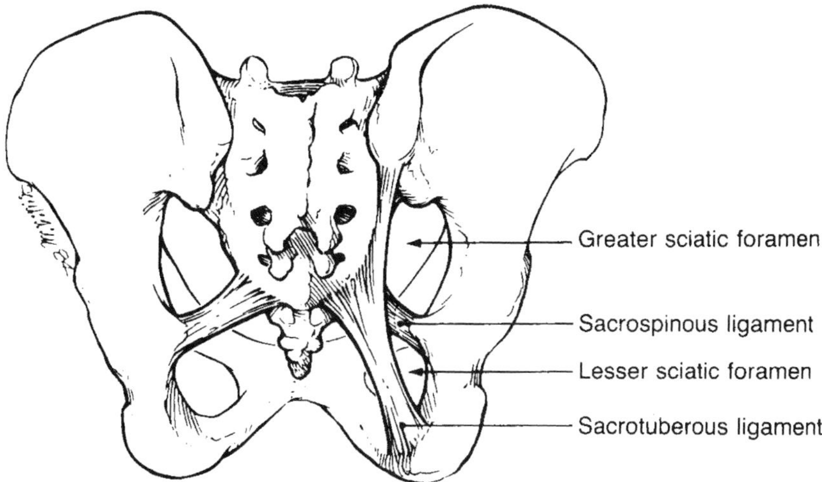

Fig. 6-2. Osseous and ligamentous anatomy of the pelvic girdle. (From Gould,[2] with permission.)

result in prolapse of bladder or rectal structures into the vagina. The internal female genital organs are palpable during a routine gynecologic bimanual pelvic examination. Unless the anatomy is altered by pregnancy or pathologic enlargement, they should not be palpable by abdominal palpation.

The nerves of the pelvis are illustrated in Figure 6-12. The lateral pelvic wall is the site of the nerve plexuses that supply the pelvic structures. Table 6-1 illustrates the nerve root values for innervation of the pelvic viscera and related structures as well as potential sites of referred pain from each structure.

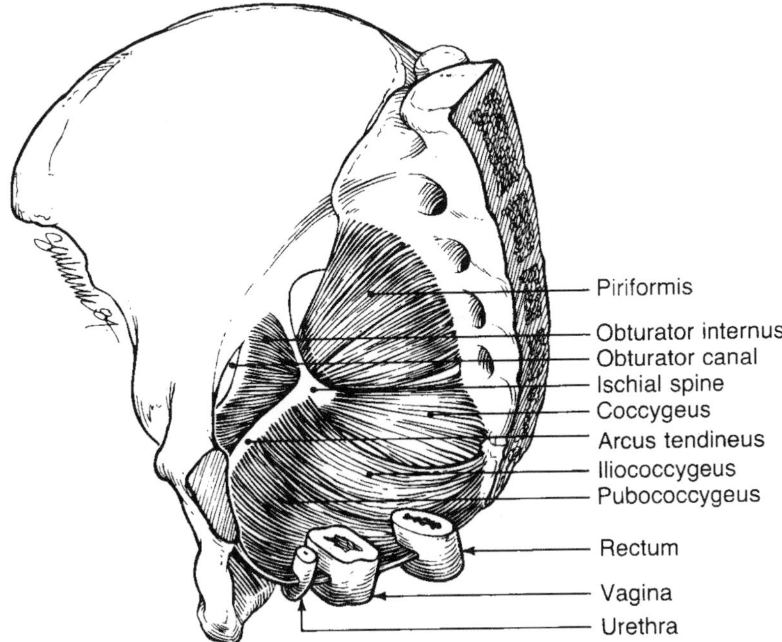

Fig. 6-3. Muscles of the pelvic diaphragm, oblique view. (From Gould,[2] with permission.)

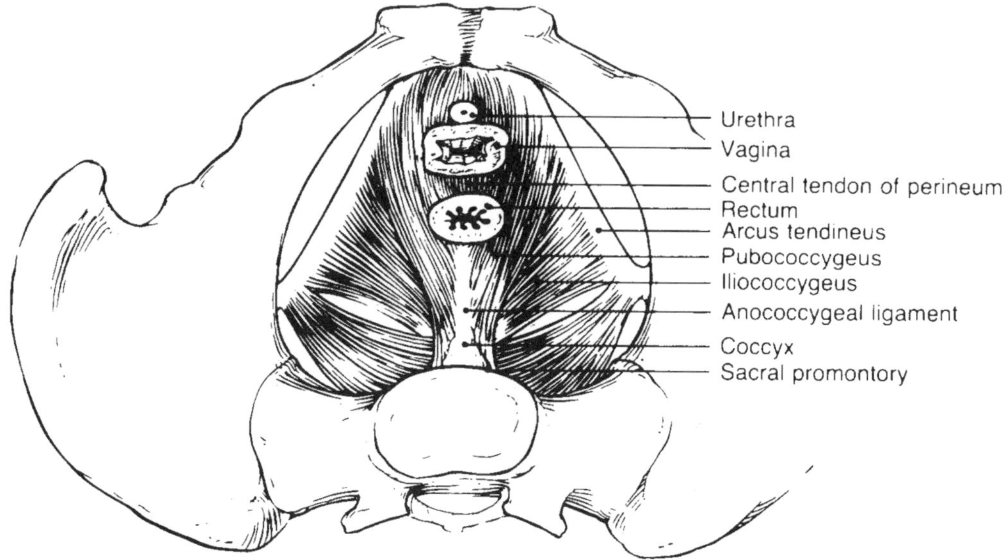

Fig. 6-4. Muscles of the pelvic diaphragm, superior view. (From Gould,[2] with permission.)

Menstrual Physiology

The normal menstrual cycle and its hormones are depicted in Figure 6-13.[4] The menstrual cycle is functionally divided into three phases: the menstrual phase (when menses occurs), the proliferative phase (during which time the ovarian follicle develops in preparation for ovulation), and the luteal phase (during which time the endometrium of the uterus is prepared for possible implantation of a pregnancy). The entire cycle lasts an average of 28 days. Ovulation occurs at what is termed the midcycle, an event that occurs typically 2 weeks before any subsequent menstrual flow.

The primary hormone of the follicular (proliferative) phase is estrogen, specifically estradiol, produced by the ovary. Progesterone is the predominant hormone of the

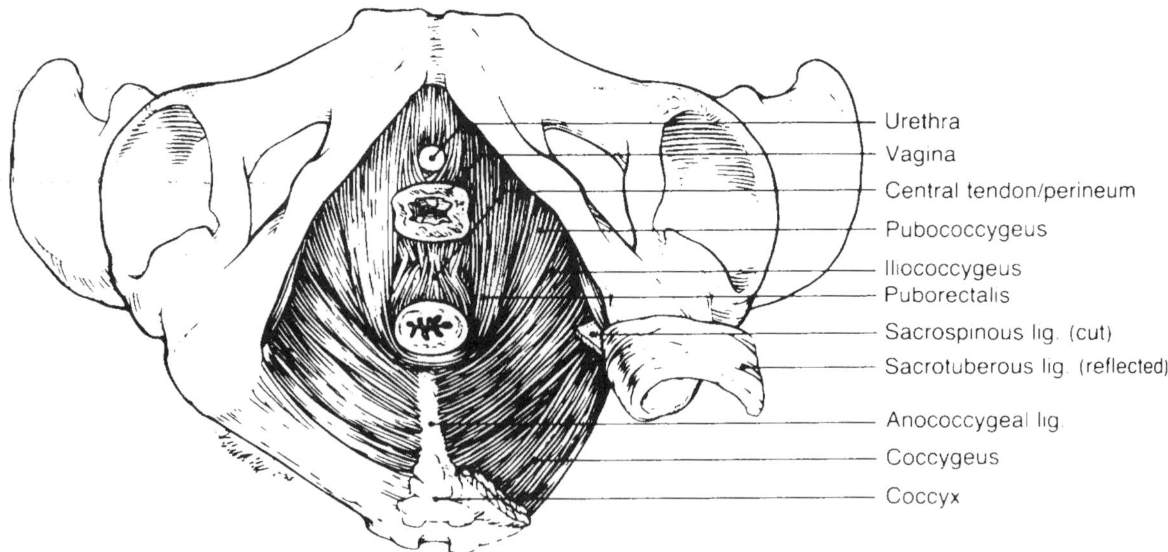

Fig. 6-5. Muscles of the pelvic diaphragm, inferior view. (From Gould,[2] with permission.)

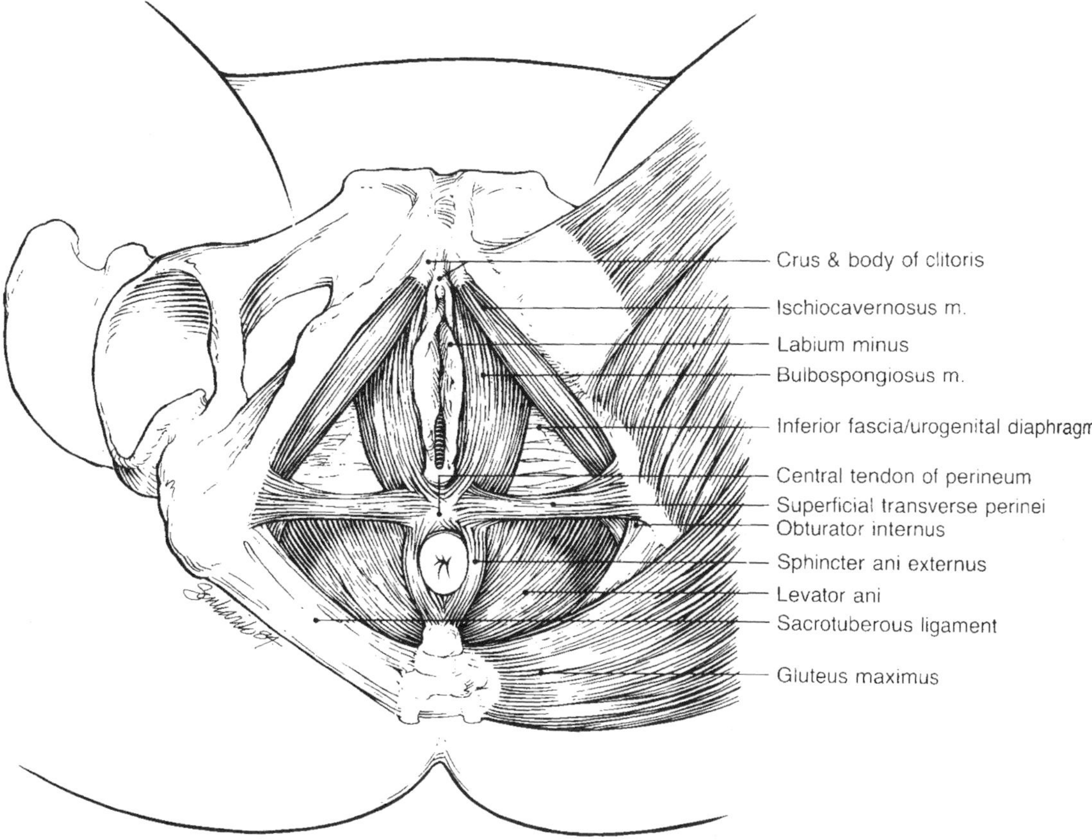

Fig. 6-6. Muscles of the perineum, inferior view. (From Gould,[2] with permission.)

luteal phase and is produced by the corpus luteum of the ovary. Relaxin is also produced in the corpus luteum during the luteal phase and is responsible for the ligamentous laxity noted primarily in the pelvic articulations during this phase.[5,6] This is significant information for physical therapists managing female patients for any musculoskeletal dysfunction but particularly those of the lumbar spine and pelvis. The presence of relaxin in the luteal phase of all normally menstruating women may enhance laxity and reduce a patient's tolerance to stretch and exercise. A physical therapist unaware of the female patient's status in the menstrual cycle may progress that patient to a more difficult or strenuous level of active or passive exercise in what is a logical sequence based on the patient's previous response. The therapist may be surprised at an unexpected negative response to treatment such as increased pain and/or inflammation that could result from the effects of relaxin on the articulations combined with an increase in stress on the tissue.

If no pregnancy occurs, hormonal support of the lining of the uterus (endometrium) is withdrawn, and a menstrual flow results. If pregnancy does occur,

Table 6-1. Referred Pain: Female Urogenital System

Structure	Segmental Innervation	Potential Site of Local Referred Pain
Ovaries	T10–T11	Lower abdomen, low back
Uterus	T10–L1	Lower abdomen, low back
Fallopian tubes	T10–L1	Lower abdomen, low back
Perineum	S2–S4	Sacral apex, suprapubic, rectum
External genitalia	L1–L2, S3–S4	Lower abdomen, medial anterior thigh, sacrum
Kidney	T10–L1	Ipsilateral low back and upper abdominal
Urinary bladder	T11–L2, S2–S4	Thoracolumbar, sacrococcygeal, suprapubic
Ureters	T11–L2, S2–S4	Groin, upper and lower abdomen, suprapubic, anterior-medial thigh, thoracolumbar

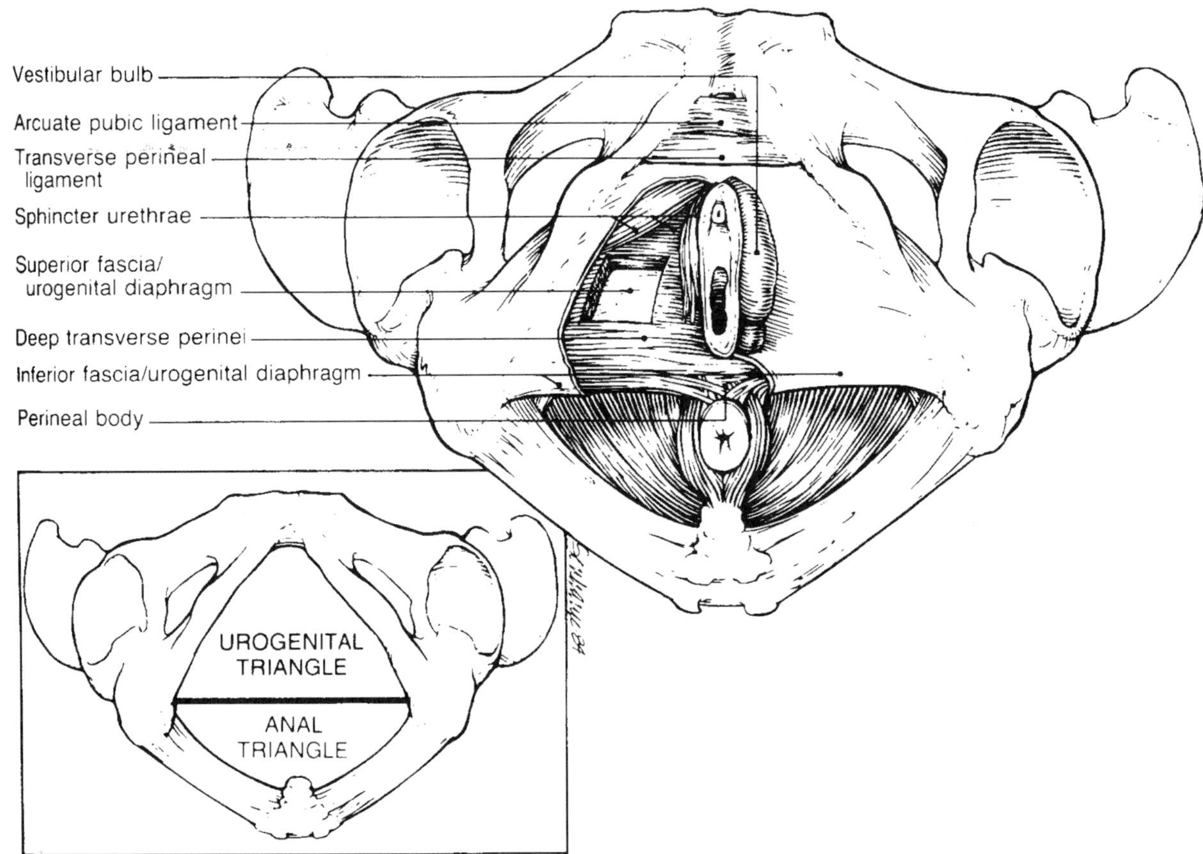

Fig. 6-7. Muscles of the perineum, inferior view; urogenital triangle. (From Gould,[2] with permission.)

hormonal support for the endometrium is provided by the placenta.

Signs and Symptoms of Normal Pregnancy

- Nausea and vomiting
- Frequent urination
- Supine hypotension
- Posture and mobility changes
- Thoracic outlet syndromes
- Carpal tunnel syndrome
- Edema in hands and feet
- Breast tenderness
- Fatigue
- Dyspnea

Physiology of Pregnancy

Anatomy and physiology are markedly altered during pregnancy to support the growth and development of the fetus. The mother must adapt both physically as well as physiologically and emotionally to these changes.

The Spine

The increasing girth of the abdomen contributes to the progressive development of lumbar lordosis posture during pregnancy. Of particular interest to the physical therapist is a noted increase in mobility of the pubic, sacrococcygeal, and sacroiliac joints that manifests during pregnancy apparently in response to increased progesterone and relaxin levels.[6] This increased mobility appears to contribute to the typical maternal posture, which is dominated by the development of an anterior pelvic tilt, exaggerated lumbar lordotic curve, and out-

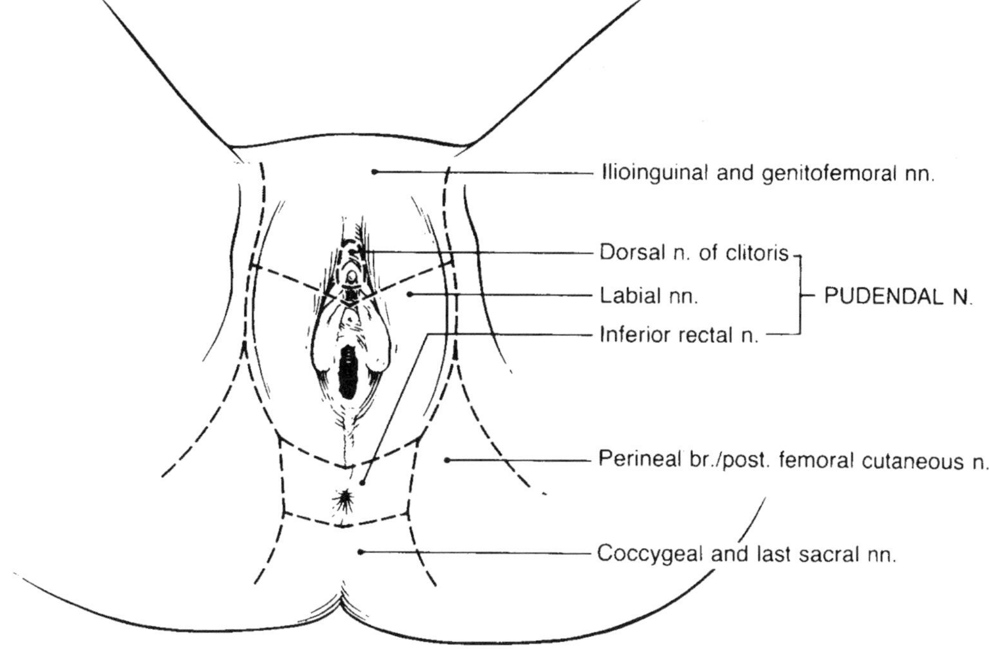

Fig. 6-8. Neurologic supply to the perineum. (From Gould,[2] with permission.)

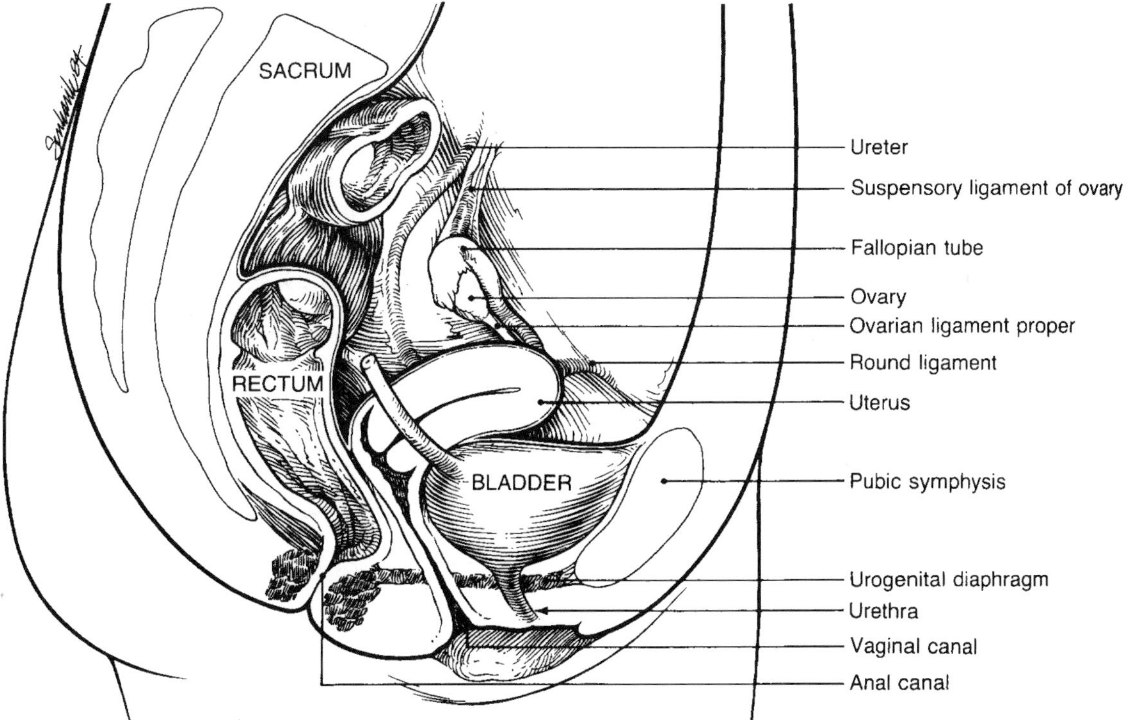

Fig. 6-9. Urogenital organs, sagittal section. (From Gould,[2] with permission.)

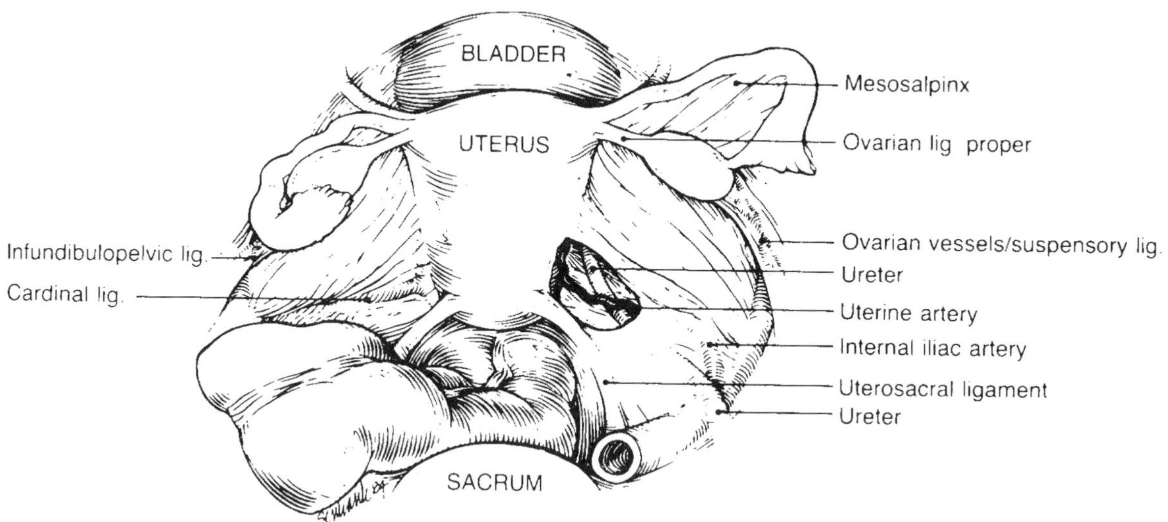

Fig. 6-10. Urogenital organs, posterior view. (From Gould,[2] with permission.)

flare of the ilium. The outflare of the ilium and the abdominal girth tend to place the patient in external rotation of the hips—a position of capsular shortening for the hip—during pregnancy. The patient's center of gravity is altered by the expanding abdominal girth and posture changes that may result in a sense of awkwardness during gait and other functional activities. Discomfort in the low back is a common symptom throughout pregnancy associated with these changes. Exercise programs that emphasize posture, strength, and

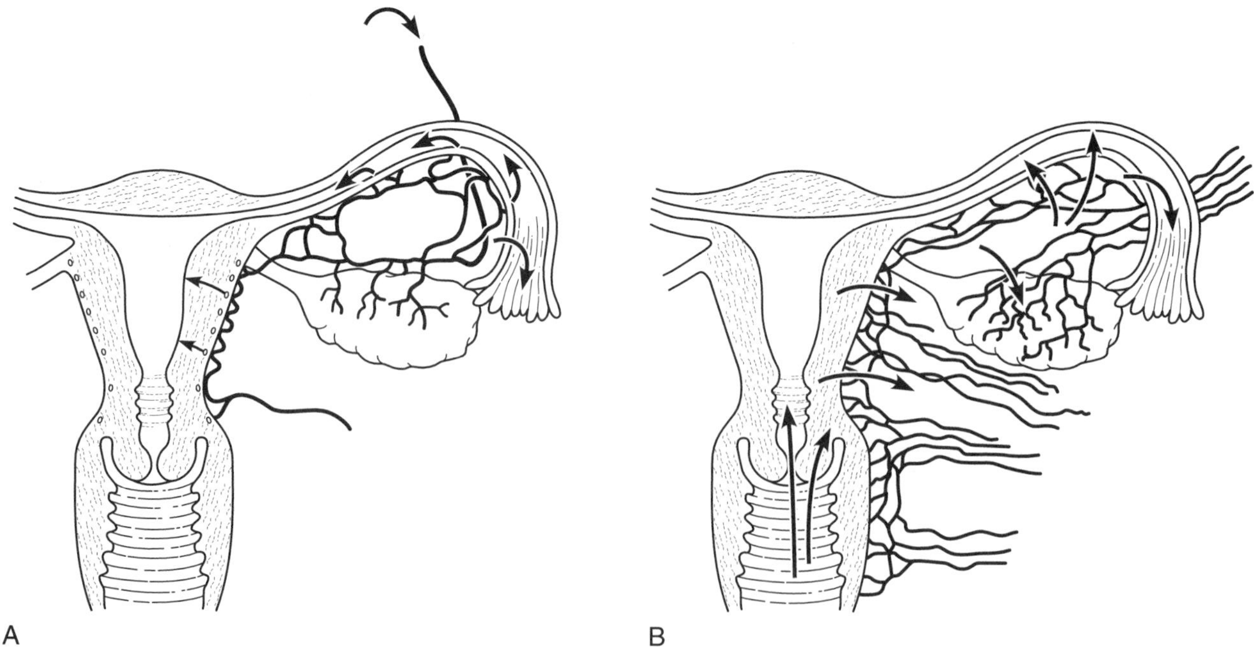

Fig. 6-11. (A) Hematogenous spread of bacterial infection. **(B)** Lymphatic spread of bacterial infection. (From Pernoll and Benson,[5] with permission.)

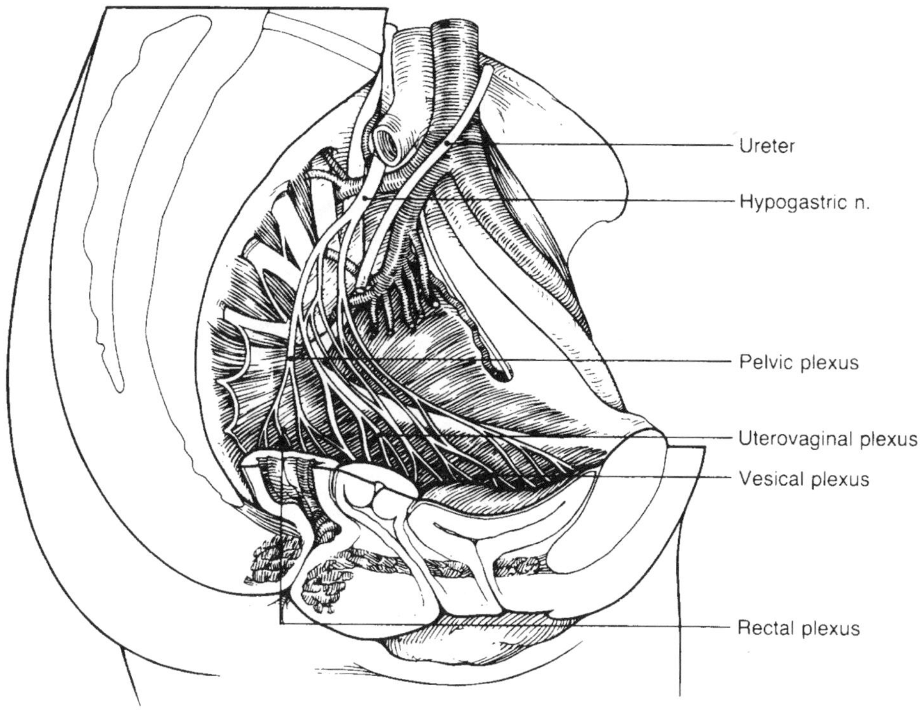

Ureter
Hypogastric n.
Pelvic plexus
Uterovaginal plexus
Vesical plexus
Rectal plexus

Fig. 6-12. Neurologic supply to the urogenital organs, lateral view. (From Gould,[2] with permission.)

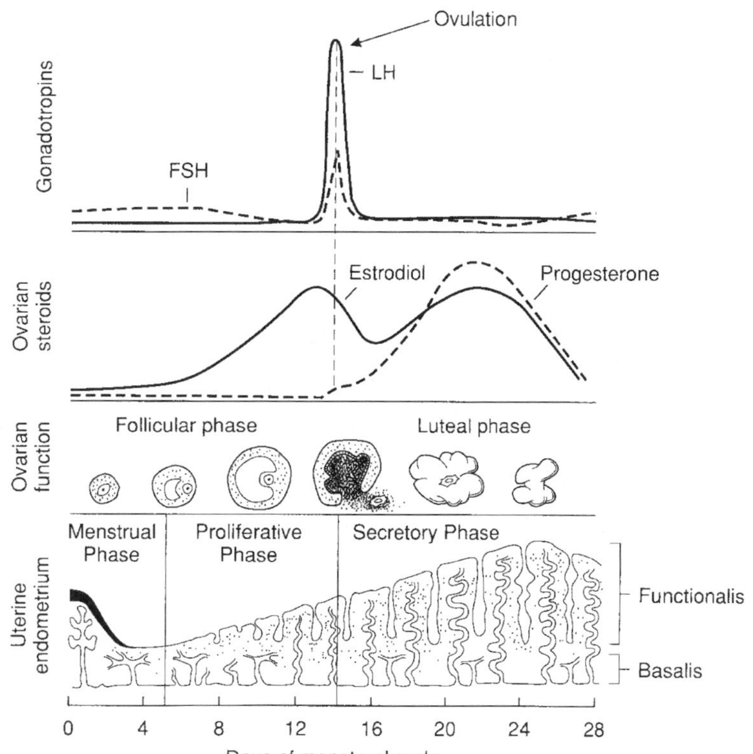

Fig. 6-13. Normal menstrual cycle. (From Hacker and Moore,[4] with permission.)

flexibility are an important aspect of prenatal care that may minimize symptoms from musculoskeletal dysfunction. Attention should be given to maintaining abdominal muscle strength as well as trunk and extremity flexibility and strength. The goal of exercise programs directed to these areas is not to prevent the increasing lordosis but to maintain strength that will be needed for delivery and postpartum child care.[3]

Late in pregnancy, weakness and paresthesia of the upper extremities are also frequently reported. This may partially result from musculoskeletal changes associated with the forward head/thoracic kyphotic posture that often develops along with lumbar and pelvic postural changes. This posture may cause compression of the neurovascular structures of the thoracic outlet region. Fluid retention is common throughout pregnancy and may also contribute to the development of nerve compression syndromes, particularly in the distal extremities. Physical therapists are familiar with the sensory and motor changes associated with thoracic outlet and carpal tunnel syndromes, both of which may manifest during pregnancy and should respond to posture, active exercise, and soft tissue stretching treatment programs.

Weight Gain

The average weight gain during pregnancy is 25 to 30 pounds, with individual variations commonly seen. The sheer weight increase is manifest as easy fatigability and pressure sensations of the lower abdomen and lower back. Diastasis of the abdominal wall musculature may also occur in the second or third trimester as a result of abdominal musculature stretch from the increased abdominal size and the tissue relaxation that occurs in response to hormonal changes.

Diastasis Recti Abdominis

Diastasis recti abdominis results from separation of the abdominal musculature in the midline of the linea alba that is thought to be associated with both mechanical stretch and tissue relaxation during pregnancy (Fig. 6-14).[5] Diastasis of the abdominal wall has been shown to be more common in the third trimester and also occurs in the second trimester and postpartum.[6,7] Specific complaints of discomfort are not usually associated with this dysfunction. It is, however, expected that a significant abdominal separation will negatively affect abdominal muscle functioning in posture, respiration, and childbirth. A severe diastasis may result in the herniation of abdominal viscera.

It is important during pregnancy and postpartum to identify the presence of a diastasis so the abdominals may be protected from further stress. To check for the presence of diastasis recti, patients should be positioned in hooklying and asked to lift the head and shoulders off the examining table with arms extended towards the knees. The clinician should palpate horizontally across the linea alba

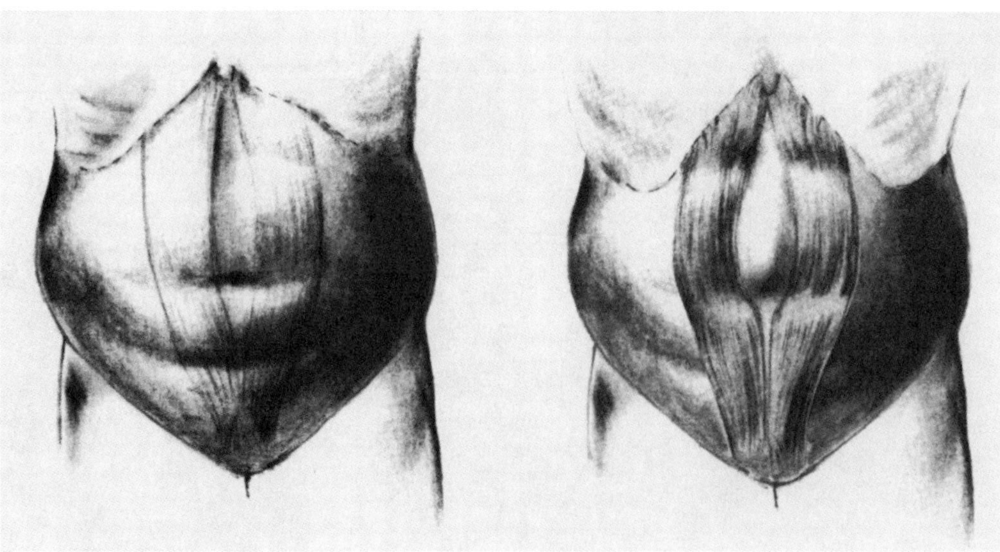

Fig. 6-14. Diagrammatic representations of diastasis recti. (From Boissonnault and Kotarinos,[19] with permission.)

with fingertips to determine how many fingers can be placed between the borders of the right and left rectus abdominis. Measurements of less than two fingers, which correlates with the normal anatomic separation of approximately 2 cm, are considered normal. Measurements should be taken through the full length of the linea alba.[3,6] Patients with abnormal rectus separation should modify abdominal strengthening exercises so that arms are crossed on the trunk with hands supporting the abdomen. Only the head should be cleared from the supporting surface in abdominal exercise until the gap has been noted to close. All abdominal strengthening exercises should be coordinated with exhale on exertion to allow more efficient muscle action.

Vascular and Skin Changes

During pregnancy, ovulation obviously ceases, and the corpus luteum of the ovary supports the pregnancy only during the first 6 to 7 weeks of the pregnancy. Hormonal support thereafter is provided by the placenta. During pregnancy, there is increased blood flow and vascularity in the skin of the vagina and the perineum. The skin becomes markedly pigmented in the midline (linea nigra), and angiomas (vascular spiders) develop in many patients.

The physiologic effects of pregnancy result in an intravascular volume increased 50 percent, with the plasma component increasing approximately twice as much as the red cell mass, resulting in a physiologic fall in hematocrit during pregnancy. This increased vascular volume is partially responsible for the weight gain and edema associated with pregnancy.

Blood Pressure

During pregnancy, blood pressure typically drops, with a maximum change seen at 20 to 24 weeks. A gradual rise to prepregnancy levels occurs as the patient approaches term. The mean drop in blood pressure is approximately 8 to 10 mmHg. Heart rate typically increases 12 to 18 bpm, and cardiac output is increased by approximately one third. Many biochemical and hematologic blood indices are changed during normal pregnancy. These include the urine chemistries, serum chemistries, serum enzymes, and serum hormones.

The enlarging uterus also compresses the iliac veins and inferior vena cava, thereby reducing venous return from the lower extremities. Supine hypotension is of significant concern, as fetal and uterine weight gain increase throughout pregnancy. There is some disagreement as to the point in pregnancy at which the supine position becomes a significant risk. The guidelines for exercise published by the American College of Obstetricians and Gynecologists[8] suggest that exercise should not be performed in the supine position after completion of the fourth month of gestation. Others suggest that exercising in the supine position is not a risk until after the seventh month of pregnancy, when supine positioning does not need to be completely avoided but monitored.[9,10] All pregnant women should be advised, however, to change positions if they become faint, dizzy, or nauseous while in the supine position. Physical therapists should be aware of this when positioning patients for treatment and advising them regarding home positions for rest and exercise. Lying on the left side with pillow support between the lower extremities is the preferred rest position, especially late in pregnancy, for reducing lower extremity edema and other problems associated with vascular congestion.

Increases in the pressure in the veins of the pelvis and legs also result from venous compression in the trunk. In response to these changes, an increase in the incidence of hemorrhoids and varicose veins is seen during pregnancy. Maintenance of pelvic floor strength as well as regular exercise and attention to diet may reduce the severity and/or incidence of hemorrhoids.

Urinary Tract

The urinary tract is dilated during pregnancy, more prominently on the right than on the left. This probably occurs secondary to both hormonal and biomechanical factors. Progesterone relaxes the smooth muscle of these organs and others throughout the body and is therefore responsible for part of the distension. Partial obstruction of the ureter is also induced by the enlarging uterus. Urinary frequency is a common occurrence throughout pregnancy. Women should be encouraged to empty the bladder completely before and after exercise. Maintenance of pelvic floor muscle strength should be emphasized throughout pregnancy to maintain support of these distended structures and to avoid unnecessarily severe symptoms of pelvic relaxation postpartum. Recent research indicates that the most efficient pelvic floor contractions are achieved when combined with simultaneous abdominal contraction as in the posterior pelvic tilt position.[11]

Diabetes

Pregnancy is also a diabetogenic state. Insulin resistance occurs after the first trimester of pregnancy, so that there is prolonged elevation of glucose after meals. A series of hormonal factors have been implicated, with the resultant increased need for the use of insulin in pregnant patients who do not display a predisposing factor for diabetes in the nonpregnant state. Although the thyroid gland normally enlarges during pregnancy, the free, biologically active concentration of both T_3 and T_4 is unchanged from the nonpregnant state.

Some pregnant women demonstrate abnormal carbohydrate metabolism, arbitrarily defined as a 2-hour postprandial glucose level greater than 129 mg/dL following 100 g carbohydrate. These women may be diagnosed as manifesting pregnancy-induced glucose intolerance—a term that is often favored over the more commonly used gestational diabetes, which has been associated with negative psychological connotations, problems with insurance coverage, and other issues associated with a diagnosis of diabetes. Risk factors identified with glucose intolerance during pregnancy include the following: previous glucose intolerance; maternal age of 25 or more; family history of diabetes; obesity; birth weight above 9 pounds in previous baby; death in previous fetus or newborn; glycosuria (glucose in the urine—fasting); recurrent infections—general or urinary tract.[5]

Nonweight-bearing exercising has been suggested in the management of gestational diabetes or pregnancy-induced glucose intolerance due to the preferential carbohydrate use that has been noted in nonweight-bearing versus weight-bearing exercise.[12] Nonweight-bearing exercise has also been suggested to be advantageous in pregnancy as a lower injury risk activity than many weight-bearing activities, which may be more difficult due to weight gain and center of gravity of changes associated with pregnancy. Chapter 7 provides more information on the topic of diabetes.

Respiration

Respiratory changes occur during pregnancy as a result of the mechanical effects of the enlarging uterus, the increase in oxygen consumption, and the stimulatory effect of progesterone on respiration. The enlarging uterus interferes with the activity of the diaphragm, particularly during the last trimester, causing an increased demand on the accessory muscles of respiration such as the scalenes and pectoralis minor. The increased activity in these muscles may contribute to the development of thoracic outlet syndrome symptoms, along with the postural changes previously mentioned. Dyspnea is a common complaint, and although pregnant women are encouraged to remain physically active they may need to make modifications in the intensity of exercise in response to hyperventilation and dyspnea.

Osteonecrosis and Osteoporosis

Rare cases of transient osteoporosis of the hip during pregnancy have been reported with no risk factors identified other than pregnancy.[13] Hip and leg pain progressively worsening and increased by weight bearing are the chief complaints reported. These complaints may be confused with the symptoms of the other common and less serious musculoskeletal changes of pregnancy. The onset of symptoms secondary to osteoporosis is reported to occur in the third trimester. The symptoms and bone density changes usually resolve shortly after delivery. Physical therapy is suggested to maintain strength and prevent contractures as treatment-involved activity decreases during the remainder of the pregnancy.

Osteonecrosis of the femoral head and of the humerus have been reported to occur during pregnancy with no other known associated risk factors.[14,15] This condition is also rare yet serious. The rehabilitation phase for osteonecrosis is much longer than for osteoporosis, extending several months postpartum, and may involve surgical intervention as well as limited functional return depending on the severity of the condition. The symptoms are of the same character as those described for osteoporosis and are also reported to manifest during the third trimester.

The etiology of both osteonecrosis and osteoporosis during pregnancy is unclear, although many factors associated with pregnancy, including hormonal effects on bone metabolism as well as vascular and neurologic compression syndrome, have been suggested as possibilities. Maintenance of physical activity, joint flexibility, and strength could play a role in prevention of both of these conditions. The intracapsular location of the blood supply to the head of the humerus may make it particularly susceptible to necrosis in any condition that increases capsular compression as does pregnancy posture. So, although they occur rarely, it is important for the clinician to be aware that these pathologies may occur in patients exhibiting third-trimester joint pain that is worsened by activity and unresolved with usual treatment interventions. Referral to a physician is of course recommended if either of these conditions is suspected. Osteoporosis is discussed further in Chapter 10.

Summary of Pregnancy Signs and Symptoms

Nausea and vomiting are common during the first trimester. Small, frequent meals with bland foods are a typical solution to the problem. Bland snacks such as soda crackers are also helpful. These symptoms typically resolve after the first trimester. Urinary frequency is seen throughout pregnancy, especially later in pregnancy, as the enlarging uterus and fetus impinge on the bladder. Supine hypotension is also common as pregnancy progresses. Low back pain, hip pain, and leg pain are caused by the increasing abdominal girth and extra weight that the patient must endure. Posture and mobility changes in these areas associated with the normal physiology of pregnancy may contribute to these symptoms. When these symptoms do not respond to typical treatment, more serious conditions such as transient osteoporosis and osteonecrosis should be considered, although their incidence is rare. Signs and symptoms associated with thoracic outlet and carpal tunnel syndromes also occur in pregnancy in response to vascular and postural changes. Edema of both the hands and the feet are common complaints. Breast tenderness is an early sign of pregnancy; later in pregnancy, it may be due to engorgement of the breasts. Generalized fatigue is a common finding throughout pregnancy and is best managed with additional rest and participation in a regular exercise program. Dyspnea is also a common complaint during pregnancy as a result of biomechanic and physiologic changes.

PHYSICAL THERAPY EVALUATION

As the physical therapist evaluates a patient, historical and/or physical findings are often elicited in addition to those communicated from the referring practitioner. Knowledge of the fundamental changes that occur in a woman's menstrual cycle and during normal pregnancy will help the physical therapist determine what may be pathologic as opposed to what may be physiologic.

Common Physical Findings

Pain
Bleeding
Vaginal discharge or burning
Breast tenderness
Urinary changes
Dyspareunia
Nausea and vomiting

Pain

Pain is the most common complaint presenting to the physical therapist. With regard to the normal menstrual cycle, the pattern of pain must be determined, that is, whether the pain is chronic or periodic. If periodic, it is useful to determine whether it is cyclic and predictable or whether it is unpredictable and noncyclic. Often a calendar of symptoms helps the patient determine when the pain becomes bothersome. Mild discomfort associated with the menstrual period (dysmenorrhea) is common. Pain that lasts 1 or 2 days at ovulation (*Mittelschmerz*) is normal and is associated with peritoneal irritation caused by ovulation. Pain that cannot be attributed to either of these entities (e.g., excessive dysmenorrhea) should be looked on as pathologic and requires further investigation. If pain is aggravated by particular activities and relieved by rest, a musculoskeletal component may be suspected as either a primary or a secondary factor. Aching in the low back, buttocks, and posterior and anterior thighs is a common complaint during the luteal phase, apparently associated with the hormone-induced musculoskeletal laxity, and this pain, like musculoskeletal pain, is often aggravated by activity, better with rest but follows a cyclic pattern. Many patients are diagnostically labeled as having chronic pelvic pain by the gynecologist.[16] This usually refers to the presence of lower abdominal pain that is either cyclic or noncyclic for a period of more than 6 months. Endometriosis, pelvic relaxation disorders, pelvic inflammatory disease, musculoskeletal dysfunction, and other conditions may be responsible for such symptoms.

Bleeding

Bleeding is considered normal only as part of the normal menstrual cycle. There should, therefore, be a cyclic predictability of the timing, amount, and duration of bleeding. The number of days from the first day of one period to the first day of the next period should be fairly constant. Women occasionally have anovulatory cycles in which a period is delayed or skipped because she failed to ovulate that month. There may, occasionally, be midcycle spotting just after ovulation. This is due to the sudden drop in estrogen at the time of ovulation (shown in Fig. 6-13).

Bleeding that does not conform to these guidelines, sudden changes in a patient's bleeding pattern, or any bleeding during pregnancy should be looked on as abnormal. It should be remembered that anovulatory cycles are more common and frequent in women during adolescence as well as during the years when ovarian function is waning, a time of life also known as the *perimenopause*.

Menopause, the permanent cessation of menses, typically occurs after the age of 40, leading to menopause at an average age of 51. A decrease in cycle length and quantity of bleeding typically leads to complete cessation of vaginal bleeding. It is most unusual for women to report vaginal bleeding 6 months after menopause. Women who report increase in frequency and intensity of vaginal bleeding after menopause should be referred to a gynecologist for assessment for the presence of organic disease. Outpatient endometrial biopsy or inpatient D & C are the typical approaches.[3]

Vaginal Discharge or Burning

Vaginal discharge is also a common complaint. Occasionally, patients complain of a discharge that is actually physiologic. Physiologic leukorrhea is an exaggeration of the normal moisture in the vagina. This is common in the second trimester of pregnancy. Physiologic discharge is produced by a combination of mucus secreted from the glands of the cervix mixed with the desquamated cells from the vaginal walls. This appears as a white, curdlike discharge that reaches a maximum at the time of ovulation, when there is a maximum of mucus stimulated by estrogen production. This decreases during the luteal phase of the cycle and becomes more sticky and opaque because of the effects of progesterone.

Vaginal burning and vaginal discharge are commonly associated with one another. Patients often describe a yellow or greenish discharge which may be foul smelling. These symptoms are commonly associated with urinary symptoms as the discharge irritates the urethral meatus. *Vaginal dryness* in menopausal patients is often associated with a lack of estrogen support. The vaginal dryness can also be seen in conjunction with urinary frequency and dysuria in the postmenopausal patient.

Breast Tenderness/ Abdominal Bloating

Breast tenderness is occasionally seen in women with fibrocystic breasts. Because of the hormonal changes of the menstrual cycle, there is an exaggeration in tenderness of the breast tissue during the luteal phase of the menstrual cycle. Typically, this pain should resolve shortly after the onset of the menstrual flow. Similarly, some women complain of lower abdominal swelling and bloating on a cyclic basis. Again, these typically occur in the luteal phase and resolve after the onset of menses. Breast tenderness is also an early sign of pregnancy. Breast symptoms or lower abdominal swelling that do not follow a cyclic pattern or are not associated with pregnancy should be investigated as possible manifestations of significant pathology.

Breast pain other than the cyclic pain of fibrocystic breasts or that associated with pregnancy should be looked on as abnormal. Often, however, patients are unable to differentiate breast pain from chest wall pain. Palpation of the affected area can often differentiate musculoskeletal pain from the pain of the primarily fatty tissue and glands of the breasts in female patients. The thoracic spine and costochondral and costovertebral articulations may all refer pain into the anterior chest. These articulations should be evaluated by the physical therapist in patients who have been cleared of breast disease or normal breast tenderness but continue to complain of anterior chest wall pain. All women should participate in a monthly breast self-examination routine to screen for breast cancer. Routine gynecologic consultation includes instruction in breast self-examination.

Urinary Changes

Urinary signs and symptoms should always suggest a possible problem, with the exception of those described as a normal part of pregnancy. Urinary tract disorders frequently refer pain to the low back and abdomen (Table 6-1) and should be considered in patients presenting with complaints in those areas.

The following symptoms may suggest a urinary tract infection that should be evaluated using urinalysis and possible culture and sensitivity: pyuria (cloudy urine), dysuria (pain with urination), hematuria (bloody urine), frequency (frequent need to urinate), urgency (immediate sense of the need to void), and incontinence (loss of the normal control of micturition). Incontinence can also be evidence of symptomatic pelvic relaxation (see under Specific Disorders) or of a loss of neurologic control of the bladder. In addition, it is seen in patients with urethral diverticula (outpouching of the urethra). Because of the proximity of the vagina and the urethra, patients with pathologic vaginal discharge can also present with symptoms simulating a urinary tract infection.

Dyspareunia

Dyspareunia (painful intercourse) is associated with both physiologic and psychological factors. Superficial or "entrance" dyspareunia is most commonly associated with a lack of arousal, as manifested by a lack of vaginal lubrication. This type of dyspareunia may also be associated with vaginitis, urethritis, vaginismus (an involuntary contraction of the pelvic musculature), or other dysfunctions of the pelvic floor. Significant problems of the urethra or bladder can be associated with entrance dyspareunia. Deep thrust dyspareunia is seen with conditions of the pelvis, such as endometriosis, pelvic infection, fibroid tumors, or ovarian cysts. In addition, dyspareunia that occurs in specific positions and not present in other coitus positions is more likely related to mechanical or musculoskeletal dysfunction than gynecologic disease.

Nausea and Vomiting

Nausea and vomiting are most commonly associated with early pregnancy. If pregnancy is not a possibility or has been ruled out, it should be remembered that nausea may be associated with any significant pain. Nausea may also present as a symptom of supine hypotension along with faintness and fatigue. Nausea and vomiting should otherwise be looked upon as a manifestation of gastrointestinal disease, and appropriate referral for medical evaluation of such symptoms is indicated (see Ch. 4).

SPECIFIC DISEASES

Endometriosis

Endometriosis is a condition typically confined to the pelvis in which tissue from the endometrium is present outside the endometrial cavity, typically in the peritoneum, around the fallopian tubes, ovaries, and rectum. The cause is unknown. Symptoms attributed to endometriosis include bilateral or unilateral lower abdominal or low sacral pain, dysmenorrhea, painful intercourse (dyspareunia), abnormal bleeding, premenstrual staining, and infertility. This history in a woman in her 20s or 30s should suggest the diagnosis. Clinical suspicion based on symptoms leads to the diagnosis, which can only be confirmed by direct observation of endometriotic lesions. These lesions are classically described as brownish, bluish, or black lesions, the color a result of recurrent hemorrhage in the area. Intense fibrosis is also associated with these lesions. Since the lesions are typically in the pelvis, visualization by means of a surgical operation is usually necessary. Under unusual circumstances, endometriosis can be visualized externally, for example, on the perineum or at the site of a previous abdominal incision. Other than visualization or histologic confirmation on biopsy, or both, no other tests are available to make this diagnosis.

Pain from endometriosis is thought to be produced by pressure or perhaps infection associated with the endometrial adhesions. There are many women, however, with extrauterine endometrial tissue who have no complaints of pain. The diagnosis of endometriosis should not therefore preclude screening for musculoskeletal dysfunction, as physical therapy has been found to be effective in the management of chronic pelvic pain associated with endometriosis.[16]

Pelvic Inflammatory Disease

Pelvic inflammatory disease (PID), either acute or chronic, is infection of the reproductive tract. The two most widely reported organisms causing the infection are *Neisseria gonorrhoea* and *Chlamydia trachomatis*. Either of these organisms can be cultured from the cervix or from the pelvic cavity if surgery is necessary. Viral, fungal, and parasitic infections also occur. The infection is typically a sexually transmitted disease (STD), although pelvic infections do occur postsurgically and postpartum and have been associated with tampon use (i.e., toxic shock syndrome). PID is diagnosed as patients present with acute bilateral lower abdominal tenderness, fever, and an elevated white blood cell (WBC) count. The tenderness is commonly rebound tenderness, an indication of peritoneal irritation, found when there is active infection or blood in the abdomen. By pressing and then suddenly releasing the pressure, intense pain can be elicited. Possible pathways for dissemination of microorganisms in pelvic infections are depicted in Figure 6-11.

All sexually active women from the teenage years through the fifth decade are at risk, but those who have sex with multiple partners and those with a previous history of pelvic infection are at highest risk. The residua of acute infection are primarily adhesions that can cause chronic pelvic pain as well as infertility. Chronic pain caused by adhesions either from PID or endometriosis cannot be diagnosed except by visualization during surgery, specifically laparoscopy. Laparoscopy permits visualization of the pelvic cavity through a fiberoptic instrument through a small subumbilical incision; this technique avoids the risks, expense, and morbidity of laparotomy.

Pelvic infections may be complicated by abscess development, which if ruptured can lead to pelvic and general peritonitis and in rare cases septic shock. Patients with pelvic abscess generally complain of more serious symptoms, although large abscesses have been found that were asymptomatic. A ruptured tubo-ovarian abscess is a surgical emergency frequently complicated by septic shock and intra-abdominal abscess and the spread of infection.

Fibroids

Leiomyomata uteri, or fibroids, are benign muscle tumors most commonly found in the uterus. They are found more commonly in blacks than in whites, in approximately one-third of all reproductive age women, and are commonly associated with symptoms such as heavy menstrual bleeding (menorrhagia), irregular bleeding (metrorrhagia), and intermenstrual bleeding. Women in their 30s and 40s are more likely to have fibroid tumors. Fibroids can also cause acute pain at the site of the tumor if they undergo cellular degeneration. They may also be a source of chronic pelvic pain, particularly when they reach larger sizes. A sense of pelvic heaviness, abdominal bloating, or pressure symptoms on the rectum or bladder, or both, are not uncommon with large fibroid tumors. Fibroid tumors are also an occasional source of back or sacral pain as well as abdominal pain.

Physical examination of the abdomen can palpate these masses if they are greater than the size of a 4-month pregnancy. Vaginal examination will demonstrate the presence of these fibroid tumors if they are smaller than that. Ultrasound is the most commonly used imaging technique to determine the size and location of these tumors.

Hormonal Dysfunction

Hormonal dysfunction is a vague term that does not have a specific diagnosis tied to it. It does, however, tend to be a catchall for any female problems that may even remotely be associated with the menstrual cycle. As a result, should the physical therapist encounter problems that appear to be limited to a history of abnormal uterine bleeding, it would not be uncommon for the patient to have had a physician evaluate her hormonal status. Because the normal menstrual cycle is regular and predictable, irregular and unpredictable periods are indicative of anovulation. Most commonly, this is due to stress or a temporary failure of the intricate neuroendocrine feedback loops. Occasionally, other endocrine abnormalities may affect ovulation (e.g., thyroid or adrenal dysfunction or a pituitary tumor). A patient will typically have sought out medical evaluation long before an impact would be expected on the musculoskeletal system. An example is premature menopause, a condition in which the patient is no longer producing any estrogen as the ovaries have, for whatever reason, ceased to function. Long-standing lack of estrogen could result in a significant decrease in bone density (osteoporosis), increasing the risk of pathologic fractures. It is for this reason that women who have undergone a surgical or natural menopause are often given exogenous estrogen replacement therapy.

Symptomatic Pelvic Relaxation

Symptomatic pelvic relaxation is typically manifested by uterine prolapse or stress urinary incontinence or both. Loss of pelvic floor muscular and ligamentous support is attributed to childbirth trauma, lack of adequate prenatal or postpartum physical conditioning, the aging process, or any combination of these factors. With relaxation of the pelvic floor the pelvic organs can begin a descent through the vagina and possibly be visible from the outside. This may result in low back pain or the sensation of pressure or "falling out" in the pelvic floor. "Heaviness" of the upper thighs is also often reported by patients.

The physical examination reveals findings compatible with a loss of the normal ligaments and muscular support for the bladder, uterus, and/or rectum. No blood tests or radiographs are necessary to make this diagnosis. The gynecologic approach to management is usually surgical repair, although supportive mechanisms such as pessaries are also utilized. Strengthening of the pelvic floor musculature and posture correction should be beneficial in the management of these patients and are suggested as the initial course of conservative treatment.[3,17] Recent research regarding the most efficient means of exercise for pelvic floor contraction are discussed earlier in this chapter under Urinary Tract.

Neoplasms

Neoplasms of the female reproductive tract present in various fashions, depending on the organ from which they arise. A general rule of thumb suggests that the older the patient, the more likely it is to be a neoplasm. Tumors of the ovary are often asymptomatic and are found only incidentally on pelvic examination. These tumors can present as acute pain if they happen to rupture, twist, or bleed. Advanced ovarian malignancies will present with vague symptoms, such as abdominal bloating or early satiety or if the patient's clothes no longer fit.

Ultrasound of the pelvis is the typical fashion in which ovarian neoplasms are visualized. Malignancies of the uterine lining usually present as abnormal bleeding, especially in the postmenopausal patient. A biopsy of the endometrial lining in any postmenopausal bleeding patient is necessary to rule out this condition. Cancer of the cervix also presents as bleeding, classically described as postcoital. These lesions are visualized on speculum examination of the cervix, where biopsy reveals the diagnosis without difficulty. Preinvasive cervical lesions are often asymptomatic and are initially picked up by routine Papanicolaou smears and by biopsies often performed under colposcopic visualization. The diagnosis of cancer of the vulva is made by biopsy of the affected area. Patients often present with subtle symptoms, such as vulvar itching or irritation. On gross inspection, these areas may look normal, appear red and inflamed or pale and thin, or have gross lesions visible. Unfortunately, cancer only infrequently presents with pain as a symptom.

Ectopic Pregnancy

Ectopic pregnancy is a pregnancy that implants and grows outside the uterine cavity. More than 95 percent of ectopic pregnancies are in the fallopian tube. Ectopic pregnancy is responsible for approximately 15 percent of all obstetric caused maternal deaths in the United States. Most maternal deaths occur secondary to hemorrhage and are thought to be preventable. Risk factors include infertility, IUD use, prior tubal sterilization or reconstructive surgery, as well as previous ectopic pregnancy. Smoking and douching have also been implicated.

The typical presentation is menstrual irregularity associated with unilateral or bilateral acute "cramping" abdominal pain. Sharp or lacerating pain associated with fainting frequently presents with acute rupture of an ectopic pregnancy. Dull, aching pain may present in patients with hematoma surrounding an unruptured ectopic pregnancy.[18] In approximately 10 percent of cases there is also referred shoulder pain, which indicates intraperitoneal spill of blood and associated diaphragmatic irritation. A positive pregnancy test in association with any of these symptoms warrants immediate gynecologic evaluation. The physical therapist is also advised to refer a patient with these symptoms to the gynecologic physician for evaluation even if the patient has not yet undergone pregnancy testing. Laparoscopy is the diagnostic procedure for suspected unruptured ectopic pregnancy. Treatment is surgical removal.

SUMMARY

Normal anatomy and physiology of the female urogenital system have been reviewed along with the clinical signs and symptoms that may be seen as a result of normal physiologic activity in this system. Clearly, the hormonal influences on muscle tone and ligamentous laxity during the normal course of pregnancy and in the luteal phase of the menstrual cycle are of concern to the physical therapist, as they may reduce musculoskeletal stability. Physical therapists have not traditionally questioned patients regarding the onset of last menstrual period or the characteristics of the menstrual cycle. This information should be collected, as it may be beneficial in physical therapy treatment of musculoskeletal dysfunction. Exercise should be modified during times of "normal" decreased stability. It is also important to note whether a patient is undergoing hormone therapy and, if so, which specific hormones are involved.

In addition to the signs and symptoms associated with normal physiology, signs and symptoms that indicate pathology in the female urogenital system are presented in this chapter. It is clear that female patients with abdominal pain or anterior pelvic pain (or persisting pain in any of the referred areas noted in Table 6-1) should be questioned about abnormal bleeding, dyspareunia, dysuria, and other signs and symptoms listed in Figure 6-15. The signs and symptoms presented in Figure 6-15 are most commonly associated with pathology in the urogenital system. Their presence indicates the need for gynecologic evaluation. Therapists working under physician referral should provide the referring practitioner with any new information collected with regard to the urogenital system. Therapists in practice without referral situations should refer patients presenting with such signs and symptoms for gynecologic evaluation.

Many trunk, pelvic, and lower-extremity structures share innervation with the structures of the female urogenital system and are potential sites of referred pain (Table 6-1). Certain pathologic processes may mimic the musculoskeletal pain pattern of symptomatic relief with rest and worsening with specific activities. It is important that physical therapists managing patients with pain complaints in these areas have knowledge of normal gynecologic and pregnancy physiology and of common pathologic signs and symptoms, so that pertinent information can be elicited from patients and appropriate referrals made to other practitioners.

Figure 6-15 should assist the physical therapist in developing historical questions to be included in their clinical evaluation and re-evaluation of patients who present with signs and symptoms related to the female urogenital system.

PATIENT CASE STUDY 1*

History

The patient was a 39-year-old housewife who came to the clinic with a diagnosis of mechanical low back pain syndrome with left gluteal muscle trigger points. Her chief complaint was constant left buttock aching and intermittent sharp pain in the left posterior superior iliac spine (PSIS) area. The left buttock aching intensity varied little but seemed to increase slightly if she was in any single position for more than 30 minutes. She stated that she was forced to change positions constantly. The sharp pain was provoked immediately with weight-bearing on the left lower extremity during both standing and ambulation. The sharp pain could be relieved within minutes by lying down in any position. The patient woke up in the morning with the left buttock aching and severe left hip stiffness. After soaking in a hot shower, the stiffness, but not the aching, resolved.

The left buttock aching began insidiously 10 weeks before the initial evaluation. She had experienced similar symptoms periodically for the past 2 years. The initial episode also began insidiously. The sharp pain had begun 3 weeks before the initial evaluation. The patient described a fall on her left buttock that preceded the onset of the sharp pain. Until this recent flare up, her symptoms had gradually improved with bed rest and heat.

The patient's general medical and surgical history was negative, and the patient was taking naproxen (Naprosyn). The patient stated that she had been constipated and had noted increased frequency of urination during the past 8 weeks. Upon specific questioning, she indicated that there was an increase in the aching of the left buttock when she was severely constipated and a concurrent decrease in the aching after a bowel movement. She stated that the referring physician was aware of the bowel and bladder dysfunction.

Physical Examination

When standing, the patient had difficulty with unilateral weightbearing on the left lower extremity caused by provocation of the sharp pain. There was a significant increase in muscle tone of the left lumbar paraspinals and gluteals with weight shift onto the left lower extremity. There was a decreased lumbar lordosis in the low lumbar spine, and the bony landmarks of the iliac and greater trochanters were symmetric. There was significant tenderness with palpation from the left inferior lateral angle of the sacrum to the caudal aspect of the left PSIS. Active movement testing of the trunk on standing revealed decreased low lumbar spine motion during backward bending with provocation of sharp discomfort medial to the left PSIS. Also, a significant pulling sensation extending from the left low lumbar

* From Boissonnault and Bass,[20] with permission.

Review of Systems: Urogenital

Sign/Symptom	Yes	No	Comments
1. Dyspareunia	______	______	____________________
2. Dysmenorrhea	______	______	____________________
3. Amenorrhea	______	______	____________________
4. Abnormally heavy menstrual bleeding	______	______	____________________
5. Abnormal bleeding pattern	______	______	____________________
6. Vaginal discharge	______	______	____________________
7. Vaginal burning/itching	______	______	____________________
8. Dysuria	______	______	____________________
9. Urinary frequency	______	______	____________________
10. Urinary urgency	______	______	____________________
11. Urinary incontinence	______	______	____________________
12. Abnormal pain not associated with menstruation	______	______	____________________
13. Abdominal bloating	______	______	____________________
14. Postural hypotension	______	______	____________________
15. History of infertility	______	______	____________________
16. History of infection	______	______	____________________

Fig. 6-15. Review of systems checklist for female urogenital system.

spine to the left buttock was noted at the end range of right-side bending. The patient had a positive sitting-forward bending test on the left for sacroiliac joint mobility. Left ilial shear test (passive spring test) provoked sharp left PSIS pain and a spasm end feel. Palpation revealed a significant left-on-right sacral torsion lesion and increased muscle tone of the left hip flexor and buttock musculature. Moderate to severe tightness was noted in the left hamstring and rectus femoris muscles.

Assessment and Outcome

The physical examination indicated that an apparent left sacroiliac joint dysfunction was responsible for the sharp left buttock symptoms. The aching pain was not altered during any of the components of the physical examination. Also of concern was the recent onset of constipation and urinary frequency and the insidious onset of the aching pain, in addition to the apparent correlation between severe constipation and increased buttock aching. After the left sacral base was mobilized, the sharp pain associated with the left lower-extremity weightbearing resolved almost immediately, as did the sharp pain noted during active backward bending. The next two sessions consisted primarily of treating the muscle imbalances and residual increased muscle tone of the left hip flexors and buttock muscles. At the end of the 2-week period, the patient noted an 80 percent decrease in the intensity of the buttock aching, no sharp pain with standing and ambulation, and a significant improvement of the constipation and urinary frequency problems. After a weekend, the patient returned to the clinic, stating that all her symptoms had returned, as severe as ever. Specific questioning indicated that only the aching pain had worsened and the constipation and dysuria had returned to the pre-evaluation level. No sharp PSIS pain had returned. The patient could not relate the return of symptoms to any incident or accident. Physical examination revealed virtually no change in signs from her last visit when she was doing so well, and again the symptoms could not be altered.

It was recommended that the patient see her internist because of the clinical findings. She called 6 weeks later to report that she had undergone abdominal surgery to remove an ovarian cyst. She stated she had been completely asymptomatic for the past 4 weeks.

PATIENT CASE STUDY 2

History

A 31-year-old black female, nullipare, was referred to outpatient physical therapy by an orthopaedic surgeon with a diagnosis of left shoulder impingement. The chief complaint was intermittent sharp left shoulder and anterior chest pain aggravated by overhead movements and deep breathing. Pain was also reported to occur occasionally at rest and often awakened her from sleep several times a night. The patient was able to return to sleep after being awakened by pain but denied the night pain to be associated with any particular position and denied any exacerbation of symptoms by left sidelying. The patient was employed as a hospital housekeeper and reported that the pain often interfered with her daily activities. She was able to relieve the sharp pain by placing her hand on her sternum and applying pressure at that contact while forward bending the trunk. She also reported that the pain would decrease if she attempted to breathe shallowly.

The patient reported that the current complaints were preceded by complaints of right lower quadrant discomfort and irregular menstruation for 5 months prior to the physical therapy referral. The lower quadrant symptoms had been followed by severe left anterior chest and shoulder pain for which she had been hospitalized. She was cleared for cardiovascular disease during that hospitalization and also evaluated with cervical and shoulder x-rays and magnetic resonance imaging. No diagnosis was made during that course of hospitalization. The pain soon subsided, with mild intermittent shoulder pain remaining for the last 4 months before physical therapy evaluation. The patient reported during the last 4 months that she had been able to relieve the pain with Hydrocodon until worsening of intensity 2 weeks prior to physical therapy referral.

Past medical history was otherwise unremarkable.

Physical Examination

Posture examination revealed a slight forward head, round shoulder posture with a reduction of the expected thoracic kyphotic curve. Active movement of the left shoulder was slightly limited in diagonal abduction and sagittal abduction at end range by complaints of pain in the anterior chest and lower left rib cage. Active elevation of the left upper extremity also revealed significant reduction in anterior expansion of the rib cage. Strength of the left shoulder musculature was within normal limits. Resisted abduction produced mild left shoulder pain but did not reproduce the patient's complaint. Passive left glenohumeral ROM was essentially within normal limits, with only slight restrictions of the pectoralis major and minor muscle lengths noted. Palpation of the left shoulder structures was negative. Palpation of the left upper abdominal quadrant revealed moderate muscle guarding and edema. Palpation of the right lower quadrant provoked abdominal rebound and reproduction of the left shoulder pain. It is significant to note that the patient did not present complaining of lower quadrant pain; it was only through the physical therapist's attempt to clear this area through provocation testing that these symptoms were manifested.

Assessment

The patient's physician was contacted and presented with the findings, which did not indicate musculoskeletal dysfunction. The physician requested the patient be sent immediately for further testing but also requested that physical therapy continue to monitor the patient and provide treatment for pain control until further notice.

Treatment

The patient was treated twice the same week as the referral with moist heat, posture instruction and positioning for pain relief. No changes were noted in objective or subjective findings with treatment.

Outcome

One week later the patient was referred to a gynecologist who diagnosed a right ovarian fibroid tumor. Physical therapy was discontinued, and gynecologic treatment was instated.

REFERENCES

1. Williams PL, Warwick R: Gray's Anatomy. 36th Ed. WB Saunders, Philadelphia, 1980
2. Gould SF: Anatomy. p. 3. In Gabbe SG, Niebyl JR, Simpson JL (eds): Obstetrics: Normal and Problem Pregnancies. 2nd Ed. Churchill Livingstone, New York, 1991
3. Noble E: Essential Exercises for the Childbearing Years. 3rd Ed. Houghton Mifflin, Boston, 1988
4. Hacker N, Moore GJ: Essentials of Obstetrics and Gynaecology. WB Saunders, Philadelphia, 1986
5. Pernoll ML, Benson RC (eds): Current Obstetric and Gynelogic Diagnosis and Treatment. 6th Ed. Appleton & Lange, E. Norwalk, CT, 1991
6. Boissonnault JS, Blaschak MJ: Incidence of diastasis recti abdominis during the childbearing year. Phys Ther 68:1082, 1988
7. Kotarinos RK: Diastasis recti and review of the abdominal wall. J Obstet Gynecol Phys Ther 14:4, 1990
8. Pre- and Post-Partum Exercise Guidelines. American College of Obstetricians and Gynecologists, Washington, DC, 1985
9. Riczo DB: ACOG's guidelines for exercise during pregnancy and postpartum: accepted or contested? J Obstet Gynecol Phys Ther 13:6, 1989
10. Perinatal Exercise Guidelines. Obstetrics and Gynecology Section. American Physical Therapy Association, Alexander, VA, 1994
11. Frahm J: Abdominal and pelvic floor muscle synergy in normal women. Research Platform Presentation, Combined Sections Meeting, American Physical Therapy Association, New Orleans, February 1994
12. Artal R, Masak DI, Khodiguidan N et al: Exercise prescription in pregnancy: weight-bearing versus non-weight bearing exercise. Am J Obstet Gynecol 162:1464, 1989
13. Lose G, Lindholm P: Transient painful osteoporosis of the hip in pregnancy. Int J Gynaecol Obstet 24:13, 1986
14. McGuigin L, Fleming A: Osteonecrosis of the humerus related to pregnancy. Ann Rheum Dis 42:597, 1983
15. Pellici PM, Zolla-Pazner S, Rahhan WN, Wilson PD: Osteonecrosis of the femoral head associated with pregnancy. Clin Orthop Rel Res 185:59, 1984
16. King Baker P: Musculoskeletal origins of chronic pelvic pain. Obstet Gynecol Clin North Am 20:719, 1993
17. Delancy OL (ed): Pelvic organ prolapse: clinical management and scientific foundations. Clin Obstet Gynecol 36:903, 1993
18. Ryan KJ, Verkowitz R, Barbieri RL: Kistner's Gynecology Principles and Practice. Yearbook Medical Publisher, Chicago, 1990
19. Boissonault JS, Kotarinos RK: Diastasis recti. p. 63. In Wilder E (ed): Obstetric and Gynecologic Physical Therapy. Churchill Livingstone, New York, 1988
20. Boissonault WG, Bass C: Pathological origin of trunk and neck pain: part I—pelvic and abdominal visceral disorders. J Orthop Sports Phys Ther 12:206, 1990.

Suggested Readings

Benson JT: Female Pelvic Floor Disorders. 1st Ed. Norton Medical Books, New York, 1992

Noble E: Marie Osmond's Exercises for Mother's and Babies. New American Library, New York, 1985

Noble E: Marie Osmond's Exercises for Mothers To Be. New American Library, New York, 1985

U.S. DHEW: Urinary Incontinence in Adults. Public Health Service, Agency for Health Care Policy and Research, U.S. Department of Health and Human Services, Washington, DC, 1992

7 SCREENING FOR ENDOCRINE SYSTEM DISEASE

Jill S. Boissonnault, M.S., P.T
Diane Madlon-Kay, M.D.

The impact of disease within the endocrine system on physical therapy practice may be considerable or relatively uncommon, depending on the physical therapy setting. The therapist practicing within a rehabilitation or geriatric setting may have a large caseload of diabetic patients with a wide variety of complications necessitating physical therapy intervention: cerebrovascular accident (CVA), amputation, diabetic ulcers, and peripheral neuropathies. The signs and symptoms are overt and the conditions prediagnosed. This endocrine system disease presents challenges to the therapist with regard to exercise physiology, wound healing, and sensory integration. Other diseases of the endocrine system are less common but, when present, may also have an impact on physical therapy. Previously undiagnosed, signs and symptoms of these diseases may be discovered during subjective and objective portions of the physical therapy evaluation, thus requiring referral to the physician. Endocrine system diseases include dysfunction of the thyroid gland, parathyroid glands, adrenal glands, and pituitary gland.

Therapists working primarily in an outpatient setting, especially in those states that allow direct access, may encounter a patient who presents with symptoms of weakness, arthralgias, paresthesias, or diffuse pain, the actual etiology of which is metabolic in nature. The therapist may be the patient's sole contact with the medical community. This chapter assists the therapist in differentiating symptoms and signs of metabolic disease from those of musculoskeletal origin, as well as learning the cardinal signs of the more common metabolic diseases. The effects of endocrine system disease are systemic in nature, resulting in an often diverse and confusing clinical picture. A delay in diagnosis of primary endocrine system disease may occur when patients are mistakenly referred to Physical Therapy for a vast array of symptoms common to many musculoskeletal dysfunctions or diseases.

Two patient case studies are presented, both dealing with the diabetic patient. These case illustrations demonstrate the confusion over the presentation of symptoms and their etiology. Although the discovery of metabolic disease rarely prevents a fatality, it can be tremendously gratifying for both the patient and the therapist. The quality of life is surely diminished when one suffers from diseases such as Graves, Cushing, or acromegaly. Therapists must avoid mistakenly treating what appear to be dysfunctions of the musculoskeletal system but that are in fact symptoms or signs of metabolic disease. The goal of this chapter is to help avoid that scenario, to aid in differentiation of signs and symptoms of metabolic disease from primary dysfunction of the neuromusculoskeletal system, and to understand the implications of these diseases on physical therapy practice, should they be prediagnosed in a patient.

PHYSIOLOGY OF THE ENDOCRINE SYSTEM

The endocrine system is composed of various glands that secrete substances called hormones into the bloodstream. The hormones are transported to their sites of

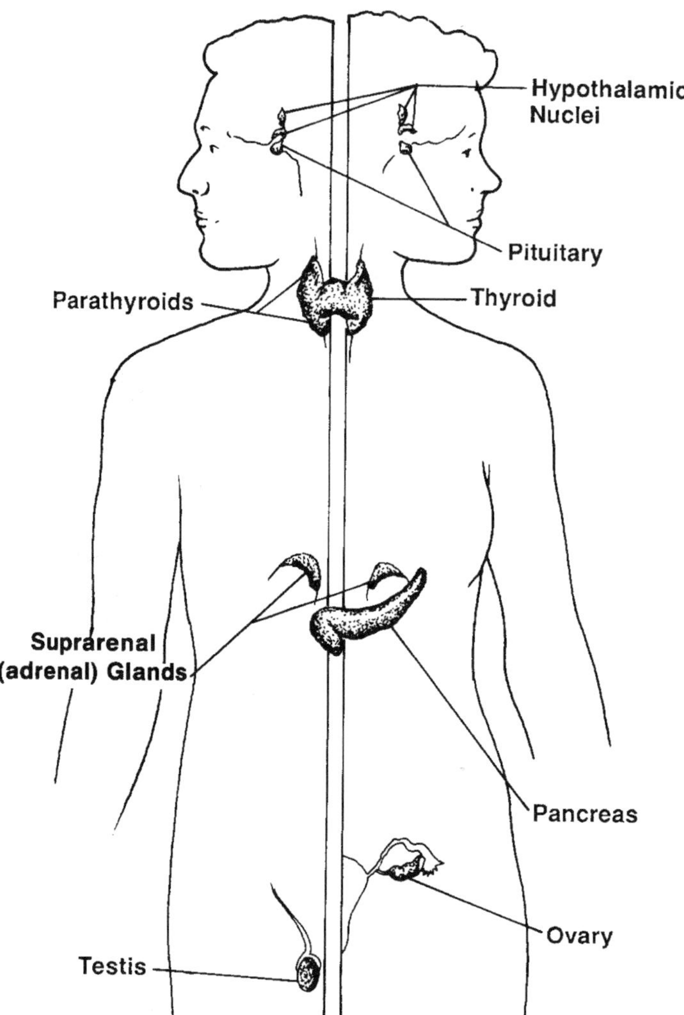

Fig. 7-1. Location of the major endocrine glands, male and female. Not shown are the liver, gastrointestinal tract, pineal gland, thymus, and placenta, all of which secrete hormones.

action elsewhere in the body. The hormones then act on other cells to regulate their functions. Hormones may act on the cells of a specific organ or on cells widely distributed throughout the body. Figure 7-1 shows the location of the major endocrine glands. Table 7-1 summarizes the major endocrine glands, the hormones they secrete, and the hormonal functions.

The release of a hormone is often triggered by a change in the concentration of some substance in the body fluids. The hormone has a corrective effect, eliminating the stimulus, which then leads to a reduction in hormone secretion. This process is called a negative feedback homeostatic control system. Hormones control and integrate many body functions with this system. In general, hormonal control regulates the metabolic functions of the body, such as moderating chemical reactions in the cells, controlling the transport of substances through cell membranes, and partaking in various aspects of cellular metabolism. The types of effects that occur inside the cell are determined by the character of the cell itself. For example, when the kidneys are stimulated by vasopressin, or antidiuretic hormone (ADH), the vasopressin binds with a receptor causing a biochemical reaction resulting in a conversion of cytoplasmic adenosine triphosphatase (ATP) into cyclic adenosine monophosphate (cAMP). This reaction is believed to be the common process for many hormones and target organs. It is the cAMP that causes the hormonal effects

Table 7-1. Summary of Hormonal Function[a]

Site Produced (Endocrine Gland)	Hormone[b]	Major Function
Hypothalamus	Releasing hormones	Secretion of hormones by the anterior pituitary
	Oxytocin	See posterior pituitary
	Vasopressin	See posterior pituitary
Anterior pituitary	Growth hormone (somatotropin, GH)	Growth: secretion of IGF-I; organic metabolism
	Thyroid-stimulating hormone (TSH, thyrotropin)	Thyroid gland
	Adrenocorticotropic hormone (ACTH, corticotropin)	Adrenal cortex
	Prolactin	Breast growth and milk synthesis; permissive for certain reproductive functions in the male
	Gonadotropic hormones: follicle-stimulating hormone (FSH); luteinizing hormone (LH)	Gonads (gamete production and sex hormone secretion)
	β-Lipotropin	Unknown
	β-Endorphin	Unknown
Posterior pituitary	Oxytocin[c]	Milk "let-down"; uterine motility
	Vasopressin (antidiuretic hormone, ADH)[c]	Water excretion by the kidneys; blood pressure
Adrenal cortex	Cortisol	Organic metabolism; response to stresses; immune system
	Androgens	Sex drive in women
	Aldosterone	Sodiums, potassium, and acid excretion by kidneys
Adrenal medulla	Epinephrine	Organic metabolism; cardiovascular function; response to stress
		Norepinephrine
Thyroid	Thyroxine (T_4)	Metabolic rate; growth; brain development and function
	Triiodothyronine (T_3)	
	Calcitonin	Plasma calcium
Parathyroids	Parathyroid hormone (parathormone, PTH, PH)	Plasma calcium and phosphate
Gonads		
Female: ovaries	Estrogen	Reproductive system; breast; growth and development
	Progesterone	
	Inhibin	FSH secretin
	Relaxin	Relaxation of cervix and pubic ligaments
Male: testes	Testosterone	Reproductive system; growth and development
	Inhibin	FSH secretion
	Müllerian-inhibiting hormone	Regression of müllerian ducts
Pancreas	Insulin	Organic metabolism; plasma glucose
	Glucagon	
	Somatostatin	
	Pancreatic polypeptide	
Kidney	Renin (→angiotensin II)[d]	Aldosterone secretion; blood pressure
	Erythropoietin	Erythrocyte production
	1,25-Dihydroxyvitamin D_3	Calcium absorption by the intestine
Gastrointestinal tract	Gastrin	Gastrointestinal tract; liver; pancreas; gallbladder
	Secretin	
	Cholecystokinin	
	Glucose-dependent insulinotropic peptide (GIP)	
	Somatostatin	
Liver (and other cells)	Insulin-like growth factors (IGF-I and -II)	Growth
Thymus	Thymosin (thymopoietin)	T-lymphocyte function
Pineal	Melatonin	? Sexual maturity; body rhythms
Placenta	Chorionic gonadotropin (CG)	Secretion by corpus luteum
	Estrogens	See ovaries
	Progesterone	
	Placental lactogen	Breast development; organic metabolism
Heart	Atrial natriuretic factor (ANF, atriopeptin, auriculin)	Sodium excretion by kidneys; blood pressure
Monocytes and macrophages	Interleukin-1 (IL-1)	See Ch. 19 in Vander et al.[27]
	Tumor necrosis factor (TNF)	
	Other monokines	
Multiple cell types	Growth factors (e.g., nerve growth factor)	Growth of specific tissues

[a]Not all functions of the hormones are listed here.
[b]Names and abbreviations in parentheses are synonyms.
[c]The posterior pituitary stores and secretes these hormones; they are made in the hypothalamus.
[d]Renin is an enzyme that initiates reactions in blood that generate angiotensin II.
(From Vander et al.,[27] with permission.)

inside the cell, such as increasing the number of enzymes in a cell or changing cell permeability. In the case of vasopressin, the cAMP affects the epithelial cells of the renal tubules by increasing their permeability to water.[1]

Many of the body's metabolic functions are under the influence of the pituitary gland, or hypophysis, which in turn is influenced by the hypothalamus. The pituitary gland is connected to the hypothalamus by the pituitary stalk. Connections to the posterior pituitary or neurohypophysis from the hypothalamus occur through a nerve tract. The hormones released through hypothalamic–neurohypophyseal interaction are vasopressin, which controls the rate of water excretion into the urine, and oxytocin, which, among other functions, helps deliver milk from the glands of the breast. The anterior pituitary gland, or the adenohypophysis, is connected to the hypothalamus by the hypothalamic–hypophyseal portal vessels. Six major hormones are secreted by the anterior pituitary gland: growth hormone, corticotropin (influencing the adrenocortical hormones), thyrotropin (controlling the rate of thyroxine secretions by the thyroid), and the three gonadotropins follicle-stimulating hormone, luteinizing hormone, and luteotropic hormone.[1]

DISEASES OF THE ENDOCRINE SYSTEM

This chapter covers those diseases of the endocrine system that have an impact on physical therapy, with the exception of metabolic disease of the female genitourinary system (see discussion in Ch. 6; further information about metabolic disease of the female genitourinary system can also be found in the texts listed under Suggested Readings). The information presented on the diseases discussed here is intended as an overview of pathology and treatment as relevant to physical therapy. The diseases covered include diabetes mellitus, hypothyroidism and thyrotoxicosis (hyperthyroidism), hypoparathyroidism and hyperparathyroidism, Cushing's disease, Addison's disease, and acromegaly.

Disease of the pituitary gland itself is limited to discussion of acromegaly. The pituitary gland secretes many tropic hormones, which in turn cause secretion of hormones from target glands. Interference with the pituitary can cause many of the same signs and symptoms as those resulting from actual disease of the target gland. For example, a benign tumor of the pituitary, the most common pathology seen in this gland, could result in diminished secretion of thyrotropin. Since this hormone stimulates production of thyroxine, decreased secretion results in hypothyroidism. Blood tests can distinguish the source of the pathology, so that treatment can be instituted. Occasionally, pituitary enlargement is great enough to cause headaches and may interfere with the optic nerve as it courses by the gland. This would result in visual field disturbances. The headache or visual problems would aid the physician in diagnosing pituitary versus target gland disease.

While reading this section of the chapter, the therapist will note the common subjective patient complaints of lethargy, fatigue, and muscle weakness. Many of our patients complain of such symptoms, and we tend to pay them little heed. It is important to realize that they can be symptoms of real pathology, as evidenced by their presence in many of the following metabolic diseases.

Diabetes Mellitus

Diabetes mellitus is a chronic disease characterized by abnormal glucose utilization with inappropriately elevated blood glucose levels. Most diabetic patients have abnormal insulin secretion, leading to deranged metabolism of carbohydrates, fats, and proteins. Insulin deficiency results in decreased utilization of glucose by the body cells, with a resultant increase in blood glucose concentration. Abnormal metabolism of lipids and proteins results in increased deposition of lipids in the vascular walls and decreased deposition of proteins in the body tissues. The former leads to atherosclerosis and the latter to microangiopathy secondary to basement membranes thickened from excess glycoprotein. Over time, this leads to complications involving the eyes, kidneys, nerves, and blood vessels.

Diabetes is classified into two major categories. Type I or insulin-dependent diabetes mellitus (IDDM) is characterized by an absolute insulin deficiency and a dependence on insulin therapy for the preservation of life. About 10 percent of cases of diabetes are type I. The onset is generally in childhood or early adulthood. Patients with type II, or noninsulin-dependent diabetes mellitus (NIDDM), do not require insulin therapy for the maintenance of life. However, insulin may be necessary to control symptoms or to correct disordered metabolism. Most type II diabetics are obese.

The prevalence of diabetes is thought to be about 1 percent. The diagnosis can be made in several ways: (1) unequivocal elevation of plasma glucose levels associated with classic symptoms of diabetes mellitus, (2) elevation of fasting plasma glucose on more than one occasion, and (3) elevation of plasma glucose after an oral glucose challenge on more than one occasion.

Treatment may be a combination of diet, oral hypoglycemic medications, and insulin. For the obese NIDDM patient, the immediate and long-term goals are weight reduction. NIDDM patients whose condition cannot be controlled by diet often respond to oral hypoglycemic medications. However, a high percentage of NIDDM patients will require insulin to control their symptoms. Insulin is required for the treatment of all type I patients.

Clinical Features

Diabetes is now most often diagnosed when the patient is asymptomatic as a result of routine blood tests showing an elevated glucose level. Most patients who are symptomatic complain of increased frequency of urination and excessive thirst with increased fluid intake. In severe cases, the patient may have increased appetite and food consumption with weight loss. Symptoms are usually present for weeks or months and have an insidious onset. Occasionally, patients present with no diabetic symptoms, but complications have already developed such as neuropathy or vascular disease.

Subjective and/or objective examination by the physical therapist might pick up previously undiagnosed diabetes. For example, a patient may have been referred for physical therapy for a misdiagnosed diabetic peripheral neuropathy. A patient's diabetic symptoms may be subtle enough not to have aroused concern on the part of the patient. A patient may be referred for a separate problem, such as low back pain, with diabetes picked up as an incidental finding. In any case, a careful history and thorough objective examination may yield findings suggestive of diabetes, with necessary referral to a physician.

In the subjective examination, complaints of orthostatic hypotension, blurred vision, sensory deficits, extremity pain, weakness, diarrhea, various bladder problems, impotence, or dysphagia can all be related to diabetes. They can also be signs and symptoms of other disease processes of sequelae of primary neuromusculoskeletal dysfunction. Response of these complaints to physical therapy treatment will help determine which of these possibilities is truly the culprit. Should any of these symptoms remain unchanged with physical therapy, referral to a physician would be indicated. Certainly a therapist would want a referring physician to be aware of some of the more viscerally related complaints right away.

Findings on objective examination that might warrant referral back to a physician would be foot ulcerations, muscle atrophy, elevated resting heart rate, or signs of cranial nerve involvement (see Chs. 8, 9). Other findings, such as absent or diminished ankle jerk, edema, impaired vibratory sense, or decreased muscle strength, if found to be unrelated to the therapist's working diagnosis, should also be cause for referral.

The chronic complications of diabetes are now the major source of morbidity and mortality in both type I and type II diabetics. A broad spectrum of clinical syndromes are potential sequelae. This discussion focuses on the peripheral neuropathy and vascular complications.

Diabetic Neuropathy

Diabetic neuropathies pose considerable challenge to the clinician in terms of differentiation between mechanically and metabolically induced signs and symptoms. It is easy to overlook the possibility of mechanical sources of lower-extremity symptoms, such as numbness and tingling, when the patient presents with a diagnosis of diabetes because peripheral neuropathy is so common in this population. These neuropathies can be responsible for a wide range of symptoms. A case study presented at the end of this chapter illustrates this point.

Diabetic neuropathies are uncommon in young patients, and the incidence rises with the duration of the disease. The liability to neuropathy appears to be similar in both sexes. This discussion classifies diabetic neuropathies by division between symmetric and focal or multifocal lesions, according to the system adapted from Thomas[2] and presented by Dyke et al.[3]

The cause of diabetic peripheral neuropathy is neither well understood nor agreed upon. There is also disagreement in the literature regarding the primary site of pathology, be it peripheral nerve, dorsal root ganglion, or spinal cord.[3] There is a relationship between the degree of control of the disease and occurrence of neuropathy. Some of the signs and symptoms can abate or diminish in intensity once control is restored or attained. The symptoms and signs of diabetic neuropathy that might be found in a physical therapy assessment are summarized in Table 7-2.

Symmetric Polyneuropathies

Peripheral Sensory Neuropathy

The most common form of diabetic neuropathy is a distal symmetric, predominantly sensory polyneuropathy. In most cases, symptoms are absent. Routine physical examination demonstrates a loss of vibratory sense, of tactile or proprioceptive sensation, or of ankle reflexes. When symptoms are present, patients complain of paresthesias described as numbness, coldness, or tingling, mainly of the feet. The sensory symptoms can be distinguished from those of peripheral nerve or segmental spinal nerve injury as the distribution does not follow dermatomal or peripheral nerve patterns. If pain is present, it may be disabling. The pain is typically worse at night.

Neuropathic arthropathies (Charcot's joint) are also possible but uncommon and are present only in association with established sensory polyneuropathy. Possible sites of joint pathology include interphalangeal and metatarsophalangeal joints of the foot, less commonly the ankle joints, knee joints, and rarely the joints of the spine.[3] Most commonly, the patient presents with a swollen foot that may be painful. The foot is deformed with "rocker-bottom" subluxation of the mid-tarsal region or subluxation of the metatarsophalangeal joints. The foot is usually erythematous and warm. An infected neuropathic ulcer may be present. In the early stages, radiographs show severe arthritis. As the disease progresses, there is complete destruction of the involved joints with resorption of the metatarsal heads. Fractures and joint effusions occur as well.[4]

The decreased sensory perception of diabetic neuropathy may lead to unperceived injury to the skin and joints. Insensitivity to heat can result in severe burns. Caution must be used by the therapist when applying physical agents. Unrecognized pressure from poorly fitting shoes can lead to ulcers and infection.

The diabetic patient may benefit from custom-fit foot orthoses. Chronic foot ulcers are generally found over the metatarsal heads. Loss of sensation and pain may be primarily responsible for their development, but ischemia, motor weakness (see peripheral motor neuropathy), the liability of diabetic tissues to infection, and anatomic deformity may also contribute to their development.[3]

Table 7-2. Signs and Symptoms of Diabetic Neuropathy

Classification of Diabetic Neuropathy	Subjective Complaints Commonly Found in Physical Therapy Evaluation	Objective Signs Commonly Found in Physical Therapy Evaluation
Symmetric polyneuropathies		
Peripheral sensory polyneuropathy	Paresthesias: numbness, coldness, tingling (mainly in the feet) Pain, often disabling, worse at night	Absent ankle jerk Impairment of vibration sense in feet Foot ulcers—often over metatarsal heads
Peripheral motor neuropathy	Complaints of weakness	Bilateral Interosseous muscle atrophy Claw or hammer toes Decreased grip strength Decreased muscle strength on manual muscle testing
Autonomic neuropathy	Orthostatic hypotension PM diarrhea, after meals Bladder problems Distal anhidrosis–symmetric Impotence Dysphagia	Elevated resting heart rate Peripheral edema
Focal and multifocal neuropathies		
Cranial neuropathy	Pain behind or above the eye Headaches Facial pain	Palpebral ptosis Inward deviation of one eye
Trunk and limb mononeuropathy	Abrupt onset of cramping or lancinating pain, hyperalgesia with hyperesthesia Cutaneous hyperesthesia of the trunk	Peripheral nerve specific motor loss Abdominal wall weakness
Proximal motor neuropathy or diabetic amyotrophy	Pain in proximal lower limbs—worse at night	Asymmetric proximal weakness, atrophy in lower limbs Absent or diminished knee jerk

Peripheral Motor Neuropathy

Motor abnormalities are much less common than sensory abnormalities. The small muscles of the feet and hands are most commonly involved. Interosseous muscle atrophy allows the foot to assume abnormal positions with "claw" or "hammer" toes. New pressure points develop, leading to callus formation and ulceration. Hand involvement leads to weakness of grip. Diffuse weakness of the legs and upper extremities may also occur.

Autonomic Neuropathy

Diabetic autonomic neuropathy, like symmetric sensory polyneuropathy, is also probably length related; the longer fibers are initially affected. Thus, the earliest changes affect the lower extremities rather than innervation to the heart or great vessels.[3] Segmental demyelination is the predominant pathologic change. Disturbances of autonomic function often occur late in the disease process and pose an increased risk of mortality. The more common clinical manifestations of diabetic autonomic neuropathy include abnormal pupillary findings, such as a reduction in pupillary size and reduction in pupillary response to light, and the cardiovascular disturbances of orthostatic hypotension, elevated resting heart rate, and peripheral edema. Other common findings of diabetic autonomic neuropathy include poor thermoregulatory function, such as anhidrosis and abnormal vasomotor responses (the patient loses the normal reflex vasoconstriction and vasodilation of skin vessels to elevation or reduction of central body temperature), and atony of the esophagus, stomach, gallbladder, colon, and bladder. Gastrointestinal disturbance may include diabetic diarrhea,[3] which usually occurs at night or after meals. Bladder disturbances usually begin with lengthening intervals between voiding and progress to problems of micturition with straining, weakness, and intermittency of stream, as well as postmicturition dribbling. The final stage involves overflow incontinence.

Focal and Multifocal Neuropathies

Cranial Nerve Lesions

It is possible to see isolated or multiple palsies of the nerves to the external ocular muscles in older diabetics. The most common disturbance is of an isolated 3rd nerve lesion resulting in palpebral ptosis that may be partial or total. The 6th nerve is less commonly affected and presents with an inward deviation of the eye on the affected side. The onset is generally abrupt and may be painless, though pain has been reported to occur in about half the cases and may precede paralysis by several days. The pain may be quite intense and can be felt behind or above the eye. Headaches may also occur. Other cranial nerves may be affected, but less frequently than those to the external ocular muscles. In almost all cases the paralyzed extraocular muscle recovers function in 4 to 8 weeks with improved diabetic control and symptomatic treatment.

Facial nerve paralysis is also possible secondary to diabetic cranial neuropathy, although less common than paralysis to ocular musculature. Clinical progress is similar to lesions of nerves III and VI.

Trunk and Limb Mononeuropathies

Mononeuropathies can affect any part of the body. This complication is characterized by involvement of a single nerve or its branches. The lower extremities are more commonly involved, specifically the femoral, lateral cutaneous or peroneal nerve. In the upper extremity, the ulnar, median, and radial nerves are most commonly affected. The onset is usually sudden with intense cramping or lancinating pain. Symptoms can involve sensory, motor, or mixed manifestations. The pain is typically worse at night and may be relieved by pacing when the lower extremities are involved. Sensory loss produces a clinical picture of hyperalgesia with hyperesthesia.

A diabetic truncal mononeuropathy has also been seen. Presentation is of abdominal wall weakness or cutaneous hyperesthesia with electromyographic evidence of paraspinal denervation. The prognosis for recovery is reported to be good for both the trunk and peripheral mononeuropathies.[3,5]

Proximal Motor Neuropathy or Diabetic Amyotrophy

Amyotrophy is a form of neuropathy that resembles a primary muscle disease. Severe proximal asymmetric muscle weakness and pain usually affect the pelvic girdle and thigh muscles through a disturbance of the lumbosacral plexus. The knee jerk is depressed or abolished, but sensory loss is not prominent. The condition primarily affects the iliopsoas, quadriceps, and adductor musculature. The anterolateral muscle group in the lower leg may simultaneously be involved, producing what has been termed the anterior compartment syndrome.[3] The typical patient is an elderly NIDDM male patient with mild disease. The onset may be rapid and accompanied by low-grade fever. Patients may have profound weight loss and severe depression. Function is often recovered spontaneously with the aid of good diabetic control.[6,7]

Diabetic Vascular Disease

Macrovascular or Macroangiopathy

The pathology of atherosclerosis in the diabetic patient is quite similar to that in the general population; however, it's rate is severely accelerated. Complications due to macrovascular disease in the diabetic include myocardial infarction (MI), which is more likely to be painless in a diabetic due to associated autonomic neuropathy affecting the pain fibers to the heart, CVA, and peripheral vascular disease. (Further reading on signs and symptoms of these processes can be found in Ch. 2.)

Microvascular or Microangiopathy

Microangiopathy is considered to be a lesion of the capillaries unique to diabetics. The basement membranes of the capillaries thicken. This is seen primarily in the retina, glomeruli, skin, and muscle. Increased permeability occurs, and eventually ischemic and hemorrhagic complications occur. These lesions are particularly threatening to the type I diabetic. (See Ch. 5 for a discussion of the signs of kidney disease and Chs. 8, 9 for a further assessment of vision in relationship to cranial nerve function.)

Diseases of the Thyroid Gland

The thyroid gland is composed of two lobes lying on either side of the trachea and connected in the midline by a thin isthmus. The isthmus lies just below the cricoid cartilage of the larynx. The examination of the thyroid begins with inspection. The patient is asked to extend his neck. The normal thyroid is barely visible. If sufficiently enlarged, a mass may be observable within the jugular notch, rendering the borders of the notch indistinct. The patient is asked to swallow. Normally, the thyroid rises during swallowing. Any mass or enlargement that moves upward is likely to be within the thyroid. Any enlargement of the thyroid gland is termed a goiter, except in pregnancy or menstruation, when enlargement is normal. The parathyroid glands are usually related to the posterior borders of the lobes of the thyroid gland.

Palpation is best done from behind the patient. The posterior approach involves placing the examiner's hand around the neck of the patient whose neck is slightly extended. The index finger is placed just below the cricoid (Fig. 7-2). As the patient swallows, the thyroid isthmus should rise under the finger. The finger is then rotated slightly downward and laterally, so that one can feel as much of the lateral lobe as possible. The normal thyroid is often not palpable.

The size, shape, and consistency of the gland, as well as any nodules or tenderness, should be noted. The normal thyroid gland has the consistency of muscle tissue. Unusual hardness may be due to cancer or scarring. A toxic goiter may be soft or spongy. Tenderness of the gland may be due to infection or hemorrhage into the gland. Local symptoms may be provoked as the therapist assesses adjacent musculoskeletal structures. For example, performing anteroposterior glides to assess mobility of the sternoclavicular joint or palpating over the caudal aspect of the sternocleidomastoid-muscles may sufficiently stress the thyroid to provoke complaints of tenderness or pain. Palpation of local structures may help the therapist determine the origin of the tenderness. If the thyroid is enlarged, it should also be auscultated. The bell of the stethoscope is placed over the lobes. A systolic bruit suggests a toxic goiter.

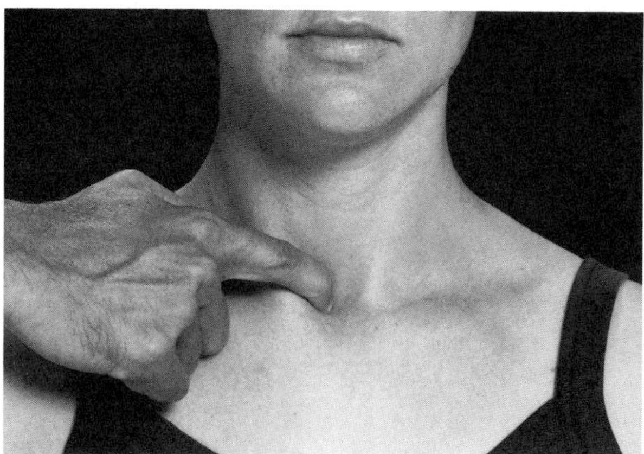

Fig. 7-2. Palpation of the thyroid gland. The examiner's finger is placed below the cricoid cartilage in the space just above the sternal notch and medial to the sternocleidomastoid muscle.

Physical examination of the thyroid reveals little about the function of the gland. Symptoms and signs elsewhere in the body provide clues to the functional status of the thyroid.

Thyrotoxicosis

Thyrotoxicosis (hyperthyroidism) is a syndrome that results from an excess of thyroid hormone. Thyrotoxicosis has several causes, the most common of which is Graves disease, an autoimmune disease. Thyrotoxicosis is also commonly caused by a hyperfunctioning nodular goiter. Less frequently, the cause is a solitary hyperfunctioning adenoma, thyroiditis, or related to iodine.

The incidence of thyrotoxicosis in the United States is 2 per 10,000 cases, with a strong female predominance. The diagnosis is made by thyroid function blood tests. Treatment varies with the etiology and may include antithyroid medications (propylthiouracil or methimazole), adjunctive medications (iodine, adrenergic antagonists), radioactive iodine, or surgery.

Table 7-3. Incidence of Symptoms and Signs Observed in 247 Patients with Thyrotoxicosis

Symptom	%	Symptom	%
Nervousness	99	Increased appetite	65
Increased sweating	91	Eye complaints	54
Hypersensitivity to heat	89	Swelling of legs	35
Palpitation	89	Hyperdefecation (without diarrhea)	33
Fatigue	88		
Weight loss	85	Diarrhea	23
Tachycardia	82	Anorexia	9
Dyspnea	75	Constipation	4
Weakness	70	Weight gain	2
Sign	**%**	**Sign**	**%**
Tachycardia[a]	100	Eye signs	71
Goiter[b]	100	Atrial fibrillation	10
Skin changes	97	Splenomegaly	10
Tremor	97	Gynecomastia	10
Bruit over thyroid	77	Liver palms	8

[a]In other studies, thyrotoxic patients, patients with normal pulse rate have been observed.

[b]Enlargement of thyroid is reported lacking in approximately 3 percent of patients with thyrotoxicosis in other studies.

(From Wilson and Foster,[28] with permission.)

Clinical Features

The clinical presentation of thyrotoxicosis is variable and dependent on the degree of hormone excess, rapidity of onset, duration, and age of the patient (Table 7-3). The typical patient presents with at least one of the following complaints: nervousness, weight loss, palpitations, enlarging neck mass, change in the appearance of the eyes, or symptoms of heart failure or fatigue. Muscle weakness and trophic changes such as thin, silky skin, hair loss and heat intolerance[8] also occur and, along with fatigue, are the signs and symptoms most likely to be picked up in physical therapy evaluation. Since these findings are also representative of many other diseases and dysfunctions, the therapist would probably need to rely on the patient's response to therapy for guidance regarding further medical evaluation; that is, if muscle strength were to return to normal levels after a conditioning program, no further referral would be necessary, but unchanged or worsening complaints would warrant referral to a physician.

Weakness and fatigability are frequent symptoms. Usually there is no evidence of local muscle disease other than a general wasting associated with weight loss. The weakness is most prominent in the proximal muscles of the extremities. Occasionally proximal muscle wasting may be seen. The myopathy affects men more than women and may be the most prominent symptom. The contraction and relaxation phases of deep tendon reflexes are shortened due to weak contractions of skeletal muscles.[9,10]

Hypokalemic periodic paralysis (resulting from abnormally small concentrations of potassium ions in the circulation) may occur, particularly in Oriental patients. The attack of paralysis may be generalized or localized and may be precipitated by exercise or high carbohydrate or high sodium meals. The attack may last for minutes to days and is associated with a lowering of the serum potassium level.[9,10]

Thyrotoxicosis may be associated with demineralization of bone and pathologic fractures, particularly in elderly women. Though not a contraindication to passively stretching a patient, this condition would warrant caution on the therapist's part when using passive accessory or physiologic techniques. Osteopathy with subperiosteal bone formation and swelling is rare but, when present, may be particularly evident in the metacarpal bones.

Thyroid dermopathy consists of a thickening of the skin, particularly over the lower tibia. Occasionally it also involves the entire lower leg and may extend into the feet. It is caused by an accumulation of glycosaminoglycans and is found in only 2 to 3 percent of patients with Graves disease. Onycholysis, separation of the nail from its bed, is a much more common finding.[11]

Hypothyroidism

Hypothyroidism results from decreased thyroid hormone production. In about 95 percent of cases, the hormone deficiency is caused by a disease within the thyroid gland itself. Only 5 percent of cases are caused by pituitary or hypothalamic disease. The most common single cause is treatment of hyperthyroidism with radioiodine or surgery. Another common cause is autoimmune destruction of the thyroid, such as in Hashimoto's thyroiditis.

Hypothyroidism is very common. Community surveys find that about 8 percent of women and 1 percent of men have subclinical hypothyroidism. Overt hypothyroidism is reported in about 1 percent of patients seeking medical care. The diagnosis is made by thyroid function blood tests. Treatment is with synthetic thyroid hormone. The symptoms of hypothyroidism in adults are largely reversible with this medication.

Clinical Features

The clinical manifestations of hypothyroidism are variable, depending on its cause, duration, and severity (Table 7-4). Thyroid hormone is required for the normal functioning of most organ systems. Therefore thyroid hormone deficiency results in slowing of physical and mental activity, cardiovascular, gastrointestinal, and neuromuscular function. Deposition of glycoaminoglycans in the intracellular spaces, particularly in skin and muscle, along with the generalized slowing down of the organism result in the clinical picture of myxedema.

Table 7-4. Frequency of Signs and Symptoms of Hypothyroidism[a]

	Frequency (%)	Diagnostic Weight	
		Present	Absent
Symptoms			
Dry skin	60–100	+3	−6
Cold intolerance	60–95	+4	−5
Hoarseness	50–75	+5	−6
Weight gain	50–75	+5	−1
Constipation	35–65	+2	−1
Decreased sweating	10–65	+3	−6
Paresthesias	50	+5	−4
Decreased hearing	5–30	+2	0
Weakness	90		
Signs			
Slow movements	70–90	+11	−3
Coarse skin and hair	70–100	+7	−7
Cold skin	70–90	+3	−2
Periorbital puffiness	40–90	+4	−6
Bradycardia	10–15	+4	−4
Slow reflex relaxation	50	+15	−6

[a]In patients with no other illness and receiving no medication, a total score of +19 or greater indicates hypothyroidism and a score of −24 or less excludes it.

(From DeGroot et al.,[29] with permission.)

Many of the symptoms and signs of hypothyroidism, such as fatigue, lethargy, constipation, and dry skin, are nonspecific. The most helpful symptoms and signs that aid in the diagnosis are slow movements, coarse skin, decreased sweating, hoarseness, paresthesias, cold intolerance, periorbital edema, and slow reflex relaxation. The thyroid gland may be diffusely enlarged or may not be palpable, depending on the etiology. Since the incidence of hypothyroidism is so great, especially in women, it is not unlikely that therapists would come upon this either previously diagnosed or undiagnosed. The trophic changes of dry skin or periorbital puffiness may be observed during the objective examination, and reflex testing might elicit the slowed relaxation response. Muscle testing might reveal a pattern of weakness (see below). The subjective examination would probably elicit the complaints of fatigue and possibly complaints of arthralgias or specific weakness.

Patients often complain of extremity paresthesias but usually have no objective neurologic abnormalities other than slow deep tendon reflexes. These characteristic "hung-up" reflexes result from a decrease in the rate of muscle contraction and relaxation. Carpal tunnel syndrome may occur because of mucinous edema of the wrist. Some patients have a polyneuropathy because of myxedema of peripheral nerves. Movements are slow and clumsy. Signs of cerebellar dysfunction may occur, such as ataxia and intention tremor.[10,12]

Muscle cramps, myalgias, and stiffness are frequent symptoms. Subjective weakness and fatigability are common. Some objective muscle weakness may be noted in the shoulder and pelvic regions. Muscle mass may be slightly increased, and the muscles tend to be firmer than normal. Rarely, a large increase in muscle mass accompanied by slowness of muscular activity may be the predominant finding. Elevated serum creatine phosphokinase (CPK) levels are commonly found even in patients without muscle symptoms.[10,13,14] Patients may have arthralgias with synovial thickening and effusions, usually of the knees or small joints of the hands and feet.[15]

Diseases of the Parathyroid Gland

Hyperparathyroidism

Hyperparathyroidism is caused by an increased secretion of parathyroid hormone by the parathyroid gland. Parathyroid adenomas or, less commonly, carcinomas are the cause. The incidence is about 1 per 1,000 persons. The excess hormone usually leads to elevated calcium and decreased phosphate levels in the blood. With the widespread use of multiphasic screening blood tests, most patients have no symptoms, but are diagnosed on the basis of elevated calcium. Other patients present with recurrent kidney stones, peptic ulcers, mental changes, or extensive bone resorption.

The diagnosis of hyperparathyroidism is confirmed by an elevated blood parathyroid hormone level. Treatment varies with the severity of the hypercalcemia. Medical management followed by surgery is required for patients with severe symptomatic hypercalcemia. Many patients can be followed with periodic testing of bone and kidney function and no specific therapy.

Clinical Features

Osteitis fibrosa cystica is the classic skeletal disorder of hyperparathyroidism. Patients may have subperiosteal resorption, bone cysts, brown tumors, fractures, deformities, and marked replacement of bone marrow by fibrous tissue. In mild cases, the subperiosteal resorption may be limited to the radial side of the middle phalanges. The skull is the next most frequently involved area. Increased bone resorption in the skull leads to a salt-and-pepper appearance on skull radiographs. Later resorption may be seen close to the acromioclavicular joint, symphysis pubis, and sacroiliac joints. Patients may also have diffuse osteopenia that is indistinguishable from postmenopausal osteoporosis.[16,17]

Several joint disorders are frequently associated with hyperparathyroidism: chondrocalcinosis, gout, juxtaarticular erosions, subchondral fractures, traumatic synovitis, and calcific periarthritis.[16] Symptoms also include proximal muscle weakness and easy fatigability, particularly in the lower extremities. Gross motor atrophy may be present on biopsy. Electromyograms are abnormal.

Occasionally patients complain of dysesthesias. The patient may have abnormal tongue movements and atrophy. The neurologic examination may show decreased vibratory sense in the feet and glove-and-stocking sensory loss.[18,19] As seen in patients with thyroid disease, hyperparathyroid disease presents with muscle weakness and fatigue. Bony loss may be present, similar to the demineralization of hyperthyroidism. Physical therapy evaluation should reveal the reflex changes, muscle weakness, and sensory changes. Most patients are asymptomatic, and the disease is found during a routine physical examination through blood work.

Hypoparathyroidism

Hypoparathyroidism is caused by a decreased or absent secretion of parathyroid hormone by the parathyroid gland. Hypoparathyroidism may be hereditary or acquired. The hereditary form may first become manifest in adult life. It may be an isolated abnormality or associated with other endocrine and skin disorders. Acquired hypoparathyroidism is usually the result of inadvertent surgical removal of all of the parathyroid glands. This may occur during surgery for hyperthyroidism or hyperparathyroidism.

The reported incidence of permanent hypoparathyroidism after thyroidectomy ranges from 0.2 to 33 percent. The incidence is 1 percent after surgery for hypoparathyroidism. The diagnosis is made by finding a low serum calcium level with a low serum parathyroid hormone level. Patients are treated with calcium and vitamin D.

Clinical Features

Mild symptoms are nonspecific and include psychological symptoms, such as irritability and depression, paresthesias, and muscle cramps. More severe symptoms are delirium, psychosis, tetany, and seizures. Left untreated, the severe form can lead to death.

The most common manifestations of hypoparathyroidism are neurologic. A typical attack of overt tetany begins with tingling in the fingertips and around the mouth. This gradually increases in severity and spreads proximally along the limbs and over the face. The muscles of the extremities and face feel tense and then go into spasm. Pain may be very severe, depending on the degree of tension developed in the muscle.

Provocative tests may demonstrate the presence of latent tetany. A positive Chvostek's sign is obtained by a sharp tap given over the facial nerve just anterior to the ear, which produces a contraction of the facial muscle around the lip. The sign may be noticed by the patient during shaving. This test is also positive in up to 25 percent of normal people.[19]

Another diagnostic maneuver, Trousseau's sign, is compression of the upper arm by a blood pressure cuff with the pressure elevated above the systolic pressure. The test is positive when spasm of the hand occurs within 3 minutes (Fig. 7-3). This test is more reliable but may occur in about 4 percent of normal people. When the cuff is released, the muscles take about 5 to 10 seconds to relax.[19]

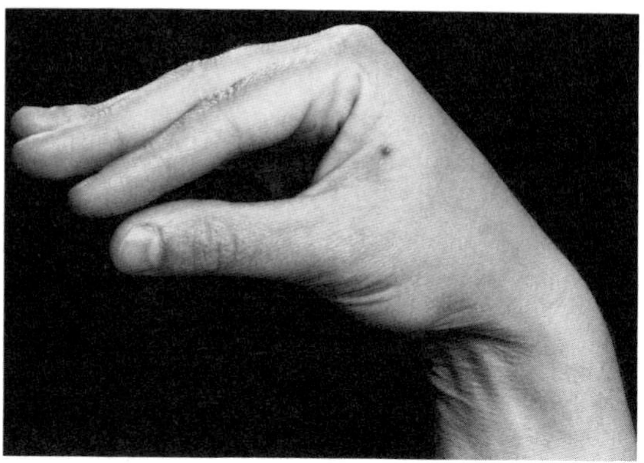

Fig. 7-3. Hand of a patient with a positive Trousseau's sign.

Many variations in clinical expression of tetany are possible. The patient may describe the muscle spasm as a cramp or stiffness or clumsiness. The patient may have continuous mild paresthesias or cramps rather than clearly defined attacks of tetany. Some patients develop carpal spasm only during prolonged use of the hand. If the spasm is more severe in the legs, the patient may have a limp or difficulty walking or fall frequently. Only one side of the body may be affected in some patients.[19]

Calcification of the basal ganglia may occur. There may be no neurologic disability associated or a variety of extrapyramidal symptoms such as chorea, tremors, dystonia, spasms, oculogyric crises, and parkinsonism. Age-related bone loss proceeds more slowly. Paravertebral ligamentous ossification can cause spinal nerve root compression and back stiffness.[20]

Fatigue and weakness are common symptoms. Rare patients may have a true myopathy.[19,21]

Patients with hypoparathyroidism would normally proceed to a physician with their complaints rather than seeking assistance from a physical therapist. Should a patient present first to a therapist, the objective and subjective signs and symptoms mentioned above would be unusual enough to immediately suggest a disease process and warrant referral to a physician.

Diseases of the Adrenal Gland

Cushing Syndrome

In Cushing syndrome (adrenocortical hyperactivity), an excess amount of glucocorticoid is secreted by the adrenal gland, along with a varying amount of adrenal androgens. Most cases are due to oversecretion of adrenocorticotropic hormone (ACTH) from a pituitary tumor, which then leads to adrenal hyperplasia. This etiology is termed Cushing syndrome. Other less common causes of adrenal hyperactivity are adrenal adenomas or carcinomas or a malignant tumor elsewhere in the body that produces ACTH. The incidence is 10 cases per 1 million people per year.

Patients with suspected Cushing syndrome can be screened by an overnight dexamethasone suppression test or measurement of the 24-hour urinary excretion of cortisol. Treatment varies with the cause of the syndrome. Adrenal adenomas are surgically removed. Pituitary tumors can also be surgically removed. An alternative treatment is pituitary irradiation in combination with an adrenal suppressing medication.

Clinical Features

The typical patient with Cushing syndrome is a middle-aged woman with truncal obesity, hirsutism (the presence of excessive body or facial hair, especially in women), a ruddy round face, and hypertension. Almost every organ system can be affected. Personality disorders are quite common (see Ch. 12).

The effect on the muscles is variable. Patients may have marked muscle wasting, especially proximally in the pelvic and shoulder girdle. Weakness may also be due to low serum potassium. Patients with long-standing Cushing syndrome will have demineralization of bone. Osteoporosis produces back pain, kyphosis, and loss of height. As many as 40 percent of patients have pathologic fractures of the ribs or vertebrae. Occasionally patients develop avascular necrosis of the femoral and humeral heads.

Dilatation and thinning of blood vessel walls occur, increasing their fragility and leading to a significant increase in bruisability. Poor wound healing is a particular problem for postsurgical patients. Signs and Symptoms are summarized in Table 7.5.

The significance of this disease to a manual therapist is the necessity to avoid techniques that might cause pathologic fractures secondary to osteoporosis. Here the emphasis should be placed on understanding and respecting the disease process in a previously diagnosed patient who presents to the clinic for pain management or for any other physical therapy intervention.

Table 7-5. Signs and Symptoms of Adrenal Gland Disease

Adrenocortical Hyperactivity (Cushing Syndrome)	Adrenocortical insufficiency (Addison's disease)
Truncal obesity	Weakness, fatigue
Hirsutism	Anorexia
	Vomiting, diahrrea
Round face	Weight loss
Hypertension	Hyperpigmentation
Proximal muscle wasting	Cartilage calcification
Osteoporosis	Neuropathy
Back pain	Myopathy
Kyphosis	Paraplegia
Height	Quadriplegia
Poor wound healing	Personality changes
Easily bruised	Organic brain syndromes
Personality changes	
Irritability	
Emotional lability	
Depression	
Paranoia	
Decreased libido	
Oligomenorrhea	
Impotence	

Addison's Disease

Addison's disease (adrenocortical insufficiency) is the primary inability of the adrenal gland to make sufficient quantities of adrenal steroid hormones. It is most commonly due to an autoimmune process, with antibodies present in adrenal tissue. Addison's disease is uncommon, with a prevalence of 4 per 100,000 persons.

It is difficult to diagnose early Addison's disease because nonspecific weakness and fatigue are the most frequent symptoms. Screening for Addison's disease may be done by ACTH stimulation testing, which measures the reserve capacity of the adrenal for steroid production. Treatment is specific hormone replacement with cortisol and often fludrocortisone.

Clinical Features

All patients with Addison's disease complain of weakness and fatigue. Gastrointestinal symptoms such as anorexia, vomiting, and diarrhea are common, and most patients will have a history of weight loss. Most patients will have signs of hyperpigmentation, most noticeably on the extensor surfaces, the creases of the palm, and the buccal mucosa. Personality changes and even organic brain syndromes are often exhibited.

Serum calcium is frequently elevated, leading to calcification of cartilage. The ears may be hardened to a stonelike consistency. The costal cartilage may also be calcified. Serum potassium elevation may produce an ascending neuromyopathy that ultimately causes flaccid paraplegia or quadriplegia. Addison's disease may also be associated with spastic paraplegia and polyneuropathy, called adrenomyeloneuropathy. Signs and symptoms are summarized in Table 7.5.

Once again, weakness and fatigue are the symptoms most relevant to diagnosis and most likely to be found on physical therapy assessment. Response to treatment, as mentioned with regard to disorders of other endocrine glands, is a key to deciding on referral of the patient for further physician follow-up.

Diseases of the Pituitary Gland

Acromegaly

Acromegaly is a disease caused by an excess production of growth hormone after adolescence. Pituitary tumors are the most common cause. This chronic, slowly progressive, debilitating disease is characterized by overgrowth of the skeleton and enlargement of soft tissues. Acromegaly occurs most often in middle age. The annual incidence is estimated to be 3 cases per 1 million persons.

Patients with acromegaly often have symptoms for many years before the diagnosis is made. The diagnosis is confirmed by an elevated serum growth hormone level that does not suppress with an oral glucose load. Treatment options include surgery, radiation, and medical therapy with bromocriptine.

Clinical Features

The most common clinical feature suggesting the diagnosis is a coarsening of facial features over many years. Multiple organ systems can be adversely affected by acromegaly. Hypertension, congestive heart failure, visceral hypertrophy, diabetes, and renal stones may all be part of the clinical picture.[2] The physical therapist rarely has the opportunity to see a patient over a course of years and therefore would not notice this coarsening of features. The symptoms and signs of skeletal changes with associated weakness and pain should clue the therapist to the possibility of acromegaly if these skeletal changes are overtly observable.

Patients with acromegaly tend to be tall. The mandible enlarges, resulting in prognathism (an underbite). The frontal, malar, and nasal bones are overgrown.

As the metacarpals, metatarsals, and phalanges increase in thickness, the patient may notice an increased glove and shoe size. The ribs elongate and result in a barrel-shaped chest. The vertebral bodies of the spine elongate and widen and develop hypertrophic spurs. Thoracic kyphosis is common. Joint symptoms are prominent and vary from backaches and arthralgias to severe degenerative osseous overgrowth. As the disease progresses, degenerative arthritis of the hips, knees, shoulders, and elbows may develop.[22] Muscle weakness is primarily due to neuropathies. There may also be a proximal muscle myopathy.[23,24]

Patients may have compression of the nerve roots at the vertebral foramina with resultant spinal stenosis from overgrowth of the bony canal. Acroparesthesias are due to entrapment of nerves by bone or connective tissue overgrowth. Paresthesias of the hand are particularly common, resulting from compression of the median nerve at the wrist.[24–26]

SUMMARY

This chapter covers those diseases of the endocrine system that might have an impact on physical therapy care or outcome. Diabetes mellitus, thyrotoxicosis (hyperthyroidism) and hypothyroidism, hyperparathyroidism and hypoparathyroidism, Cushing syndrome, Addison's disease, and acromegaly have been discussed. The most common subjective and objective changes found in patients suffering from these diseases are summarized in Table 7-6. Many of these diseases present with common subjective complaints of weakness, fatigue, and lethargy. It is therefore important to pay heed to these complaints, especially if they are accompanied by unexplained objective findings or when seemingly explainable objective findings do not respond to physical therapy. A screening checklist for review of the endocrine system is presented in Figure 7-4.

The goals of this chapter have been to provide the physical therapist with the information necessary to determine when referral to a physician might be warranted in the case of metabolic disease. Additionally, the discussion of these diseases and their signs and symptoms should aid the clinician in appropriate treatment planning and goal setting.

PATIENT CASE STUDY 1

History

A 52-year-old male tool and dye worker was referred by physician to physical therapy with a diagnosis of cervical and lumbar spondylosis. His chief complaints were of right neck, posterior shoulder, and low back pain. He was seen a year after involvement in a motor vehicle accident. He had been in another vehicle accident 1 year before this second one and suffered a work-related low back injury 9 years before therapy. Previous physical therapy did help but did not relieve his symptoms. In addition to the neck, shoulder, and arm symptoms, he complained of some dizziness and discomfort in the medial aspect of both great toes.

The patient's neck pain was aggravated by pulling, picking things up, or turning his head too fast. The low back discomfort was brought on by quick forward bending or by sitting in a car for more than 1 hour. The patient was unaware of what increased or brought on his dizziness. Medications and assuming a nonweight-bearing position diminished his neck and back symptoms. The patient denied any general medical problems and had a surgical history of tonsillectomy and vasectomy.

Objective Examination

Observation demonstrated the patient's head to be slightly rotated to the right and presence of scoliosis of the lumbar spine convex to the right. Increased muscle tone was noted throughout the paraspinal musculature: motion testing revealed restriction in C1–C2 joint mobility and decreased anterior glide at the cervicothoracic junction. Various muscle length restrictions were found, including bilateral tightness of gastrocsoleus, hip flexors, rectus femoris, hamstrings, and hip adductors. Disruption of normal mechanics was found at the L5–S1 motion segment. Neurologic examination was negative.

Assessment and Outcome

The patient was seen for 10 physical therapy visits. He was treated with soft tissue mobilization, joint mobilization, muscle energy techniques, muscle stretching, and strengthening. He was provided with a home program for stretching and strengthening and given guidance regarding a previously established general conditioning program. The patient's low back and neck pain abated after the 10 visits to physical therapy. His dizziness remained. During the course of treatment the patient complained of blurred vision, which came on while doing push-ups, bicycling, and a home exercise program. The therapist suggested the patient contact his physician, which he did. He was then diagnosed with diabetes and when discharged was working to get it under control

Review of Systems: Endocrine Disease

Item	Yes	No	Comments
1. Constitutional symptoms (fatigue, weight loss, weakness)	_____	_____	_____
2. Psycho/cognitive changes (depression, personality changes, memory loss, confusion, irritability)	_____	_____	_____
3. Gastrointestinal symptoms (diarrhea, dysphasia, constipation, nausea, vomiting, anorexia)	_____	_____	_____
4. Musculoskeletal symptoms (muscle weakness, arthralgias, myalgias, stiffness, muscle cramps, bone pain)	_____	_____	_____
5. Sensory impairment (paresthesias, numbness, tingling in fingertips/mouth)	_____	_____	_____
6. Urogenital symptoms (impotence, intermittent stream, dribbling, straining to void)	_____	_____	_____
7. Dermatologic signs (foot ulcerations, edema, dry/course skin, impaired wound healing)	_____	_____	_____
8. Miscellaneous complaints (temperature intolerances, visual changes, orthostatic hypotension, increased bruising)	_____	_____	_____

Fig. 7-4. Screening checklist for endocrine system disease.

Table 7-6. Subjective and Objective Changes Associated with Common Endocrine Disease

Disorder	Subjective	Objective
Diabetes mellitus	Orthostatic hypotension Blurred vision Sensory deficits Extremity or truncal pain Weakness Diarrhea Bladder complaints Impotence Dysphagia	Edema Foot ulcerations Muscle atrophy Elevated resting heart rate Deviation of the eye inward Diminished ankle jerk Impaired vibratory sense Decreased muscle strength
Thyrotoxicosis (hyperthyroidism)	Nervousness Weight loss Palpitations Muscle weakness Fatigue Heat intolerance	Enlarging neck mass Decreased muscle strength Trophic changes—thickening of the skin Pathologic fractures
Hypothyroidism	Fatigue, lethargy Constipation Paresthesias Cold intolerance Arthralgias, myalgias Stiffness, muscle cramps	Dry, coarse skin Slowed movements Decreased sweating Hoarseness Periorbital edema Slowed reflex relaxation Decreased muscle strength
Hyperparathyroidism	Weakness Fatigue Nausea, vomiting Joint complaints, bone aches Memory loss, confusion	Decreased muscle strength Glove and stocking sensory loss Ostopenia, subperiosteal resorption, bone cysts
Hypoparathyroidism	Irritability Depression Paresthesias Back stiffness Muscle cramps	Tetany (initially tingling in fingertips and mouth) Seizures Stiffness upon passive spinal mobilization
Cushing syndrome (adrenocortical hyperactivity)	Back pain Increased bruising	Truncal obesity Hirsutism Hypertension Muscle atrophy Decreased muscle strength Osteoporosis with increased thoracic kyphosis and pathologic fractures of ribs or vertebrae Poor wound healing
Addison's disease (adrenocortical insufficiency)	Weakness Fatigue Weight loss GI symptoms	Hyperpigmentation Decreased muscle strength
Acromegaly	Backache Arthralgias Muscle weakness Paresthesias of the hand	Coarsening of facial features over many years Overgrowth of mandible, frontal, and nasal bones Thickening of metacarpals, metatarsals, and phalanges Barrel-shaped chest Increased thoracic kyphosis Decreased muscle strength Sensory changes

through insulin injections and diet. He was still having dizziness and blurred vision when discharged.

The patient's diabetic complications did interfere with his physical therapy treatment in that his exercise program had to be postponed due to his inability to regulate his insulin during these periods, at least initially. The important point of this case is that the therapist initially paid little attention to the dizziness because the patient had a cervical problem that could have been responsible for this symptom. Fortunately, the therapist recognized the complaint of blurred vision with exercise as being unexpected and referred him back to a physician. The dizziness did not change with manual therapy even though the cervical pain and dysfunction abated. Had the blurred vision not signaled the diabetes, at the end of treatment the therapist might have realized that the dizziness did not fit a musculoskeletal diagnosis and referred him back to the physician in any case.

PATIENT CASE STUDY 2

History

A 54-year-old man was seen in October 1989 by physician referral with a diagnosis of degenerative disc disease at L5–S1 and a small herniated nucleus pulposis on the left. When initially evaluated in physical therapy he was not working his light-duty airport commission job secondary to uncontrolled diabetes. The patient complained of constant deep aching in the central low lumbar spine, sometimes spreading into the buttocks, left greater than right. In addition, he complained of a constant numblike sensation in the lateral aspect of the left thigh and calf extending to the left heel. The patient noted an increase in the lower-extremity symptoms with an increase in the low back ache. The low back and buttock symptoms were aggravated by sitting greater than 60 to 90 minutes or with walking greater than two blocks. Forward bending or reaching activities also increased his low back pain. Diminishment of the low back ache could be attained through self-traction achieved by putting his weight on his arms in the sitting or standing positions, through a constant change of position, or by assuming any recumbent position. His symptoms began in 1985 when he was pulling on a heavy wrench trying to loosen a lock and felt a sharp stabbing pain in the low back. The next morning he could not get out of bed. He stated that he had progressively gotten worse as the pain had spread into his buttock and left leg, and he felt stiffness up through the trunk to the cervical region.

The patient was a diabetic under the care of a physician for the condition. When initially seen, his diabetes was out of control and he was attempting to remedy this. The patient also suffered from high blood pressure. He had been told by another physician that his low back and buttock pain were the result of his herniated disc and that his left lower extremity complaints were the results of his diabetes. The patient denied any previous surgeries of any kind.

Objective Examination

Observation in the standing position revealed a loss of lumbar lordosis, moderate lateral shift to the right, and an increase in cervicothoracic junction kyphosis. A compensatory lateral curvature was present in the thoracic spine, convexity to the right. The patient was unable to forward bend without pain, and backward bending provoked sharp pain in the low back and numbness in the left lower extremity. Straight leg raising was positive on the left at 45 degrees for increased buttock and low back pain. There was a slight hyposensitivity to pin prick in the left lateral calf, and the S1 ankle jerk reflex was slightly decreased as well. Myotome testing for the lower quarter was negative. Central pressures at L5 and prone press-ups both provoked his symptoms at the lumbosacral area and into the left buttock. There was extensive muscle guarding in the left lumbar paraspinals from S1 to L3 and on the right from S1 to L4.

Treatment

On the first visit the patient was treated by attempting to correct his lateral shift in standing against the wall. This alleviated all of the patient's symptoms, including the "numbness" of the left leg. He was fit with a lumbar support with a hard insert and given a home program for the shift correction. Follow-up visits included a progression through extension exercises; he was given soft tissue mobilization to the right lateral trunk, buttock, and hip flexors.

Assessment and Outcome

At discharge the patient was back at work, wearing the lumbar support, and complaining only of some intermittent left lateral thigh numbness and occasional low back ache. His lower leg numbness had subsided. This case demonstrates the need to pursue conservative care, including physical therapy, for complaints of distal pain or altered sensation, even when systemic disease might seem conveniently to explain away those symptoms. Diabetic peripheral neuropathy can explain many lower extremity and, less commonly, upper extremity complaints, but not all. Provocation of this patient's lower extremity symptoms through movement of the lumbar spine and by direct pressures at the L5–S1 motion segment established a direct correlation between the patient's low back and leg complaints. In this case, the patient was already under the therapist's care and was going to receive therapy, regardless of this correlation. However, when we as therapists have the opportunity to screen patients for physical therapy without prior physician referral, we should always maintain the possibility that symptoms common to the patient's known disease process may not be a result of that disease, but may instead result from a neuromusculoskeletal dysfunction amenable to our care.

REFERENCES

1. Guyton A: Textbook of Medical Physiology. WB Saunders, Philadelphia, 1991
2. Thomas P: Metabolic neuropathy. JR Coll Physicians Lond 7:154, 1973
3. Dyck P, Thomas P, Lambert E et al (eds): Peripheral Neuropathy. 2nd Ed. Vol. II. WB Saunders, Philadelphia, 1984
4. Sinha S, Munichoodappa CS, Kozak GP: Neuro-arthropathy (Charcot joints) in diabetes mellitus. (Clinical study of 101 cases.) Medicine (Baltimore) 51:191, 1972
5. Podolsky S: Clinical Diabetes: Modern Management. Appleton & Lange, E. Norwalk, CT, 1980
6. Chokroverty S, Reyes MG, Rubino FA, Tonaki H: The syndrome of diabetic amyotrophy. Ann Neurol 2:181, 1977
7. Asbury AK: Proximal diabetic neuropathy. Ann Neurol 2:179, 1977
8. Rubin E, Farber J (eds): Pathology. 2nd Ed. JB Lippincott Co, Philadelphia, 1994
9. Engel AG: Neuromuscular manifestations of Graves' disease. Mayo Clinic Proc 47:919, 1972
10. Swanson JW, Kelly JJ, McConahey WM: Neurologic aspects of thyroid dysfunction. May Clin Proc 56:504, 1981
11. Greenspan F, Forsham P: Basic and Clinical Endocrinology. 2nd Ed. Lange Medical Publications, Los Altos, CA, 1986
12. Sanders V: Neurologic manifestations of myxedema. N Engl J Med 266:547, 1962
13. Khaleeli AA, Griffith DG, Edwards RHT: The clinical presentation of hypothyroid myopathy and its relationship to abnormalities in structure and function of skeletal muscle. Clin Endocrinol (Oxf) 19:365, 1983
14. Klein I, Parker M, Shebert R et al: Hypothyroidism presenting as muscle stiffness and pseudohypertrophy: Hoffmann's syndrome. Am J Med 70:891, 1981
15. Dorwart BB, Schumacher HR: Joint effusions, chondrocalcinosis and other rheumatic manifestations in hypothyroidism: a clinicopathologic study. Am J Med 59:780, 1975
16. Steinbach HL, Gordan GS, Eisenberg E et al: Primary hyperparathyroidism: a correlation of roentgen, clinical, and pathologic features. AJR 86:329, 1961
17. Dauphine RT, Riggs BL, Scholz DA: Back pain and vertebral crush fractures: an unemphasized mode of presentation for primary hyperparathyroidism. Ann Intern Med 83:365, 1975
18. Patten BM, Bilezikian JP, Mallette LE et al: Neuromuscular disease in primary hyperparathyroidism. Ann Intern Med 80:182, 1974
19. Frame B: Neuromuscular manifestations of parathyroid disease. In Vinken PJ, Bruyn GW (eds): Handbook of Clinical Neurology. Vol. 27. North-Holland, Amsterdam, 1976
20. Okazaki T, Takuwa Y, Yamamoto M et al: Ossification of the paravertebral ligaments: a frequent complication of hypoparathyroidism. Metabolism 33:710, 1984
21. Kruse K, Scheunemann W, Baier W, Schaub J: Hypocalcemic myopathy in idiopathic hypoparathyroidism. Eur J Pediatr 138:280, 1982
22. Detenbeck LC, Tressler HU, O'Duffy JD, Randall RV: Peripheral joint manifestations of acromegaly. Clin Orthop 91:119, 1972
23. Mastaglia FL, Barwick DD, Hall R: Myopathy in acromegaly. Lancet 2:907, 1970
24. Pickett JBE, Layzer RB, Levin SR et al: Neuromuscular complications of acromegaly. Neurology (NY) 25:638, 1975
25. Epstein N, Whelan M, Benjamin V: Acromegaly and spinal stenosis. J Neurosurg 56:145, 1982
26. O'Duffy JD, Randall RV, MacCarty CS: Median neuropathy (carpal-tunnel syndrome) in acromegaly. Ann Intern Med 78:379, 1973
27. Vander AJ, Sherman JH, Luciano DS: Human Physiology–The Mechanism of Body Function. 5th Ed. McGraw-Hill, New York, 1990
28. Wilson JD, Foster DW (eds): Williams Textbook of Endocrinology. 8th Ed. WB Saunders, Philadelphia, 1992
29. DeGroot LJ, Besser GM, Cahill GF et al (eds): Endocrinology. 2nd Ed. WB Saunders, Philadelphia, 1989

SUGGESTED READINGS

Barker LR, Burton JR,Zieve PD (eds): Principals of Ambulatory Medicine. 3rd Ed. Williams & Wilkins, Baltimore, 1991

Bates B: A Guide to Physical Examination and History Taking. 5th Ed. JB Lippincott, Philadelphia, 1991

Berkow R (ed): The Merck Manual. 16th Ed. Merck & Co, Rahway, NJ, 1992

Isselbacher KH, Braunwald E, Wilson JD et al (eds): Harrison's Principles of Internal Medicine. 13th Ed. McGraw-Hill, New York 1994

Kohler PO, Jordan RM (eds): Clinical Endocrinology. John Wiley & Sons, New York, 1986

8 SCREENING FOR PATHOLOGIC ORIGINS OF HEAD AND FACIAL PAIN

Edward R. Isaacs, M.D., F.A.A.N.
Mark R. Bookhout, M.S., P.T.

Physical therapists are increasingly confronted by patients with headache or facial pain as a consequence of musculoskeletal system dysfunction. During this era of direct access, patients may not be screened by a physician before treatment is initiated by a physical therapist. Patients who have been referred by a physician may develop new medical conditions during a course of physical therapy treatment that require a physician's attention. It has therefore become mandatory to broaden the knowledge of the therapist to consider other diseases involving the cranial structures and nervous system that may manifest as head or facial pain, such as tumors, vascular diseases, infections, neuralgias, and endocrine and ophthalmologic disorders. The goal of this chapter is to provide the physical therapist with a means of identifying those potentially serious conditions that are beyond the scope of physical therapy practice. Once a disease of this sort is suspected, an appropriate referral to a physician can be made in a fashion that would enhance meaningful communication.

Although headache is a very common affliction, only recently has the role of the physical therapist been recognized in its treatment. In 1944 Campbell and Parsons[1] demonstrated that irritation of both joint and ligamentous structures of the upper cervical spine resulted in referral of symptoms to the cranium and therefore can be a potential source of head and facial pain (Fig. 8-1). Edeling[2] and Jull[3] have described the use of manual therapy directed to the upper cervical spine in the treatment of chronic headaches. The following characteristics have been associated with headaches related to cervical spine dysfunction[4,5]:

1. Headaches precipitated by movements of the neck or pressure on trigger points in the neck
2. Pain, stiffness, and decreased range of motion (ROM) of the cervical spine
3. Asymmetric or unilateral symptoms
4. Occasional associated ipsilateral shoulder or arm pain

Myofascial spray and stretch techniques directed toward the skeletal muscles that refer pain into the head or the facial area have been extensively documented by Travell and Simons.[6] Any multidisciplinary approach to the evaluation and treatment of pain caused by temporomandibular joint dysfunction now includes the participation of a physical therapist.

According to Butler,[7] headaches from dural irritation are now a recognizable clinical entity and nearly always are associated with a previous history of nervous system injury (i.e., whiplash, postepidural and/or postlumbar puncture). Symptoms of a dural headache may include the following: (1) symptoms may be nondermatomal (i.e., patients may complain of caps of pain, nondermatomal strips, "tightness" and "fullness" of the head), (2) symptoms will often alternate sides and are commonly bilateral and central, (3) symptoms may be brought on by neurodynamic tension testing of the nervous system (i.e., slump sitting), and (4) symptoms continue despite adequate manual therapy treatment to zygapophyseal joints and muscles.

When the patient's signs and symptoms are atypical for head pain arising from mechanical dysfunction, or if the response to treatment is not as expected, a pathologic origin of head and facial pain should be considered.

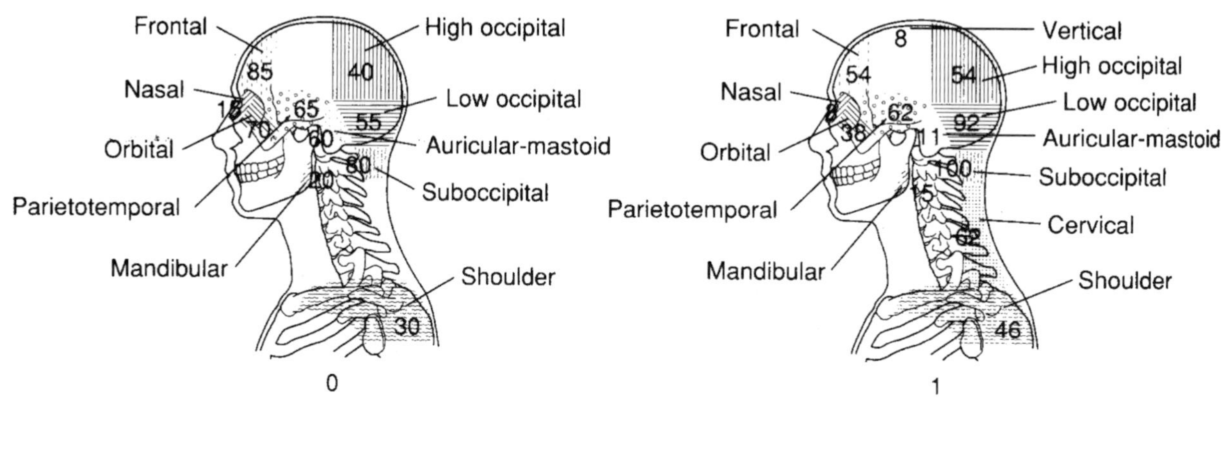

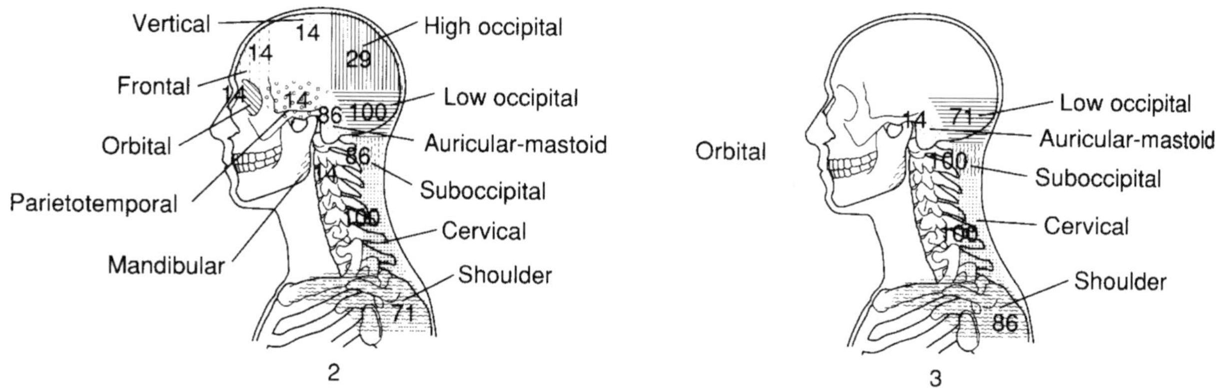

Fig. 8-1. Charts of head, neck, and shoulder regions, illustrating schematically the distribution and frequency of pains referred from the following sites: 0, basal occipital region; 1, occipitoatlanto region; 2, interspinous space C2; 3, interspinous space C3. (From Campbell and Parsons,[1] with permission.)

PHYSICAL THERAPY EVALUATION FOR DISEASES OF THE CRANIUM THAT PRESENT AS HEAD OR FACIAL PAIN

Subjective Examination

History of Present Illness

The patient's history with regard to head pain is especially important, since many diseases of the cranium and cranial nerves can only be diagnosed on the basis of history, as there may be no physical or laboratory manifestations to rely on. While taking the history, the examiner also has an opportunity to assess cognitive and language ability, speech patterns and articulation, and mannerisms. Descriptions of head pain should be directed to include location, quality, frequency, duration, progression, peak intensity, and consistency of symptoms, when pain is recurrent. Associated symptoms that are important include loss of concentration and memory ability, numbness, weakness, incoordination, and any cranial nerve dysfunction affecting vision, smell, hearing, taste, swallowing, and speech (Table 8-1). Any determination of an alteration of mentation or cognitive ability, especially when associated with nausea, vomiting, and/or loss of consciousness, indicates the need for referral to a physician.

Symptoms that emerge with postural or positional change may sound mechanical in nature but may also be caused by changes in intracranial pressure, which, when abnormally elevated, can be further increased during a strenuous activity or when the patient is lying down. Pathologic processes within the cranium produce symptoms by disturbing blood vessels, dura, periosteum, sinus

Table 8-1. Questions To Ask During the Subjective Examination Pertaining to Cranial Nerve Function

Question	Cranial Nerve(s) Involved
Any loss of smell?	I
Any loss of taste?	VII, IX
Any loss of vision or visual acuity?	II
Double vision?	III, IV, VI
Numbness of face or frontal scalp?	V
Hypersensitivity to sound?	VII
Any loss of hearing or ringing in the ears?	VIII
Difficulty swallowing?	IX, X
Chronic cough, loss or impairment of voice?	X

membranes, and cranial nerves. Screening of the nervous system should be a priority during the initial evaluation, especially if the patient describes any of the following symptoms (see Ch. 9):

1. Headaches that worsen with activity or exertion
2. Headaches that begin suddenly and that are immediately severe and generalized in location
3. Headaches that begin after lying down, especially if they awaken the patient from sleep
4. Headaches associated with projectile vomiting, but no nausea
5. Headaches that begin with, or remain as, unilateral pulsating pain in synchrony with the heartbeat
6. Focal tenderness over the temporal artery in any patient past the age of 60 (Fig. 8-2)
7. Sudden, intense, lancinating, brief pain that is either spontaneous or triggered by a mild stimulus
8. Intense pain localized over a sinus or around the teeth
9. Headaches associated with other symptoms
   a. Altered ability to think or personality change
   b. Visual disturbance (i.e., blindness, double vision, distortions, spots, or jagged scotoma; loss of vision on one side)
   c. Numbness or altered sensibility defined by a cortical (hemisensory), brain stem (bilateral), or spinal (disassociated) pattern
   d. Loss of strength or coordination ability
   e. Loss or alteration of smell or taste
   f. Loss or alteration of hearing
   g. Fever or associated systemic illness

A complete history regarding the events preceding the development of head pain is just as important as the descriptive analysis of the events during and after the onset of symptoms. Any history of head or neck injury close to the time of onset should raise suspicion of subdural hematoma or undiagnosed fracture of the odontoid process and/or loss of integrity of the alar ligaments. Recent dental treatment may be a cause of focal sinus infection or temporomandibular joint dysfunction. Any previous malignancy, especially carcinomas of the breast, lung, kidney, bowel, prostate, and malignant melanoma, must be considered, as they metastasize to the skull or brain.

Past Medical History

Past medical history reviews previous as well as ongoing illnesses that might affect treatment plans or provide additional information that may not have seemed relevant to the history concerning the primary complaint. A history of heart disease becomes important when one considers that the pain of angina often is referred outside of the chest and can localize to the jaw and occasionally the forehead.[8] Patients with diabetes are more susceptible to infection, vascular disease, and cranial neuropathies. Taking a past history also gives the practitioner an additional opportunity to screen for history of malignancy and trauma that may have been missed.

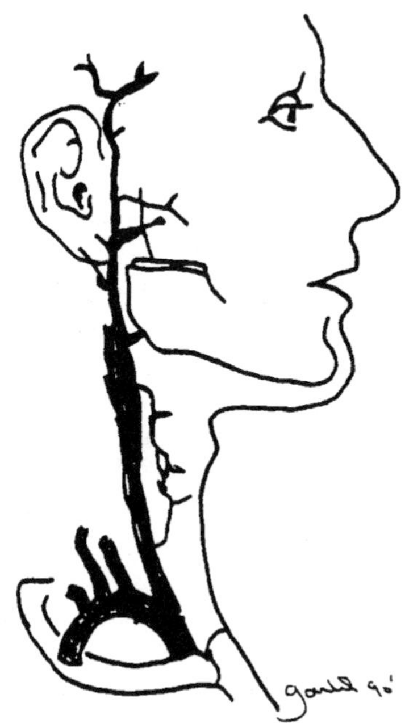

Fig. 8-2. Temporal artery distribution. Palpable anterior to the ear and in the temporal region. (From Boissonnault and Bass,[12] with permission.)

Family History

The family history is of limited value in the diagnosis of head pain outside of migraine, in which 66 percent of patients with this complaint report a history of migraine in another close family member.[8] Recurrent Bell's palsy and adult-onset diabetes also have some familial tendencies.

Social History

The social history describes habits, hobbies, work, and home environment and can provide additional useful information. Questions are directed toward detecting potential sources of support and stress. Pressures and stresses from work, marriage, and family strife, as well as other social relationships, may be disclosed. Habits concerning the use and abuse of alcohol, tobacco, or drugs not only directly affect health but also suggest deficiencies in coping mechanisms. Descriptions of work requirements and work environment provide information about potential injury, physical demands, and possible toxic exposure.

Review of Systems

As part of a complete history, the patient is asked about organ or body system functions in an organized manner designed to elicit other pertinent information. Questions about head, eyes, ears, nose, and throat should have been covered but can be asked again in regard to other problems, such as allergies. Chest function is discussed in terms of chest pain, cough, and/or shortness of breath and might uncover potential infection or malignancy. Symptoms of heart disease include chest pain, angina, shortness of breath, and edema in the extremities and may also be associated with other vascular complaints. Problems affecting the gastrointestinal system cause altered appetite, weight loss, nausea, vomiting, diarrhea, and abdominal pains. Painless bleeding from the bowel may produce red or black stools, depending on the site of bleeding. Constipation may be a cause of headache, since increased intra-abdominal pressure can be directly transmitted centrally through the paraspinal venus plexus, which is unique in its absence of intraluminal valves. Genitourinary system disorders affect bladder function in regard to either control or pain on voiding. Recurrent urinary tract infections in the male suggest neurogenic bladder dysfunction or chronic infection associated with systemic disease. An obstetric/gynecologic history can be an easy way of learning about an early pregnancy as well as endocrine function. The neurologic system review was done as part of the history of present illness. A suggested checklist of items to be covered during history taking to screen for diseases of the cranium is outlined in Table 8-2.

Physical Examination

Observation is an integral part of any physical examination and can be accomplished indirectly as the patient walks into the examination/treatment area and directly during the formal examination. Particular attention

Table 8-2. History Taking to Screen for Diseases of the Cranium

1. Date of onset
2. Mode of onset
3. Location of pain
4. Character and intensity of pain
5. Duration of pain
6. Aggravating or relieving factors
   - Postural/positional
   - Activity/rest
   - Medication
   - Previous therapy or treatment
   - Diet
   - Associated complaints (i.e., numbness, pins-and-needles sensation, tingling)
7. Special senses
   - Vision
   - Hearing
   - Smell
   - Taste
8. Past medical history
   - Cancer
   - Head injury
   - Heart disease
   - Stroke
   - Allergy
   - Ease in frequency of infection
   - Dental history
   - Surgical history
9. Family history
10. Social history
    - Work
    - Toxic exposure
    - Habits (tobacco, alcohol, drugs)
    - Marital status or living arrangement
11. Review of systems
    - Chest pain
    - Shortness of breath
    - Chronic cough
    - Edema in extremities
    - Weight loss
    - Abdominal pain/vomiting
    - Bloody stool
    - Pain on voiding
    - Ob/gyn problems

should be paid to head and neck posture, which provides the first suggestion of dysfunctional cervical spine mechanics. A head tilt might also be the result of diplopia (double vision) or extraocular eye muscle weakness (cranial nerve IV). Drooping of an eyelid and lateral eye deviation are indicative of oculomotor dysfunction (cranial nerve III). Viewing the open mouth is a part of the assessment of the temporomandibular joint, and it provides an opportunity to visualize the tongue for atrophy and the health of the gums and teeth. Missing teeth and malocclusion should be noted, as well as unhealthy gum tissue that does not appear to be a firm or a pink fleshy color. Drooping of one shoulder may be the consequence of abnormal thoracic or scapular mechanics or may be due to atrophy of the trapezius secondary to a peripheral lesion of cranial nerve XI.

Active and passive ROM of the cervical and thoracic spines should be assessed, with an attempt made to provoke the patient's symptoms either partially or wholly while searching for a musculoskeletal cause for this complaint. Particular attention should be paid to the upper cervical spine segments, since these are most commonly the origin of referred pain to the cranium.[2,3] Functional mobility of the temporomandibular joint should also be examined.

A neurologic screening examination may be necessary to confirm suspicions of serious illness or simply to satisfy the therapist that there are no obvious contraindications to proceeding with therapy directed toward the patient's complaint (refer to Ch. 9).

The examination includes palpation of the cranium, seeking painful areas, especially over blood vessels, or for enlarged and possibly tender lymph nodes, which may reflect local infection or systemic disease (see Ch. 1 for a description of the characteristics associated with lymph node abnormalities). Areas to be palpated for lymph nodes include the submental, submandibular, periauricular, and posterior cervical regions (Fig. 8-3).

DISEASES OR DISORDERS THAT CAN CAUSE HEAD OR FACIAL PAIN

After taking the history and completing an examination of a patient with head pain, therapy is initiated unless there is concern about a disease or disorder that is not amenable to physical therapy. The following section is not meant to provide information from which the physical therapist might make a diagnosis. Greater difficulties might arise if the patient is referred to the physician with a particular diagnosis rather than a report outlining concerns about particular history and/or findings on examination.

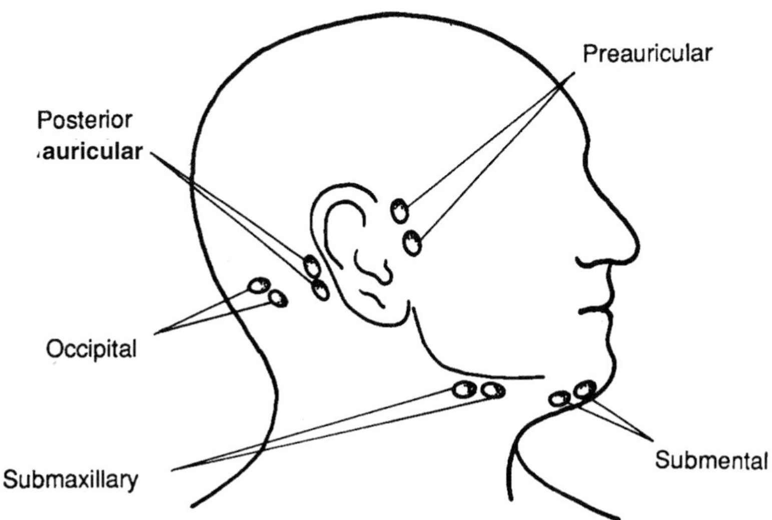

Fig. 8-3. Lymph nodes of the head and neck.

Headache: General Considerations

The most common headache types are migraines, tension headaches, and headaches arising from either mechanical cervical or cranial dysfunction, or both. Despite overlap of these categories, it is possible to define these types of headaches within a diagnostic framework that would encourage the most appropriate therapy. Any text or paper that reviews headache emphasizes the need to consider what structures are pain sensitive (i.e., have nociceptor innervation). Generally those structures with the capability of generating painful sensation include blood vessels, dura, ligaments, fascia, periosteum, muscles, joints, skin, subcutaneous tissues, glandular tissue, sinus and nasal mucosa, dental pulp, gums in the lining of the oropharynx, endoneurium, epineurium, and perineurium of the cranial and cervical nerves.[8] Pain can also be referred into the cranium from structures located elsewhere, but pain-sensitive structures are still primarily involved.

The term *migraine* refers to headaches believed to be of vascular origin. The name itself derives from the term hemicrania, suggesting an asymmetric, unilateral location of the pain. This derivation can be appreciated if the "he" is dropped from the hemicrania, leaving "micrania" from which emerges *migraine*. Migraines may be associated with a severe tension headache especially if there is photophobia, nausea, and vomiting. More recent research and theories would suggest that migraine is really a brain stem dysfunction involving serotinergic pain pathways with the vascular changes reflecting only epiphenomena.[9] True migraine is further classified into subcategories of typical, classic, and complicated forms, depending on the presence of an aura and associated symptoms. Migraine is a familial disorder, with fairly stereotypical headaches recurring at various frequencies, often before or during menstrual periods or after periods of stress or precipitated by certain foods containing tyramine (aged cheese, red wine) or other vasoactive substances (e.g., chocolate). The typical migraine begins with unilateral discomfort, which is pulsatile and associated early on with nausea, often followed by vomiting. The pain usually increases, and the sense of illness pervades and incapacitates. Some patients with typical migraine note inexplicable alterations of mood beginning about 1 day before onset. Interestingly, in support of the central brain stem dysfunction theory, many migraineurs find relief of symptoms after sleeping. This usually requires assistance from some medication. There may be some underlying cervical mechanical dysfunction that can be treated, but treatment will not significantly reduce the discomfort. Classic migraine differs from typical migraine by the occurrence of a preceding or associated aura that usually affects vision with perception of a central or peripheral bright scotoma that may have a geometric configuration. Occasionally the aura is olfactory, with a migraineur sensing a peculiar, usually unpleasant, aromatic hallucination. Complicated migraine is noteworthy in that the aura consists of more significant neurologic dysfunction, including ophthalmoplegia, hemisensory loss, and even hemiplegia. Often the epiphenomena persist well into the headache and occasionally occur without associated headache, nausea, or vomiting and are then called "migraine equivalents."

In 1962 the ad hoc committee on the classification of headache adopted the term *muscle contraction headache* for conditions previously referred to as tension or nervous headaches.[10] Pain generation is then defined as being derived from sustained contraction of skeletal muscles of the head and neck as the primary source of pain. Trott[11] believes that the diagnosis of a tension headache or muscle contraction headache presents a problem to clinicians, as it is often clouded by either a vascular element or a triggering mechanism, or both. She defines underlying trigger factors as anxiety, depression, poor posture, occlusal problems, and disorders of the upper cervical spine. It is not clear whether frequent tension in the suboccipital muscles leads to stiffness in the underlying joints or whether the muscle tension is secondary (reflexive) to dysfunction of the cervical joints. Typically the pain is described as a dull ache that may be located frontally or in the occipital and posterior upper neck regions; it then builds in intensity while spreading in distribution around the scalp and neck. The pain builds slowly and steadily, usually over hours and sometimes days. At its peak there is usually some throbbing or pulsatile quality noted especially with motion, and, if severe enough, nausea, vomiting, and fainting can occur. With intense pain, the ciliospinal reflex adds blurred vision and photophobia by causing pupillary dilatation. Tension headaches can last hours to days, being most responsive to nonprescription drugs if taken early or close to the onset.

Stress is often cited as one of the major causes of the pain, but it would seem more appropriate to consider the alerting response as the mechanism that first tightens the posterior neck, frontal, and periaurical muscles as noted in other mammals.[8] Once these muscles cause discomfort, the alerting response continues and a self-aggravating situation ensues. Adding to the building headache is a tendency to be more concerned and distracted by the headache as well as becoming increasingly more irritable and less tolerant of environmental stress, which again feeds into the alerting response. Some of this behavior is a consequence of "psychic investment" in the head, which is a measure of importance placed on the structure that is most closely identified with personality and self-image. A similar pain located in the leg, for instance, would not be as distracting or disabling. As with migraine, underlying mechanical restrictions subjected to the stress of increased muscle tone and shortening might well further decompensate and predispose to a more asymmetric presentation that will require some direct manual therapy treatment.

Edeling[2] argues that tension or muscular contraction headaches and headaches of cervical origin are one and the same. Physical therapy directed at treating the muscle is ineffective, since the reflex muscle contraction is in response to abnormal and dysfunctional upper cervical spinal mechanics. Patients with headaches of cervical origin often have a history of preceding cervical strain. In a retrospective study of 96 patients with headache complaints, Jull[3] found that the onset of headache was directly related to a neck injury in 40 percent of the patients studied, 16 of the patients having been involved in motor vehicle accidents. Headaches of cervical origin are usually sensitive to positions of sustained neck flexion or changes in posture. Pain is most commonly referred into the frontal, retro-orbital, occipital, or suboccipital areas, with neck pain as a frequent accompaniment of the headache.[3] Edeling[2] and Jull,[3] among others, have found that manual therapy treatment directed at restoring the accessory movements of the upper cervical spine, specifically C0–C1, C1–C2, and C2–C3, have been very effective in successfully managing headaches of cervical origin. Temporomandibular joint pain must be also considered as a special form of head pain of musculoskeletal origin and treated appropriately.

Tumors and Headaches

Perhaps the greatest fear among patients and those not trained in the neurosciences is that a persistent, recurrent, or severe headache is associated with a brain tumor. Actually brain tumors rarely cause headaches either early on or even after they are well established and diagnosed. Brain tumors produce symptoms of neurologic dysfunction far more often and consistently than they do headache. The absence of pain should be of no surprise, since brain tissue is not a pain-sensitive structure, there being no nociceptors within the central nervous system (CNS). When it occurs, pain is due to a distortion of the supportive pain-sensitive structures, such as dural membranes, blood vessels, and periosteum. Intracranial brain tumors cause symptoms of brain or CNS dysfunction either by directly compressing or destroying tissue or by interfering with blood supply to brain tissue. Irritation of the brain tissue is not uncommon and may lead to the onset of seizures.

As the tumor increases in size and the surrounding cerebral edema produces increased intracranial pressure, alterations in mentation and progressive neurologic dysfunction develop, but usually without head pain. Head pain as a result of increased intracranial pressure occurs as a consequence of pressure elevations at a rate that is faster than accommodating mechanisms. Any further increase in pressure caused by physical exertion, postural changes, or lying down (which eliminates the negative intracranial pressure affects of gravity) will not be tolerated, and the headache will increase in severity. The increase in intracranial pressure causes reduced mentation, vomiting without nausea, nonlocalized dull headache, blurred vision, and a loss of lateral gaze with the eyes deviated medially (cranial nerve VI).

Tumors that are considered benign include meningiomas and neurofibromas. They grow relatively slowly and do not invade brain tissue but grow by displacing and pushing normal tissue aside. This characteristic enables potential total removal without disrupting brain tissue. Meningiomas are troublesome because they are usually highly vascular and may calcify because they are slow growing. These tumors may also grow around vital arteries or venous sinuses, making removal difficult. Meningiomas arise from arachnoid villi and can grow from any surface area or from the sagittal sinus. Those that grow under the brain tend to invade bone and may be impossible to remove. One such tumor tends to grow in the olfactory groove, causing an ipsilateral loss of sense of smell long before frontal headache develops. Meningiomas are most commonly found incidentally during the examination of a brain scan or as part of an evaluation for adult-onset seizures with little in the way of neurologic deficit.

Neurofibromas are most commonly diagnosed as acoustic neuromas and first cause unilateral hearing loss (bilateral if they are present at multiple sites). Growth begins in the internal auditory canal expanding into the cerebellopontine angle. Large tumors compress cranial nerve VII and then V but eventually compress the brain stem and cause increased intracranial pressure as a result of noncommunicating hydrocephalus. Head pain is not common before this late stage. Interestingly, there is a decreased incidence of multiple intracranial tumor formation when the patient has a preponderance of external skin lesions and tumors.

Tumors that grow within the pituitary gland can affect the endocrine system either by producing hormones or by destroying the functioning part of the gland. As these tumors grow, sudden swelling can occur with rapid onset of dysfunction. Because the tumors grow into the bone and up into the dura, pain is not uncommon, referring to the occiput or frontal regions. As these tumors grow upward, pressure is applied to the underside of the middle of the optic chiasm. The result is compression that directly affects the crossing nerve fibers that provide lateral peripheral vision for each eye. The visual field deficit affecting bilateral lateral vision is therefore very specific for a lesion affecting the optic chiasm. Plain lateral skull radiographs may demonstrate an enlarging sella turcica.

Primary malignant brain tumors are graded on the basis of local invasiveness and rapidity of growth and usually originate from the supporting glial tissues rather than the neurons. These tumors grow within the substance of the brain, destroying neurons and interrupting connecting pathways. Headache is an extremely rare complaint attributed to these tumors. The diagnosis is usually made as part of an evaluation for seizures with the development of neurologic dysfunction. Metastatic brain tumors from outside the nervous system behave in much the same way and also generally do not cause headaches. The onset of neurologic dysfunction in a patient with a history of carcinoma of the breast, lung, kidney, bowel, or oropharynx necessitates diagnostic scanning of the brain.

Tumors that originate within sinuses or oropharynx may cause local or referred pain before their presence is obvious. Early diagnosis is best made by skilled examination and by radiographic scanning techniques.

Although not a neoplasm, subdural hematomas develop as extracortical masses after head trauma and act like rapidly growing tumors. By the time symptoms develop, cognitive dysfunction may interfere with the ability to present an accurate history. Usually there is a headache, fluctuating focal neurologic signs including dysfunction of cranial nerves III or VII, excessive drowsiness, worsening of symptoms on lying down, and occasionally scalp tenderness to percussion over the region of the hematoma. Because of the unstable nature of the condition and the erratic growth pattern, the sooner diagnosis is made and proper management instituted, the better the outcome. When it is difficult to obtain a reasonable history from the patient, it is best to try to obtain some history from anyone who knows the patient and who can at least describe the usual level of mentation and ability.

Increased intracranial pressure associated with severe headache and transient visual loss, especially with postural changes and without any focal neurologic deficit except for weakness of the lateral rectus muscle (cranial nerve VI), can occur without the ability to demonstrate any intracranial tumor or mass. This condition is known as pseudotumor cerebri. The pain characteristics conform to the consequence of rapidly increasing intracranial pressure. Blindness is a possible outcome in the untreated patient as a result of increasing pressure on the optic nerve. The condition can be suspected during periods of rapid weight gain, especially pregnancy.

Vascular Disease Causing Headache

Aside from brain tumor, stroke is also often feared as a cause of recurrent or chronic severe headache. Most feared is the possibility of an aneurysm and intracranial headache. The headache associated with aneurysmal rupture is sudden, immediately severe, and often associated with a transient loss of consciousness, followed by reduced mentation, drowsiness, and usually nausea and vomiting. Nuchal rigidity is usually too severe to permit neck flexion, but this may not be true when there is depressed mental function or coma. There may or may not be any other neurologic signs, except for a positive Babinski or loss of either cranial nerve III or VI, because of the close proximity to the aneurysm or because of hematoma formation and/or increased intracranial pressure. There are no signs, clues, or reliable noninvasive ways to diagnose this type of aneurysm before rupture;

even if diagnosed before hemorrhage, there is no way to predict if and when the rupture will occur. It is not uncommon to find other aneurysms that have not ruptured during diagnostic arteriography of the intracranial vessels. The aneurysm remains fairly asymptomatic until rupture.

Arteriovenous malformations are capable of causing severe recurrent headaches, especially if there is recurrent leakage of blood into the subarachnoid space. These malformations tend to cause some form of neurologic dysfunction and seizures, affecting brain function and tissue by altered local blood supply as well as by small hemorrhages. As with any cause of meningeal irritation, neck stiffness to flexion far exceeds resistance to neck rotation, thereby differentiating meningeal irritation from mechanical dysfunction of the cervical spine.

Migraine headaches were well described earlier. Other forms of vascular headaches include cluster headaches and lower-half headaches. Cluster headaches usually occur in males who smoke cigarettes. The headache lasts less than 2 hours and localizes behind one eye with associated redness and tearing and occasionally Horner syndrome (small pupil, mild ptosis, and shrinkage of the globe). Cluster headaches are excruciating and usually begin in the early morning, awakening the patient from sleep. They may occur more than once a day and recur daily for weeks to months. Between these clusters of headaches, the patient is headache free, except for the common tension type. Lower-half headaches usually occur in women with many of the features of migraine except that the pain is localized to the lower half of the face extending into the anterior neck and associated with tenderness over the carotid artery.

Extremely rare before the age of 60, temporal arteritis is always of concern when headaches begin later in life. This syndrome is usually associated with diffuse muscle and joint pains typified as polymyalgia rheumatica. It is similar to migraine in that unilateral throbbing head pain recurs. Tenderness may be palpated over the temporal artery. The danger of delayed diagnosis or misdiagnosis by failure to obtain an erythrocyte sedimentation rate and/or biopsy of the artery with subsequent appropriate steroid therapy is progression to retinal ischemia and blindness or cerebral ischemia and stroke, or both. Therefore, immediate referral of the patient to a physician is warranted if the therapist suspects the presence of this condition.

Neck pain and headaches have been reported during carotid artery occlusion or after emboli, but the neurologic deficit will be obvious and will overshadow this complaint. Atherosclerotic disease or stenosis of either carotid or vertebral arteries does not cause headache, nor can headache be generated by a mechanical distortion of these structures alone.

Throbbing, severe, focal, or generalized headaches occasionally will follow a convulsive or nonconvulsive seizure and may last for hours. The headaches probably result from postictal alterations of pain pathways perhaps in a way similar to migraine. These headaches occur in the absence of any obvious head trauma and do not respond to physical treatment.

Infection

Probably the most commonly self-diagnosed cause of headache is sinus headache, especially if a painful fullness is located over, between, or below the eyes and worsens with head flexion (see Figs. 8-4 and 8-5). That many patients find relief with over-the-counter "sinus remedies" further substantiates a belief in the notion that chronic headaches are sinus in origin rather than from "tension" or from something more serious.

True sinus infection is quite rare and is accompanied by fever, severe localized pain, and systemic generalized aches, pains, and malaise. Such conditions are usually diagnosed by plain radiographs and are not the cause of recurrent or chronic headache. Sinus infection is a serious and debilitating illness that usually requires surgical drainage along with antibiotic therapy. Sinuses can be seen to contain fluid, cysts, and even thickened mucous membranes when viewed incidentally by computerized tomography or magnetic resonance imaging. When diseased, the maxillary sinus membranes report painful sensations along the first and second branches of the trigeminal nerve locally and refer pain to the teeth, upper jaw, temporomandibular joint, ear, and supraorbital and retro-orbital areas. When pain is referred from the sphenoid sinus, it is typically located at the vertex of the skull, while pain from the frontal sinus remains localized.

Confusing the issue of sinus head pain is the tendency of cervical and other cranial structures to refer along the trigeminal pathways to the sinuses. Pain originating from the nasal turbinates usually localizes either to the frontal or maxillary sinuses and the upper jaw and teeth, ear, and temporal regions. Such pain may originate from

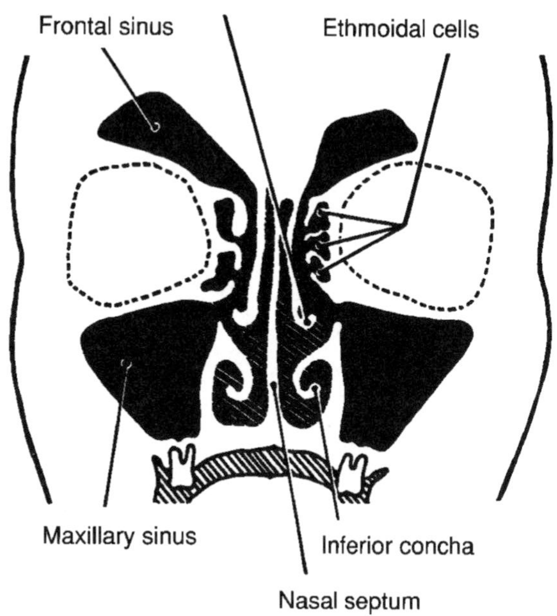

Fig. 8-4. Anterior view illustrating the location of the frontal and maxillary sinuses.

nasal membrane congestion, from allergens or infections, and also from dry membranes as a result of forced dry air heating systems or from overuse of antihistamines found in nonprescription sinus headache remedies, diet aids, sleep aids, and cold or allergy formulas. "Allergic" headaches probably originate from both the turbinates and sinuses when all such membranes are inflamed by pollen or fumes. Stimulation of nociceptors in the soft palate by ingesting cold fluids or foods, as experienced by the so-called ice cream headache, refers to both frontal and vertex regions.

Pain originating from dental disease from upper teeth can refer back to the sinuses, as can any diseases causing destruction of tissues innervated by the fifth cranial nerve, such as infection or cancerous growths in the oropharynx or anterior neck. In addition, mechanical dysfunction affecting the upper cervical vertebrae, and especially the craniocervical junction, can cause frontal and retro-orbital pain. Lower cervical dysfunctions are seen in association with temporomandibular dysfunction and pain that can be felt in the ear as well.

Cranial infection caused by a virus or bacteria is an acute or subacute illness with severe pain, nausea, vomiting, and signs of meningeal irritation. On examination, varying degrees of resistance to neck flexion will be palpated, yet no such resistance will accompany neck rotation. Associated fever and systemic signs usually require evaluation at a local emergency room. Chronic meningi-

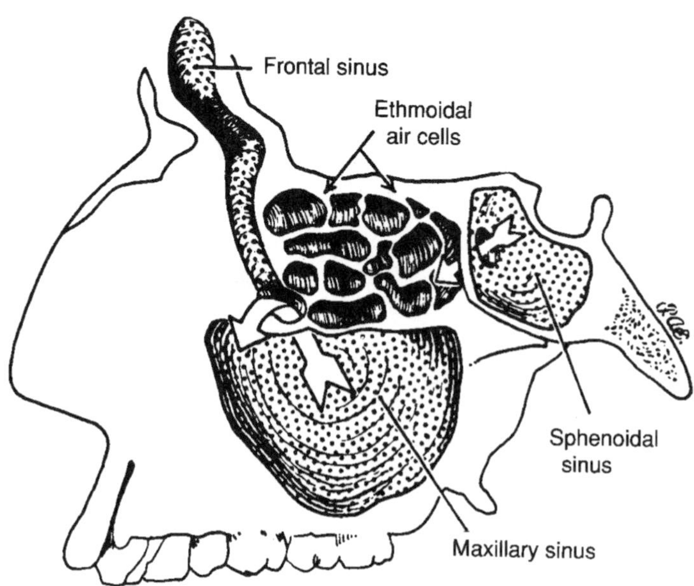

Fig. 8-5. Sagittal view illustrating the location of the frontal, sphenoidal, and maxillary sinuses.

tis caused by fungal infection leads to chronic headache but little early on in the way of focal findings or neck stiffness. Such infections occasionally present in diabetics and in immunocompromised patients, now much more frequently seen in those patients suffering from acquired immune deficiency syndrome (AIDS). Any form of meningitis may also result in increased intracranial pressure and present with additional signs and symptoms appropriate to this condition. Encephalitis is not usually associated with neck stiffness, but instead presents with headache and varying degrees of neurologic deficit, usually nonfocal and cognitive in nature.

Vertigo

Another common complaint originating from cervical and cranial structures is dizziness. As with any nonspecific complaint, it is important first to determine the patient's definition of the symptom rather than assume the dictionary's. Dizziness can be either a sensation of lightheadedness or weakness or of an impending loss of consciousness caused by fainting, or a sense of spinning, loss of balance and unsteadiness, and propensity to fall down. The sense of dizziness can then be further defined as a sense of fainting versus a sense of vertigo. Otolaryngologic and craniocervical disorders tend to cause vertigo, while cardiovascular or gastroenterologic disorders are associated with a sense of fainting, lightheadedness, or weakness.

Vertigo is best defined as a sense of spinning, either of the individual or the environment. The direction can be left or right, and, if both, it is usually in the vertical plane. In addition to a sense of motion, vertigo is associated with a sense of imbalance with nausea and, if severe enough, vomiting. True vertigo is the consequence of a loss of concordant information regarding the actual position of the head as determined by visual, vestibular, and cervical proprioceptive sensory input to the CNS. If cervical and vestibular mechanisms are activated while the visual system reports stability, a sense of vertigo develops, commonly experienced as "sea sickness," "car sickness," and "air sickness." Similar experiences can occur while viewing a motion picture, especially with 360 degree screens in which the individual views the scene from a moving object yet remains positioned stationary. "Cervical vertigo" is also observed in those patients with abnormal tone in cervical musculature or after mobilization of the cervical spine, when proprioceptive feedback does not match ocular and vestibular sensations. Diseases affecting vestibular structures or the nerve pathways from them, or the central brain stem integrating circuits, can cause a sense of vertigo, again due to an unmatched input of information from visual and cervical receptors. As long as there remains intact cortical structures and the absence of congenital retinal disease, the presence of nystagmus indicates a dysfunction in the vestibular system or brain stem, since the vestibular-ocular reflex will cause a deviation of the eyes and the oculomotor cortex will seek to correct for this involuntary ocular motion. Nystagmus is not usually observed when a sense of vertigo originates from cervical dysfunction or from a sense of faintness due to hypotension.

SUMMARY

During the evaluation and treatment of patients presenting with head and facial pain, the physical therapist must be aware of the signs and symptoms of conditions that are not of musculoskeletal origin.

The following conditions require referral to a physician:

1. Head or facial pain associated with trauma not responding to therapy and associated with focal neurologic signs or symptoms or an alteration of personality and mental status
2. Head pain preceded by or associated with a loss of consciousness
3. Head pain associated with tenderness of a scalp artery in any patient past the age of 60 years
4. Head or facial pain in any patient with focal cranial nerve dysfunction
5. Head or facial pain in any patient with neurologic dysfunction involving corticospinal, extrapyramidal, cerebellar, and spinal or radicular dysfunction

PATIENT CASE STUDY 1

History

The patient was a 46-year-old bookkeeper who came to the clinic with a diagnosis of spastic torticolis. She had been treated previously at the physical therapy clinic, with the last visit occurring 4 months before her return. At the end of her previous physical therapy program, her chief complaint of left posterolateral cervical pain and stiffness and left occipital and temporal headaches had improved considerably. She had returned to the clinic stating that her headaches had returned and were much more severe than before. She had not seen her physician since this recent flare-up, having called his office only. The patient had spoken to someone on the physician's staff, stating, "My headache came back. Can I see my physical therapist, since the treatment helped last time?" Permission was granted.

The patient's current chief complaint was daily, constant headaches. This was in contrast to her previously described chief complaint of left cervical pain and stiffness. When asked about the location of symptoms, she stated that it was primarily facial pain, specifically in the frontal and orbital regions bilaterally. She described the headaches as being a deep pressure sensation, severe at times. Again, this was in contrast to her previous description of headaches located in the left occipital and temporal region and described as tension or tightness.

The current headaches were constant, but the intensity quickly increased with the assumption of a forward-flexed head and neck posture when sitting or standing. The facial pressure subsided within a few minutes of returning the head and neck to an upright position. She noted a slight decrease in the pressure and intensity when she would lie down supine or on her side. The previously described left temporal and occipital headaches were aggravated by sitting more than 90 to 120 minutes, including driving. Forward-flexed postures had not influenced these headaches.

The facial pain had begun insidiously 3 weeks before re-evaluation. The patient could not recall any incident or accident that may have precipitated the onset of these symptoms. She noted there had not been a concurrent increase in left cervical symptoms. She recalled having similar pressurelike symptoms in the frontal and orbital regions two to three times in the past, although this pain was much more intense. The previous facial headaches seemed to have disappeared when the patient was given medication for sinus infections.

The patient's medical history had not changed over the 4 months between physical therapy sessions. She had not seen a physician for a medical condition, nor had her medications changed. She acknowledged a past history of recurrent sinus infection; in fact, she felt as though she had had a cold for the past month.

Objective Examination

The objective examination findings were very similar to the presentation 4 months earlier regarding postural assessment, active and passive ROM findings, and special tests. Differences were noted, however, including swelling in the orbital regions, the eyes being red and teary, and the patient sounding very congested. Forward-bending ROM had not changed, but a sustained forward-flexed posture caused a significant increase in facial pressure within 10 to 15 seconds. The patient's previous left-sided headaches did not change in the past with cervical active ROM or sustained head and neck postures. Specific palpation or other active or passive cervical or cranial maneuvers did not alter the patient's current chief complaint. Cranial nerve assessment was negative.

Assessment and Outcome

The pattern of evaluation findings suggested that the patient's current chief complaint was probably unrelated to what she had been treated for previously. In fact, the symptoms noted in the past had remained significantly improved over the previous 4 months. The referring physician was called regarding the patient's current status and the concern about the origin of these new complaints. It was communicated to the physician that the headaches were of new location and description as compared to what she had been treated for previously, and the previous symptoms remained improved from when she was last treated; also reported were insidious onset of the new headaches, inability to alter the facial pain except with sustained forward-flexed postures during the objective examination, swelling noted around the eyes and redness of the eyes, the feeling that the patient had a cold for 4 weeks, and the fact that she has had similar symptoms previously that had resolved with taking medications for sinus infections. The physician saw the patient immediately, made the diagnosis of sinus infection, and placed the patient on antibiotics. The patient was called in 2 weeks later, and she reported complete relief of the facial pain and had resumed all normal activities. She did not feel the need to return for physical therapy.

The main point of this patient case presentation is that it represents a common mechanism of how certain medical conditions can arrive at the doorstep of the physical therapy clinic. This patient had developed new symptoms and failed to relate this information to the physician's office when she called. She did not realize that they were unrelated to her previous condition treated by the physical therapist and physician. She also did not realize that these new symptoms were similar to the type of pain she had experienced previously and subsequently treated with antibiotics. Therefore, the patient called the physician stating that her headaches were back and could she go see her physical therapist again. In her case, the condition was not life threatening and was easily diagnosed and treated by the physician.

True sinus infections are relatively rare, but they should be considered if orbital or maxillary pain is noted; if the pain is described as aching, throbbing, or pressure; if the pain is accompanied by fever; if local edema in the area of the sinus is noted; and if a sense of nasal congestion or copious amounts of nasal discharge are noted by the patient. Allergic rhinitis (e.g., hay fever) may result in similar symptoms, such as nasal congestion, watery eyes, and nasal discharge. The congestion may lead to complaints of pressure or tension in the facial or frontal regions. The frontal, orbital, and maxillary regions are not uncommon referral areas for cervical structures. A patient may present with a chief complaint of headaches with discomfort located in the occipital, temporal, and frontal regions. The therapist must consider all local structures, as well as structures from adjacent regions (cervical area), as a source of symptoms. In this case, the left temporal and occipital headaches were related to cervical mechanical dysfunction, while the facial pain was related to involvement of local structures—the sinuses.

PATIENT CASE STUDY 2

History

The patient was a 47-year-old receptionist who came to the physical therapy clinic on the recommendation of a friend. Her chief complaint was intermittent but severe right-sided headaches. The aching and throbbing pain was most intense in the right parietal, temporal, and frontal regions of the cranium. The headache seemed to start in the right cervicothoracic and upper scapular regions and spread to the cranial areas described above. In the past 6 months, the headache would be present and severe for 3 to 4 days; the patient would then be pain free for up to 7 to 10 days. The patient could not relate the onset of the headaches to any particular incident or accident, nor could she explain why the headaches disappeared.

When present, the headaches were most intense when the patient would lie down. She woke up two to three times per night due to the severity of the headaches. The intensity of the throbbing and aching would decrease when she got up to walk around. Neck movements and activities such as tennis would increase the stiffness in the right cervical spine and cause a slight increase in the headache intensity.

The patient stated that the headaches began years ago following an automobile accident. During the past 18 months, the headaches had increased in frequency and severity, and seemed more intense in the temporal and frontal regions. Soon after the automobile accident, the headaches were more localized to the cervical and occipital regions. The patient could not relate the increase in headache frequency or severity to a particular incident or accident that might have happened 18 months ago. During the 12 months prior to the physical therapy evaluation, the patient went to a chiropractor and received adjustments of the cervical spine and shoulder girdle exercises. She had also gone to a dentist and was fitted with a mouth appliance for a temporomandibular joint condition. Neither the chiropractic care nor the appliance helped the patient's condition.

Besides the chief complaint, the patient also described left-sided headaches similar to the right-sided symptoms, but they were very infrequent and not intense. They were only present when the right-sided symptoms were at their worst. She stated that both arms felt weak even though she had been exercising them for months using free weights. Although she denied problems with vision, taste, smell, or swallowing, she had noticed a decrease in her hearing ability, especially the right side, over the past 12 months. She had not seen a physician for her current condition.

The patient stated that her current medical history was negative. The only medication she was taking was estrogen replacement, which she had taken since her hysterectomy. Surgical history also included a craniotomy to remove a benign cyst from the right frontal lobe region. When asked about symptoms leading up to the craniotomy, the patient described headaches and cervical pain very similar to her current symptoms. After the surgery, the headaches were significantly reduced.

Physical Examination

Postural assessment revealed that the occiput was side bent left and right rotated on the cervical spine. The right shoulder girdle was elevated compared with the left. There was moderate muscle guarding noted in the right posterior suboccipital, upper trapezius, and levator scapulae regions. Cervical spine active ROM testing revealed right upper cervical spine discomfort (posterior aspect) with forward and backward bending and right rotation. Left rotation and backward bending were the most restricted. Vertical cervical compression and distraction were negative. Mandibular depression was of functional ROM and caused slight discomfort in the right temporomandibular joint region.

Passive accessory vertebral motion (PAVM) testing revealed significant hypomobility of C1, right and left side, and of C7, T1, and T2 centrally. Symptoms were not altered with the PAVM testing of the temporomandibular joint and the cervical and upper thoracic spine. Sensory and motor testing of the upper extremities revealed no abnormalities, but cranial nerve assessment revealed a significant deficit in hearing of the right ear. There was also slight weakness noted when assessing cranial nerve XII.

Assessment and Outcome

Despite the dysfunction noted during the evaluation (i.e., segmental vertebral hypomobility, postural faults, muscle guarding, etc.), the patient was advised to see a neurologist before any further physical therapy was administered. Numerous findings (described earlier in this chapter) caused concern, and the therapist had more questions than answers regarding the patient's condition after the evaluation. The history revealed a condition marked by intermittent but severe headaches, aching and throbbing in nature, which insidiously worsened 18 months ago. The onset and cessation of the headaches could not be explained mechanically. When present, the headaches were most intense when the patient was lying down, and they woke her at night. She had a previous history of craniotomy for a benign cyst, and, with specific questioning, the patient admitted her current symptoms were similar to symptoms she experienced prior to the craniotomy. After the surgery, she had noted a dramatic decrease in the intensity and frequency of her symptoms.

Raising concern in the physical examination was the significant hearing loss on the right side and possible weakness of the tongue. Also of importance was the inability of the therapist to alter the headache during the physical examination. Being unable to alter the patient's headache by stressing musculoskeletal structures locally or in the cervical/thoracic region raised questions regarding the relevance of the findings of mechanical dysfunction as they related to the patient's complaints.

The patient scheduled an appointment with a neurologist and was instructed to contact the therapist after her visit. The therapist contacted the neurologist and the above information was communicated. After not hearing from the patient 3 weeks after her scheduled physician visit, the therapist called the patient. She stated that she had to cancel her physician appointment because of her busy schedule. The therapist encouraged the patient to reschedule the appointment as soon as possible, and the reasons for the referral to the neurologist were reviewed with her. Three months later, the therapist met the friend who initially referred the patient to the physical therapy clinic. The friend stated that since the physical therapist's evaluation the patient had been hospitalized for depression and further testing had been done by a neurologist. The test revealed the presence of numerous brain tumors.

REFERENCES

1. Campbell DG, Parsons DM: Referred head pain and its concomitants. J Nerv Ment Dis 99:544, 1944
2. Edeling J: Manual Therapy for Chronic Headache. Butterworths, London, 1988
3. Jull GA: Headaches associated with the cervical spine—a clinical review. p. 322. In Grieve GP (ed): Modern Manual Therapy of the Vertebral Column. Churchill Livingstone, Edinburgh, 1986
4. Fredriksen TA, Sjaastad O: Cervicogenic headache: a clinical entity. Cephalgia 7(suppl 6):171, 1987
5. Jaeger B: Cervicogenic headache: relationship to cervical spine dysfunction and myofascial trigger points. Cephalgia 7(suppl 6):398, 1987
6. Travell JG, Simons DG: Myofascial Pain and Dysfunction. The Trigger Point Manual. Williams & Wilkins, Baltimore, 1983
7. Butler DS: Mobilisation of the Nervous System. Churchill Livingstone, Melbourne, 1991
8. Dalessio DJ (ed): Wolff's Headache and Other Head Pain. 5th Ed. Oxford University Press, New York, 1987

9. Raskin N, Appenzeller O: Major Problems in Internal Medicine. Vol. XIX: Headache. WB Saunders, Philadelphia, 1980
10. Blumenthal LS: Tension headache. p. 157. In Vinken PJ, Bruyn GW (eds): Headaches and Cranial Neuralgias: Handbook of Clinical Neurology. Vol. 5. John Wiley & Sons, New York, 1968
11. Trott PH: Tension headache. p. 336. In Grieve GP (ed): Modern Manual Therapy of the Vertebral Column. Churchill Livingstone, Edinburgh, 1986
12. Boissonnault W, Bass C: Pathological origins of trunk and neck pain. Part 2. JOSPT 12:208, 1990

SUGGESTED READINGS

Abramson M: Dizziness and hearing loss. p. 31. In Rowland LP (ed): Merritt's Textbook of Neurology. 8th Ed. Lee & Febiger, Philadelphia, 1989

Dalessio DJ: Wolff's Headache and Other Head Pain. 5th Ed. Oxford University Press, New York, 1987

Friedman AP: Headache. p. 13-1. In Joynt RJ (ed): Clinical Neurology. JB Lippincott, Philadelphia, 1993

Ryan RE Jr, Ryan RE Sr: Headache and Facial Pain Seen by the Otorhinolaryngologist, Part II. p. 17. J.C.E.O.R.L. and Allergy. CV Mosby, St. Louis, 1978

9 Screening for Nervous System Disease

Susan Barker, M.S., P.T., N.C.S.

Physical therapists in many settings work with patients who have primary diagnoses involving the nervous system. For example, pediatric therapists working in educational settings work with children with cerebral palsy, those in rehabilitation centers work with persons following spinal cord injury, and those in acute care hospitals work with individuals following surgery for brain tumor resection. For these patients, there is obviously no need for the physical therapist to screen for nervous system injury or disease. For these patients, the physical therapy evaluation is geared toward defining the sources of the patient's functional limitations in order to develop the physical therapy treatment plan while monitoring the patient's neurologic status.

Physical therapists also work with many patients who do not present with primary neurologic diagnoses. It is possible that undetected nervous system pathology can produce these patients' symptoms or exist independently of the primary problem. For these patients, the physical therapy evaluation should initially screen for nervous system dysfunction. Then, if the screening examination gives the physical therapist reason to suspect involvement of the nervous system, the therapist should examine the nervous system in more detail, with referral to a physician possibly warranted. An easily identifiable example of this type of situation is the physical therapist who evaluates a patient referred to physical therapy for a lumbosacral sprain/strain and finds muscle weakness, sensory deficit, and tendon reflex evidence of nerve root involvement. This type of situation is readily determined while performing an upper-quarter or lower-quarter screening examination (see Appendices II and III). In addition to performing this type of examination, physical therapists are trained to detect other sometimes more subtle types of evidence of neurologic dysfunction, particularly with regard to the patient's movement and gait patterns.

This chapter provides a review of neuroanatomy and neurophysiology with respect primarily to the motor and sensory systems, followed by a discussion of some common forms of injury and disease to these systems. Practical methods are presented for examining the various components of the nervous system. Two case studies are included that exemplify physical therapy cooperation in the recognition of neurologic dysfunction.

ANATOMY

A review of the general anatomy and function of the human nervous system is included to provide a basis for discussion of the effects of lesions to its various components. The primary organizational division that can be made is between the central and peripheral nervous systems (CNS and PNS).

The CNS consists of the brain and spinal cord. Various schemes have been used to organize the components of the CNS. The central nervous system can be divided into six main regions: the spinal cord; medulla; pons and cerebellum; midbrain; diencephalon; and cerebral hemispheres. The medulla, pons, and midbrain are often collectively referred to as the brain stem (see Fig. 9-1).[1]

The PNS is made up of the ganglia and peripheral nerves that lie outside the brain and spinal cord. The PNS can be further divided into somatic and autonomic divisions.

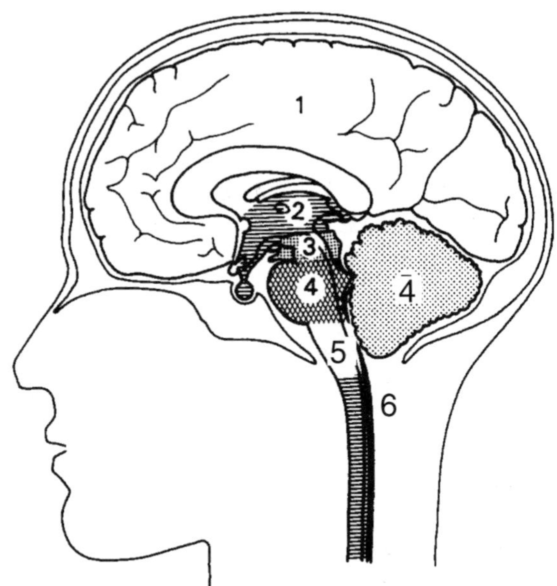

Fig. 9-1. The central nervous system is divided into six main parts: (1) cerebral hemispheres; (2) diencephalon; (3) midbrain; (4) pons and cerebellum; (5) medulla oblongata; (6) spinal cord. (Modified from Romero-Sierra,[14] with permission.)

Central Nervous System

Spinal Cord

The spinal cord is the most caudal portion of the CNS. It contains central gray matter made up of neuronal cell bodies, surrounded by white matter made up of ascending and descending axons. The gray matter forms bilateral ventral (or anterior) horns, dorsal horns, and intermediate zones. The ventral horns contain the cell bodies of motor neurons and give rise to the ventral roots, the dorsal horns contain sensory neurons that receive input from the periphery via the dorsal roots, and the intermediate zones contain interneurons and autonomic neurons. The white matter can be divided into dorsal, lateral, and ventral columns. The dorsal and lateral columns contain axons carrying both ascending somatosensory and descending information, and the ventral columns carry descending efferent information.

There are regional differences in the exact configuration of the spinal cord. The size of the gray matter is related to the number of structures innervated in a region. Therefore there are cervical and lumbosacral enlargements of the gray matter, because the upper and lower extremities receive their innervation from these segments. The size of the white matter is related to the flow of information between the periphery and the brain. In the lumbar region, the white matter is made up of axons carrying information to and from the lower extremities only; in the cervical region, the white matter contains not only the axons related to the lower extremities, but also those to and from the upper extremities. Therefore the white matter increases in size as more rostral segments are examined.

At the vicinity of the first lumbar vertebra, the spinal cord tapers to form the conus medullaris. Below this, the remaining nerve fibers are referred to as the cauda equina.

Brain Stem

The brain stem is made up of the medulla, pons, and midbrain. The medulla is most caudal, and the midbrain is most rostral. All three components contain three types of structures compactly intermingled in the relatively small area making up the brain stem: axonal tracts, the reticular formation, and collections of cell bodies referred to as nuclei. The long axonal tracts found in the brain stem convey all somatic and visceral information between the periphery and brain. Embedded between the tracts and nuclei are the neurons of the reticular formation. This neuronal network is involved in regulating alertness, modulating muscle tone, controlling cardiac and respiratory function, and modulating pain sensation. The brain stem nuclei involved in the control of movement are of two types: those giving rise to cranial nerves and those giving rise to ascending and descending pathways.

Diencephalon

The term *diencephalon* means *between-brain*. This name refers to the fact that the diencephalon lies between the brain stem and the cerebral hemispheres. The structures included in the diencephalon are the thalamus and hypothalamus. The thalamus receives and integrates almost all motor and sensory information ascending to the cerebral cortex. The hypothalamus regulates the autonomic nervous system.

Cerebral Hemispheres

Each cerebral hemisphere is made up of the cerebral cortex and the underlying white matter in which three nuclei are embedded: the hippocampus, amygdala, and basal ganglia. The cerebral cortex is divided into four lobes: frontal, parietal, temporal, and occipital. Each lobe is responsible for different functions: emotion, cognition, memory, sensory input processing, and motor activity planning and implementation.

The nuclei embedded in the cerebral cortex are responsible for diverse functions. The hippocampus and amygdala are part of the limbic system. The hippocampus is involved in memory storage, and the amygdala plays a role in emotions and control of autonomic nervous system responses. The basal ganglia include the caudate nucleus, putamen, globus pallidus, substantia nigra, and subthalamic nucleus.[1] They are involved in the control of movement.

Peripheral Nervous System

The somatic division of the PNS conveys motor information to and sensory information from the trunk and limbs (see Fig. 9-2). Sensory information enters the spinal cord through the dorsal root, and all output exits the spinal cord through the ventral root. The ventral and dorsal roots join to form the radicular nerves, carrying motor information outward from the CNS and sen-

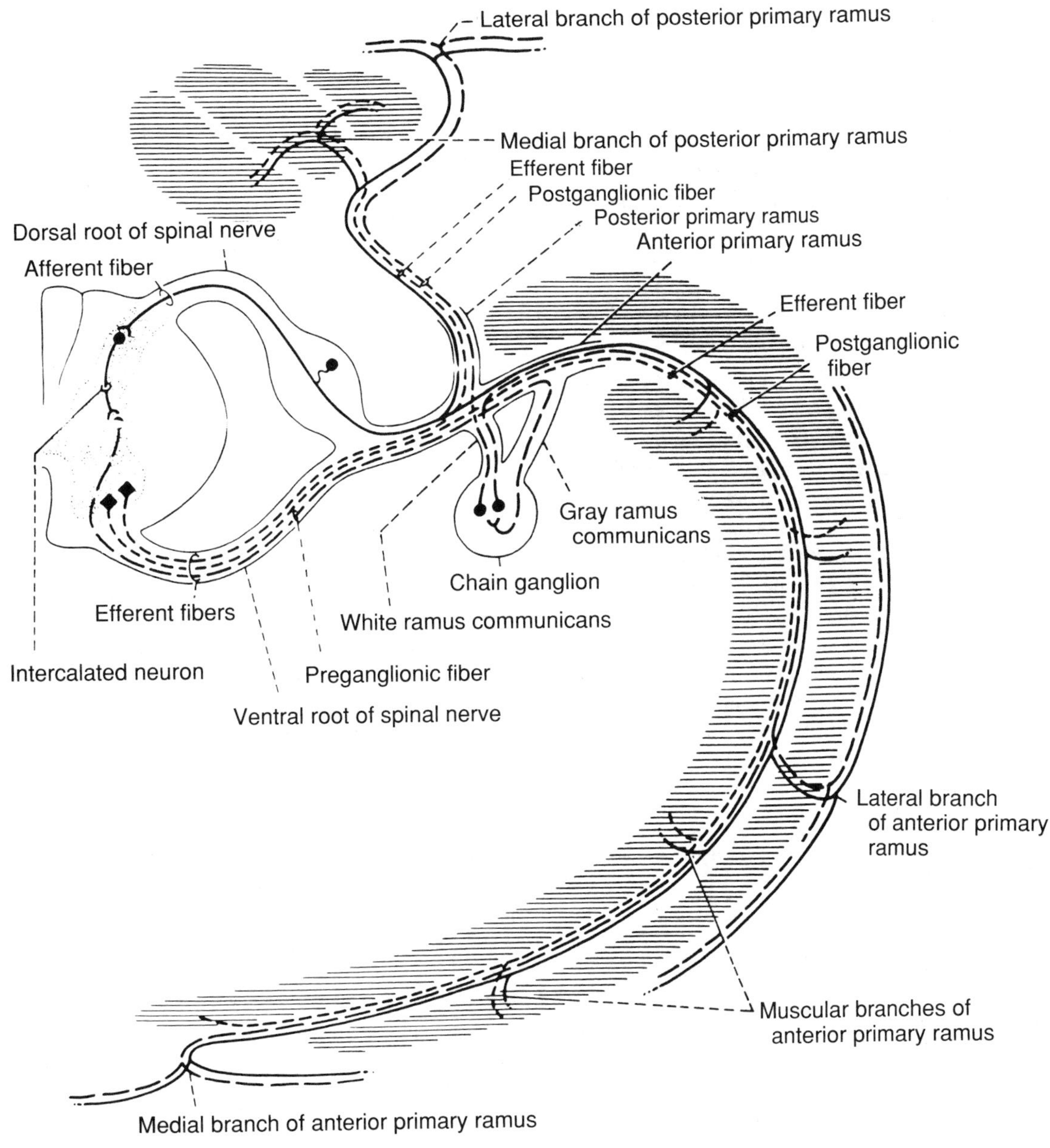

Fig. 9-2. Segmental spinal nerve showing the course of motor, sensory, and preganglionic and postganglionic sympathetic fibers. (From Haerer,[8] with permission.)

sory information inward toward the CNS. Shortly distal to this junction, the radicular nerve divides into anterior and posterior primary rami. The anterior ramus segmentally innervates the limbs and the anterior and lateral thorax; the posterior ramus segmentally innervates the posterior structures of the trunk. Distal to the formation of the anterior and posterior rami, the radicular nerves subdivide to form plexi in the cervical and lumbosacral areas (see Figs. 9-3, 9-4). Any branches from the plexus as well as the nerves created by the plexus are peripheral nerves, and each innervates distinctly different patterns of skin, muscles, and bone.

The 12 paired cranial nerves represent another portion of the somatic PNS. They provide motor and sensory innervation for the head and neck and function as modified spinal nerves. They arise from different portions of the brain and exit the cranium through various fossae. In contrast to spinal nerves, not all of the cranial nerves are mixed. Some are purely motor and others purely sensory.

The autonomic nervous system (ANS) has three main divisions: sympathetic, parasympathetic, and enteric. Ganglia located outside the CNS play a major role in the ANS. The preganglionic neuron located in the brain stem or spinal cord projects to a ganglion, where the postganglionic neuron is located. The postganglionic neuron then projects to the target organ. The sympathetic system includes the paravertebral chain ganglia and several prevertebral ganglia. The ganglia in the parasympathetic system are located close to or are embedded in the target organ. The enteric system ganglia are embedded in the walls of the gastrointestinal tract, pancreas, and gallbladder and are regulated by preganglionic fibers of both the sympathetic and parasympathetic systems. The sympathetic system is also called the thoracolumbar division of the ANS, since the cell bodies of its preganglionic neurons are located in the thoracic and lumbar regions of the spinal cord. The parasympathetic system is called the craniosacral division of the ANS, since the cell bodies of its preganglionic fibers are located in several brain stem nuclei giving rise to cranial nerves or in the sacral segments of the spinal cord.

FUNCTIONAL SYSTEMS

Numerous functional systems can be defined as operating in the normal adult human nervous system. For the purpose of physical therapy screening, however, only the somatosensory and motor systems will be outlined.

Somatosensory Systems

Somatosensory input from the neck and face is transmitted into the CNS by way of several cranial nerves. Input from the trunk and extremities is transmitted to the CNS by way of sensory neurons whose cell bodies are located in segmental dorsal root ganglia. The neurons of the dorsal root ganglia are one of the few instances of bipolar neurons found in the human nervous system; that is, they have two axons. One axon projects into the periphery via a peripheral nerve to supply a sensory receptor. The second axon enters the spinal cord via the dorsal root to convey information into the CNS. There are two major divisions of the somatosensory system: the dorsal column–medial lemniscal (DCML) pathway and the spinothalamic pathway. The DCML transmits information primarily about discriminatory touch and body part position and movement, as well as some pain input. The spinothalamic tract transmits pain, temperature, and discrete touch input. Because of this arrangement, there is some overlap of function. Both systems are involved in pain and touch sensation, providing a form of biological insurance.

Dorsal Column–Medial Lemniscal Pathway

The DCML's main function is to provide the CNS with information about touch, vibration, and joint position and movement. This information appears to be important in interpreting complex patterns of sensory input. Stereognosis is an example of such an activity. When we hold an object in our hand, we are able to combine information about how an object touches the hand with information about the configuration of the fingers needed to hold the object, and then we identify the object. In the spinal cord, the dorsal columns can be divided into two fiber bundles, the medially located fasciculus cuneatus and the more lateral fasciculus gracilis (see Fig. 9-5). Sensory information from the lower limb is carried by the fasciculus gracilis, and information from the upper limb is carried by the fasciculus cuneatus. When proprioceptive, touch, or vibratory sensation is detected by the appropriate sensory receptors, the input travels along the afferent fibers that enter the dorsal horn of the spinal cord. Some of these fibers travel directly to the dorsal columns, where they ascend ipsilaterally. Those that do not directly enter the dorsal columns synapse on neurons located in the dorsal horn. The axons of these dorsal horn neurons also ascend ipsilaterally in the dorsal columns. When the fibers reach

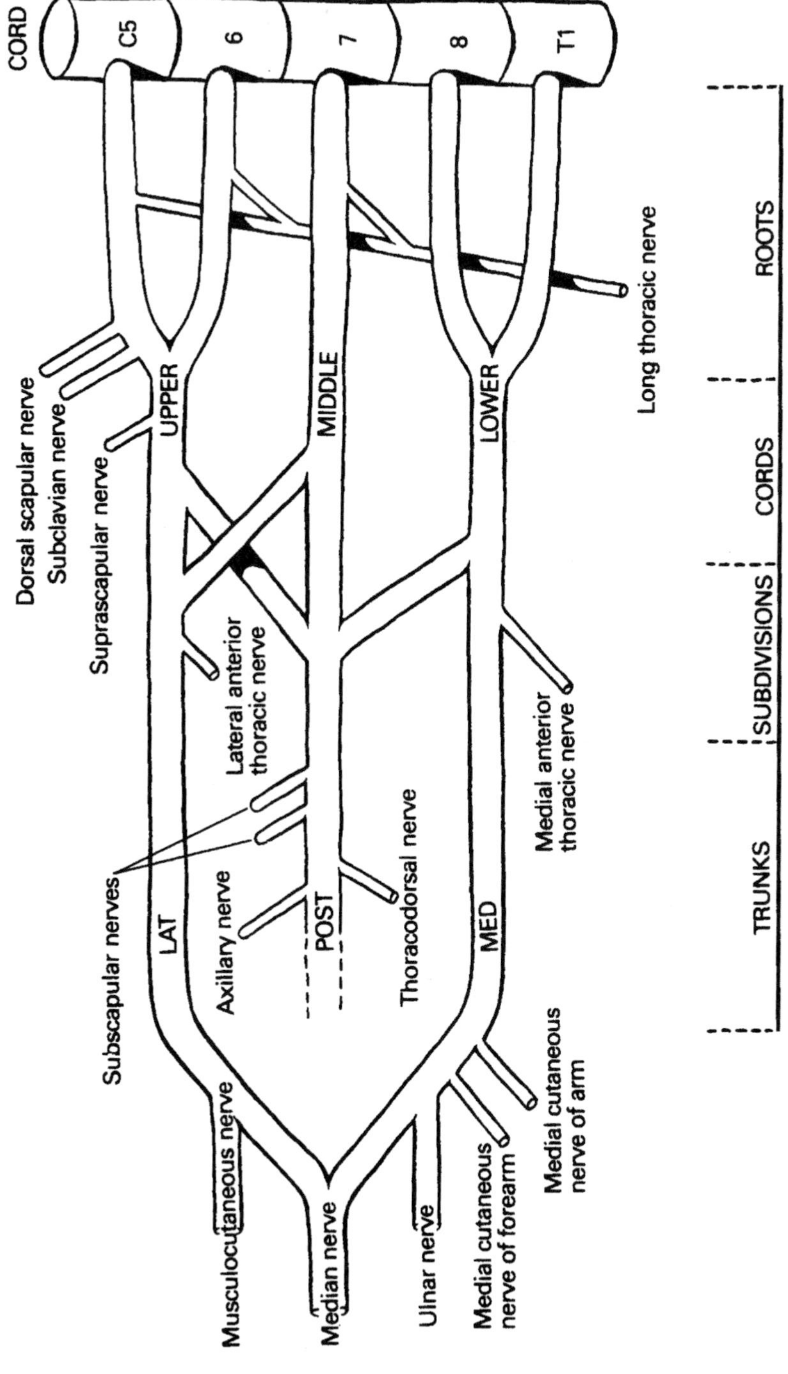

Fig. 9-3. The brachial plexus. (From Devinsky and Feldmann,[9] with permission.)

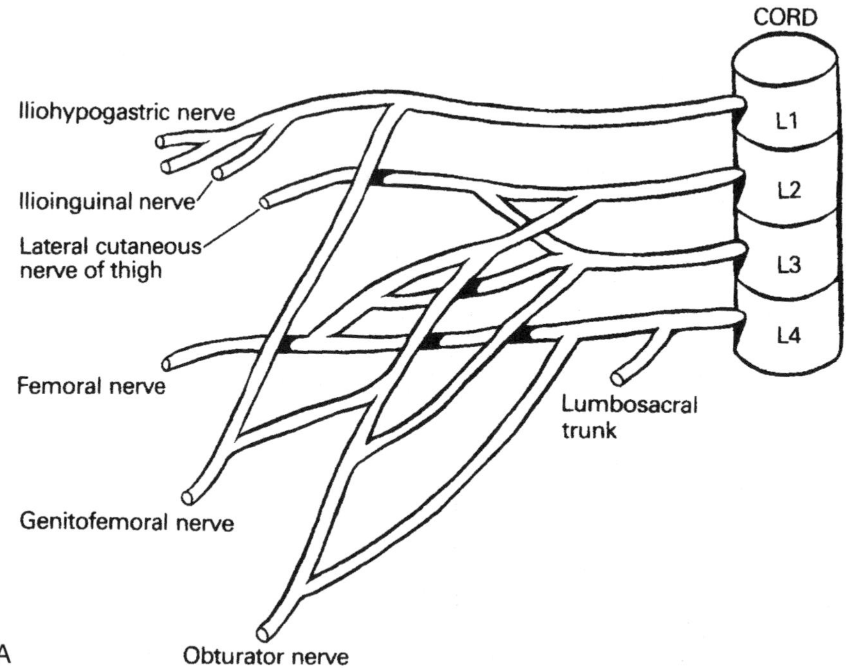

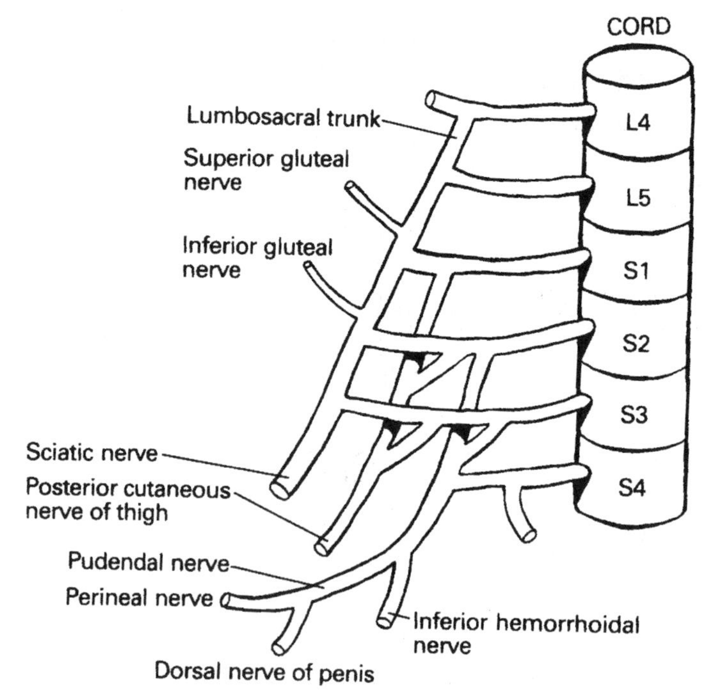

Fig. 9-4. (A) The lumbar plexus. **(B)** The sacral plexus. (From Devinsky and Feldmann,[9] with permission.)

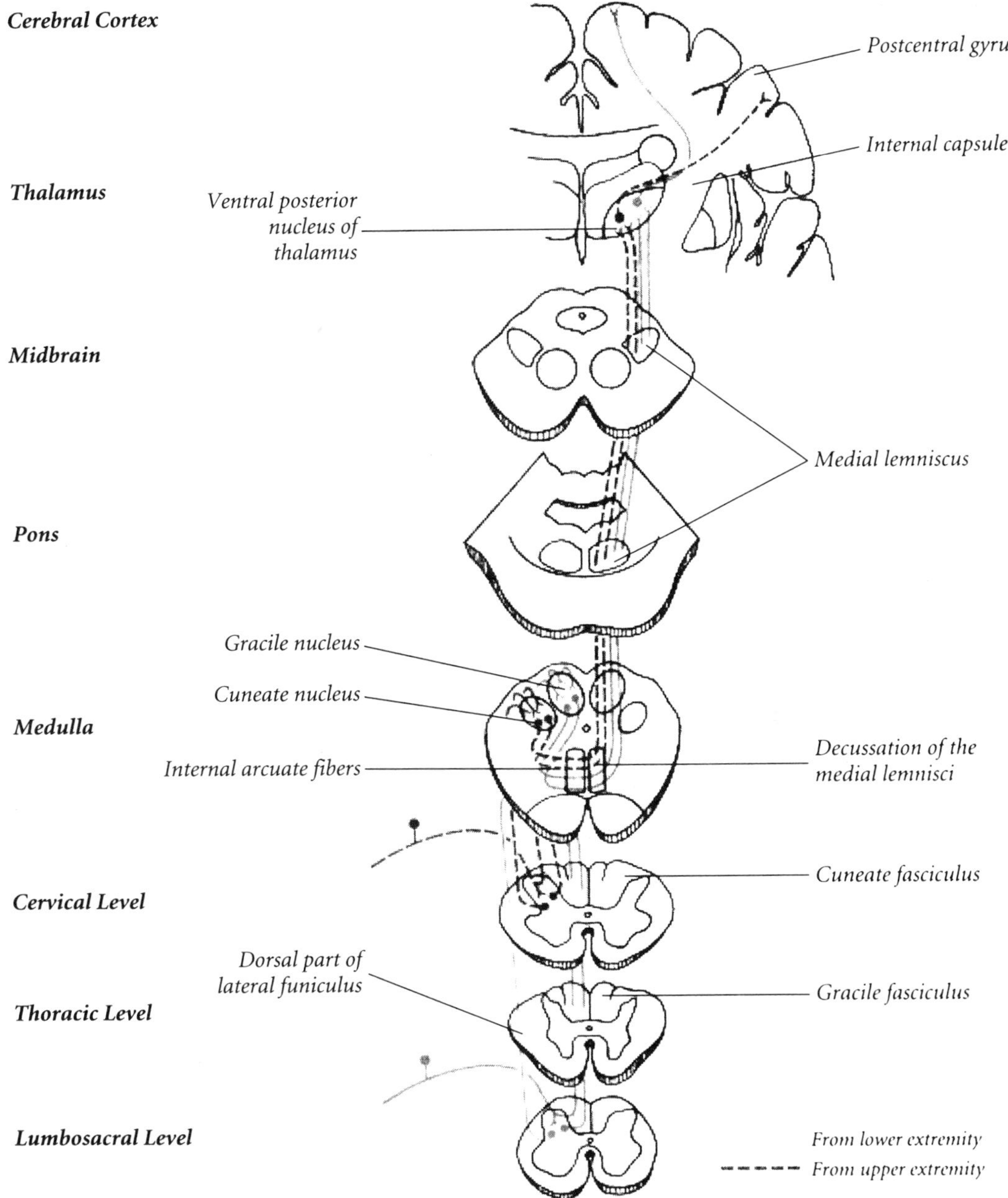

Fig. 9-5. The dorsal column–medial lemniscal (DCML) pathways mediating the epicritic sensations. Lower extremity proprioceptive input is shown traveling via Clarke's nucleus. (From Barr and Kiernan,[10] with permission.)

the lower medulla, they synapse on neurons in either the nucleus cuneatus or nucleus gracilis, collectively called the dorsal column nuclei. The axons of these neurons then form the medial lemniscus, a tract that decussates then ascends to the thalamus. The fibers of the medial lemniscus synapse on cell bodies in the thalamus. These cells relay the information to the primary somatic sensory cortex. Collateral branches also supply somatosensory information from the DCML to the cerebellum.

Spinothalamic Pathway

When pain or temperature sensation is detected by the appropriate sensory receptors, the input travels along the

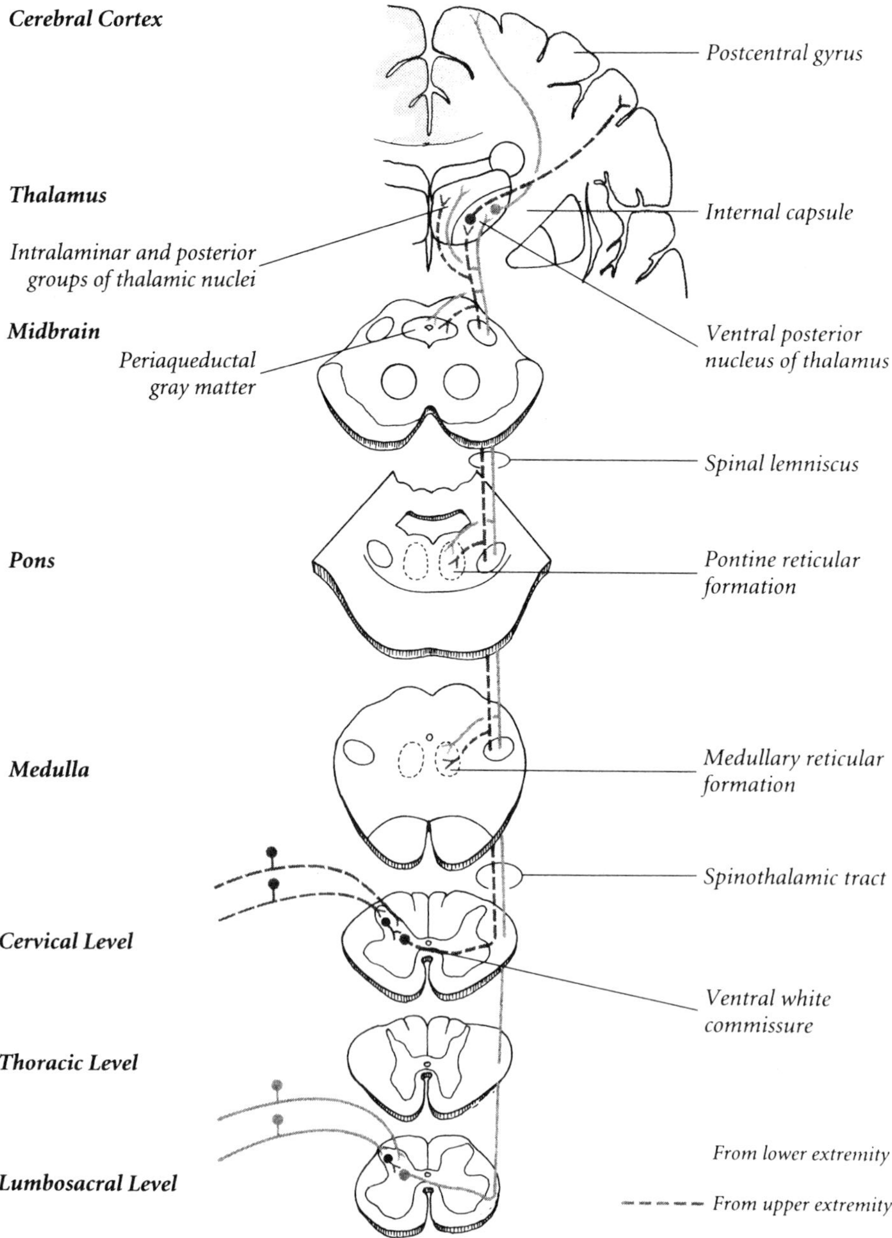

Fig. 9-6. The spinothalamic pathway, which mediates pain, touch, and temperature. (From Barr and Kiernan,[10] with permission.)

afferent fibers that enter the spinal cord to synapse on sensory neurons in the dorsal horn (see Fig. 9-6). The axons of the dorsal horn cells ascend in the spinal cord, but decussate within one to several segments to travel in the ventral or lateral columns. Like the DCML, there is topographic representation in the spinothalamic pathway. Fibers from distal body parts are located medially, and those from proximal body parts are located laterally. Most of the fibers in the DCML terminate in one nucleus of the thalamus, but the termination of the fibers in the spinothalamic pathway ranges throughout the brain stem and in three different nuclei in the thalamus. These thalamic cells then project to the somatosensory cortex and also to other cortical regions.

Motor System

In the trunk and extremities, the event necessary to produce muscle fiber contraction is depolarization of the cell membrane of an alpha motor neuron located in the ventral horn of the spinal cord. Similarly, in the head and face, the membrane of a motor neuron located in a cranial nerve nucleus must be depolarized in order for muscle fiber contraction to occur. When the neuron's membrane reaches its threshold, an action potential is generated. The action potential travels along the neuron's axon, resulting in contraction of the muscle fibers supplied by the neuron. Inputs to these motor neurons can be from the periphery or from various elements within the nervous system.

Neurons involved in the control and production of movement can be classified into two categories: upper motor neurons and lower motor neurons. Lower motor neurons include the neurons whose axons directly innervate muscle fibers. These are the anterior horn cells and the cell bodies in brain stem nuclei whose axons form cranial nerves. Upper motor neurons are those neurons whose axons carry the descending flow of motor information. An example of upper motor neurons are cortical cells whose axons make up the corticospinal and corticobulbar pathways (see Fig. 9-7).

There are three areas in the CNS that have direct connections with motor neurons: the spinal cord, brain stem, and cerebral cortex. Two other important areas exert an indirect influence over motor neurons: the basal ganglia and cerebellum.

Spinal Cord

The spinal cord contains various neuron circuits that are capable of activating motor neurons. The simplest of these circuits is the monosynaptic stretch reflex arc, which is responsible for deep tendon reflexes (DTRs). Other spinal circuitry is quite complex, controlling the activation of motor neurons at several spinal levels. Perhaps the most complex spinal neural circuitry may activate the oscillating bilateral movements responsible for walking.

Brain Stem

The brain stem contains two types of neurons that are involved in the motor system. The first are the cranial nerve motor neurons, which receive both ascending and descending input. The second are neurons in other nuclei such as the vestibular nuclei that project to spinal motor neurons. These brain stem descending pathways are involved in posture control and in the coordination of head and eye movements.

Cerebral Cortex

The cerebral cortex has several areas containing neurons whose axons descend through the nervous system to innervate spinal motor neurons directly. On the ventral surface of the medulla, these axons form an anatomic landmark, the medullary pyramids. For this reason, the corticospinal tract is often referred to as the pyramidal tract. At the junction between the medulla and spinal cord about three-fourths of these axons decussate and descend in the lateral columns of the spinal cord as the lateral corticospinal tract. The remaining one-quarter of the fibers do not cross to the contralateral side, but continue to descend in the ipsilateral ventral columns as the ventral corticospinal tract (see Fig. 9-8).

The cortex is responsible for activating cranial nerve motor neurons by way of the corticobulbar tract. Many projections in the corticobulbar tract to motor neurons are bilateral. That is, neurons in the right cerebral hemisphere involved in control of cranial nerve muscles send their axons to activate motor neurons in both the right and left brain stem nuclei. Left-sided cortical cells would also project to motor neurons in both the right and left sides of the brain stem. Two cranial nerves do not receive bilateral innervation from the cerebral cortex: VII (facial) and XII (hypoglossal). The motor neurons giving rise to the facial nerve receive split innervation; that is, those supplying the upper face have bilateral innervation, while those of the lower face receive contralateral innervation only. The motor neurons giving rise to the hypoglossal nerve receive contralateral innervation only.

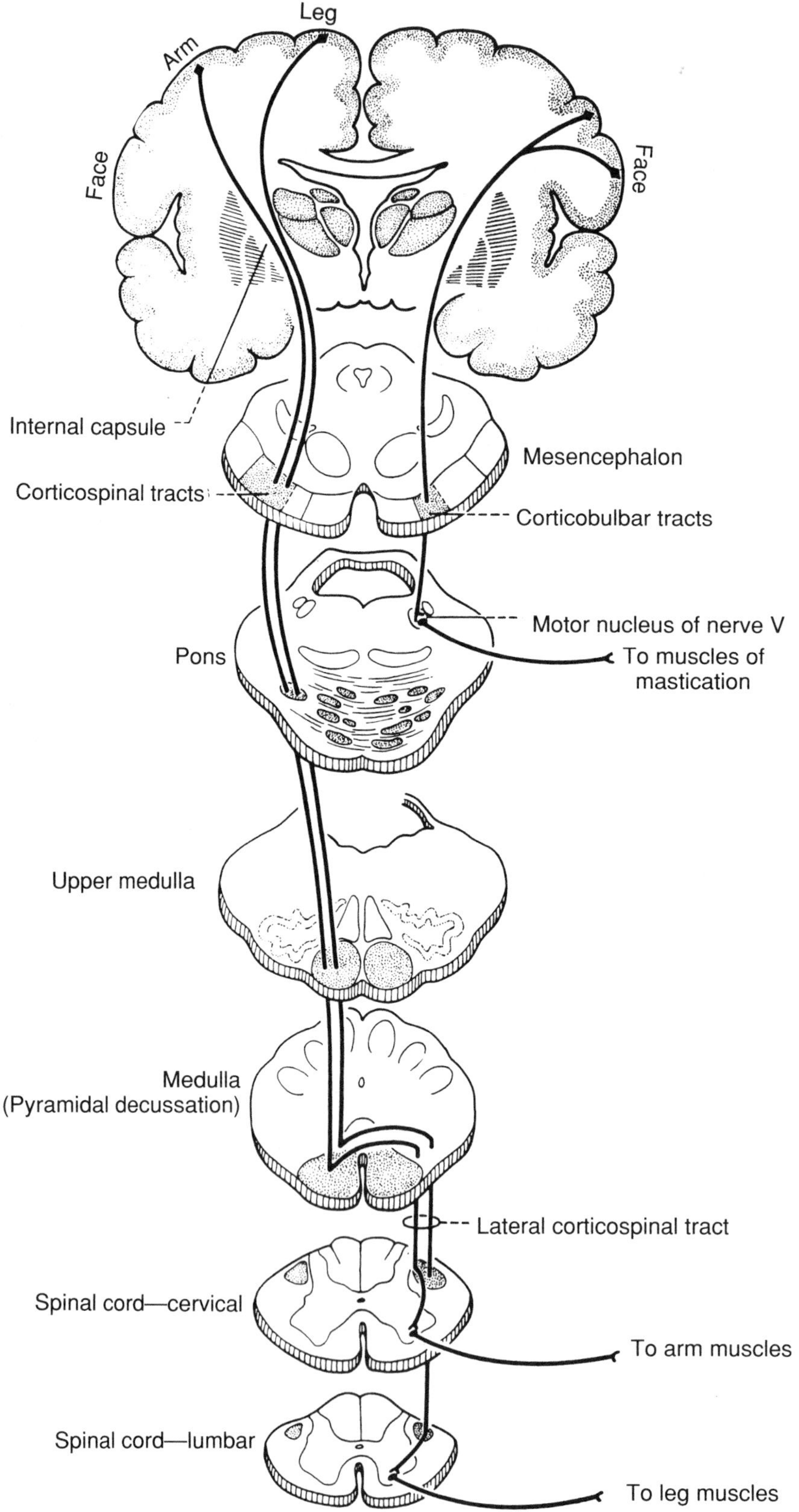

Fig. 9-7. The corticobulbar and corticospinal pathways. (From Haerer,[8] with permission.)

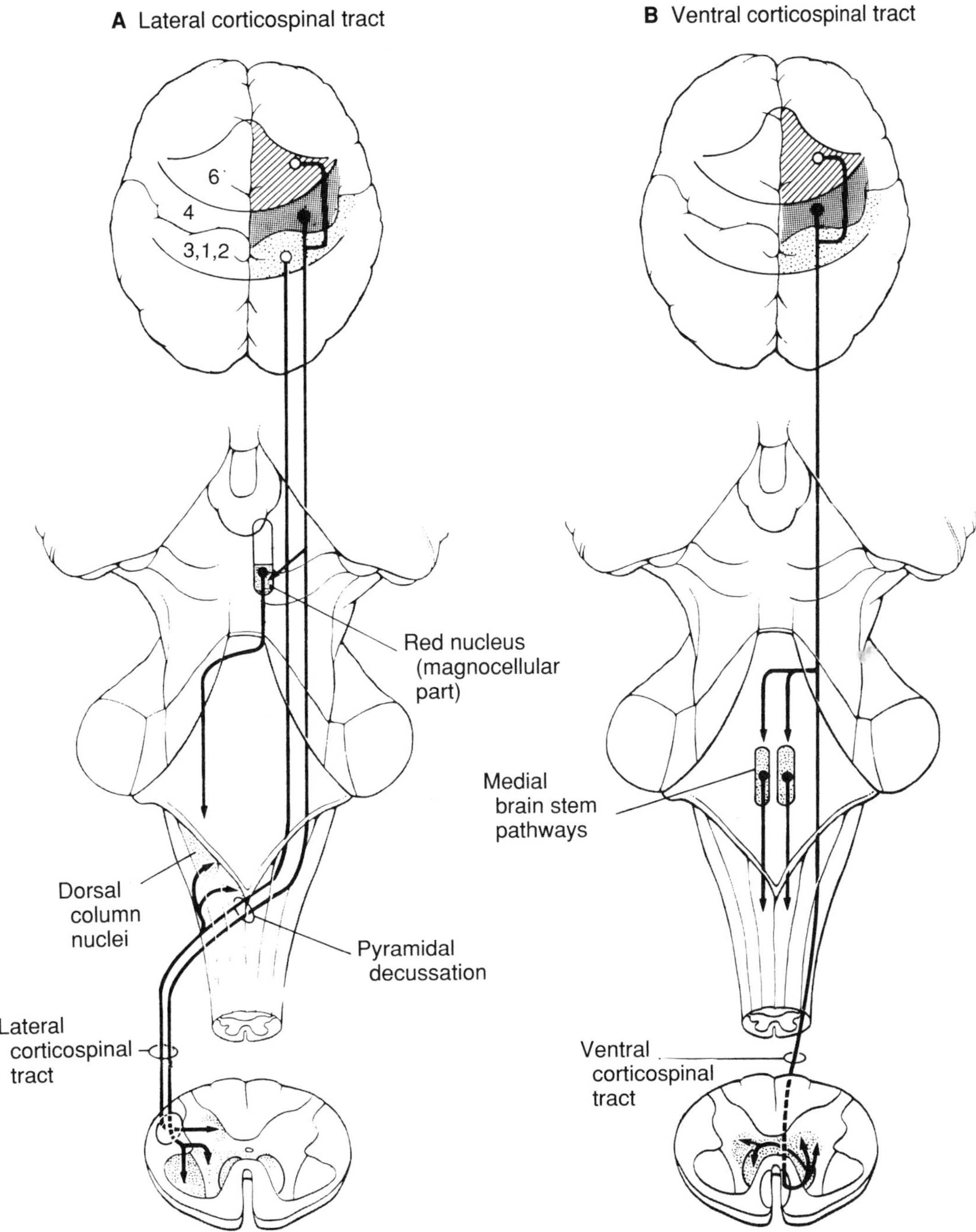

Fig. 9-8. The descending cortical pathways to the spinal segments. **(A)** The crossed lateral corticospinal tract originates from Brodmann's areas 4 and 6 and sensory areas 3, 2, and 1. The tract then crosses at the pyramidal decussation, descends in the dorsolateral column, and terminates in the shaded area of the spinal gray matter. Corticorubral neurons are mainly located in area 6. The principal area of termination of the corticospinal neurons originating from the sensory cortex is the medial portion of the dorsal horn. Collaterals project to dorsal column nuclei. **(B)** Uncrossed pathways (ventral corticospinal tract) originate principally in Brodmann's area 6 and in zones controlling the neck and trunk in area 4. Terminations are bilateral, and collaterals project to the medial brain stem pathways. (From Kandel et al.,[1] with permission.)

Basal Ganglia

As mentioned previously, the basal ganglia do not directly activate motor neurons but do play an important role in motor control. The basal ganglia receive input from the entire cerebral cortex and from a portion of the thalamus. Output from the basal ganglia is projected to motor planning areas of the cerebral cortex. The exact role of the basal ganglia in the control of movement is not yet known, but it is clear that persons with basal ganglia disease have specific motor control abnormalities. Historically, when researchers first discovered the basal ganglia's participation in motor control, they referred to these pathways as the extrapyramidal system. At the time, it was believed that the motor system consisted of only the pyramidal and extrapyramidal systems. We now know that other areas of the nervous system are involved in movement; therefore, this classification is no longer accurate.

Cerebellum

The cerebellum is another portion of the nervous system that does not directly activate lower motor neurons, yet is extremely important for the production of normal movement. The cerebellum receives two types of input: motor planning information from the cerebral cortex and sensory information from the periphery. The output from the cerebellum is projected to the descending motor systems of the brain stem and cortex. The cerebellum ensures that movement is carried out as planned, by comparing the intended with the actual movement and modifying the output of the descending motor systems as needed.

Effects of Lesions to or Disease of the Motor and Sensory Systems

To screen for nervous system disease, the physical therapist must be familiar with the effects of lesions to its various components, as well as the manifestations of common neurologic diseases. This discussion is not meant to be an exhaustive list of all possible nervous system disorders, but rather includes those lesions and diseases that are most commonly seen by the general practice physical therapist working with adult patients. It is important to remember that the immature nervous system responds differently, is subject to different disorders, and is evaluated differently than the adult nervous system. Especially when there is suspicion of a central nervous system dysfunction, it is best to refer children to a pediatric specialist.

Lesions in the nervous system can be the result of numerous factors, including direct trauma, compression, ischemia, toxicity, and various disease processes.

Upper Versus Lower Motor Neuron Symptoms

Before considering lesions affecting the motor system, it is important to differentiate between upper motor neuron and lower motor neuron lesions. Any insult that disrupts the flow of information from higher centers to lower motor neurons is considered an upper motor neuron lesion. An upper motor neuron lesion is characterized by a group of symptoms that can include hyperactive DTRs, increased muscle tone, clonus, presence of abnormal reflexes, abnormal posturing of body parts, and the presence of abnormal muscle force production in nonmyotomal groups of muscles. A patient with an upper motor neuron lesion may have difficulty contracting individual muscles in an isolated manner, but be able to contract the same muscles in a mass pattern of movement. Physical therapists often refer to these patterns as synergies.

Any damage to the motor neuron or its axon is defined as a lower motor neuron lesion. A lower motor neuron lesion affects only the muscles innervated by the lesioned nerve fiber. The findings include muscle weakness and atrophy, fasciculations, and diminished or absent DTRs.[2]

A disease that affects both upper and lower motor neurons is amyotrophic lateral sclerosis (ALS). ALS is a progressive disorder, with onset usually in the later adult years. Common initial complaints include gait problems, limb weakness, dysarthria (speech difficulty caused by weakness), and dysphagia (swallowing difficulties caused by weakness). Deep tendon reflexes may be either exaggerated or diminished, depending on the balance between upper and lower motor neuron involvement. Prognosis is poor, with death usually occurring within 5 years of onset.[3]

Lower Motor Neurons

Damage to lower motor neurons can occur because of direct trauma or vascular disorders affecting the ventral horn of the spinal cord or the brain stem nuclei, where lower motor neurons are located. Several diseases target lower motor neurons.

Poliomyelitis is one such disease. It is a viral infection that often affects the spinal cord and brain stem, causing degeneration of lower motor neurons. In the United States, the incidence of this disease is extremely low and usually occurs in areas where vaccination is not practiced. Postpolio syndrome occurs in rare individuals who had developed muscle paralysis/weakness early in life. These persons, whose neurologic deficit had remained stable for many years, experience increasing weakness in the affected muscles. Weakness can progress to previously unaffected muscles.

Upper Motor Neurons

Multiple sclerosis (MS) is a disease that affects upper motor neurons, as well as any other portion of the central nervous system. MS is a disease of young adults, leading to scattered demyelination and the formation of plaques throughout the CNS. Areas that tend to develop lesions more frequently include the optic chiasm and nerves, brain stem, cerebellum, and the corticospinal tracts and posterior columns of the spinal cord.[4] Onset is usually either acute or subacute, with several symptoms occurring initially. The disease is often characterized by exacerbations and remissions. Diagnosis is based on the presence of multiple neurologic symptoms with periods of exacerbation and remission. Many persons with MS have easy fatigability and report that warm temperatures worsen their symptoms.

Peripheral Nerves

Lesions to peripheral nerves are frequently caused by penetrating injury, traction, fractures, pressure, or entrapment. Because peripheral nerves are mixed, symptoms include both motor and sensory deficits. Motor deficits are consistent with a lower motor neuron lesion and affect only the muscles supplied by the affected nerve. Sensory deficits are present in the cutaneous distribution for the affected nerve (see Fig. 9-9).

Guillain-Barré syndrome is a disease process that affects spinal and cranial nerve motor neurons, causing scattered demyelination. Symptoms usually occur within days or weeks of a viral infection and include symmetric limb weakness, often with paresthesia. Eventually, muscle weakness progresses, and DTRs can become absent. The extent of sensory deficit varies, and recovery is generally slow, taking many months. Early treatment with plasmapheresis has been shown to accelerate recovery and diminish the incidence of permanent neurologic deficits.

Plexus Injuries

The roots or trunks of the brachial plexus may be damaged by penetrating trauma, tumors, and by traction during falls, shoulder dislocation, in delivery at birth, or by neoplasm. The location of the injury will determine which roots or trunks are involved. The muscles innervated by the involved nerve fibers will demonstrate motor deficits (see Tables 9-1, 9-2), and regions of skin supplied by the involved nerve fibers will exhibit sensory loss (see Fig. 9-10). Dysfunction can be located in a combination of several segmental or peripheral nerve dermatomes and myotomes, because a trunk injury involves several roots that become several peripheral nerves. Identifying the site of lesion in this type of injury can be a formidable task, and a thorough familiarity with the anatomy of the plexus is critical.

Radicular Nerves

Injuries to the radicular nerves are another example of lower motor neuron lesion. They can occur by the same mechanisms as injury to the brachial plexus, as well as by displaced spinal fracture, spinal dislocation, or compression by osteophytes or herniated intervertebral discs. The resultant motor symptoms are present only in the muscles supplied by the affected roots, and sensory disturbances are located in the segmental distributions for the involved roots.

Spinal Cord

In adults, lesions to the spinal cord are caused most often by major trauma.[5] However, nontraumatic damage can also occur. Nontraumatic causes can include vascular malfunctions leading to ischemia, vertebral subluxation secondary to rheumatoid arthritis, spinal cord infection, diseases such as multiple sclerosis, and tumors.

Traumatic Lesions

Spinal cord injury can result either from direct damage to the tissues of the cord or from cord compression. Compression first affects the tissues lying in the periphery of the spinal cord. Early signs can include spastic weakness and sensory impairment below the level of the

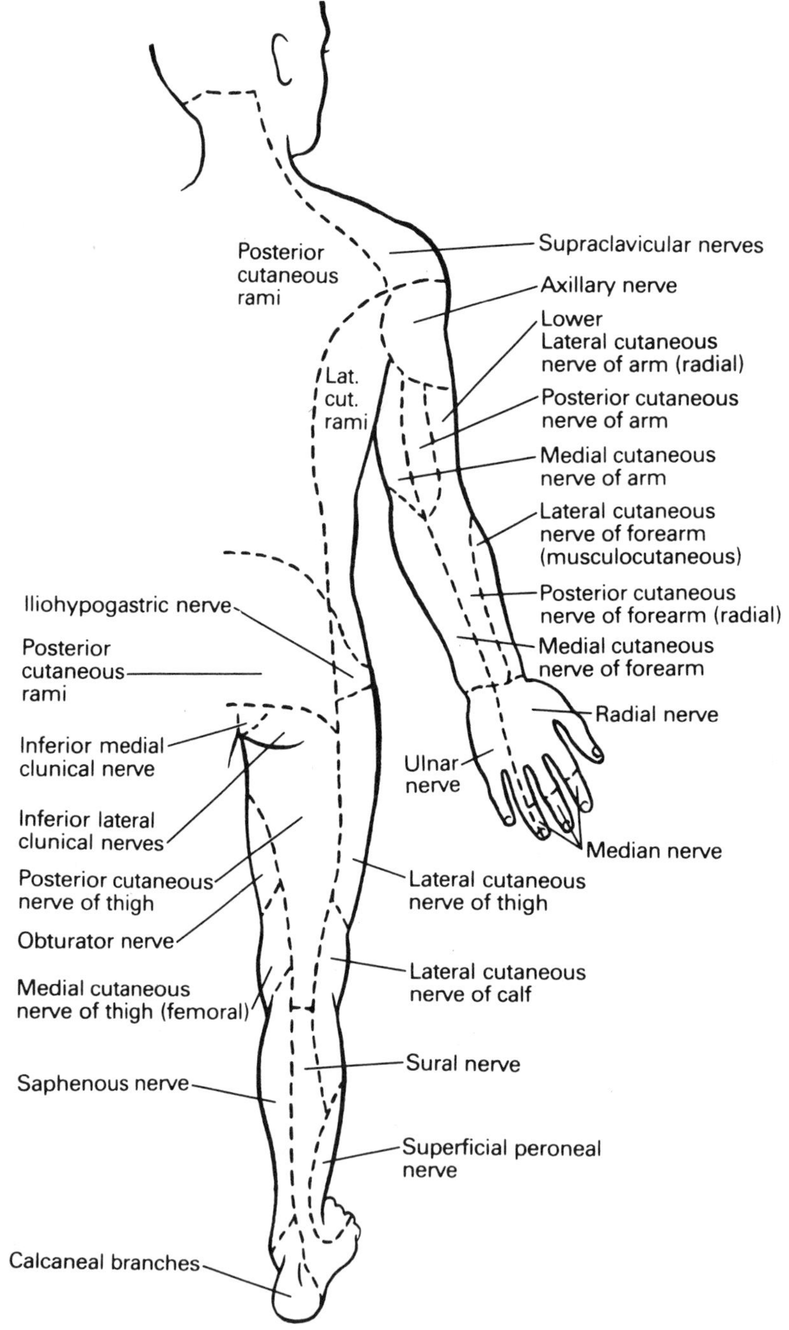

Fig. 9-9. Peripheral nerve sensory distribution. **(A)** Posterior view. *(Continues.)*

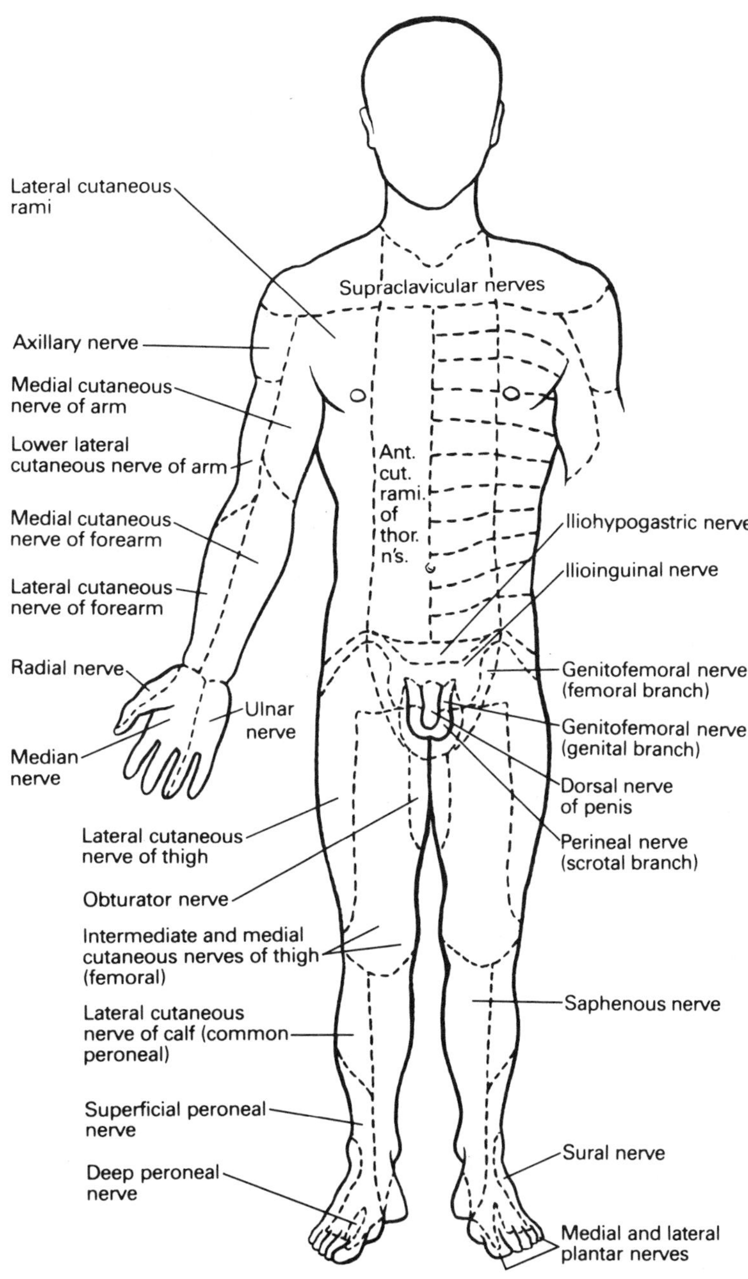

Fig. 9-9 *(Continued).* **(B)** Anterior view. (From Devinsky and Feldmann, as modified from Haymaker and Woodhall,[11] with permission.)

Table 9-1. Innervation of Muscles Responsible for Movements of the Shoulder Girdle and Upper Extremity

Muscle	Segmental Innervation	Peripheral Nerve
Trapezius	Cranial XI; C (2) 3–4	Spinal accessory nerve
	C 3–4	Nerves to levator scapulae
Levator scapulae	C 4–5	Dorsal scapular nerve
Rhomboideus major	C 4–5	Dorsal scapular nerve
Rhomboideus minor	C 4–5	Dorsal scapular nerve
Serratus anterior	C 5–7	Long thoracic nerve
Deltoid	C 5–6	Axillary nerve
Teres minor	C 5–6	Axillary nerve
Supraspinatus	C (4) 5–6	Suprascapular nerve
Infraspinatus	C (4) 5–6	Suprascapular nerve
Latissimus dorsi	C 6–8	Thoracodorsal nerve (long subscapular)
Pectoralis major	C 5–Th 1	Lateral and medial anterior thoracic
Pectoralis minor	C 7–Th 1	Medial anterior thoracic
Subscapularis	C 5–7	Subscapular nerves
Teres major	C 5–7	Lower subscapular nerve
Subclavius	C 5–6	Nerve to subclavius
Coracobrachialis	C 6–7	Musculocutaneous nerve
Biceps brachii	C 5–6	Musculocutaneous nerve
Brachialis	C 5–6	Musculocutaneous nerve
Brachioradialis	C 5–6	Radial nerve
Triceps brachii	C 6–8 (Th 1)	Radial nerve
Anconeus	C 7–8	Radial nerve
Supinator brevis	C 5–7	Radial nerve
Extensor carpi radialis longus	C (5) 6–7 (8)	Radial nerve
Extensor carpi radialis brevis	C (5) 6–7 (8)	Radial nerve
Extensor carpi ulnaris	C 6–8	Radial nerve
Extensor digitorum communis	C 6–8	Radial nerve
Extensor indicis proprius	C 6–8	Radial nerve
Extensor digiti minimi	C 6–8	Radial nerve
Extensor pollicis longus	C 6–8	Radial nerve
Extensor pollicis brevis	C 6–8	Radial nerve
Abductor pollicis longus	C 6–8	Radial nerve
Pronator teres	C 6–7	Median nerve
Flexor carpi radialis	C 6–7 (8)	Median nerve
Pronator quadratus	C 7–Th 1	Median nerve
Palmaris longus	C 7–Th 1	Median nerve
Flexor digitorum sublimis	C 7–Th 1	Median nerve
Flexor digitorum profundus (radial half)	C 7–Th 1	Median nerve
Lumbricales 1 and 2	C 7–Th 1	Median nerve
Flexor pollicis longus	C 8–Th 1	Median nerve
Flexor pollicis brevis (lateral head)	C 8–Th 1	Median nerve
Abductor pollicis brevis	C 8–Th 1	Median nerve
Opponens pollicis	C 8–Th 1	Median nerve
Flexor carpi ulnaris	C 7–Th 1	Ulnar nerve
Flexor digitorum profundus (ulnar half)	C 7–Th 1	Ulnar nerve
Interossei	C 8–Th 1	Ulnar nerve
Lumbricales 3 and 4	C 8–Th 1	Ulnar nerve
Flexor pollicis brevis (medial head)	C 8–Th 1	Ulnar nerve
Flexor digiti minimi brevis	C 8–Th 1	Ulnar nerve
Abductor digiti minimi	C 8–Th 1	Ulnar nerve
Opponens digiti minimi	C 8–Th 1	Ulnar nerve
Palmaris brevis	C 8–Th 1	Ulnar nerve
Adductor pollicis	C 8–Th 1	Ulnar nerve

Table 9-2. Innervation of Muscles Responsible for Movements of the Lower Extremities

Muscle	Segmental Innervation	Peripheral Nerve
Psoas major	L (1) 2–4	Nerve to psoas major
Psoas minor	L 1–2	Nerve to psoas minor
Iliacus	L 2–4	Femoral nerve
Quadriceps femoris	L 2–4	Femoral nerve
Sartorius	L 2–4	Femoral nerve
Pectineus	L 2–4	Femoral nerve
Gluteus maximus	L 5–S 2	Inferior gluteal nerve
Gluteus medius	L 4–S 1	Superior gluteal nerve
Gluteus minimus	L 4–S 1	Superior gluteal nerve
Tensor fasciae latae	L 4–S 1	Superior gluteal nerve
Piriformis	S 1–2	Nerve to piriformis
Adductor longus	L 2–4	Obturator nerve
Adductor brevis	L 2–4	Obturator nerve
Adductor magnus	{L 2–4 L 4–5	Obturator nerve Sciatic nerve
Gracilis	L 2–4	Obturator nerve
Obturator externus	L 2–4	Obturator nerve
Obturator internus	L 5–S 3	Nerve to obturator internus
Gemellus superior	L 5–S 3	Nerve to obturator internus
Gemellus inferior	L 4–S 1	Nerve to quadratus femoris
Quadratus femoris	L 4–S 1	Nerve to quadratus femoris
Biceps femoris (long head)	L 5–S 1	Tibial nerve
Semimembranosus	L 4–S 1	Tibial nerve
Semitendinosus	L 5–S 2	Tibial nerve
Popliteus	L 5–S 1	Tibial nerve
Gastrocnemius	L 5–S 2	Tibial nerve
Soleus	L 5–S 2	Tibial nerve
Plantaris	L 5–S 1	Tibial nerve
Tibialis posterior	L 5–S 1	Tibial nerve
Flexor digitorum longus	L 5–S 1	Tibial nerve
Flexor hallucis longus	L 5–S 1	Tibial nerve
Biceps femoris (short head)	L 5–S 2	Common peroneal nerve
Tibialis anterior	L 4–S 1	Deep peroneal nerve
Peroneus tertius	L 4–S 1	Deep peroneal nerve
Extensor digitorum longus	L 4–S 1	Deep peroneal nerve
Extensor hallucis longus	L 4–S 1	Deep peroneal nerve
Extensor digitorum brevis	L 4–S 1	Deep peroneal nerve
Extensor hallucis brevis	L 4–S 1	Deep peroneal nerve
Peroneus longus	L 4–S 1	Superficial peroneal nerve
Peroneus brevis	L 4–S 1	Superficial peroneal nerve
Flexor digitorum brevis	L 4–S 1	Medial plantar nerve
Flexor hallucis brevis	L 5–S 1	Medial plantar nerve
Abductor hallucis	L 4–S 1	Medial plantar nerve
Lumbricales (medial 1 or 2)	L 4–S 1	Medial plantar nerve
Quadratus plantae	S 1–2	Lateral plantar nerve
Adductor hallucis	L 5–S 2	Lateral plantar nerve
Abductor digiti quinti	S 1–2	Lateral plantar nerve
Flexor digiti quinti brevis	S 1–2	Lateral plantar nerve
Lumbricales (lateral 2 or 3)	S 1–2	Lateral plantar nerve
Interossei	S 1–2	Lateral plantar nerve

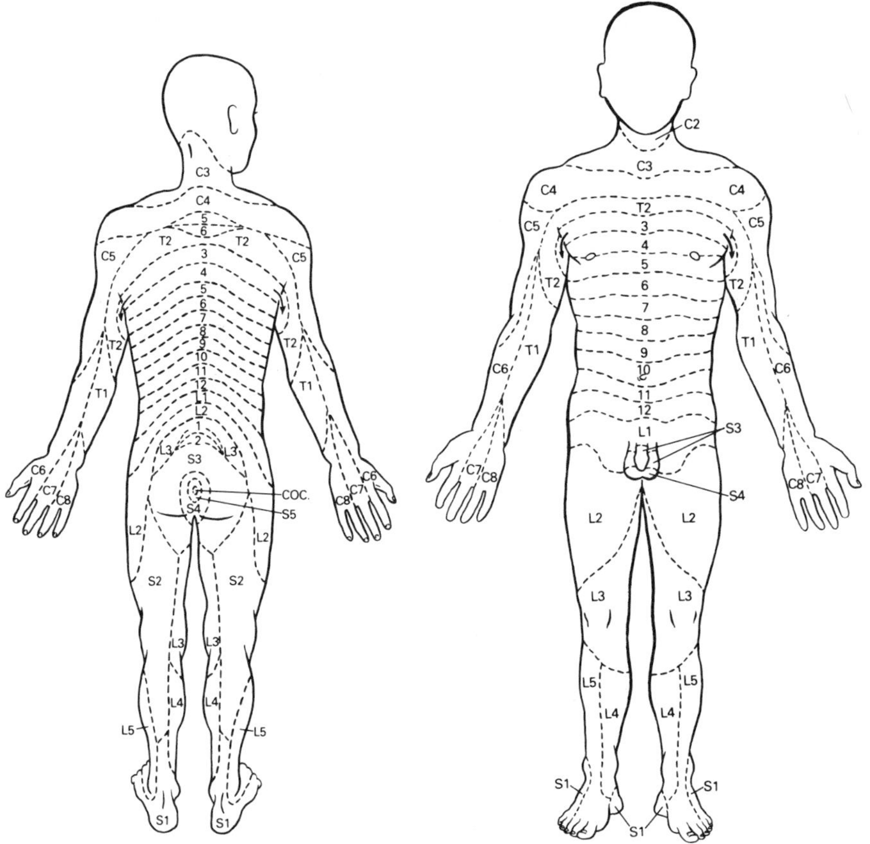

Fig. 9-10. Dermatome charts. (From Devinsky and Feldmann, as modified from Haymaker and Woodhall,[11] with permission.)

lesion, impaired bowel and bladder control, increased lower extremity DTRs, and a positive Babinski response. If untreated, the compression can lead to a complete spinal cord transection.

The findings upon examination are dependent on the spinal cord structures damaged. Damage to the gray matter causes local dysfunction, while damage to the tracts causes more widespread symptoms. In a complete spinal cord transection, there are lower motor neuron signs at the level of lesion (because of the gray matter damage) and upper motor neuron signs below the level of lesion (because of the axonal tract disruption), with no sensory function below the level of injury. Incomplete lesions affect only those spinal cord structures that are damaged. Patterns of dysfunction following incomplete spinal cord lesion have been defined, based on the area of the spinal cord that is injured.

Incomplete Syndromes

A hemisection of the cord results in the Brown-Sequard syndrome, resulting in loss of voluntary motor function with signs of upper motor neuron lesion below the level of lesion ipsilaterally, with normal motor function contralaterally. These findings are due to the disruption of the anterior and lateral corticospinal tracts. Below the level of the lesion, sensory function is lost ipsilaterally for position, tactile discrimination, and vibration and contralaterally for pain and temperature. The different sensory deficits occur because of the difference in decussation level between the DCML and spinothalamic systems.

The central cord syndrome causes more motor dysfunction in the upper than the lower extremities, with proximal muscles more involved than distal. These findings occur because cervical tracts are medial to lumbosacral tracts, and proximal tracts are medial to distal tracts. Sensory loss is variable and can be minimal, depending on the extent and location of damage to ascending tracts.

The anterior cord syndrome causes loss of motor function below the level of the lesion, because it disrupts the corticospinal tracts. There will also be loss of pain and temperature sensation below the injury because of damage to the spinothalamic system. However, joint position and vibration will be unimpaired.

In a posterior cord syndrome, motor function is preserved because the corticospinal tracts are located in the anterior and lateral columns. Damage to the posterior columns results in loss of function in the DCML pathway, with subsequent deficits in position sense, discriminatory touch, and vibratory sensation. These sensory deficits often lead to a wide-based gait even though motor function is normal.

Lesions to the cauda equina are often incomplete and result in lower motor neuron symptoms, because these fibers represent the axons of peripheral nerves. These roots are the most caudal in the nervous system; therefore, findings can include paralysis of the bowel and bladder sphincters, problems with erection and ejaculation in men, paralysis of the pelvic floor muscles, and absence of ankle DTRs.

Nontraumatic Causes of Spinal Cord Damage

Infections can reach the spinal epidural space by direct extension from adjacent tissues, through the blood from infection in a distant site, and through perforating wounds, spinal surgery, or lumbar puncture. The midthoracic area is the most frequently affected. Symptoms develop suddenly, with severe back pain as the usual presenting symptom, often accompanied by malaise, fever, headache, and neck pain. Shortly afterward, radicular pain and motor paralysis occur distal to the infection. Treatment should occur as soon as possible, to minimize permanent motor and sensory deficits, and can include antibiotics and surgical drainage.

Spinal cord tumors can occur either as primary spinal tumors or as metastasis, mainly from the lung, breast, and prostate. They can be classified as intramedullary or extramedullary[6] (see Ch. 10). Intramedullary tumors arise in the tissue of the spinal cord itself. These tumors cause symptoms because of direct disruption of the function of spinal cord structures. Extramedullary tumors are located either between the cord and dura mater or within the spinal canal, outside the dura mater. They cause symptoms by involving nerve roots or by compressing the spinal cord or its blood vessels. Initial symptoms of spinal cord tumors usually include paresthesias, followed by the development of lower extremity weakness and sensory loss. There is often an early loss of bowel and bladder control. The motor symptoms in the lower extremities are consistent with upper motor neuron syndrome, including hyperreflexia, positive Babinski, and spasticity.

Brain Stem

Lesions to the medulla, pons, and midbrain usually occur because of vascular events, but can also be caused by trauma or disease, such as ALS, or by tumors. Motor deficits can occur because of (1) disruption of corticospinal pathways, (2) disruption of corticobulbar pathways, (3) damage to motor neurons in cranial nerve nuclei, or (4) damage to nuclei giving rise to descending pathways. Sensory deficits can occur because of disruption of sensory pathways ascending from the body or from damage to cranial nerve sensory neurons. Numerous syndromes resulting from lesions to various portions of the brain stem have been described, depending on the location of the lesion. Common clinical signs include contralateral hemiparesis and sensory deficit. Cranial nerve deficits can include extraocular muscle paralysis, facial paralysis, tongue weakness, hearing deficits, hoarseness secondary to vocal cord paralysis, chewing difficulties, and sensory deficits of the face and head. Parasympathetic nervous system control can be affected by lesions to cranial nerves III, IX, and X. Vertigo or balance deficits can occur because of damage to the vestibular nuclei. Severe lesions can damage respiratory centers or cause coma.

Diencephalon

The diencephalon is made up of the thalamus and hypothalamus. Damage to the thalamus is usually of vascular origin. Because the thalamus is primarily a relay center for sensory information, a lesion can cause severe contralateral sensory deficits. Another manifestation of lesions to the thalamus is "thalamic pain," a condition characterized by intractable, persistent contralateral pain.

Damage to the hypothalamus can lead to problems with physical development, alterations of the sleep–wake cycle, changes in eating patterns, autonomic disorders, and affective problems such as depression and bipolar disorder.

Cerebral Cortex

Lesions to the cerebral cortex can be the result of trauma, ischemia, or neoplasm. Symptoms can vary greatly, ranging from headaches, dizziness, and cognitive and language deficits to motor and sensory deficits.

Trauma

Lesions to the cerebral cortex can occur whenever a patient has a history of head injury. More severe cases can result in coma and may require surgical intervention. Less severe cases can cause diffuse cognitive and memory deficits, balance and coordination deficits, or paresis.

Ischemia

For normal function the brain requires that oxygen and glucose be present constantly and can function for only a few minutes if these substances are not provided. Any event that disrupts the flow of blood through cerebral arteries can cause ischemic death, or infarction, of neural tissues. Occlusion of cerebral arteries is caused by atherosclerosis, thrombus, or embolus. Neuronal damage can also be caused by intracerebral hemorrhage.

In general, infarction in the region supplied by the middle cerebral artery causes contralateral weakness, sensory loss, and homonymous hemianopsia (or visual field cut). If the lesion is to the right hemisphere, language disturbance is common. When a lesion affects the left hemisphere, spatial perception is often disturbed.

Infarction of the anterior cerebral artery causes weakness, clumsiness, and sensory loss of the distal contralateral leg. Also occurring can be anomia (a language disturbance), urinary incontinence, and facial weakness.

The posterior cerebral artery supplies numerous regions, including the temporal lobe, thalamus, and brain stem. Occlusion of this artery can lead to a variety of clinical problems, including hemianesthesia, thalamic sensory syndrome, homonymous hemianopsia, amnesia, and hemiballismus.

Neoplasm

Intracranial tumors can be primary or the result of metastasis from another site. They usually grow slowly, and patients usually develop symptoms somewhat insidiously. These symptoms occur because tumors have one or more of the following effects:

1. Pressure effects because of the size of the tumor
2. Irritation of the neural tissue
3. Impairment or destruction of brain tissue or cranial nerves
4. Endocrine effects

Pressure effects are manifested by headache, nausea and vomiting, mental changes, and double vision. Headache is the most common complaint of a patient with increased intracranial pressure. It may awaken the patient from sleep and is often worse on waking, but improves as he remains upright. Coughing, straining, or bending over increases the headache. Vomiting caused by increased intracranial pressure is projectile and causes an immediate decrease in complaints of headache. The mental changes commonly seen with increased pressure are irritability or a generalized dulling of the intellect. Diplopia, or double vision, is frequent, especially with lateral gaze.[6]

The irritation caused by intracranial neoplasm usually manifests itself via pain or seizure. As a tumor grows and compresses a pain-sensitive structure, the patient may experience pain. An example is facial pain caused by irritation of the fifth cranial nerve. In addition, as a tumor grows, it can irritate the electrically excitable nerve tissues long before damage is caused. This irritation can lead to focal seizures.

When the tumor causes decreased function or damage in the surrounding tissues, it can result in weakness, sensory changes, visual field defects, decreased auditory acuity, and incoordination. The specific deficits vary greatly, depending on the location of the tumor.

The endocrine effects listed above usually occur because of pituitary dysfunction. This can occur because compression of the pituitary by adjacent tumors leads to damage and decreased function. In addition, when some pituitary cell types become neoplastic, they secrete excessively, leading to increased function (see Ch. 7).

Basal Ganglia

The most common disease involving the basal ganglia is Parkinson's disease. The most common form is idiopathic, but symptoms can be the result of therapy with certain drugs or they can occur following encephalitis or manganese poisoning. The idiopathic type is a progressive disease, with onset usually in middle age. The motor problems associated with Parkinson's disease include the classic triad of tremor, rigidity, and akinesia. Tremor is an involuntary rhythmic joint motion. In Parkinson's disease, it occurs when the patient is at rest and is the initial symptom noted by a majority of those diagnosed with this disease. It can affect any area of the body. The rigidity seen in these patients can occur in any muscle and often has a cogwheel- or ratchet-like characteristic. It is not necessarily related to motor control problems; one can occur in the absence of the other. Akinesia refers to the motor control problems seen: the patient has difficulty initiating movement, and there is a lack of normal automatic motions or a poverty of movement. The problems with initiation are frequently seen when the patient attempts to rise to standing or, once standing, in starting to walk. Poverty of movement can lead to diminished facial expression, or masking, which can lead an observer to suspect the presence of clinical depression. Other examples of automatic muscle activity that are missing in many persons with Parkinson's disease are arm swing during ambulation, occasional weight shifting, and gestures or other subtle forms of nonverbal communication.

Another characteristic motor control problem frequently seen in Parkinson's disease is bradykinesia, or slowness of movement. It can seriously interfere with functional activities and postural reactions. Persons with Parkinson's disease also tend to develop a characteristic posture, with a forward head, increased thoracic kyphosis, and flexed knees and elbows. This posture brings the center of mass significantly anterior to normal. The gait pattern in these patients is referred to as a festinating gait. It involves small shuffling steps, with an increased cadence as walking continues. It appears as if the patient is attempting to "catch up" with his center of mass. Many patients with Parkinson's disease also develop cognitive deficits, even though the basal ganglia are subcortical structures.

Other basal ganglia disorders include Huntington's disease, ballism, and tardive dyskinesia. Huntington's disease is a hereditary disorder characterized by progressive chorea, which is another form of involuntary movement. There is also progressive dementia. The disease is usually fatal within 10 to 15 years after diagnosis. Ballism is a flailing involuntary limb movement, usually occurring after a vascular lesion to the subthalamic nucleus. Tardive dyskinesia is caused by long-term treatment with certain drugs and is characterized by abnormal involuntary movements, especially of the face and tongue. It usually subsides after administration of the causative agent is stopped, but can be permanent.

Cerebellum

Cerebellar lesions can occur because of trauma, ischemia, tumor, cerebellar disease, or systemic disorders, such as malnutrition associated with alcoholism. Unilateral cerebellar lesions produce dysfunction in the ipsilateral limbs. The clinical features of cerebellar dysfunction reflect its roles in ensuring accurate and smooth limb movement, in the control of posture and muscle tone, and in the coordination of eye and head movements. *Hypotonia* with decreased DTRs is often seen in patients with cerebellar dysfunction. *Tremor* is a common clinical finding in persons with cerebellar lesions. Tremor is an involuntary oscillatory movement that can take two general forms in cerebellar dysfunction: *intention* tremor that occurs during the execution of volitional limb movements and *titubation*, a back-and-forth motion of the trunk that occurs when the patient attempts to hold the body upright against gravity. Force and accuracy control problems are also frequently seen in patients with cerebellar lesions and are referred to by the general term *ataxia*. Two motor disturbances contribute to ataxia: *dysmetria* and *decomposition of movement*. Dysmetria is a disturbance in the ability to judge the distance or range of a movement, leading to overshooting or undershooting the desired target. Movement decomposition describes a movement performed as a sequence of discreet motions rather than as a smooth integrated action. An *ataxic gait* has also been described, consisting of a wide base of support with an unsteady, irregular, staggering gait pattern. Another clinical finding in persons with cerebellar damage is *nystagmus*, an involuntary rhythmic oscillatory movement of the eyes.

Physical Therapy Evaluation of Nervous System Dysfunction

For the purpose of this chapter, the components of evaluating the nervous system are divided into separate entities, but in reality they are inseparable. Data collection should begin the moment the therapist first sees the patient. Observations made while the patient is preparing for the evaluation and during the interview can be as important as the findings on objective examination in suggesting the presence of nervous system disease.

Often the physical therapist is the first health care provider to observe and analyze the patient's gait pattern or other movement patterns. Because disturbances of the nervous system can seriously affect motor control, the physical therapist's observation of the patient's movement can lead to further examination of nervous system function during the objective evaluation.

When the physical therapist evaluates a patient with a non-neurologic diagnosis, a neurologic screening examination should be performed to determine the need for a more detailed nervous system examination. See Table 9-3 for a general screening of the nervous system. Conditions may exist at the outset though that direct the therapist to proceed with a more complete examination, including a history of previous nervous system involvement or a history of trauma to the head and neck region.

Patient Interview

Past Medical History

The patient should be asked about the presence of previous or ongoing medical conditions, whether or not they have been treated medically. These conditions may affect the treatment of the current problem or may relate to the chief complaint. All body systems should be addressed in this process, including the nervous system.

Table 9-3. General Screening of the Nervous System

General observation
Gait pattern
Gross movement patterns
Asymmetric facial features
Facial contour
Pupil size
Mentation disturbances (i.e., confusion, memory deficits)
Tremor
History
Complaints of
Weakness
Sensory abnormalities
Tremor
Dizziness
Headache
Visual disturbances
Hearing disturbances
Gait/balance disturbances
Peripheralization of symptoms
Physical examination
Observed muscle atrophy
Muscle weakness
Palpable clonus

History of Present Illness

The purpose of this portion of the subjective examination is to determine the patient's chief complaint and its nature. A problem in obtaining a worthwhile history is clarifying what patients mean when they use specific terms to describe their symptoms.[7] When patients complain of "dizziness," they can be referring to anything from vertigo to lightheadedness. It is important to ask sufficient questions to clarify the nature of the complaint, without guiding the patient into a decision biased by the examiner's suspicions.

Common chief complaints that indicate problems with the nervous system include headache, dizziness, tremor, weakness, and sensory, visual, or gait disturbances. See Chapter 8 for a thorough review of examination of patients with headache. A complaint of dizziness can refer to *vertigo*, a sense of spinning of the person or environment. This symptom is indicative of a lesion of the vestibular system. *Lightheadedness* can indicate a cardiac or other problem leading to decreased brain oxygenation. *Tremor* can be related to anxiety or to an organic nervous system condition. If the tremor occurs at rest, it can indicate Parkinson's disease. If the tremor worsens with movement, it can indicate cerebellar disease. Patients often use the term *weakness* to refer to general fatigue, not to specific muscular weakness.[6] Whether or not true lack of muscle strength exists can often be elicited by asking functional questions, such as "Can you get up from a chair without pushing with your arms?"

Social History

An examination of the patient's work and life habits can provide insight into the nature of the problem. Drug or alcohol abuse should be discussed, since these habits can directly affect the nervous system (see Ch. 12). The physical therapist can also determine the patient's goals and expectations for treatment and knowledge of the medical condition, both of which can influence the effectiveness of physical therapy treatment.

Physical Examination

To evaluate the nervous system, the following should be included in the physical examination: mental status, cranial nerves, motor function, sensory function, coordination, and reflexes.

Mental Status

A screening examination of a patient's mental status should assess alertness, orientation, memory, and general cognitive function. The patient being evaluated by a general practice physical therapist will most often be fully conscious, so the evaluation of alertness is not usually an issue. For further information, a text discussing physical therapy treatment of persons with traumatic brain injury should be consulted. Orientation should be established as to person, time, and place. This should be accomplished indirectly during routine conversation without embarrassing the patient by asking these questions directly. Other aspects of memory and cognitive functioning can be evaluated by self-report from the patient. The patient may note that he is less able to concentrate on his work or has memory problems, but it is best if the patient's family can corroborate these reports. If a more detailed evaluation is needed, the patient should be referred to a neuropsychologist or other qualified professional.

Cranial Nerves

Cranial nerve I (olfactory) is tested by presenting a familiar aromatic odor such as coffee, orange, or vanilla, to each nostril individually, which the patient is asked to identify. Abnormal findings are frequently the result of obstructed nasal passages or the normal decline in smell that occurs with aging. However, if there is a frontal lobe lesion, there can be a decrease in the patient's sense of smell as well as a visual loss. These deficits occur because the olfactory pathways run under the frontal lobe near the optic chiasm.

To evaluate cranial nerve II (optic), two functions can be tested by the physical therapist: central visual acuity and peripheral vision. If further testing is warranted, an ophthalmoscopic examination can be conducted by a qualified medical practitioner. Visual acuity testing can be approximated by asking the patient to read signs or other printed materials located across the room. Peripheral vision is tested by asking the patient to cover one eye and maintain gaze on the therapist's face, while the therapist stands a few feet in front of the patient, with the therapist's arms abducted. The therapist then randomly wiggles the fingers on one or both of his or her hands, making sure to test both the upper and lower portions of both visual fields. The patient is asked to indicate the side on which the therapist's fingers are moving. This procedure is then repeated for the other eye. Lesions of the eye and optic tract produce visual defects in one eye only (see Fig. 9-11). Lesions of the medial optic chiasm produce bilateral defects of the temporal visual fields (see Fig. 9-12). Lesions of the lateral optic chiasm produce bilateral defects of the nasal visual fields (see Fig. 9-13). Lesions posterior to the chiasm produce *homonymous hemianopsia*, a loss of input from the contralateral visual fields of both eyes (see Fig. 9-14).

Cranial nerves III, IV, and VI (oculomotor, trochlear, abducens) are usually assessed together, since they work together to control eye movements. Two aspects of eye motor function must be evaluated: pupillary reaction to

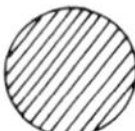

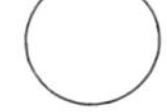

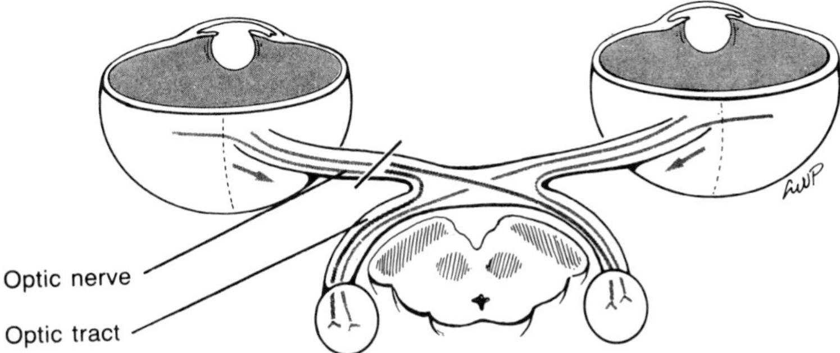

Fig. 9-11. Lesion to optic nerve causing ipsilateral blindness. (From Wilson-Pauwels et al.,[12] with permission.)

light, and lateral and vertical movements of the eyes. The pupils should be equally dilated in normal lighting and constrict equally when tested with a penlight. Both pupils should constrict when the light is directed at one eye while the therapist's hand shields one eye from the other. The normal range includes up to a 20 percent difference between the right and left pupil sizes. To evaluate eye motion, a target (the therapist's finger or a pen) is slowly moved laterally left to right and right to left. The patient is asked to follow the target with the eyes while holding the head still. The target is then moved vertically and obliquely (see Figs. 9-15, 9-16, and 9-17). During testing, the patient's eyes should be observed for symmetry and speed of motion and for the presence of nystagmus. Also important to note is whether the patient complains of diplopia (double vision) during testing and, if so, with which motions it occurs.

Cranial nerve V (trigeminal) is responsible for sensation of the face and anterior scalp and for motor innervation of the muscles of mastication. When performing sensory assessment, it is important to test the three branches of the trigeminal nerve: ophthalmic, maxillary, and mandibular. Light touch can be utilized comparing the left and right sides of the face (see Fig. 9-18). Motor testing of the muscles of mastication is somewhat difficult. It is possible to palpate the temporalis and masseter muscles bilaterally while the patient forcefully bites, comparing the degree of tone, one side versus the other. This procedure though provides little objective information. An equally nonobjective option is to ask the patient to bite forcefully on several tongue blades placed between the molars, first on the right and then on the left, and ask the patient if a subjective difference exists between the sides.

Cranial nerve VII (facial) is responsible for motor innervation to the muscles of facial expression. When testing, it is important to ask the patient to use muscles of both the upper and lower portions of the face, because upper motor neuron lesions affect only the lower half of the face, while lower motor neuron lesions affect the whole face. An activity for the upper face is wrinkling the brow and for the lower face, smiling.[11] This nerve also supplies the sense of taste to the anterior two-thirds of the tongue.

Cranial nerve VIII (vestibulocochlear) carries the special sensations of hearing and the vestibular apparatus, important for the maintenance of balance and the coordination of eye and head movements. Patients with lesions of the vestibular component often complain of dizziness, nausea, and balance disorder.

A patient with a lesion of the cochlear component of this nerve may complain of *tinnitus* (ringing in the ear) or complain of a hearing deficit. To screen the patient's hearing the therapist can use air conduction and/or bone conduction tests. For air conduction, the therapist rubs the thumbs and index fingers together in front of the patient's ears. The therapist gradually moves the hands away from the patient's ears. The patient tells the therapist when the noise is no longer heard. The therapist can judge the distance between the hands and the patient's ears, comparing left and right sides (see Fig. 9-19). For

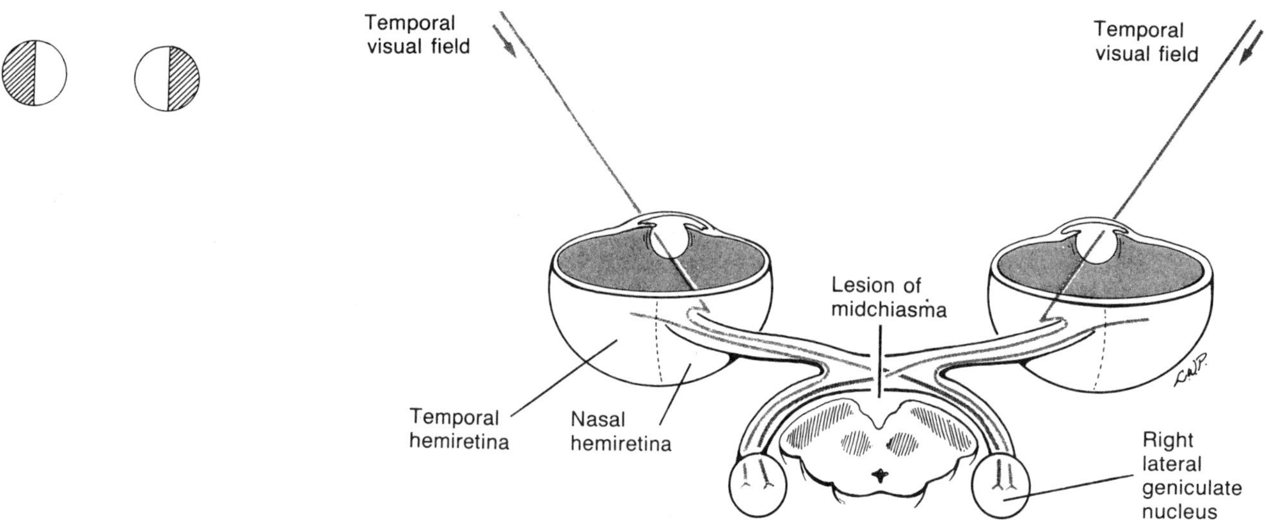

Fig. 9-12. Loss of peripheral vision (bitemporal hemianopsia). (From Wilson-Pauwels et al.,[12] with permission.)

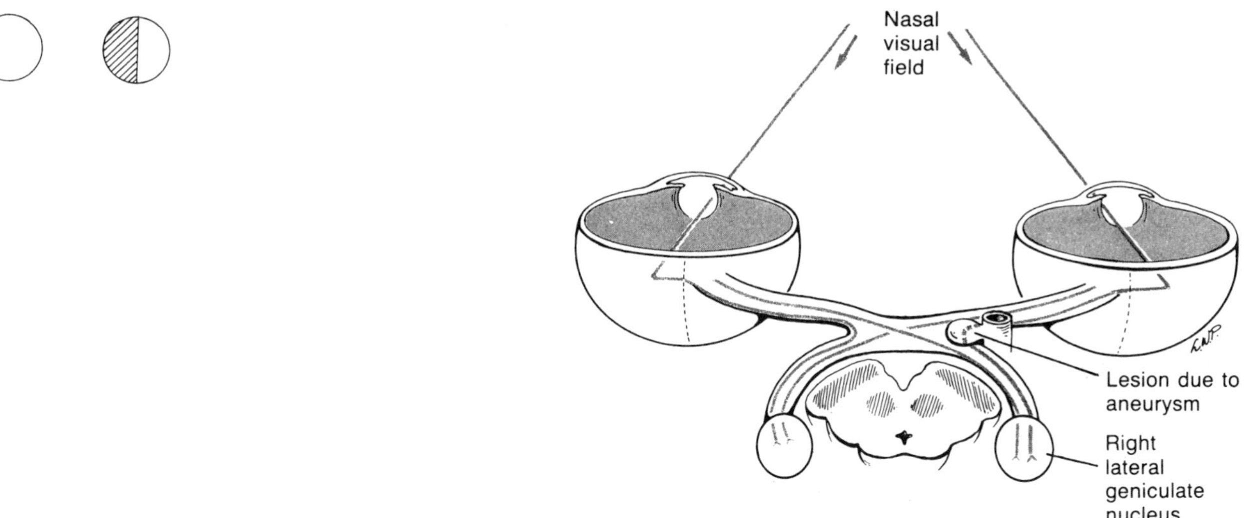

Fig. 9-13. Loss of nasal visual field in right eye only. (From Wilson-Pauwels et al.,[12] with permission.)

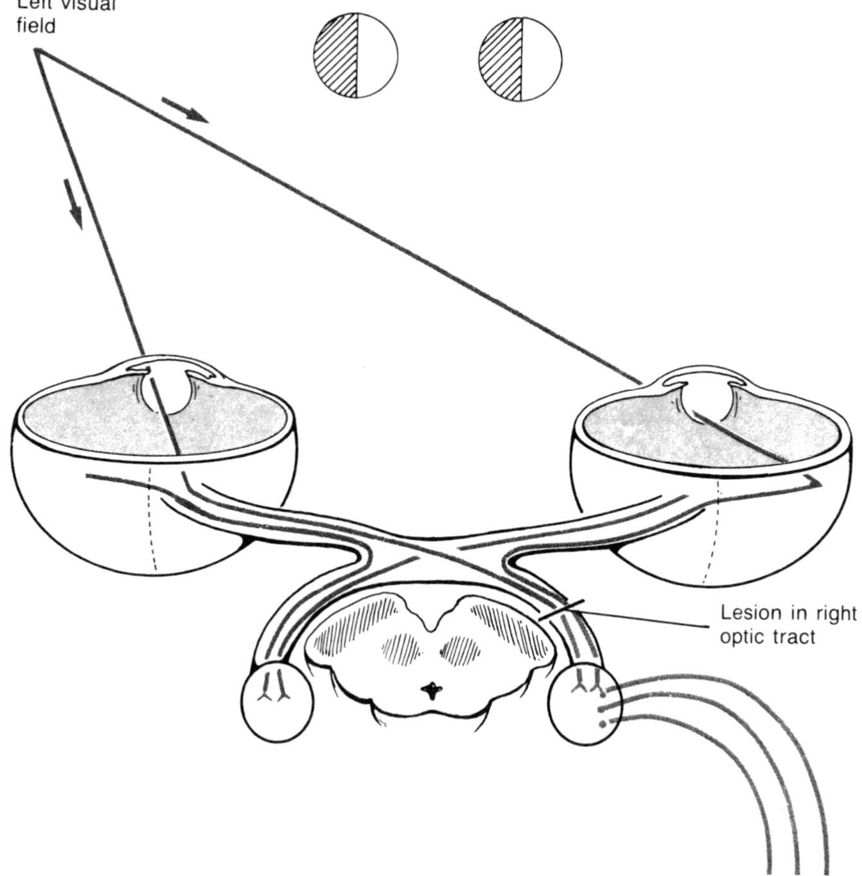

Fig. 9-14. Damage to optic tract (homonymous hemianopsia). (From Wilson-Pauwels et al.,[12] with permission.)

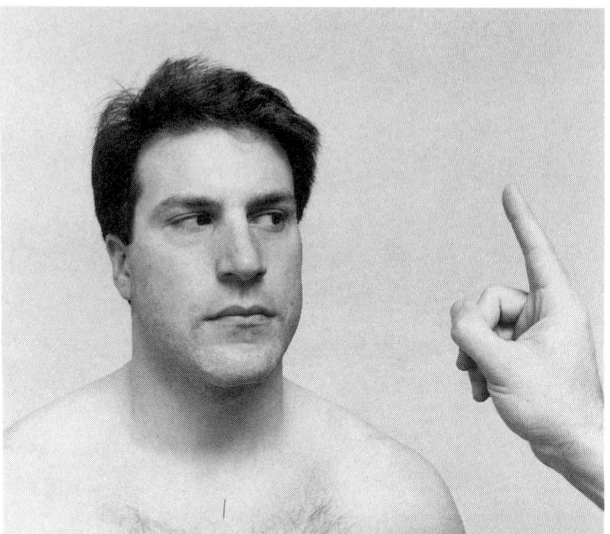

Fig. 9-15. Eyes following the target laterally to the right. Assessment of intact cranial nerve VI (right) and cranial nerve III (left).

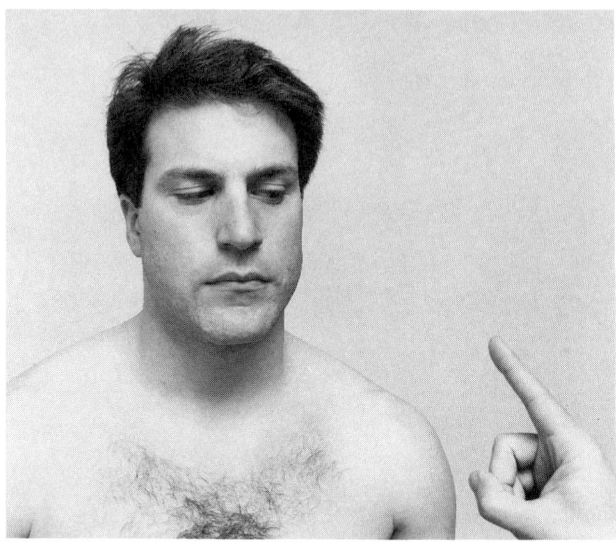

Fig. 9-17. Eyes following the target laterally and inferiorly. Assessment of intact cranial nerve III (right) and cranial nerve IV (left).

bone conduction, a 256 Hz tuning fork can be used. After striking the fork the therapist places the stem on the cranial vertex (see Fig. 9-20). The patient should hear the noise equally with the left and right ears (Weber's test). With positive findings of the above tests, the patient should be referred to a specialist for objective evaluation.

Cranial nerves IX and X (glossopharyngeal and vagus) are located closely together, so a lesion of one usually also affects the other. They also work together in the function of swallowing. The glossopharyngeal nerve supplies the sense of taste to the posterior one-third of the tongue and provides the sensory component of the gag reflex. The

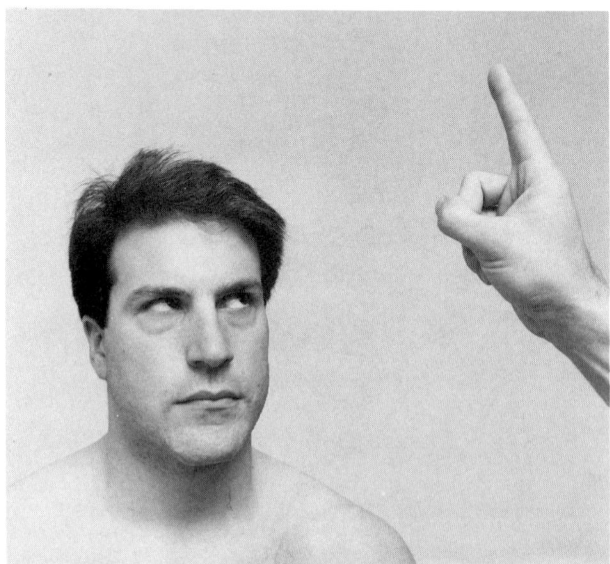

Fig. 9-16. Eyes following the target laterally and superiorly. Assessment of intact cranial nerve III (right) and cranial nerve III (left).

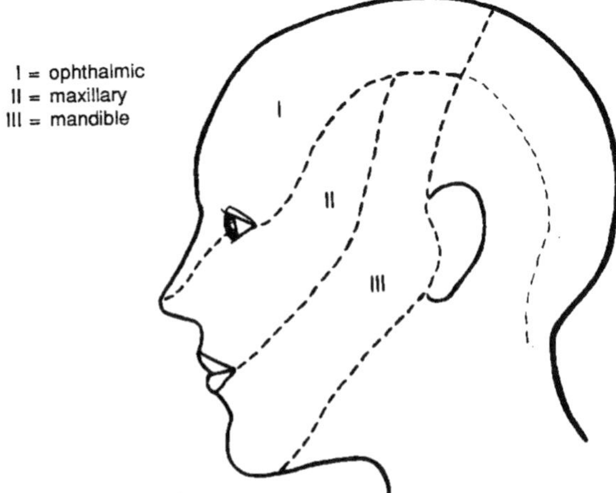

Fig. 9-18. Sensory distribution of the three divisions of the trigeminal nerve. (From Devinsky and Feldmann,[9] with permission.)

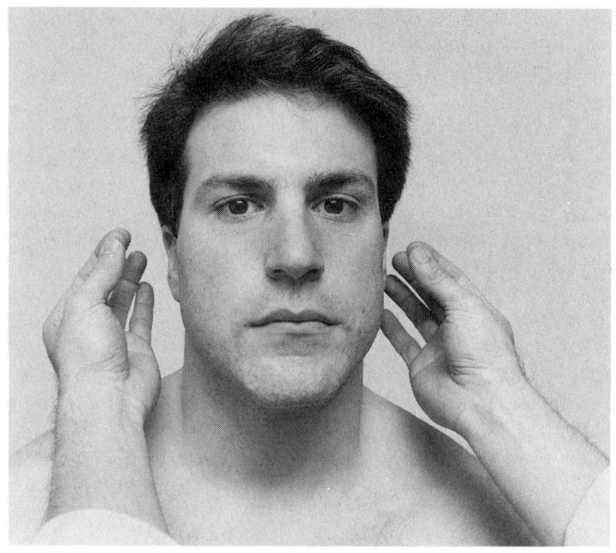

Fig. 9-19. The therapist rubs thumbs and index fingers together in front of each ear and gradually moves the hands away from each ear until the patient reports that he no longer hears the sound. The therapist compares the distance left versus right side.

vagus nerve supplies the motor component of the reflex. See Figure 9-21 for an abnormal reflex response. These

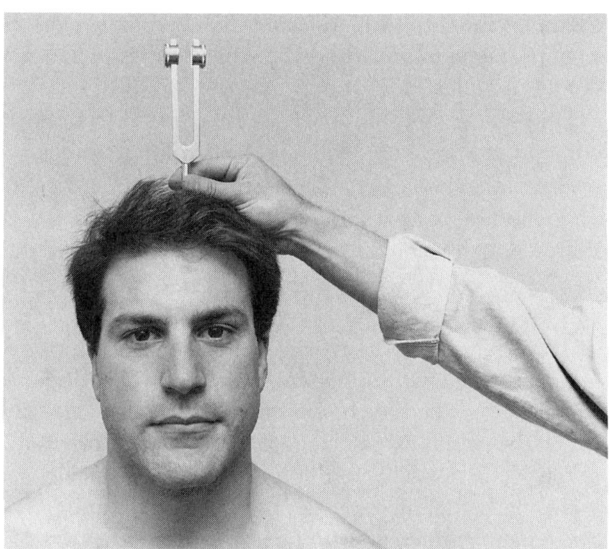

Fig. 9-20. After striking the tuning forks the therapist places the stem on the vertex of the cranium. The patient should be able to hear the noise equally in the left and right ears (Weber test).

nerves can be tested together by evaluating the patient's ability to swallow, an action that is more acceptable to most patients than testing the gag reflex.

Cranial nerve XI (accessory) supplies the motor innervation to sternocleidomastoid and upper trapezius. Testing of these muscles will test the accessory nerve. This nerve is closely related to the upper cervical lymph nodes, so extreme care must be exercised to avoid the accessory nerve in surgeries requiring dissection in this area.

Cranial nerve XII (hypoglossal) innervates the muscle of the tongue. Unilateral weakness causes deviation of the tongue toward the unaffected side when the patient protrudes the tongue. Tongue strength can be assessed by having the patient push laterally to the left, then right against a tongue blade. Observation of the tongue may also reveal atrophy or fasiculations.

Motor Function

The importance of the physical therapist's role in observing and evaluating the patient's ability to control his motor system normally cannot be sufficiently emphasized. The differences between upper and lower motor neuron lesions have previously been discussed, but aspects related to their effects on the patient's movement are again mentioned in light of the importance of motor system evaluation.

Lower motor neuron lesions lead to decreased muscle tone and localized weakness. Affected areas of the body can appear "floppy." If weakness is not severe, the most striking finding on observation can be clumsiness or incoordination with an upper extremity lesion or a tendency to trip during ambulation if the lesion affects muscles in the lower extremity. The sensory loss might cause the patient to rely more heavily on visual input during tasks.

Upper motor neuron lesions are usually accompanied by increased muscle tone. If the examiner passively moves the affected joints, he feels more resistance to movement than is normal. The extremity may appear very stiff and tend to assume an abnormal posture. The weakness often affects groups of muscles, with a decreased ability to disassociate movements (i.e., flexion or extension occurs as a mass movement at a number of joints). The patient may be unable to perform isolated movement at one joint without movement occurring at another joint.

When assessing the ability of a muscle to develop force, in addition to the amount of force produced, it is also important for the therapist to note whether the patient is able to terminate force production upon command. Resisted manual muscle testing is usually used in the clinic

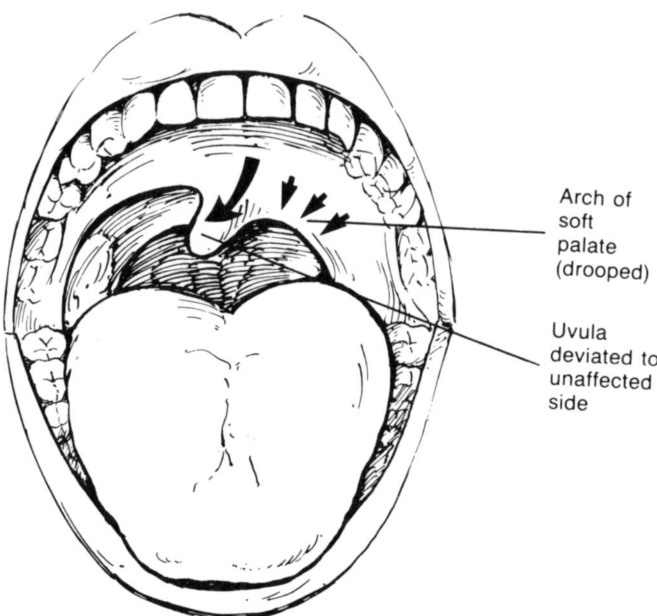

Fig. 9-21. Lower motor neuron lesion vagus nerve. The above may be noted during testing of the gag reflex or when the patient says "ah." (From Wilson-Pauwels et al.,[12] with permission.)

as a quick and relatively reliable assessment of force production. Many clinicians prefer to use a "break" test, in which the patient performs a maximal resisted isometric contraction at a midpoint in the range. This procedure is adequate for a screening examination, but, if a weakness is suspected, testing should be carried out through the full joint range. Measuring isometric action of a muscle at one point in the range of motion is hardly an indicator of the muscle's ability to function. Testing should be performed in a manner so that all myotomes are evaluated (e.g., for the upper extremities: deltoids, C5, C6; supraspinatus and infraspinatus, C7, C8; wrist extensors, C6, C7, C8; grip, C6, C7, C8, T1; finger adductors and abductors, C8, T1; and thumb opposition and flexion (C8, T1); for the lower extremities: iliopsoas, L2, L3; quadriceps, L2, L3, L4; hamstrings, L5, S1, S2; ankle dorsiflexors, L4, L5; and toe extensors, L5, S1). See Chapter 1 regarding principles related to motor testing.

Sensory Function

Patient instruction prior to a sensory assessment should include an explanation of both the purpose of the procedure and the patient's role in the process. The patient should also be instructed not to guess when uncertain of a response. A demonstration of each test should be provided before the actual procedure, to acquaint the patient with the testing. The patient's vision should be occluded during testing. Most patients are able to cooperate by keeping their eyes closed. If this is not possible, a blindfold can be used. When applying the stimulus, the therapist should follow the main dermatomes, working from proximal to distal and applying the stimuli in a random, unpredictable manner.

Pain sensation is tested with a safety pin or bent paper clip, providing sharp and dull ends. These items are preferable because they are readily disposable after use on an individual patient. The sharp end should not be sharp enough to puncture the skin. Both sharp and dull stimuli are applied in random fashion, after which the patient is asked to reply "sharp," "dull," or "don't know."

Temperature sensation can be tested using stoppered test tubes filled with hot or cold water. Both hot and cold stimuli are applied to the skin surfaces to be tested, after which the patient is asked to reply "hot," "cold," or "unable to tell." The reliability of this method is questionable, and it is somewhat cumbersome to perform as a screening tool. Since temperature and pain fibers travel together through most of the nervous system, many clinicians defer temperature testing, since a lesion that disturbs pain sensation will most likely also affect temperature sensation.

Light touch is assessed using a soft brush, piece of cotton, or tissue. The area to be tested is lightly touched, and the patient is asked to note when the light touch is felt. Touches should be randomized with trials without touch.

The proprioceptive senses include both *position sense* and *movement sense* (kinesthesia) as well as *vibration*.[7] Position sense is the awareness of the position of a joint at rest; movement sense is the awareness of movement. To test position sense, the therapist passively moves the patient's extremity and holds it in a static position, using small increments of range of motion. The therapist's grip should remain constant, to reduce tactile input. The patient is asked to describe the position of the joint or to imitate it with the opposite extremity. To test movement sense, or kinesthesia, a similar procedure is used, except that the patient is asked to identify the joint movement while it is occurring. Vibration sense is tested using a tuning fork, whose base is placed in contact with a bony prominence. The fork should be randomly applied, vibrating at some times and not at others.

A complete sensory evaluation can also include combined sensations, such as stereognosis, tactile localization, two-point discrimination, and graphesthesia. Stereognosis is the ability to recognize and identify familiar objects by touch. Tactile localization is the ability to localize touch sensation on the skin. Two-point discrimination is a measure of the smallest distance between two stimuli that can still be perceived as two stimuli. Graphesthesia is the ability to recognize and identify letters, numbers, or simple designs traced on the skin. Since these forms of sensation involve function of numerous levels of the nervous system, they are sometimes referred to as cortical sensations. A deficit in any of these sensations does not implicate any specific nervous system lesion, so, although they are important for function, they do not provide a good deal of useful information for a screening evaluation. See Chapter 1 regarding additional principles related to sensory testing.

Coordination

Coordination is the ability to execute smooth, accurate, controlled movements. Numerous tests have been used traditionally to evaluate coordination. Most of these tests have involved asking the patient to perform reciprocal or targeted movements. Simple completion of these tests does not imply that the patient has normal coordination. Several factors should be evaluated by the therapist as the patient performs the motions, including

1. Are movements direct, precise, and easily reversed?
2. Can appropriate motor adjustments be made if speed and direction are changed?
3. Can a posture of the body or extremity be maintained without swaying or oscillations?
4. Are the motor responses consistent over time?

Some common tests for the upper extremity include finger to nose, finger to therapist's finger, finger opposition, and supination/pronation. These are generally tested with the patient sitting. In *finger to nose*, the patient's arm is abducted to 90 degrees with the elbow extended. The patient is asked to maintain the shoulder position while bringing the tip of the index finger to meet his nose. In *finger to therapist's finger*, the patient is asked to bring the tip of his index finger to meet the tip of the therapist's finger at different locations. *Finger opposition* involves having the patient touch the tip of the thumb to the tip of each of his fingers in sequence. The *supination/pronation* test involves having the patient's elbows flexed to 90 degrees and held close to his sides while he alternately supinates and pronates the forearms.

Nonweight-bearing lower extremity tests performed in supine include alternate heel to knee and toe, and heel on shin. *Alternate heel to knee and toe* involves having the patient bring the heel back and forth between the opposite knee and big toe. In *heel on shin*, the patient is asked to slide the heel up and down the opposite shin.

Numerous standing tests have also been used to evaluate "coordination." These tests involve the interaction of numerous body areas functioning with input from diverse areas of the peripheral and central nervous systems, relying heavily on normal balance mechanisms. Similar to the cortical sensory tests, the actions being assessed are critical for normal function, but do little but alert the therapist that "something may be wrong." Standing coordination tests include having the person stand with feet close together, stand on one foot, walk a straight line, walk sideways or backward, or walk on heels or toes.

Reflexes

Deep tendon reflexes are tested to evaluate the integrity of the reflex arc. They should be compared on the basis of presence or absence and with regard to symmetry of response between sides of the body. After tapping the tendon directly with a reflex hammer, the therapist grades the resulting muscle contraction using a scale of

0 to 4, with a normal response being 2+. In the upper extremity, the tendons that are useful to test are the biceps (C5, C6) and triceps (C7, C8); in the lower extremity, the patellar (L2, L3, L4) and ankle (S1, S2).

In upper motor neuron lesions, tendon reflexes are commonly hyperactive. However, the presence of brisk tendon reflexes alone is not sufficient to warrant concern over the integrity of the central nervous system, since many normal persons show heightened tendon reflexes. When the response to passive stretch is marked because of an upper motor neuron lesion, *clonus* can sometimes be elicited. Clonus is a sustained phasic response to stretch that is most readily seen after applying a quick stretch to the ankle plantarflexors or wrist flexors. If clonus is elicited, it is often described in terms of the number of beats of clonus that follow a simple quick stretch.

A cutaneous reflex that *if positive* indicates an upper motor neuron lesion in an adult is the Babinski (see Fig. 9-22). A stroking stimulus is applied with the sharp end of a reflex hammer on the sole of the foot along the lateral surface of the foot and up across the ball of the foot. A normal (or negative) response consists of flexion of the big toe, sometimes the other toes, or no response at all. An abnormal response (positive Babinski) consists of extension of the big toe, sometimes with fanning of the other toes. See Chapter 1 for additional principles related to reflex testing.

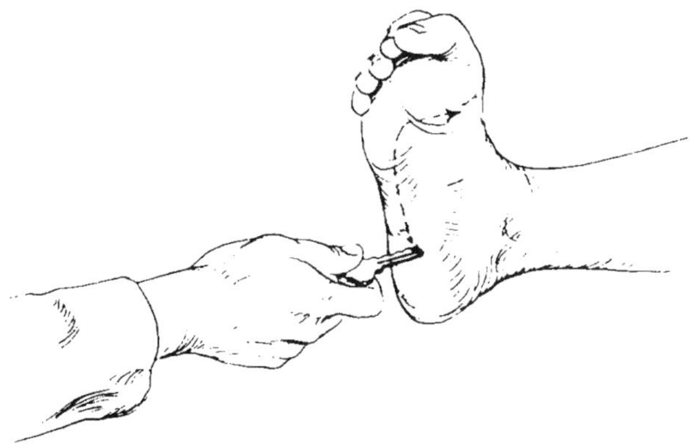

A negative Babinski

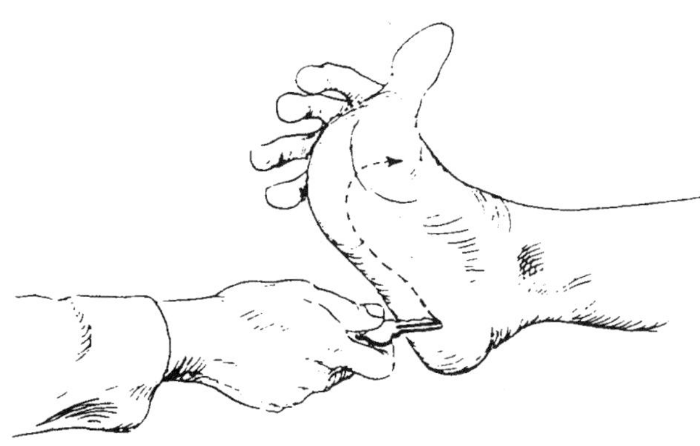

Fig. 9-22. Babinski test. (From Hoppenfeld,[13] with permission.)

SUMMARY

This chapter discusses some important aspects of the anatomy and functions of the components of the nervous system related to sensation and movement. Common pathologies of the different components are discussed. Assessment techniques that can be useful to screen for nervous system dysfunction are presented. It is important for the physical therapist to remember that evaluation of the nervous system involves more than an upper-quarter or lower-quarter screening.

PATIENT CASE STUDY 1

History

The patient was a 74-year-old man referred to physical therapy for treatment following a fracture of the surgical neck of the right humerus, sustained during a fall 4 weeks earlier. The patient stated that the fall occurred during midday as he was walking to the kitchen to get something to eat. He felt that he tripped over a bulge in the carpet.

The patient was a retired construction worker who lived by himself in a first floor apartment. He denied smoking or alcohol use. His past medical history was unremarkable; he did not take any medications on a regular basis. He stated, however, that he had fallen 6 months ago, sustaining a Colle's fracture on the right. When questioned about his overall health, he stated that he felt he was much less active than a year ago.

Physical Examination

Observation of the patient's gait revealed a small base of support, short step lengths bilaterally, and increased thoracic kyphosis. Posture analysis showed significant forward head with increased thoracic kyphosis. The right arm was still being supported in a sling; the right shoulder was higher than the left. Throughout the interview and examination, the patient appeared depressed. His face displayed little emotion, and his responses appeared slow.

Ranges of motion (ROM) of the shoulders were limited as follows:

	Active	Passive
Right shoulder		
Flexion	0–45°	0–50°
Abduction	0–40°	0–45°
Internal rotation	0–90°	0–90°
External rotation	0–30°	0–40°
Left shoulder		
Flexion	0–60°	0–115°
Abduction	0–55°	0–110°
Internal rotation	0–90°	0–90°
External rotation	0–80°	0–90°

Both passive and active ROM limitations also existed at the right wrist. Manual muscle testing of the upper extremities was 3+/5 to 4−/5 throughout.

Testing of the lower extremities revealed extremely reduced hip ROM, both actively and passively, for abduction and internal and external rotations. Passive movement of the lower extremity joints revealed increased tone, which was bidirectional and not influenced by the speed of the movement. Manual muscle testing of the lower extremities was 4−/5 to 4/5 throughout.

Outcome and Assessment

The patient's postural and movement deficits indicated that he could have Parkinson's disease. Although an orthopaedist was the referring physician, the physical therapist decided to contact the patient's general practice physician to discuss the findings of the evaluation. The general practice physician referred the patient for a neurologic consultation, at which time the patient was diagnosed with Parkinson's disease and started on pharmacologic treatment for the disorder.

The patient continued to attend physical therapy sessions, with goals of increasing active and passive ROM of both shoulders, improving posture, increasing overall muscle strength, and increasing functional endurance. Occupational therapy was also initiated, with goals of improving the patient's independence in activities of daily living.

The patient was seen for a total of 8 weeks. Upon discharge, the patient was able to perform all activities of daily living without pain. He was able to ambulate outside of the home for the first time in a year, with endurance up to 500 feet without resting. ROM of the right shoulder was limited by about 15 percent, but this did not interfere with the patient's lifestyle. Manual muscle testing was 4/5 to 4+/5 throughout.

PATIENT CASE STUDY 2

History

The patient was a 62-year-old female referred to physical therapy for rehabilitation following a shoulder arthroplasty on the right 4 weeks ago. The surgery was performed because the patient had problems performing overhead activities with her right shoulder. Her past medical history included hypertension, which was controlled with medication. Her past surgical history included carpal tunnel surgery on the right 5 months ago. When asked about the events leading up to the carpal tunnel surgery, the patient stated that she had been experiencing clumsiness in the right hand.

Physical Examination

Observation of the patient's gait showed a right–left asymmetry. Step lengths on the right were shorter than the left, and the right knee did not flex as much as the left during swing. The patient stated that the right knee felt unstable at times.

Passive ROM of the right shoulder was flexion, 0 to 70 degrees; abduction, 0 to 65 degrees; internal rotation, 0 to 80 degrees; external rotation, 0 to 30 degrees. Manual muscle testing was 3−/5. Biceps tendon reflex was 3+ on the right, 2+ on the left.

Because the patient reported right knee instability, the therapist performed a structural examination. There was no evidence of ligamentous laxity. There were no areas of tenderness upon palpation. Resisted muscle testing was 4/5 for both quadriceps and hamstrings. Patellar tendon reflexes were 3+ bilaterally, and ankle clonus was easily elicited with a quick stretch to the plantarflexor tendon.

Outcome and Assessment

The therapist was very concerned about the upper motor neuron lesion signs and contacted the patient's general practice physician to discuss them. The patient's physician referred her to an internist, who diagnosed her with degenerative joint disease and recommended a total knee replacement arthroplasty on the right. At this time, the physical therapist again contacted the patient's general practice physician, who then referred the patient for a neurologic consultation. After magnetic resonance imaging showed no brain lesions, based on the findings on examination, the neurologist diagnosed the patient with amyotrophic lateral sclerosis.

REFERENCES

1. Kandel ER, Schwartz JH, Jessell TM: Principles of Neural Science. 3rd Ed. Elsevier Science, New York, 1991
2. Cohen H (ed): Neuroscience for Rehabilitation. JB Lippincott, Philadelphia, 1993
3. Rowland LP (ed): Merritt's Textbook of Neurology. 8th Ed. Lea & Febiger, Philadelphia, 1989
4. Wiederholt WC: Neurology for Non-Neurologists. Academic Press, San Diego, 1982
5. O'Sullivan SB, Schmitz TJ: Physical Rehabilitation: Assessment and Treatment. 3rd Ed. FA Davis, Philadelphia, 1994
6. Gunderson CH: Quick Reference to Clinical Neurology. JB Lippincott, Philadelphia, 1982
7. Goldberg S: The Four-Minute Neurologic Exam. MedMaster, Miami, 1984
8. Haerer AF: DeJong's The Neurologic Examination. 5th Ed. JB Lippincott, Philadelphia, 1992
9. Devinsky O, Feldmann E: Examination of the Cranial and Peripheral Nerves. Churchill Livingstone, New York, 1988
10. Barr ML, Kiernan JA: The Human Nervous System—An Anatomical Viewpoint. 5th Ed. JB Lippincott, Philadelphia, 1988
11. Haymaker W, Woodhall B: Peripheral Nerve Injuries; WB Saunders, Philadelphia, 1953
12. Wilson-Pauwels L, Akesson EJ, Stewart PA: Cranial Nerves: Anatomy and Clinical Comments. BC Decker, Philadelphia, 1988
13. Hoppenfeld S: Physical Examination of the Spine and Extremities. Appleton & Lange, New York, 1976
14. Romero-Sierra C: Neuroanatomy: A Conceptual Approach. Churchill Livingstone, New York, 1986

SUGGESTED READINGS

Caplan LR, Kelly JJ Jr: Consultation in Neurology. BC Decker, Philadelphia, 1988

deGroot J, Chusid JG: Correlative Neuroanatomy. 21st Ed. Appleton & Lange, Norwalk, CT, 1991

Edwardson BM: Musculoskeletal Assessment: An Integrated Approach. Singular Publishing Group Inc, San Diego, 1992

Littell EH: Basic Neuroscience for the Health Professions. Slack, Thorofare, NJ, 1990

Poeck K: Diagnostic Decisions in Neurology. Springer-Verlag, Berlin, 1985

Rodnitzky RL: Van Allen's Pictorial Manual of Neurologic Tests. 3rd Ed. Year Book Medical Publishing, Chicago, 1988

Strub RL, Black FW: The Mental Status Examination in Neurology. 2nd Ed. FA Davis, Philadelphia, 1985

Weisberg LA, Strub RL, Garcia CA: Decision Making in Adult Neurology. BC Decker, Philadelphia, 1987

10 Screening for Musculoskeletal System Disease

Terry Randall, M.S., P.T., O.C.S., A.T.C.*
Kevin McMahon, M.D., F.A.A.S., F.A.C.S.

"The Scientist is not content to stop at the obvious."
Charles H. Mayo

Physical therapists devote most of their time to treating impairments of the musculoskeletal system. The evaluation of specific deficits, such as muscle strength or proprioception, is becoming increasingly sophisticated. At times it seems very difficult to keep pace with the latest innovations in rehabilitation. However, this is not the only area of practice that is changing rapidly. The development of direct access will alter the methods of the physical therapist's evaluation and scope of practice.

With expanding roles and increasing responsibilities, physical therapists must expand their knowledge base beyond that of traditional practice. Functioning in a direct access mode "assumes that we desire to achieve an even greater degree of excellence and accountability. . ."[1] Physical therapists will find themselves functioning in the role of primary care provider more often in the future. Clinicians who practice in more traditional, referral-based settings must also recognize their increasing responsibility. The quality of evaluation is not dependent on the mode of practice.

To achieve this level of excellence and practice, we must be more aware of the role of the physical therapist in view of the entire medical system. "Physical therapy is part of the health-care system, not the whole thing. If all we do is provide excellent physical therapy, the independent practitioner will not be a door into the health-care system but a dead end."[2] The expansion of the physical therapist's responsibilities must be associated with broadening the physical therapist's view of the patient. No longer can patients be viewed as just having an ankle sprain or back pain. The goal of physical therapy evaluation should be to formulate an unambiguous diagnosis that demonstrates specific impairments and disabilities.[3]

The precise terminology of this diagnosis is controversial.[4–6] However, the value of making a clinical assessment concerning the patient's complaint and basing a treatment plan on that assessment should be universally acceptable. It stands to reason that a definitive assessment will lead to a more precise treatment. Clinical evaluation models can assist in formulating a thought process to assist in making a specific diagnosis.[7,8]

This chapter provides an overview of musculoskeletal system diseases that, while not always amenable to physical therapy treatment, can be seen in our patients. Descriptions of the more common primary skeletal neoplasms, skeletal metastasis, infections, and metabolic dis-

*The opinions or assertions contained herein are the private views of the author and are not to be construed as official or as reflecting the views of the Department of the Army or the Department of Defense.

orders are included. While these musculoskeletal disorders may be relatively uncommon, they are serious conditions for which early detection is crucial to effective treatment. Information is provided concerning the pathogenesis of each disorder so that clinicians will have a common background as to their origins.

The epidemiology and clinical features of the disease are of primary importance to the physical therapist. Special attention has been given to situations in which these diseases may present as more typical or common disorders routinely treated by physical therapists. A brief description of appropriate treatment techniques is included. This book is not intended to be a treatment manual, but physical therapists do need to be familiar with the extent and forms of treatment available so they may educate their patients.

The conditions presented in this chapter require consultation or referral for further diagnostic tests. Physical therapists must develop the skills needed to function within the framework of medical specialties. For these reasons, the appropriate referral process is discussed as well.

PRIMARY SKELETAL NEOPLASMS

The diverse nature of musculoskeletal pathology makes the differential diagnosis elusive. Zohn[9] describes five pathologic conditions that can affect seven anatomic structures (Table 10-1). Cross-matching these lists produces an extensive list of musculoskeletal problems that must be considered during an evaluation. Neoplasms are but one small, albeit important, part of the spectrum.

Primary tumors of the musculoskeletal system are a very rare finding. Thus, it is easy to become complacent in our daily practice, comforted in the knowledge that the odds are against us ever seeing a primary neoplasm. From time to time, it is important to reiterate the significance of these lesions and the catastrophic ramifications that can ensue if treatment is delayed unnecessarily. For these reasons, physical therapists must be familiar with the clinical features of the more common of these lesions. In an area where clinicians claim a wide disparity of experience, it may be best to begin with commonly used terms.

Table 10-1. Summary of Cross-Matching Anatomic Structures and Pathologic Conditions

Anatomic Structures That May Be the Seat of Pain-Producing Pathology	Pathologic Changes or Conditions That May Affect These Structures
Bone and periosteum	Trauma (extrinsic and intrinsic)
Hyaline cartilage	Inflammation
Synovial capsule	Metabolic disease
Ligaments	Neoplasms
Muscles, tendons, and tendon sheaths	Congenital anomalies
Intra-articular menisci	
Bursae	

(From Zohn,[9] with permission.)

The following definitions are taken from Salter.[10] *Tumor* is a commonly used word that may be used in rather imprecise ways to describe any localized swelling or mass. *Neoplasm* has more meaning in describing a new and abnormal formation of cells. *Metastasis* refers to the ability of a neoplasm to initiate independent growth at a distant site, therefore being malignant.

Many of the symptoms that physical therapists are accustomed to dealing with on a daily basis can also be manifestations of the presence of neoplasms. Pain, swelling, and loss of function may represent the body's reaction to mild trauma. However, these same symptoms can also be the primary warning signs of far more serious pathology. For this reason, neoplasms are often missed at the initial presentation. This fact also emphasizes the importance of physical therapists continually re-evaluating their patient's response and progress to treatment. An unexpected or unexplained response to treatment should generate suspicion that may lead to further evaluation or referral. Likewise, symptoms that do not lead to a specific diagnosis must be suspect. This important concept should be an integral part of the clinician's evaluation and documentation process.[11]

Many different classifications for tumors have been used. Even the broad distinction between malignant and benign is not always straightforward. Consideration of the tissue of origin of a neoplasm can provide a useful classification. Most primary neoplasms can therefore be divided into osteogenic, chondrogenic, collagenic, and myelogenic.[12] Neoplasms can also have a neurogenic, vascular, or adipose origin.[13]

Fortunately, the malignant neoplasms are less common than benign bone lesions. Both types are serious, however, and even benign lesions can jeopardize the affected limb. It is important to know the incidence of neoplasms if one expects to avoid missing subtle physical signs. Some lesions are correlated with, but not limited to, a specific age group; for example, osteosarcoma is most commonly seen in childhood.

Clinical Features

The clinical features are of particular interest to anyone involved in evaluation of musculoskeletal conditions. While trauma is a common complaint of patients with neoplasms, this only serves to focus the evaluation to a specific area and is not associated with the type, location, or progression of the lesion.

Pain, while not universal, is by far the most common symptom in all neoplasms and, unlike trauma, may be directly linked to a neoplasm. Pain is more likely to occur with rapidly growing neoplasms, such as osteosarcoma. The characteristics of the pain, as always, can vary but may evolve from mild and intermittent to more intense and constant. In aggressive malignant lesions, the pain can be caused by the rapidly expanding mass. Pain does not occur in the same stage of development for all lesions. In some cases, pain may present very early in the course and hence be helpful in early detection. In other instances, the neoplasm may progress significantly before the development of pain. This varied response is due to the nature, location, and rate of growth of the neoplasm. It is vital, therefore, for physical therapists to be aware of the subtle differences in the description of pain and how patients react to it. It is also important to remember the patterns of referred pain. A careful examination, both distal and proximal to the painful area, must be done. Constant vigilance is required to detect causes of pain that are uncharacteristic of common musculoskeletal conditions. The expected response to treatment must also be known and monitored.

The use of percussion can also aid in the assessment of pain. Both direct and indirect methods can be used.[14] By generating a firm, sudden force from one hand, a specific bone or portion of bone can be assessed through the fingers of the other hand, or else a reflex hammer can be used to apply the force (Fig. 10-1). Joint dysfunction may cause a sharp pain of short duration, while disease may produce a deep throbbing pain that persists for several minutes.[15] These general descriptions do not apply in all situations.

Swelling can be present with many different neoplasms, but it is not always detectable clinically. The swelling can be localized or diffuse, tender or painless, warm or neutral. The nature of the swelling is a function of the vascularity, the proximity of the lesion to the surface, and the rate of growth. Palpation can also help discern whether a mass is present, as well as the consistency, mobility, location, dimensions, and growth rate of the neoplasm.[16] These ordinary clinical signs may be the only clue to the severe nature of the underlying pathology. Therefore, some of the more common neoplasms and their specific characteristics are presented.

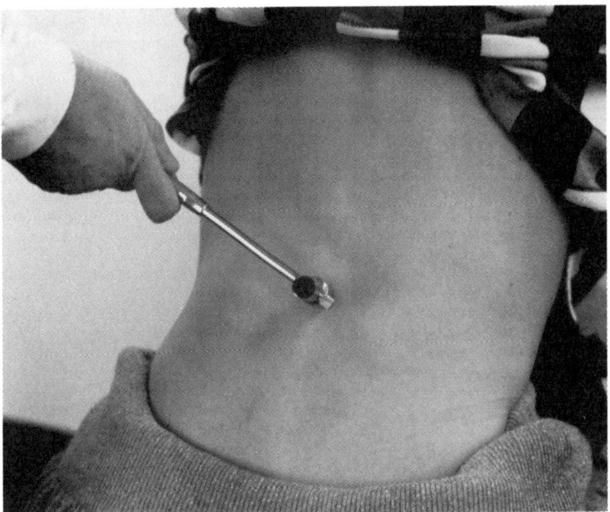

Fig. 10-1. With the patient sitting and the trunk supported, but slightly forward flexed to separate the spinous processes, a reflex hammer or the therapist's hand can be used to percuss the vertebra via the spinous process.

Most neoplasms have an age group where the incidence is highest (Table 10-2). This does not mean that a specific lesion cannot occur outside this range. In general, primary neoplasms of bone occur in children and young adults. It has been suggested that this is due in part to the higher rate of growth in the bones in this age group.

Neoplasms that are destructive to bone in weight-bearing areas may cause weakening, leading to pain. If the destruction continues, a pathologic fracture may occur. Pathologic fracture occurs when destructive characteristics of the neoplasm weaken the cortex. A history of insignificant trauma along with pain in the area before the fracture should raise suspicion.[17] In this case, the physical therapist may require further consultation to rule out a pathologic fracture.

Referral

Proper referral of the patient with a suspected neoplasm should contain some basic information that can be gathered from a thorough physical examination. The physician will be interested in the general health of the patient. A detailed history and review of all systems is appropriate[18] (see Ch. 1).

Table 10-2. Characteristics of Bone Tumors

Type of Tumor	Age of Patient (yr)	Site of Tumor	Radiographic Features	Histopathologic Features	Comments
Benign					
Osteochondroma	5–35	Metaphyseal	Cancellous and cortical	Normal bone and cartilage	Malignant transformation in <1%
Osteoid osteoma	15–30	Femur, tibia, posterior elements of spine	Sclerotic area surrounding lytic nidus	Disorganized, thin osteoid trabeculae with or without mineralization	Painful, relieved by aspirin
Osteoblastoma	10–30	Vertebrae, long bones	Destructive with or without sclerosis >2 cm	Thicker osteoid trabeculae with mineralization	Differential diagnosis includes aneurysmal bone cyst and osteosarcoma
Chondroblastoma	15–30	Epiphysis of long bones	Central bone destruction surrounded by a thin sclerotic rim	Chondroblasts in chondroid matrix	Giant cells may be present
Giant cell	20–40	Epiphysis of long bones	Eccentric expanding zone of radiolucency	Benign giant cells with oval or spindle-shaped stromal cells	7.5% may behave as a malignant lesion
Malignant					
Osteosarcoma	15–30	Metaphysis of long bone	Destructive lesion with or without an ossified matrix	Malignant connective tissue cells producing osteoid	Most common primary malignant bone tumor
Ewing sarcoma	10–20	Diaphysis of long bones	Permeative destructive lesion with or without periosteal "onion skin"	Monotonous pattern of cork staining small cells	May mimic infection
Myeloma	40–80	Spine, ribs, pelvis	"Punched-out" areas of destruction with or without cortical expansion	Sheets of closely packed plasma cells	Most common neoplasm of bone

(From Wilkins and Sim,[19] with permission.)

If a mass is present, its characteristics should be noted. Descriptions of size, location, mobility, tenderness, and texture are important in the differential diagnosis. While the size of the mass may not be an indicator of the severity of the condition, the change in size over time is very important. The location of the lesion must be determined as accurately as possible. The type of bone involved and even the specific location within the bone can provide information concerning a possible diagnosis.

If the mass is located within the muscle belly, it may become fixed when the muscle is contracted and mobile when the muscle is relaxed. Neoplasms that are deep and connected to fascia or bone are not usually mobile. In this way, palpation alone can distinguish a soft tissue neoplasm from a bone lesion.[19]

Most physical therapists cannot order radiographs, but films may be available for review. Despite many of the newer, highly sophisticated imaging equipment available today, the plain radiograph remains the standard for the initial workup in suspected neoplasms. Wilkins and Sim[19] alert the examiner to four features to be noted when a lesion is detected radiographically.

Features to Note in a Radiographically Detected Lesion

1. *Location:* The specific bone, and location within the bone (epiphysis, metaphysis, or diaphysis), can be determined.
2. *Effect on normal bone:* The effect the lesion has had on the normal bone should be checked. Both osteolytic and osteoblastic changes can be present with neoplasms.
3. *Local response:* The local response to the presence of the lesion should be assessed. Sclerotic borders and periosteal reactions give indications of the growth characteristics.
4. *Presence of a matrix:* The presence of a matrix is determined. An ossified matrix can be seen on either bone or soft tissue lesions. A more detailed description of the radiologic findings in bone lesions can be found in Madewell et al.[20]

OSTEOGENIC NEOPLASMS

Osteoid Osteoma

Jaffe[21] is credited with describing a benign, bone-forming tumor that is characteristically found in the long bones of the lower extremity. This neoplasm, like many others, is most common in boys and young adults, but the precise etiology is unknown. The lesion, like many tumors, can affect joint function, which may lead to a misdiagnosis of musculoskeletal origin on the basis of subjective complaints of pain and some loss of function in the associated joint. Because joint pain and injury are common, especially in an active population, more mundane types of problems are usually implicated as the source of pain.

Clinical Features

Pain is associated with this lesion. It can be described as a dull ache that may increase in severity over several months. An important quality of the pain is that it is often worse at night and is alleviated with salicylates. No systemic symptoms such as weight loss or fever are present. Males between the ages of 5 and 30 years are most susceptible.

This lesion is seen on radiographs, but it may not appear for several months after the onset of symptoms. Therefore, it is important to obtain repeated films when symptoms are persistent. The appearance of an osteoid osteoma is that of a small (<1-cm) translucency called a nidus[22] (Fig. 10-2). This is surrounded by sclerotic bone.[23] Treatment is usually successful but requires excision of the entire nidus. Patients can expect to return to normal function after complete excision.

Physical Therapy Evaluation

Physical therapists should be aware of the osteoid osteoma because a patient with this lesion may have had multiple evaluations that indicate few objective findings, yet the symptoms continue. The presence of associated trauma or possible overuse only confuses the presentation further. Years can pass with continued symptoms before a correct diagnosis is made.[24] The presence of gradually increasing night pain relieved with aspirin should clue the clinician to this possible alternative diagnosis. There are no reported malignant tendencies associated with this neoplasm, but it must be treated by an orthopaedic surgeon.

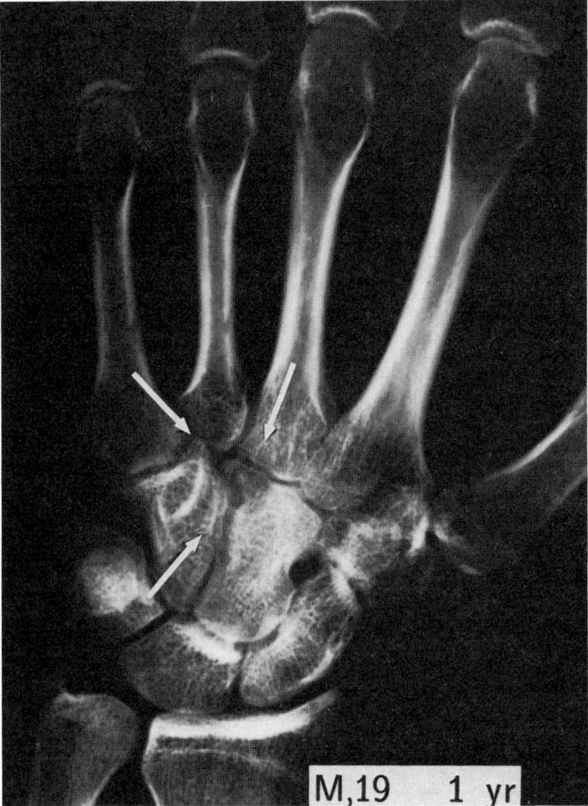

Fig. 10-2. Anteroposterior radiograph of the wrist and hand of a 19-year-old man with wrist pain and median nerve paresthesias of 1-year duration. The capitate bone shows a small area of increased density surrounded by a radiolucent area (arrows). The osteoid osteoma was excised. (From Cohen et al,[22] with permission.)

Osteoblastoma

A neoplasm that has many similarities to the osteoid osteoma is the osteoblastoma. The World Health Organization (WHO) recognizes the common characteristics and places both lesions under a common heading.[25]

Clinical Features

Most patients with osteoblastoma are under 30 years of age. Osteoblastoma differs from osteoid osteoma in that the most common location is in the spine. The posterior elements are frequently involved. Pain is common to both types of neoplasms, but the osteoblastoma is considered less painful and more difficult to localize. This may result in longer elapsed time before the lesion is detected. Typically, several months and up to 2 years may pass before the lesion is detected. Thirty-four percent of osteoblastomas are located in the spine, and of those 50 percent will cause neurologic symptoms.[26]

Radiologically, the lesion does not produce the reaction in surrounding bone seen in osteoid osteoma. Therefore, the dense sclerotic margin surrounding osteoid osteoma is not seen in the osteoblastoma. When present in the posterior elements of the spine, the affected area may appear enlarged.[27]

Treatment

Treatment principles are the same as those for osteoid osteoma in that the best prognosis occurs when the lesion can be excised. Because of the predilection for the spine, excision may be a challenging procedure.

Osteosarcoma

Osteogenic sarcoma is one of the more common primary malignant bone neoplasms, representing 25 percent of primary malignant tumors.[28] The lesion itself has an extremely rapid growth rate. It is often found in areas such as the metaphysis of long bones, which also have a rapid growth rate. The most common sites include the lower femur or upper tibia and the proximal humerus. In one series of 243 patients, 80 percent had lesions in these locations.[29]

Children and adults in their 20s and 30s are most susceptible; another rise in incidence is seen in adults over the age of 50. This may be due to an association with Paget's disease. Males are twice as likely to have osteosarcoma than are females.

Clinical Features

The most consistent clinical finding is that of pain. The pain is usually described in a classic pattern of progression from mild and intermittent to severe and continuous. Some alteration in function can be expected because this neoplasm is found in the metaphysis, hence close to the joint. A mass may be one of the initial findings. If present, it may vary from soft and fluctuant to very firm. The skin overlying the tumor may be warm to the touch because of the increased vascularity associated with the rapid growth.[10]

Radiography shows cortical destruction early during the course of the lesion,[16] predisposing the bone to pathologic fracture. Another radiologic sign associated with osteosarcoma is Codman's angle.[30] This refers to the area of periosteal bone that lifts from the cortex as a malignant tumor breaks into the surrounding soft tissue (Fig. 10-3). Further studies such as tomograms, bone scans, computed tomography (CT), and magnetic resonance (MR) imaging are used for diagnosis and staging.

Treatment

Treatment for osteosarcoma, like that for many tumors, has evolved rapidly over the past 10 years. A survival rate of less than 10 percent was the prognosis only a decade ago. Left untreated, death occurs in less than 2 years.[31,32] The poor prognosis was in part due to the fact that osteosarcoma metastasizes to the lungs through the bloodstream early in its course. With state-of-the-art treatment including better staging of the lesion, improved surgical techniques and equipment, surgery, and advances in chemotherapy, the survival rate is improving.[33]

The most widely accepted method of staging was developed by Enneking.[34] The purpose of a staging system is to enable clinicians to predict the course of disease. The most efficacious treatment can then be chosen, depending on the classification. Characteristics used to stage a neoplasm include a histologic grade, location, and presence or absence of metastasis. Histologic grade is subdivided into two categories according to the aggressiveness of the lesion. The location also has two levels: intracompartmental and extracompartmental. The presence or absence of metastasis is also an important variable in predicting outcome.

CHONDROGENIC NEOPLASMS

Osteochondroma

The most common benign primary neoplasm of the bone is osteochondroma. It is formed by an osseous outgrowth that is continuous with the host bone. The outgrowth is composed of spongy bone with a cartilaginous cap. It occurs in adolescence and rarely continues to develop once skeletal maturity is reached. The metaphysis of the long bones is affected. The knee and elbow are commonly affected.

Clinical Features

Initial symptoms may be associated with a bursitis or localized inflammatory response caused by friction

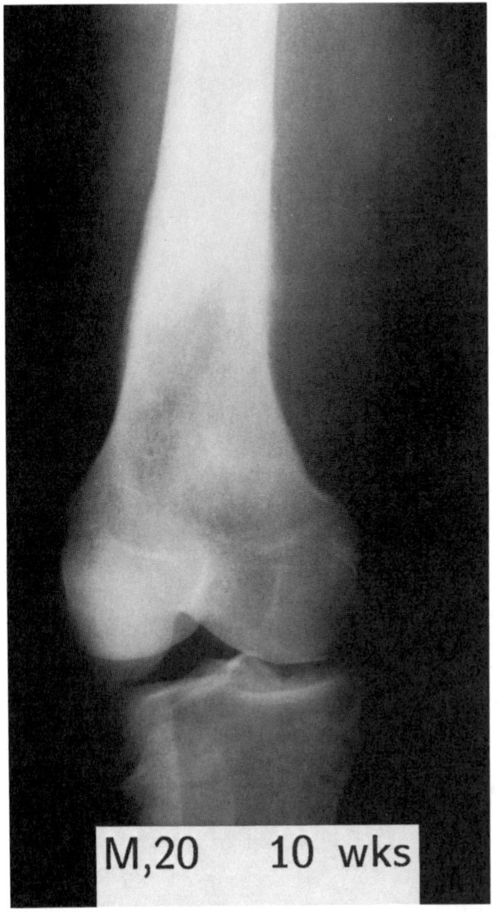

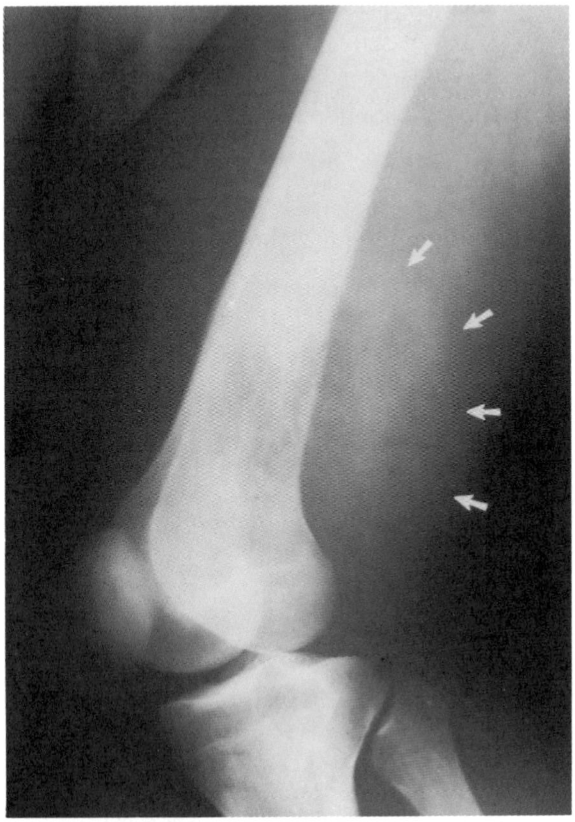

Fig. 10-3. Anteroposterior **(A)** and lateral **(B)** radiographs of the right femur showing a lytic osteosarcoma with posterior extension into soft tissue (arrows). (From Cohen et al,[22] with permission.)

from the overlying tissues. A firm, stable, nontender mass may be palpated. Because the cartilaginous cap is not visible on radiography, the mass will feel much larger than it appears on the x-ray film[35] (Fig. 10-4). The outgrowth always points away from the nearest epiphysis.[10] Trabeculated bone will be seen within the outgrowth.

Treatment

Treatment of osteochondroma is largely symptomatic. Surgical excision is considered if the lesion interferes with the normal function of the muscle-tendon units in the area. If no symptoms are present, no definitive treatment may be needed. The lesion does need to be followed because of the risk of malignant change, although this risk is very small.

Chondroblastoma

A chondroblastoma is a rare primary neoplasm of cartilaginous origin. It is most often found in the epiphyseal region of long bones, primarily the femur and humerus. Often the lesion can cross the epiphysis into the metaphysis. Most chondroblastomas are detected in males under the age of 30. Clinical symptoms include pain and tenderness, and, because the lesion is close to a joint, limitations in movement or function may be seen. A joint effusion may also be detected.[19] There have been reports of neurologic involvement; this finding is related to the location of the lesion.[36]

Clinical Features

A chondroblastoma will appear as an oval translucent area in the epiphyseal region and will have a thin scle-

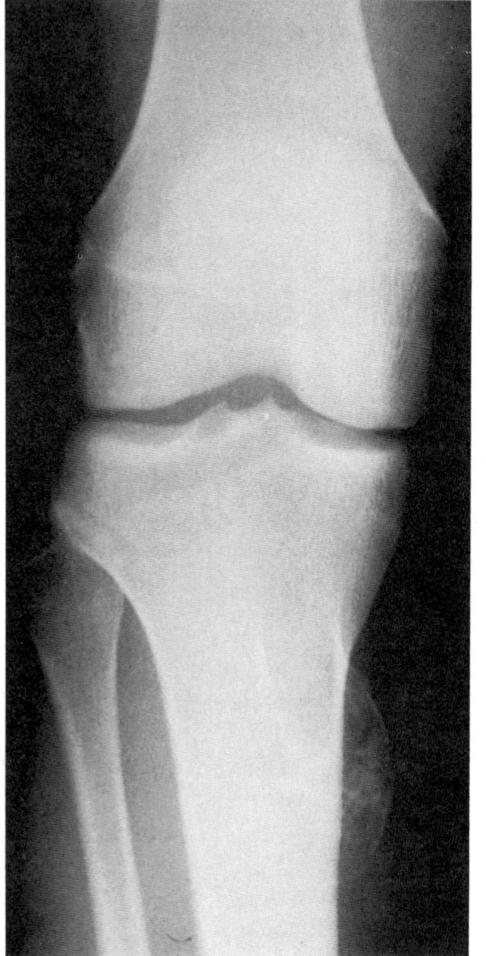

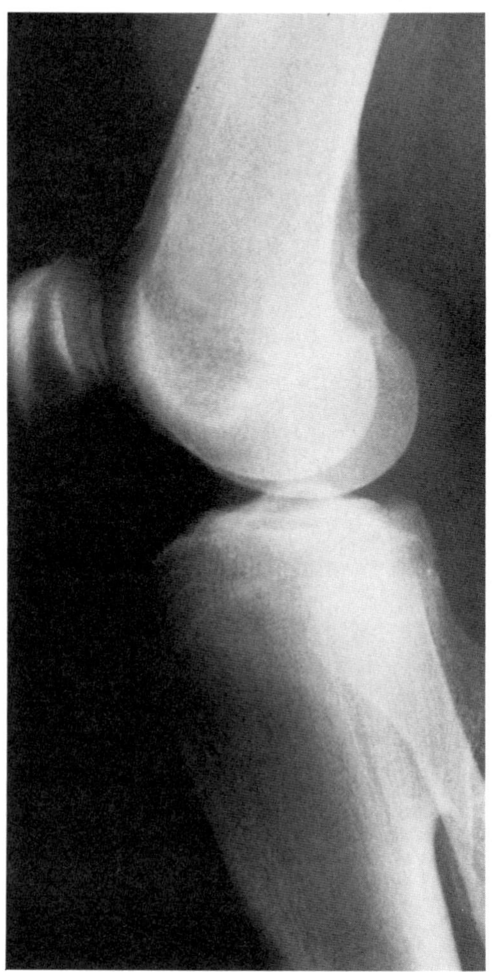

Fig. 10-4. Osteocartilaginous exostosis. A 20-year-old man presented with complaints of pain and of a mass about the proximal aspect of his right tibia. Anteroposterior **(A)** and lateral **(B)** radiographs showing an osteochondroma arising from the posterior medial aspect of the proximal tibial metaphysis with continuity of the host cortex sweeping into the cortex of the osteochondroma. (From McGuire et al,[35] with permission.)

rotic margin. This sets it apart from more malignant lesions, such as osteosarcoma, which is usually isolated in the metaphysis and has a wide sclerotic rim.[37] The lesion is contained by the cortex, but some thinning may occur.

Treatment

Treatment of chondroblastoma usually includes curettage and bone grafting. A chondroblastoma is a benign lesion that generally does not require radiation or chemotherapy. Results of treatment are generally good, and patients may eventually resume a normal activity level. In a recently reported case, a college football player returned to competitive athletics 1 year after excision and bone grafting of a chondroblastoma from the proximal humerus.[36]

Osteoclastoma/Giant Cell

Four to 5 percent of all primary neoplasms of the bone in the United States are giant cell tumors.[38] The epiphysis of the long bones, such as the distal femur, radius, and the proximal tibia, are likely areas in which it occurs. Osteoclastoma develops after the epiphysis is closed and therefore is generally seen in people over the age of 20. The incidence decreases after 40 years of age. Pain is the most prevalent symptom initially. A soft tissue mass may be palpable, and pathologic fractures do occur.[19] This type of involvement in the proximity of the joint may impair function.

There is a tendency for the neoplasm to cross the epiphyseal line to involve the subchondral bone. Radiography will show a large, osteolytic lesion that may expand the cortex outward but not penetrate it[39] (Fig. 10-5). Treatment has progressed from amputation to more functional limb- and joint-sparing procedures. Radiation is also an adjunct treatment, especially in those cases in which complete excision is not possible.

Enchondroma

A very common benign neoplasm is the enchondroma. This lesion is found in both men and women, aged 10 to 50 years. It usually occurs in the hands or feet, forming in the medullary cavity and expanding slowly. Over many years, the cancellous bone is replaced with cartilage, and the cortex thins; this will be indicated by the lucency on the radiograph.[40] Most enchondromas are asymptomatic. The difficulty in management is establishing the diagnosis. The presence of a malignant lesion must be ruled out. Eventually the patient may notice a firm swelling, which is due to the expanding bone. Pathologic fractures may also occur (Fig. 10-6). Treatment consists of curettage and packing the defect with bone. The prognosis in solitary lesions is excellent.

MYELOGENIC NEOPLASMS

Plasma Cell Myeloma

The most common primary neoplasm of bone is the plasma cell myeloma. Myeloma is a neoplastic prolifera-

A

B

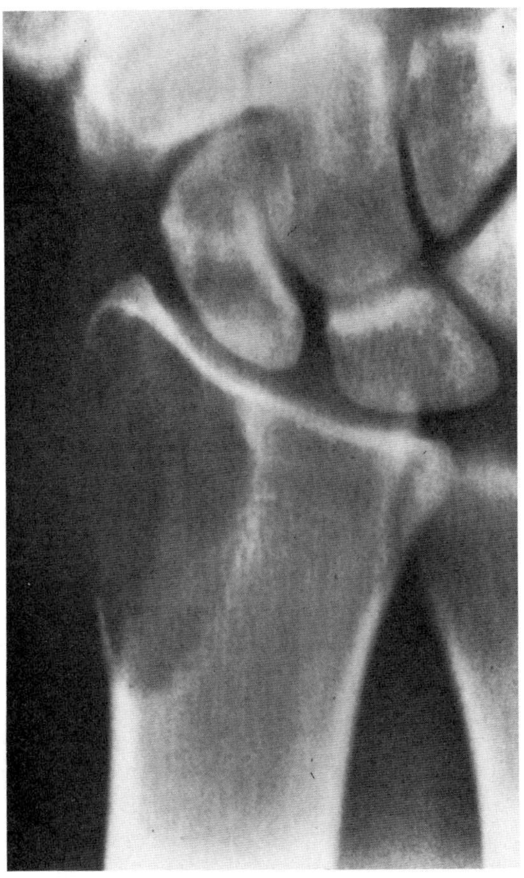

Fig. 10-5. Giant cell tumor in the distal radius of a 29-year-old man. **(A)** Plain film showing an unmarginated geographic lesion with a sharp zone of transition extending from the metaphysis into the epiphysis. **(B)** Conventional tomogram showing the lesion extending distally to the subchondral bone. *(Continues.)*

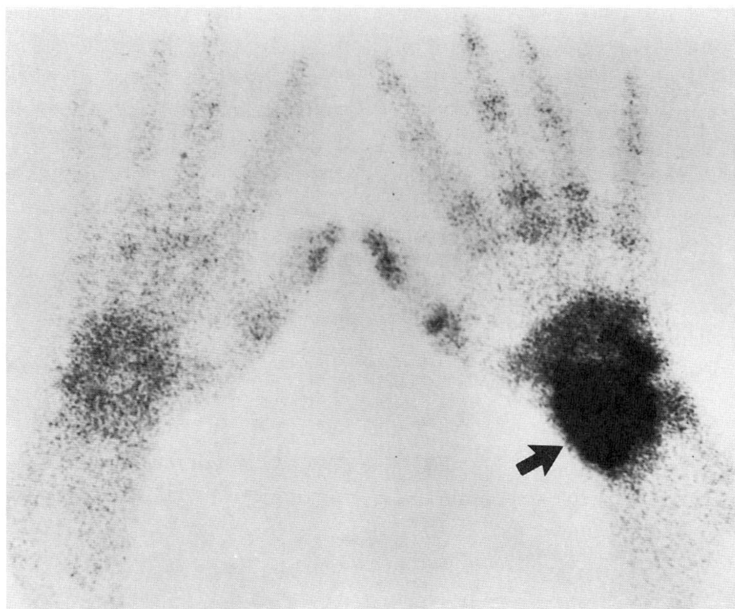

Fig. 10-5 *(continued).* **(C)** Radionuclide bone scan showing increased activity in the lesion (arrow). (From Chew,[39] with permission.)

tion of plasma cells in the bone marrow. It can be multifocal (multiple myeloma) or solitary. It is likely that the solitary lesions will become multicentric over time. This is one neoplasm that is apt to be found in people over 40 years of age. The peak incidence appears to occur during the sixth decade.[41] In this age group, the largest concentration of bone marrow is in the spine, pelvis, and skull—the most common sites of involvement.[10] Clinical findings include pain, bone tenderness, weight loss, and anemia with a normal white blood cell (WBC) count. Pathologic fractures are common.[42]

Clinical Features

The pain associated with plasma cell myeloma is described as deep and may increase with activity. Back pain is a common complaint because the location of the lesion is frequently in the spine. Compression of the cauda equina by the lesion can cause radicular symptoms. Turek[27] describes a situation in which a patient may present with symptoms very similar to those of a disc herniation. Although initially episodic, the pain eventually becomes constant.

The initial radiographic finding may be osteopenia of the spine. In the flat bones, cystic or punched-out areas may appear (Fig. 10-7). Eventually, the osteolytic effects extend to the cortex and beyond.

Treatment

Treatment for plasma cell myeloma has not proved successful. Most patients succumb to the disease within 11 to 32 months of detection.[43]

Ewing Sarcoma

Like multiple myeloma, Ewing sarcoma arises in the bone marrow. Myeloma develops directly in the marrow cells; Ewing sarcoma develops in the marrow support structure or reticuloendothelial tissue.[27]

Clinical Features

Ewing sarcoma is a highly malignant primary bone neoplasm that occurs in children and young adults. Ninety percent of these neoplasms occur between the ages of 5 and 30 years. In 25 percent of cases, metastatic disease will develop.[44] It does appear to be rare in the black population. The diaphysis of the femur is the most likely site, but the pelvis, tibia, and humerus can also be involved.[19] Pain and swelling cause these patients to seek medical care. The pain may be intermittent early in the course but usually becomes constant. A mass may be palpable and can be tender. Systemic symptoms such as fever and malaise are common.

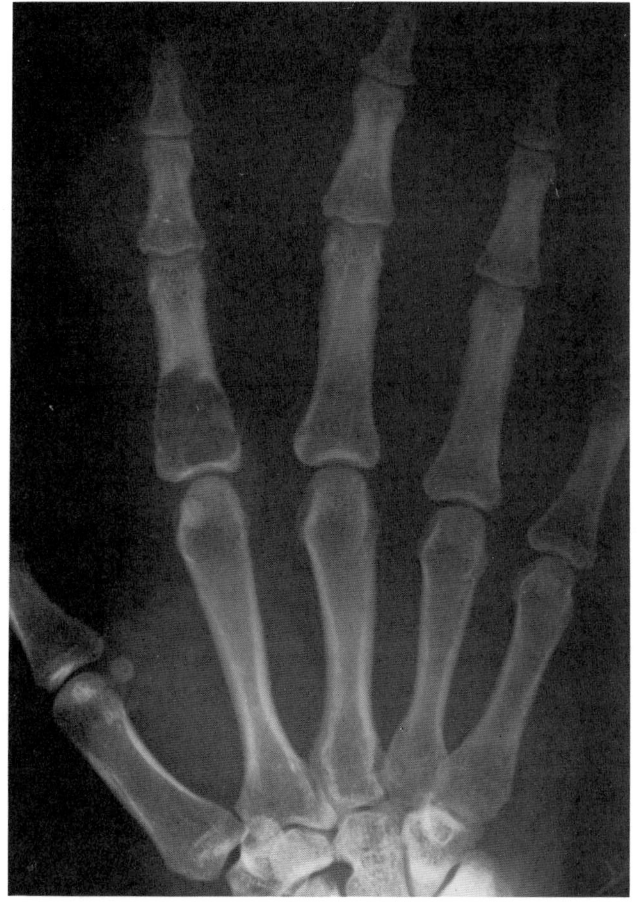

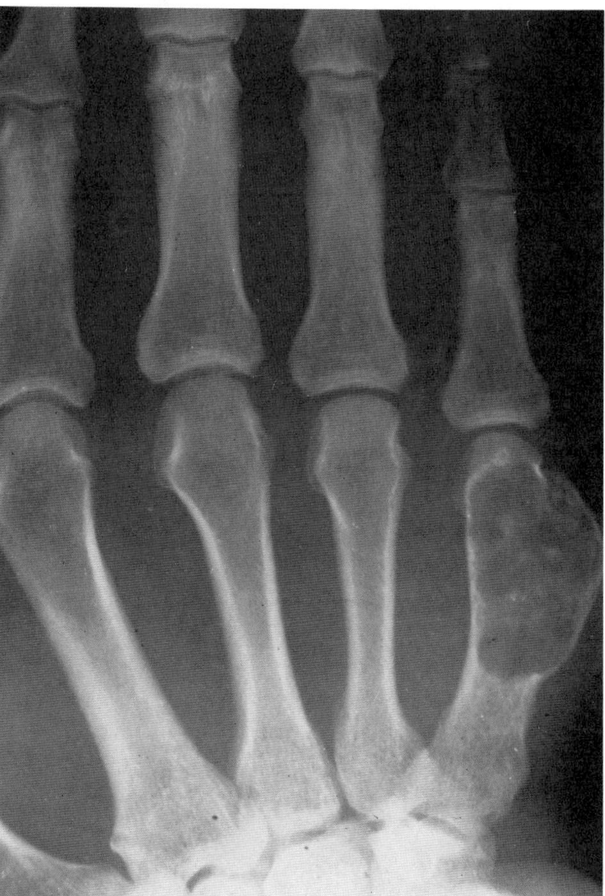

Fig. 10-6. Solitary enchondromas. **(A, B)** Radiographic appearance of solitary enchondromas of the short tubular bones of the hands. The lesion of the proximal phalanx of the index finger has thinned the cortex and is radiolucent in nature. The lesion of the fifth metacarpal has markedly expanded the cortex and has small calcific densities within the lesion itself. This picture would be considered diagnostic of enchondroma. (From McGuire et al,[35] with permission.)

The term "onion peel" is often applied to the radiographic appearance of Ewing sarcoma, attributable to the formation of new periosteal bone in multiple layers parallel to the bone shaft. The destructive nature of this lesion can lead to cortical thinning, leaving the patient susceptible to pathologic fractures (Fig. 10-8). The use of braces or crutches may be indicated during treatment if the weight-bearing bones are involved.

Treatment

Surgical treatment for Ewing sarcoma has not played as important a role as have radiation and chemotherapy. However, as more is learned about the significant limitations of chemotherapy, surgical intervention is increasing. Late effects of radiation and chemotherapy include stiffness, asymmetry, and limb shortening. These can all pose problems for the physical therapist who is trying to improve function.

MISCELLANEOUS LESIONS

Lipoma

The most common tumor of the musculoskeletal system is the lipoma. This mass of mature fat appears in adults after the second decade. The mass is usually asymptomatic, soft, and highly mobile. Physical therapists will undoubtedly palpate many lipomas during their evaluations. The mass may be noted to harden significantly after the application of ice.[19] The physical therapist should palpate the entire area of the body to be treated with any modality in order to detect post-treatment changes.

Although lipomas rarely cause problems, the patient should be questioned as to the progression of the mass. Patients who are unaware of its presence should be taught to palpate and recognize any changes that might develop. Pain is associated with lipomas only when nerve compression is involved. In these cases, excision may be required.

Dermatologic Lesions

Other lesions that physical therapists should be aware of are those affecting the skin. Physical therapists often see a large number of patients and have the opportunity to screen for skin lesions during the evaluation of the patient's musculoskeletal problem. While the presentation of skin lesions is varied, a few points must be emphasized. See chapter 13 for detailed screening of the skin.

Dermatologic Screening

1. *Know the types of lesions:* There are many different types of skin lesions. Many do not represent conditions that warrant further evaluation or treatment. But as with the neoplasms previously discussed, the value of an appropriate referral of a potential malignancy is immeasurable.
2. *Ask about the nature of skin lesions that are present:* Any change in the size, color, texture, or shape should be noted. If the lesion has changed, the rate of change may be important. Tendencies for the lesion to ulcerate or bleed may be an indication for referral. Some skin lesions, such as basal cell carcinoma, rarely metastasize, while metastasis from a melanoma is common.[45]
3. *Know skin cancer risk factors:* Certain patients are more at risk of the development of skin cancer. A fair complexion and exposure to excessive sunlight will increase the risk. Biopsies are routinely performed for definitive diagnosis. Excision may be indicated, and radiation is sometimes used in treatment.

PHYSICAL THERAPY TREATMENT

The physical therapist must proceed with caution in treating the patient with a known or suspected neoplasm. Many of the modalities frequently used in physical therapy are contraindicated in the presence of neoplasms. The more common modalities to be concerned with include ultrasound, electrical stimulation of various types, and diathermies. Various types of manual therapy and spinal traction are also contraindicated in patients in whom tumor or infections may be aggravated by the treatment.[46] The need for physical therapists to be aware of the signs related to primary neoplasms should be obvious.

It must be emphasized once again that primary tumor of the bone is a rare condition. It is estimated that only 10,000 new cases of primary bone neoplasms occur in the United States each year.[45] Therefore, most physical therapists will not have the unenviable experience of finding these lesions in their patients. This fact does not excuse them from knowing the signs and symptoms of these conditions.

SKELETAL METASTASES

Secondary neoplasms refer to the development in bone of cancerous lesions that have their origin in other organs of the body. Relative to primary tumors, skeletal metastases are much more common. All malignant tumors have the capability to metastasize to bone. Patients usually succumb to their primary cancer, but, because of advances in treatment, they are now often able to live longer, more productive lives. This has led to increased interest in the disability caused by skeletal metastases and appropriate treatment. The incidence of skeletal metastases is increasing because of increased life expectancy and improved methods of detection.

The incidence of metastases for any given type of cancer has been difficult to assess, as suggested by the wide spectrum of reported values.[47] For example, carcinoma of the breast has been reported to metastasize within a range of 47 to 85 percent of cases. The site of metastasis is somewhat predictable. Overall, the spine, particularly the lumbar vertebral body, is the most common area.

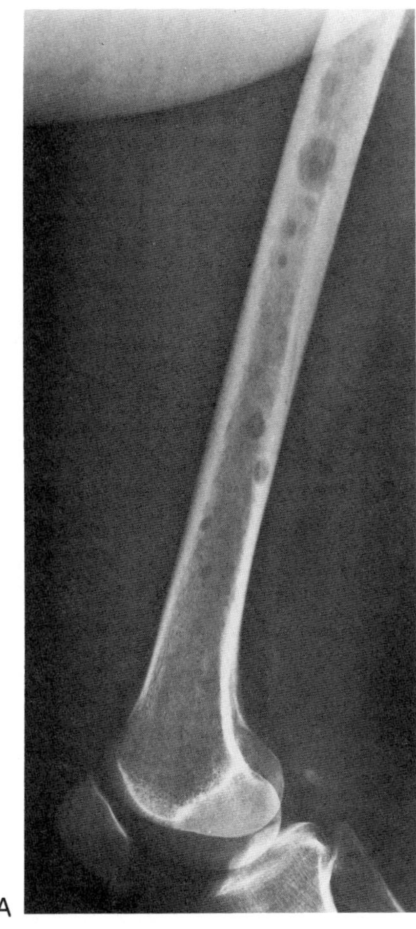

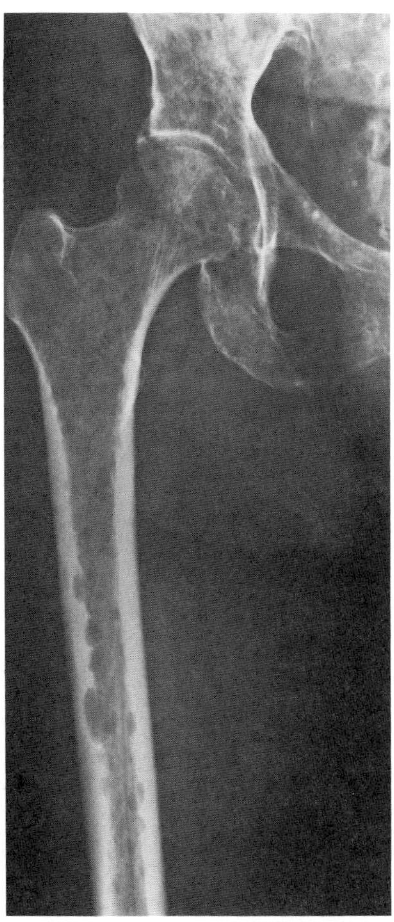

Fig. 10-7. Multiple myeloma in a 44-year-old woman. **(A, B)** Radiographs of the femur showing multiple lytic lesions of varying size throughout. Bone destruction has proceeded from the endosteal side of the cortex. The pelvis is diffusely involved. (From Chew,[39] with permission.)

Metastases to the skeleton are of interest to the physical therapist because patients may present with complaints of musculoskeletal pain that could be the first sign of an undiscovered carcinoma elsewhere in the body. If a patient is known to have cancer, it behooves the physical therapist to be aware of the incidence of metastases and the most likely site. Knowledge of the possibility of skeletal metastases in a patient could therefore dramatically affect the assessment and treatment of many musculoskeletal complaints.

Skeletal metastases are most often seen as secondary lesions from the breast, prostate, lung, kidney, and thyroid. All the factors involved in the development of metastasis in certain locations are not known. The location of a metastasis is dependent on the vascular supply to the area, proximity to the primary growth, environment of the host, and probably many other factors of both chemical and mechanical nature that are not well understood at this point.

Neoplasms can spread and develop in secondary locations by transport of the tumor emboli through the bloodstream or lymphatic system or by direct extension. It appears that the vascular system is of primary importance when considering skeletal metastases. The bloodstream is responsible for the spread of most cancerous growths. Most likely sites include those bones that have the greatest amounts of bone marrow, such as the vertebrae, pelvis, and proximal portion of the femur and humerus. Along with the many necessary functions, such as the production of antibodies and transportation of lymphatic fluid, the lymph system serves as one of the avenues for the spread of malignancy. The circulatory and lymphatic systems are intimately linked, and the method of transporting the can-

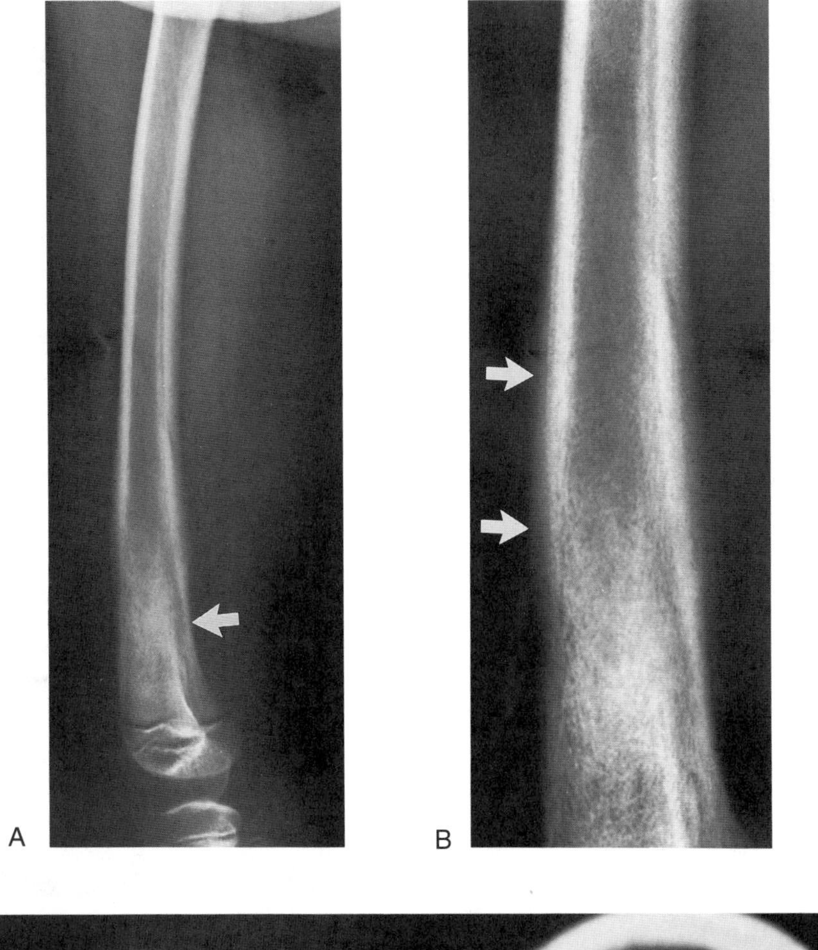

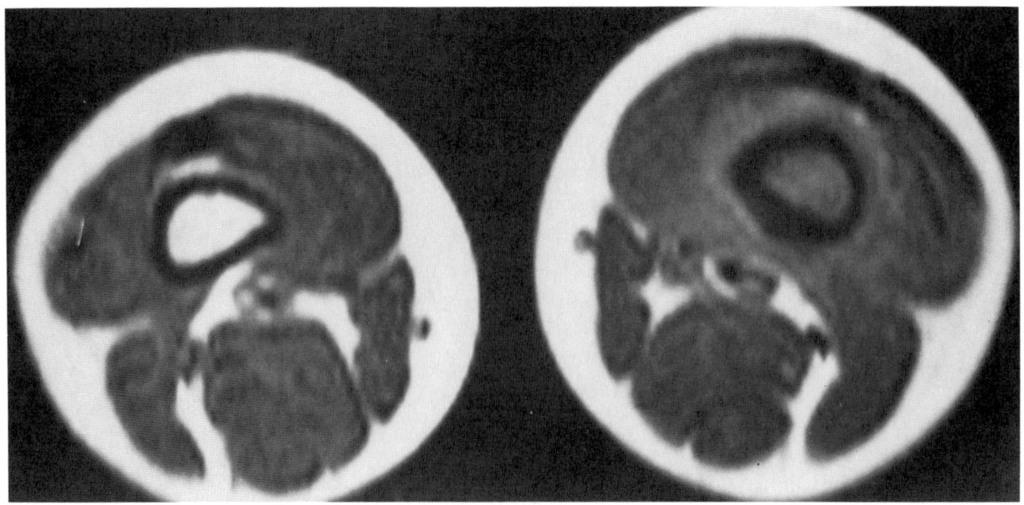

Fig. 10-8. Ewing's sarcoma in the femoral shaft. **(A)** Lateral radiograph showing a region of sclerosis in the distal femoral shaft (arrow). **(B)** Photographic enlargement showing cortex thickened by periosteal new bone (arrows). **(C)** MR scan with T_1 weighting showing abnormal marrow signal in the left femur. Soft tissues surrounding the bone also have abnormal signal. *(Continues.)*

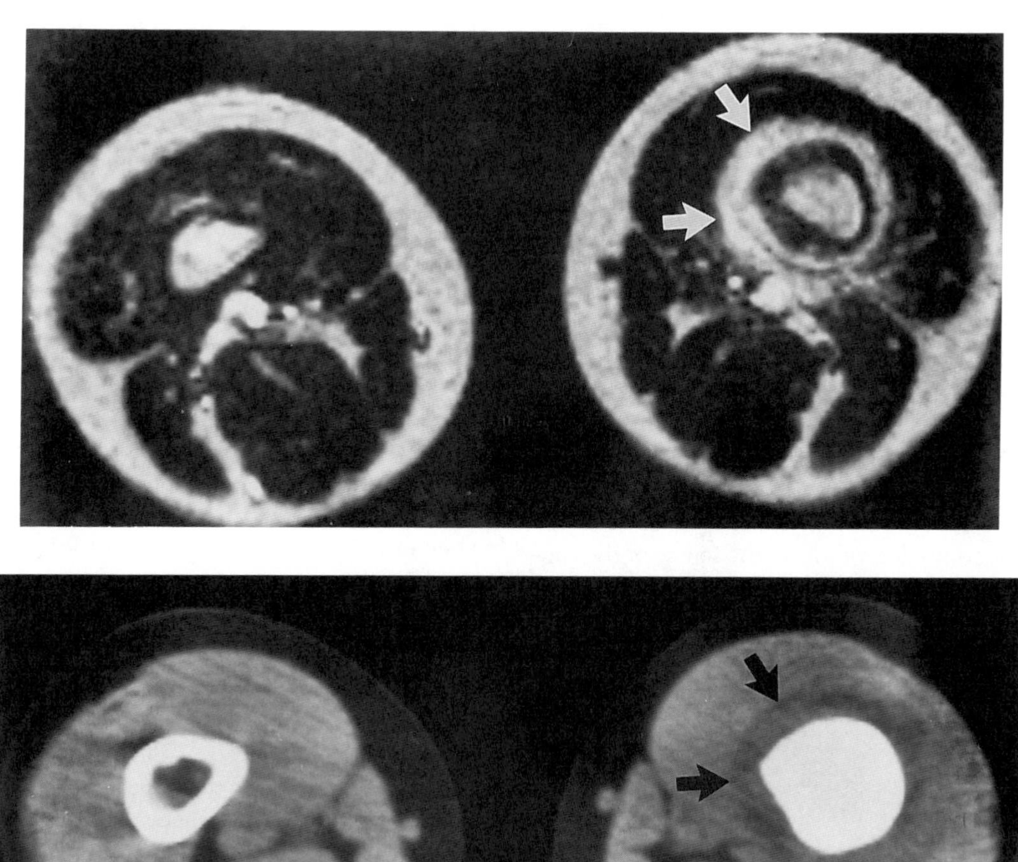

Fig. 10-8 *(continued).* **(D)** MR scan with T_2 weighting showing a rim of abnormal signal surrounding the femur (arrows) and areas of high signal in the thickened cortex. These findings correspond to cortical penetration of tumor from the marrow space into the surrounding soft tissues. **(E)** CT scan showing increased attenuation in the marrow cavity and decreased attenuation in the surrounding soft tissues (arrow), indicating marrows pace involvement and cortical penetration, respectively. (From Chew,[39] with permission.)

cerous cells is probably similar. The direct extension of neoplastic growths to the skeletal system can be seen in several locations. Breast cancer often spreads to the rib cage or the thoracic vertebrae. The pelvis and skull are also susceptible to this type of metastasis.

Clinical Findings

Although not universal, the hallmark of skeletal metastases is severe, incessant, pain. The specific characteristics of the pain depend on the bone involved. Pain can also have a variety of sources other than bone. Nerve compression, soft tissue involvement, and the viscera must be considered as possible sources of pain.[48,49] As with primary neoplasms, pathologic fractures occur when the metastasis is responsible for cortex thinning in a weight-bearing bone. This type of fracture is most often seen as a result of metastasis from mammary carcinoma. The proximal femur is the most likely location.[50]

Swelling and tenderness are less common clinical findings in patients with skeletal metastases. Radiography may show either osteolytic or osteoblastic reactions in the host bone. In reviewing spinal films, scrutiny of the pedicles may indicate destruction as an initial finding. As in primary neoplasms of bone, sophisticated studies are becoming more useful in diagnosing, staging, and planning the treatment of skeletal metastases. These studies include scintigraphy, CT, and MR imaging (see Ch. 16).

Physical therapists can have a significant effect on the outcome of many malignancies when consulted early in the treatment course.[51] For example, establishing a baseline for pulmonary status, teaching proper breathing techniques, and assessing the fitness level can provide valuable data that will aid in the rehabilitative effort. Specific evaluations depending on the source of the cancer may be appropriate. Shoulder ROM and circumferential measurements are necessary for patients undergoing treatment for breast cancer. Along with other standard contraindications for the use of modalities, caution should be exercised in the application of heat to areas that have had recent irradiation.[51]

Breast

Carcinoma of the breast is the third most common type of cancer, with 130,000 new cases diagnosed every year.[52] Only cancer involving the lung and skin is seen more frequently. Breast cancer is the most common primary lesion that will metastasize to bone. Occasionally, the metastasis will be the first indication of carcinoma.[53] When the cancer does metastasize, it will likely be seen in the pelvis, ribs, vertebrae, or proximal femur.

The etiology of breast cancer is unknown, but many risk factors have been identified. Both genetic and environmental influences are being studied. A positive family history of breast cancer and the presence of benign breast disease are two important factors that certainly increase the risk. International differences in the incidence of breast cancer implicate environmental and dietary factors.[54] Breast malignancy is seen most often in women between the ages of 40 and 60.[55] In this age group, breast cancer is the leading cause of death.[56] Many times a painless lump is detected by the patient as the initial sign. Not only masses, but nipple discharge and local skin changes, can be a sign of cancer. This underscores the importance of teaching patients self-examination and encouraging them to perform it on a monthly basis. A benign breast cyst is differentiated from a malignancy through palpation and aspiration. The aspirate can be examined if there is suspicion of malignancy.[57]

The use of screening mammograms is becoming more popular in an attempt to detect this carcinoma in an earlier stage, when treatment is more successful. The American Cancer Society currently recommends that women obtain their first screening mammography between the ages of 35 and 40.[58] For women with higher risk, mammography should be performed much earlier.

Cancer of the breast has a high rate of recurrence; therefore, patients who have had treatment should be followed on a regular basis. The opposite breast is a very likely location for the development of cancer. Physical therapists should be aware of the possibility of recurrence when examining patients with a history of breast cancer (see Ch. 6).

Treatment

Various combinations of radiation, chemotherapy, and surgery are used in the treatment of breast cancer. The extent of both surgery and radiation is dependent on many factors, including the stage of the cancer. The size, location, and number of metastases will also direct the treatment plan. Biopsy is performed to determine the characteristic of an abnormality in the breast.

The success of treatment seems to be highly correlated with the stage of the disease when detected. When found in the initial stages, treatment can be promising. In general, the earlier the diagnosis, the less extensive the surgical procedures needed to control the disease.

Prostate

In the United States, 20 percent of all new cancers in men will be found in the prostate. The distinctive characteristic of prostate cancer is its relationship to advancing age. Ninety-nine percent of prostate cancer detected is found in men over the age of 50.[59] Other risk factors have been studied, but no definitive conclusions can be made. Carcinoma of the prostate will metastasize to bone in about 50 percent of cases.[60] The lumbar vertebrae, proximal femur, and pelvis are commonly involved. If the pain from metastases is treated as a musculoskeletal complaint, progression may occur undetected. Screening is considered important for the early detection of this disease (see Ch. 5). Rectal examination should be included in all routine physical examinations for men over the age of 50.[61]

Treatment

If the cancer is detected early, radical prostatectomy can remove all of the lesion, which may cure the disease. While prostatectomy may be successful in removing the cancer, it is not without significant morbidity. Urinary incontinence and impotence are common sequelae. The use of transrectal ultrasound may offer advances in the ability to diagnose and stage prostate cancer. In more advanced cases in which the cancer has progressed, radiation or chemotherapy will be added to the treatment. When metastasis is found in bone outside the pelvis, the prognosis is poor. Bone scans will usually detect metastasis before routine radiography. Hormonal therapy is often begun in an effort to decrease the level of serum androgens.

Kidney

Renal cell carcinoma is found primarily in the 50- to 60-year-old group. The clinical presentation of renal carcinoma includes pain, hematuria, fever, and weight loss. Unfortunately, these symptoms may not occur until the disease has progressed significantly. The pain, when present, may be found directly over the kidney. The kidney can be examined with palpation and percussion.[62] Kidney tenderness can be elicited by striking the hand placed over the costovertebral angle. This should produce a solid blow to the patient, but not pain. Direct palpation can also be performed with an anterior approach. The right kidney is more often palpable than the left (see Ch. 5).

Primary neoplasms in the kidney will spread to the vertebrae, pelvis, and proximal femur in about 40 percent of cases. It can also be seen in the lung and liver. The intravenous pyelogram (IVP) and ultrasound are used to examine the kidney initially. Biopsy and CT are also used in diagnosis and staging. Renal carcinoma is unique in its unpredictability. Both the rate and pattern of growth can be erratic.[63]

Treatment

Treatment often consists of surgical excision of the tumor in conjunction with chemotherapy. Survival rates are probably related to the localization of the tumor. If the disease has spread beyond the local area or has metastasized to distant sites, the prognosis is not favorable.

Lung

Nearly 150,000 new cases of lung cancer are detected every year in the United States. It has been estimated that the incidence would be only 15 to 20 percent of the current rate if smoking were eradicated.[64] Cigarette smoking has been strongly linked to most cases of lung cancer. The strength of this correlation is seen in the dramatic rise in the incidence of lung cancer in women that corresponded with the increase in women smokers. It now ranks ahead of breast cancer as the leading cause of death in women.

Screening has not been found effective in early detection of lung cancer. Symptoms such as a change in cough, sputum production, shortness of breath, or pneumonia may not surface until the disease is advanced. It is not uncommon for the initial symptoms to be related to the presence of metastasis in the skeleton. Because metastasis occurs relatively early in the disease, treatment is often unsuccessful (see Ch. 3).

Thyroid

Cancer of the thyroid is not a common occurrence but can be associated with metastasis to bone. Two or three new cases in 100,000 are reported every year.[65] Women are affected three times more often than men. Pain is rarely associated with thyroid cancer, but hoarseness and a palpable mass may be present (see Ch. 7). Carcinoma of the thyroid typically follows a slow progression over many years. Metastases are commonly found in the skull, ribs, sternum, and spine; these metastasis are osteolytic. It is important to remember that the development of metastasis can be delayed and can even occur after removal of a cancerous thyroid.

Summary

The goals for treatment of skeletal metastasis are quite different from those directed toward primary neoplasms of bone. For metastasis, the goal shifts from affecting life expectancy to improving function and relieving pain as the primary benefits. The same methods are used: surgery, irradiation, and chemotherapy. Treatment of a pathologic fracture requires consideration of more factors than in traumatic fractures of the same type. The source of the primary tumor, stage of the cancer, and life expectancy of the patient must be weighed.

As with primary neoplasms of bone, the fundamental concept in screening patients for cancer and skeletal metastasis is that of awareness. Being cognizant of the possibility for carcinomas to mimic musculoskeletal complaints will improve evaluation and influence clinical decisions.

Physical therapists who are aware of the characteristics associated with malignant disease may easily increase their screening effectiveness using skills normally possessed by clinicians. Observation and palpation are skills that physical therapists must develop and use to the fullest. Physical therapists sometimes have the opportunity to observe their patients repeatedly over time. This allows for the identification of changes in the general condition of the patient as well as specific points such as skin lesions.

Complaints or symptoms that do not appear to be related specifically to the physical therapy problem should not be dismissed; rather, they should be investigated to ascertain their significance. Many cancers are detected during the course of a regular physical examination. Again, it must be emphasized that the physical therapist's role in medical screening is not to replace physicians, but to augment their efforts. Physical therapists can increase patient awareness relative to the benefits of screening, regular medical examinations, and self-examination. Physical therapists have a unique opportunity to intervene with their patients on a level that can lead to many health benefits.

METABOLIC BONE DISEASE

The processes of bone formation and resorption can be altered in many different disease processes. Rickets is caused by a lack of calcification of the bone matrix, which is regulated by the amount of serum calcium and phosphorus. Scurvy is a disease that decreases the osteoblastic formation of the bone matrix. The resorption rate is normal in both cases, but the change in balance causes osteopenia. Both rickets and osteomalacia can be caused by either vitamin D deficiency or malabsorption, or both. Although dietary changes have reduced the incidence of these disorders, it can still be present in mild forms in patients who do not eat a balanced diet and who have little exposure to the sun. The diffuse demineralization seen with osteomalacia can cause bone pain and tenderness. The possi-

Screening for Cancer

1. *History:* A thorough history will elicit considerable information relevant to the patient's relative risk factors for many forms of cancer. Information such as the age and sex of the patient is important. The incidence of most cancers increases with advancing age, especially with those malignancies associated with a high mortality rate. Patients must be queried specifically concerning previous detected cancer in themselves and their families. Insight regarding their lifestyle may reveal excessive exposure to sun, tobacco, or alcohol. Nutritional status may have implications both for medical screening and for physical therapy evaluation. Specific questions should address the presence of other treated illnesses or symptoms. Any changes in the patient's bowel or bladder habits (e.g., frequency, urgency, bleeding, or pain) must be noted. Recent weight loss presence of fever, and persistent fatigue may be warning signs.
2. *Characteristics of pain:* The characteristics of pain, as always, are vitally important. The clinician must obtain an exhaustive description of the location, severity, frequency, and variability of the patient's pain. Pain that increases at night or that is not associated with activity should be suspect. Migrating pain or pain of insidious onset that covers large unrelated areas can have a systemic or visceral origin.
3. *Palpation:* If possible, all structures, both superficial and deep, should be identified and palpated. However, palpation must not be restricted to the patient's area of complaint. Information from the history may warrant examination of unrelated symptoms at various locations.
4. *Additional screening:* A more thorough medical screening may include inspection of the mouth and throat, breast and pelvic examination, rectal and testicular evaluation, and appropriate laboratory studies. As in many other situations, however, it may be helpful for the physical therapist to explain procedures and their purpose. It is crucial that the physical therapist be aware of normal procedures in a physical examination. Allaying patients' fears may encourage them to seek an appropriate medical evaluation.

bility of pathologic fractures also exists. Treatment with increased vitamin D is usually effective.

Many diseases that cause hormone imbalances have their primary effect in bone. Hyperpituitarism produces various skeletal abnormalities from gigantism to acromegaly. Diseases of the adrenal cortex and thyroid can also cause generalized bone disturbances. While physical therapists may treat patients with these diseases for secondary problems, their clinical presentation is usually not mistaken for a musculoskeletal disorder.

Osteoporosis

Osteoporosis is the most common metabolic bone disease. The quality of bone present is normal, but the quantity is decreased. It is a growing concern because of the effects of the disease and the increasing number of elderly Americans who may be affected. More than 20 million Americans are affected every year. The associated fractures can lead to extreme disability or death. The costs of treatment and follow-up care are increasing annually.

Physiology of Bone

To treat osteoporosis and its effects, the underlying physiology must be understood. Cortical bone is solid and dense and is found in the outer walls of bones. It is most abundant in the shafts of the long bones. The haversian system, made up of concentric rings of lamellae arranged around a central canal, is found in the cortical bone. The trabecular, or cancellous, bone is found in the ends of long bones and is more common in the axial skeleton. It is described as porous or as resembling a honeycomb. The size and number of trabeculae are related to the magnitude and direction of force placed on the bone. The trabecular bone has a higher metabolic rate than that of cortical bone, which means that metabolic disturbances will be seen initially in the trabecular bone.

Bone consists of highly differentiated types of cells. Osteoblasts are responsible for bone formation, which is accomplished by synthesizing various collagens, alkaline phosphatase, and other chemicals. The counterpart to the osteoblast is the osteoclast. Resorption of calcified bone is accomplished by the acid produced by the osteoclasts. All bone undergoes an ongoing process of resorption and bone formation. In response to an abnormal stimulus, either the rate bone resorption or bone deposition can be altered. Localized cell death (avascular necrosis) can also occur.[66]

Osteoporosis is characterized by a decreased bone formation as well as increased resorption. The clinical symptoms of osteoporosis may include chronic back pain. This can be caused by the anterior wedge compression fractures commonly seen in the thoracic spine. In the lumbar spine, the vertebral bodies may develop a concavity on both superior and inferior surfaces. This biconcavity is called a codfish vertebra and is present when the central portion of the lumbar vertebral body is 80 percent or less than the height of the posterior aspect of the body. As the disease progresses, there is a characteristic increase of the dorsal kyphosis (Fig. 10-9). Radiographs will show the decreased bone density as well as changes in the lumbar spine. The vertebral bodies may develop a concavity on both the superior and inferior surfaces.

Etiology

There are numerous causes of osteoporosis; among these are disuse and hormonal imbalance. Two important factors determine the extent and development of the disease. One factor is the amount of peak bone mass attained early in adult life. This level is affected by dietary habits, lifestyle, and hormonal status. For this reason, adequate nutrition is important long before the earliest signs of the disease are manifested. Of particular interest is the calcium intake from early childhood. The recommended daily allowance for calcium in the young adult is 1,200 mg/day.[68]

Exercise is also a factor in the development of peak bone mass.[69] Weight-bearing activity is thought to be especially helpful in bone development. Weight lifters have been found to have increased bone density, whereas swimmers may not show this increase.[70]

A major factor in the development of osteoporosis is the rate of bone loss. When the rate of bone deposition is less than bone resorption, there will be an overall loss of bone density. If the process continues, this will be visible as a decrease in radiographic density, or rarefraction.

These rates will vary depending on the age, sex, and health of the patient, as well as on many other variables. Bone mass usually reaches its peak at about age 30. Bone density tends to decrease after the age of 40 in both sexes. In women, bone density decreases dramatically during the decade after menopause. The changes in bone density are important because density is correlated with fracture rate. Fractures are most often seen in areas that have a high percentage of trabecular bone, such as the distal radius, vertebral bodies, and femoral neck. It is the treatment and resultant disability stemming from these fractures that make osteoporosis so costly, not only in terms of dollars but in lifestyle changes as well.

There is not total agreement in the literature concerning the level of correlation of peak bone mass and resorption rates with the prevention and development of the disease or with treatment. This is due to many variables that are difficult to control in research studies. Even the method of measurement of bone density is sometimes questioned. Conventional radiography is the most frequently used method of assessing osteoporosis in clinical practice. Osteopenia is the term used to describe

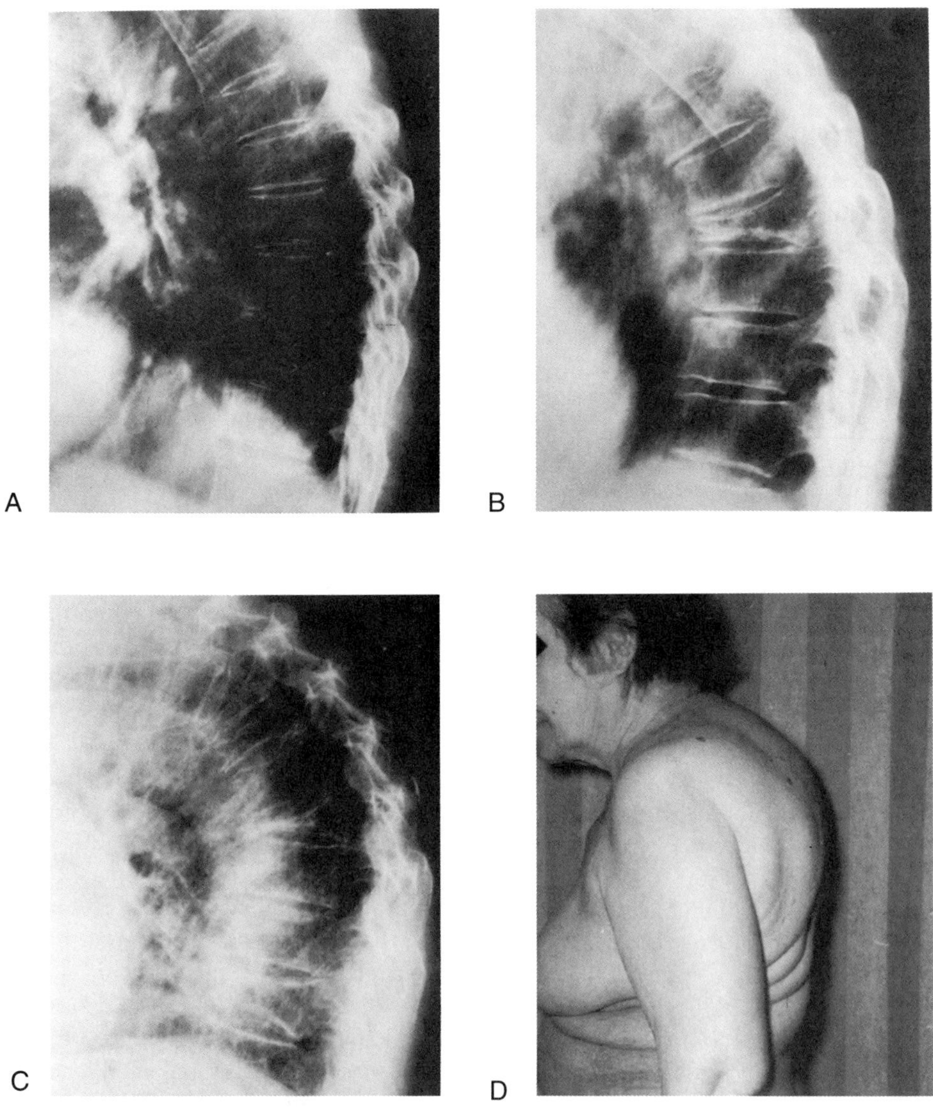

Fig. 10-9.–Progressive wedging and collapse of thoracic vertebrae **(A–C)** in a postmenopausal woman from the age of 68 over a period of 4 years. This led to marked loss of height, as well as hyphosis and **(D)** the development of abdominal creases caused by impaction of the lower ribs onto the pelvic brim. Risk factors were menopause at age 36 and smoking. (From Woolf and Dixon,[67] with permission.)

the appearance of decreased bone density on radiography. The spine is often examined radiographically; in osteoporosis, the vertebral bodies will eventually show the decreased density. There is a tendency to lose the horizontal trabeculae first; and height of the body will also decrease (Fig. 10-10). This will be evident on the lateral view, where only the faint vertical trabeculae may be seen. Unfortunately, significant bone loss has occurred before the radiograph shows osteopenia and at best should be considered a crude measurement.

Other methods of assessment using radiography include comparison of vertebral body height in the lumbar spine, noting trabecular patterns in the proximal femur, and measurement of cortical thickness of the metacarpals. These methods are easy to use clinically but have limitations.

Single- and dual-photon absorptiometry, dual-energy x-ray absorptiometry, and quantitative CT are just a few of the other common methods of assessment.[71] Of these dual-energy x-ray absorptiometry is used the most. A low beam is directed at the bone to be studied, as the absorbance of the beam is measured. The proper use of these tests in screening or treatment has not been standardized. Other discrepancies in the research can be attributed to the fact that changes in bone metabolism are multifaceted. Diet, hormones, exercise, and genetics as well as research design can affect the findings.

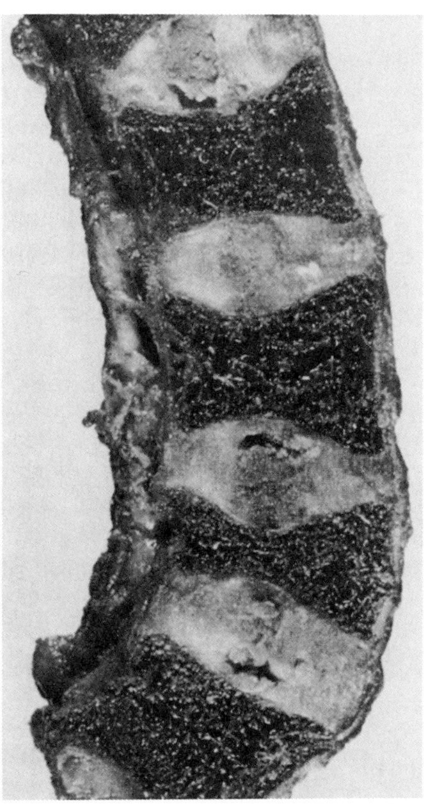

Fig. 10-10. Cross section of an osteoporotic spine showing loss of trabeculae, especially horizontally, and loss of height of vertebrae. (From Woolf and Dixon,[67] with permission.)

Physical Activity

While evidence is accumulating that physical activity and muscle strength are correlated with bone density, specific recommendations concerning intensity, duration, and frequency cannot be made with certainty.[72–74] This is an area that should be of special interest to physical therapists because exercise may play a vital role in prevention and treatment of osteoporosis. It is likely that proven principles used in cardiovascular conditioning and strengthening will be used in modified forms, depending on the individual needs of the patient.

The important factors to be considered before making recommendations are the relative risk of developing osteoporosis (Table 10-3), the extent and rate of progression, and the risk of fracture. With these factors in mind, the specific exercise program may include an emphasis on balance and strength to reduce the risk of falls for patients who have significant progression of the disease.[75] The tendency to develop compression fractures of the spine dictates that flexion exercises for the spine may not be desirable. Modifications may also be necessary in the daily routine. Avoidance of sudden forceful contractions, especially in a flexed posture, and emphasis on proper lifting techniques are indicated. For those at risk of developing osteoporosis later in life, a consistent exercise program should be initiated along with proper dietary counseling.

Identifying those at risk is extremely important because prevention will become integral to the management of this disease as further studies are analyzed. The single most important variable is the onset of menopause in women. A rapid loss of bone is seen in women near the onset of menopause. The decrease in bone density can continue at a rapid rate for a decade after menopause. Other factors that can influence the development of osteoporosis are race, nutritional status, and exercise habits.

Treatment

Trends in treatment include various recommendations concerning the use of dietary supplements, hormonal therapy, and exercise, especially weight-bearing exercise. The importance of dietary calcium appears to be greatest in the development of peak bone mass in early adulthood. The effect of dietary calcium in postmenopausal women is controversial. Combining calcium supplements with estrogen replacement therapy appears to give better results in slowing the rate of bone loss in older women.[76]

Of the many types of osteoporosis, that resulting from disuse and immobilization will be encountered most often by the physical therapist. Disuse can be a result of pain, joint pathology, paralysis, or immobilization. The bone loss will be more rapid in weight-bearing and trabecular bone. While mobility will restore bone density, the process is much slower.[77] The implications for the physical therapist should be obvious. Activity levels must be monitored and patients educated concerning appropriate limitations.

Treatment of osteoporosis is a good example of a physical therapist working concurrently with the physician to implement a total treatment regimen that will have a positive effect on the patient. Patients who have been diagnosed as having osteoporosis as well as those who have not been evaluated but who are at great risk should be encouraged to have regular follow-up visits with their physician. For these patients, it is important to have a medical evaluation before the implementation of an exercise program addressing osteoporosis. Physical therapists can take an active role in educating patients of the risks and preventive measures they might use to lessen their chance of the development of osteoporosis and to minimize the effects of the disease process. Patients who present with significant clinical risk factors should be encouraged to have further testing to ensure proper treatment and follow-up management.

Table 10-3. Risk Factors for Osteoporosis

Female	Long-term calcium deficiency
Aging	
Early menopause	Ectomorphic body type
Caucasian or Asian race	Cigarette smoking
Genetic predisposition	Long-term use of steroids

Paget's Disease

Although Paget's disease (osteitis deformans) is quite common, the actual cause is unknown. A viral origin has been implicated, but more study is needed. Males are affected more often than females. It is usually seen in patients over the age of 50.

Osteitis deformans is best considered a disease that progresses through several phases. Initially, osteoclast activity results in areas of osteolysis. These weakened areas then go on to fill with fibrous tissue. Haphazard attempts at repair leave the bone susceptible to fracture. Later the bones become enlarged and more dense. The femur, tibia, vertebral bodies, and skull are commonly affected. Conversely, the hands and feet are rarely affected.

Often the symptoms are so mild as to go unrecognized. The disease may be discovered as an incidental finding when the patient is examined for other problems. The diagnosis is made with the aid of radiographic and biochemical findings. While plain radiography may establish the initial diagnosis, a radionuclide bone scan can localize all sites of involvement. The initial symptom may be pain at the involved site, which can be a dull ache. The pain is not necessarily constant and can in fact subside spontaneously. When the skull is involved, headache is a common complaint. As the disease progresses, the enlargement of the bones may be noticed. The long bones of the lower extremities tend to bow anteriorly (Fig. 10-11). The spine will become more kyphotic. Although the disease is disabling to varying degrees, patients can expect a normal life span, unless malignant degeneration occurs. The affected bones become thicker, which is obvious in the jaw, skull, and extremities. The enlargement can also lead to nerve impingement. Hearing impairment can develop as a result of either the nerve compression or bone enlargement.[78]

The secondary development of osteosarcoma is the most serious complication of Paget's disease. It may be found in the early stages of the disease and is a very malignant type of neoplasm. The most common complication of Paget's disease is fracture of the weight-bearing bones. Successful healing depends on the stage of the disease. Fractures that occur late, when the bone is dense and vascularization is poor, may result in delayed union.

Treatment

There is no specific treatment to reverse or prevent Paget's disease. Treatment to alleviate disability as a result of fracture or pain is common. Calcitonin inhibits bone resorption and is used along with other medications that affect the osteolytic process.

INFECTIONS

Physical therapists are accustomed to treating a wide variety of inflammatory disorders and should be aware of the normal responses the body has to these reactions. There are general features common to different types of inflammation. Response to inflammation at the tissue level sets off a predictable course of events and typical symptoms. Rubor (redness) and calor (heat) are a result of the increased vascularity, which is an immediate response of the body to irritation. Vascular changes are primarily due to hemodynamic adjustments, such as arteriolar dilatation, increased blood flow, and increased permeability of the small vessels. Neurogenic and chemical mediators, such as histamine and kinins, also contribute to the vascular changes by dilating arterioles and increasing permeability.

Tumor (swelling) indicates the presence of an exudate. The characteristics of the exudate, such as duration, type, and composition, are important in classifying the inflammation. Dolor (pain) has many characteristics, and it is very important to assess both the quantity and quality of the sensation. The pain can be a result of direct pressure on nerve endings or can be caused by chemical irritation. Most infections have this inflammatory response in common. Other characteristics may differentiate the infections into very diverse types. Infections such as osteomyelitis and septic arthritis can produce pus, thereby being pyogenic. Pyogenic infec-

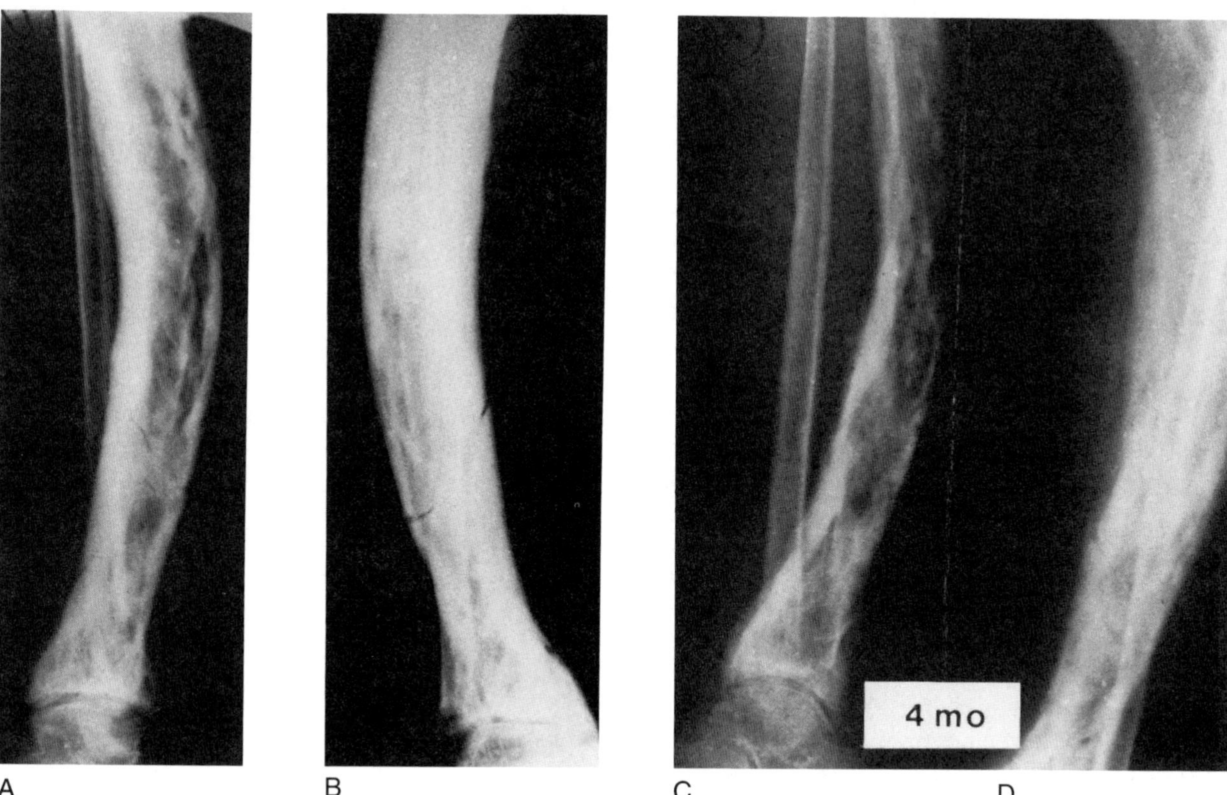

Fig. 10-11. Anterior **(A)** and lateral **(B)** radiographs showing Paget's disease of the tibia, with anterior bowing and fracture of the junction of the middle and distal thirds. **(C, D)** At 4 months, the fracture is healed. (From Cohen et al,[22] with permission.)

tions are serious conditions. Not all bacteria cause infection, but many produce toxins that can stimulate an inflammatory response. The bacteria can spread through the lymph system and eventually reach the bloodstream. If the bacteria enters the bloodstream (bacteremia), continued buildup of toxins may result in septicemia. This progression can occur quite rapidly, requiring immediate intervention. With acute pyogenic infections, surgery is often necessary to remove the pus and hasten the effect of antibiotics.

Acute Osteomyelitis

Acute osteomyelitis is a rapid, progressive infection of the medullary cavity of bone. The infection can also involve the cortex and periosteum. It is seen primarily in children and more often in boys. The metaphyses of the long bones are affected, especially the femur, tibia, and humerus.

Staphylococcus aureus is responsible for the infection in more than 90 percent of cases. This bacteria can enter the body through infected scratches on the skin or through the mucous membranes in the presence of an upper respiratory infection. If not recognized or left untreated, the infection can spread rapidly, from a small localized area of bone to the bloodstream, resulting in septicemia. Often the initial focus is in the metaphysis, which may permit direct access for the bacteria to enter the joint, producing a septic arthritis. During this process of expansion through the cortex and periosteum, pain will be the significant finding.

Diagnosis

The clinical findings are most important in this diagnosis because the radiographic and laboratory values will be normal in the early stages. Radiographic evidence of the infection may not be visible for 1 week. Symptoms may include pain, fever, local tenderness, and swelling.[79] The presentation of acute osteomyelitis usually includes a highly febrile child with intense, deep, or throbbing pain in the affected limb. Blunt trauma may be included in the history. Occasionally a patient presents with pain and decreased function or limp, but no fever. Again, the infection spreads quickly, and this will cause an associated increase in the patient's systemic symptoms of fever and fatigue.

Acute osteomyelitis can also be seen after a focal infection, which is common after surgical procedures, prosthesis implantation, puncture wounds, or comminuted fractures. After the insertion of prosthetic material, clinicians should be more alert to signs of infection. Daily inspection will indicate signs of acute osteomyelitis, such as recurrence of inflammation along the scar, discharge at a wound edge, pain with physical therapy exercise or movement, and low-grade fever. Any of these signs warrants further inspection.[80]

Treatment

Acute osteomyelitis is best evaluated and treated by collaboration between an orthopaedic surgeon and an internist. Immediate treatment with appropriate antibiotics is indicated. Some cases require early surgery if septic complications occur. Prognosis is related to the speed with which the infection is diagnosed and appropriate treatment initiated. Both early and late complications can materialize. Septic arthritis or abscess formation can occur. Chronic osteomyelitis and local growth disturbances may complicate the treatment course over the long term.

Chronic Osteomyelitis

The demarcation line between acute and chronic osteomyelitis is not well defined. Chronic osteomyelitis can be a result of a delay in the diagnosis of acute osteomyelitis or of inadequate treatment in the early phases. The classification is sometimes based on prior diagnoses, the type of organisms found, or the presence of later stage sequelae, such as radiographic changes.

Often the patient will have none of the symptoms commonly seen in acute cases. The findings are much more vague and are often mistaken for other musculoskeletal pathology. Wound drainage should always alert the clinician. Loss of function and local signs of pain and swelling may still be present but are usually less dramatic than in the acute phase. The diagnosis is made with various imaging studies, blood cultures, and biopsies.

For treatment the use of appropriate antibiotics is important. Once again, surgery may be indicated to remove all necrotic bone and infected granulation tissue. Outcomes can be good and are best when a team approach, utilizing infectious disease specialists, surgeons, and radiologists, is used.

Vertebral Osteomyelitis

Vertebral osteomyelitis is very difficult to diagnose because the primary complaint is back pain. There may be no associated fever or radiographic signs, and rest may actually improve the symptoms of pain, as in the more common musculoskeletal conditions. Vertebral osteomyelitis can also present in either acute or chronic stages. With acute pyogenic osteomyelitis, the pain is not always severe but may be continuous. The picture of fever, chills, and severe back pain is probably the exception rather than the rule. The patient may have a positive straight leg-raising test. The onset of back pain in conjunction with a history of a recent infection elsewhere, such as urinary or respiratory tract infection and folliculitis, should raise the level of suspicion. Obviously, recent surgery, intravenous catheterization, or drug abuse may also be implicated. Any procedure that might have punctured the disc space, such as acupuncture, discography, or laminectomy, should be noted. Exquisite spinal tenderness or a fluctuant mass suggests spinal epidural abscess. Chronic infections are more difficult to detect because systemic signs of illness are often absent.

Osteomyelitis of the vertebrae usually occurs through the hematogenous route, probably related to the pattern of blood supply in the vertebrae. Tiny branches of the vertebral intercostal or lumbar arteries supply the anterior body. These vessels also give branches to the anterior longitudinal ligament. The vascularity of the disc changes with age, decreasing markedly when the vessels that pass through the cartilaginous plate in children disappears. In addition, the vertebral body is mostly cancellous bone, which may be a conducive environment.

Radiographs may show symmetric destruction of two adjacent vertebral bodies with a narrowed disc space. Unfortunately, significant bone destruction may take place before radiographic documentation because visible changes may not be detected for 4 to 12 weeks after onset of symptoms. The earliest radiographic changes may be erosion or rarefaction of the cortical margin of the vertebral body.[81]

Other infections that may present as back pain are epidural abscess and tuberculosis. Both of these infections are relatively rare in the North American population. Their symptoms are quite variable and often include back pain, spinal tenderness, muscle guarding, and decreased active ROM. Early detection is therefore difficult unless systemic symptoms such as fever, weight loss, or fatigue are also present.

Infections of Bursae and Tendons

Acute infections located in the bursae and tendons are not commonplace, but the serious sequelae that can result demand attention. Infections are usually seen in the more superficial structures. Bursae and tendons lying close to the skin are susceptible to direct contact with microorganisms when even a minor insult to the skin occurs. Less commonly, the infection can begin as a result of transmission from the bloodstream.

Infections of certain bursae and tendons can be suspected quite easily from knowledge of the local anatomy. But many times the clinical picture is not clear. Aspiration and inspection of fluid must be done to rule out septic infection. The fluid is cultured and a cell count performed to determine the characteristics of the fluid. Once this is completed, appropriate treatment can be initiated.

The bursae are filled with synovial fluid and are located throughout the body. They are susceptible to inflammation and infection from many sources. In many cases, the inflammation is due to repetitive motion. The friction causes inflammation of the bursae. This type of bursitis is often seen and treated quite successfully by physical therapists. The most common site of infection of the bursae is the elbow.

The olecranon bursa is superficial and subject to trauma in many situations. Certain activities, such as wrestling, may predispose this bursa to injury. The onset of symptoms is usually sudden and may be extremely painful. The elbow will be held in a flexed position, and movement will be guarded. Swelling is localized to the bursal area rather than the elbow joint. Examination of the aspirate is necessary to determine whether the swelling is caused by a septic infection. Culture will also indicate the proper antibiotic therapy.[82] Immediate treatment is indicated. Left untreated, a bacterial olecranon bursitis may not resolve. Fortunately, the infection does not readily develop into osteomyelitis.[83]

The subdeltoid bursa plays a crucial role in the normal function of the shoulder. It is one example of a bursa that lies deep to muscle and is therefore protected from direct contact. It is still possible to have an infected subdeltoid bursa, but it may be secondary to an infection in the glenohumeral joint that reaches the bursa through a tear in the rotator cuff.

Tendon sheaths in the distal extremities can also become infected. This is a common occurrence because of the many injuries seen involving the hand. Lacerations and abrasions permit direct access for the microorganisms to pass through the skin. *Staphylococcus aureus* is a common bacterium responsible for serious infections in the hand. The reaction of the tendon

Kanavel's Four Cardinal Signs of Suppurative Tenosynovitis[84]

1. Slight flexion of finger
2. Fusiform swelling of finger
3. Pain on extension (passive or active)
4. Tenderness along tendon sheath into palm

sheath to infection is quite predictable. Because of the pyogenic nature of the infection, the tendon sheath becomes distended and the finger assumes a flexed posture. Localized swelling and severe pain that occur with passive motion are the most important clinical features. Treatment for pyogenic tenosynovitis must not be delayed and entails operative management for drainage and the use of antibacterial drugs.

The physical therapist must remember the four cardinal signs and consider consultation or referral when they are present in patients for whom a diagnosis has not been confirmed.

Differential Diagnosis of Suppurative Tenosynovitis

1. Reaction to local calcific deposits
2. Gout
3. Reiter syndrome
4. Collagen vascular diseases

Pain with passive extension of the finger is thought to be the most reliable sign of acute tenosynovitis of the flexor tendons. Patients will usually complain of swelling and pain associated with activity. Pain will soon increase, and patients often seek medical treatment within 2 to 3 days after onset. Operative intervention is commonly required. Thorough irrigation of the tendon sheath is critical. Normal motion can be expected within 1 week of drainage.[85]

Besides the tendon sheath, the paronychia and felon can be involved. The felon is primarily fat, and the infection gains access through puncture or extension of a paronychia. Treatment consists of proper antibiotics along with incision and drainage.

CONSULTATION AND REFERRAL

Physical therapists are accustomed to receiving referrals from all types of physicians and specialties. In some instances, referrals follow rigid guidelines concerning appropriateness and format. In other cases, a more informal system is employed between practitioners who use each other's services regularly. Referrals range from requests for specific treatments to open consultation and treatment as indicated.

In general terms, consultation entails asking for another opinion or point of view on a particular patient or finding. It may include collaboration and discussion. This can occur within the specialty or from another source. Generally, physical therapists work closely with their colleagues, and consultations are routine within the confines of their clinic. Consultation with other health professionals is sometimes not as convenient, and many physical therapists do not have the opportunity to engage in this beneficial process. Both parties benefit from consultation because in many instances it is a sharing of knowledge. In no way should a physical therapist feel inadequate because the expertise of a colleague is needed. On the contrary, responding to the needs of the patient in this way is exemplary.

The better the physical therapist's understanding concerning the expertise and perspective of the potential

Four Functions of a Consultant[86]

1. *Evaluation:* Diagnostic skills are applied to analyzing and assessing the problem. The need for additional data is identified.
2. *Advice:* A course of action is recommended, and additional studies of value in resolving the problem are specified. Alternative approaches to the solution and the potential outcomes of each are identified.
3. *Teaching:* The role of continuing education in the consultative process is recognized. The consultant contributes on-the-spot teaching or other appropriate approaches.
4. *Liaison:* Ongoing availability and liaison are offered with the consultant's own professional group and with other consultants in that group or elsewhere.

consultation source, the more meaningful the information will be. Many differences exist between specialities concerning evaluation and management of patients. For example, Fig 10-12 presents an algorithm that a primary care physician may consider when evaluating a patient with low back pain. It is worthwhile for the physical therapist to consider the different perspective that this algorithm reveals and to contemplate how a physical therapy evaluation could complement it.[87] Physical therapists must broaden their perspective if medical disease is to be recognized early and treatment provided by the appropriate physician.

A referral may take on a slightly different meaning. When a patient is referred to physical therapist, generally a working diagnosis has been made and the need for treatment or specialized evaluation has been recognized. Traditionally, this referral does not mean that the referral source, whether it be a physician or physical therapist, is no longer interested in the well-being of the patient. The accepting health professional may take responsibility for the specific treatment or evaluation requested, but the referring source should be kept informed. The relationship between two practitioners may dictate the exact referral process, but general guidelines are helpful. A pertinent history leading to the reason for the referral is necessary.

Results of previous examinations and tests that may aid in the evaluation must be included. At the same time, extraneous information must be eliminated to provide a succinct clinical picture. The patient must also be aware of the specific reasons this referral is being considered. Vague excuses (e.g., "I just want another opinion") may not be appropriate and will not justify the patient's trust.

Physical therapists will also find the need to refer patients to outside sources more frequently as their roles expand. Soon it may be commonplace for physical therapists to have a vast network of referral sites that will provide a wide variety of services. From a simple technical request for bracing to the complex examination for suspected musculoskeletal disease, referrals and consultations must take place efficiently and accurately if patients are to receive the highest quality care.

SUMMARY

Although the foundations of physical therapy were laid thousands of years ago, in many ways physical therapists have only just begun to realize the important role that they have in patient care. The training and expertise of physical therapists must advance along with the expectations and responsibilities if the profession is to continue to prosper and gain the esteem it deserves. Continued progress will only come with the cooperation and partnership of the entire medical community.

Medical technology has pushed life to the limits and brought to the surface ethical dilemmas that were science fiction a decade ago, yet patients with low back pain suffer daily without the proper treatment that comes from a sound understanding of the pathology. Physical therapists must foster closer working relationships with physicians not only for the treatment of their patients but also for collaboration in research. Independent practice must not develop into isolated practice. Without close ties to the medical community, the open communication necessary for the optimal treatment of patients will not be present.

Disease of the musculoskeletal system should be a familiar topic to the physical therapist. The existence of these disorders underscores the importance of a thorough evaluation. Both subjective and objective portions are extremely valuable. Expertise in conducting a thorough examination can only be developed with experience. It is recommended that the physical therapist become familiar with one examination sequence and develop the specific techniques to a high level.[88]

Supervision is also important. Direct feedback concerning techniques and methods can be of great value in developing a proficient examination. The use of intake forms and examination work sheets can also be important adjuncts to the examination process. Upper- and lower-quarter screening examinations should be required with all extremity evaluations.

Attempts should be made to gather objective and subjective data that are measurable. The more reliable the measurements, the more meaningful the data will be. It will also help the therapist assess progress or changes in patient status. Continuous re-evaluation is crucial to detection of subtle changes in a patient's symptoms or response to treatment. The following case history demonstrates the importance of these principles.

PATIENT CASE STUDY

History

The patient was a 75-year-old tool-and-die maker who was referred to the clinic with a diagnosis of mechanical low back pain syndrome. His chief complaint was intermittent sharp, stabbing pain in the right low lumbar

*(From Boissonnault and Bass, [89] with permission.)

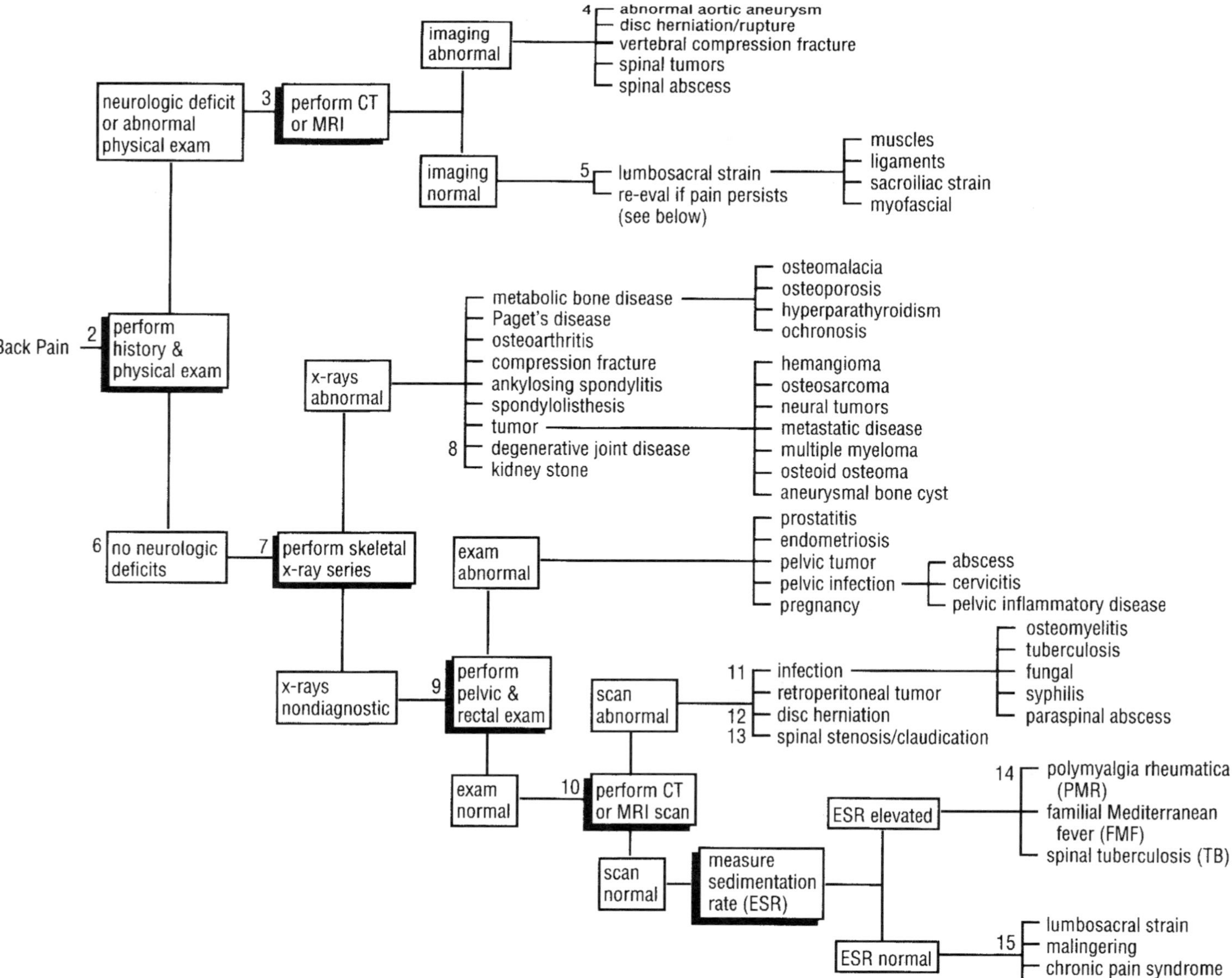

Fig. 10-12. Algorithm for low back pain. (From Healey and Jacobson,[87] with permission.)

spine and a constant throbbing pain across the lumbosacral junction. The sharp, stabbing pain was aggravated with coughing and sneezing, bending, and transitional movements such as sit-to-stand movements and bed mobility. Because the patient was unable to assume any recumbent position because of the sharp pain provoked, he had been sleeping in a lounge chair. The throbbing pain did not appear to vary in intensity, regardless of posture.

The sharp pain began approximately 4 weeks before the initial evaluation. While the patient was pulling up fence posts, he felt a tug in the low lumbar area. The sharp right lumbar pain began shortly after the incident and was primarily noted with sit-to-stand movements and bed mobility. The intensity of the sharp pain had increased steadily over the next 4 weeks. The deep throbbing pain began 1 to 2 days after the original incident and had steadily increased in intensity as well. Initially the patient went to a chiropractor for four sessions, receiving hot packs, electrical stimulation, and adjustments to the lumbar spine. After obtaining no relief from chiropractic care, the patient went to a physician and was placed on pain medication and referred for physical therapy. This patient had a 30-year history of low back pain episodes. The precipitating incident was usually repetitive lifting and bending, but the symptoms usually would be gone within a few days. The pain associated with the fence post-pulling incident was much sharper than usual and had lasted much longer. Also, the patient noted that during the previous episodes, lying down generally helped improve symptoms, but he could not lie down in any position during this most recent episode because of the excruciating pain.

The patient's medical history included current treatment for high blood pressure (medication) and a slight diabetic condition (diet controlled). He stated that he had had a stomach tumor removed surgically 1 year earlier. He was not scheduled to be checked by an oncologist for another 6 months. He had not undergone any radiologic testing following his most recent episode of low back pain. He also denied any bowel or bladder dysfunction.

Objective Examination

Observation indicated a significant reduced lumbar lordosis with significant muscle guarding noted with palpation from L2 to S2, left and right sides. Active backward bending caused immediate sharp right low lumbar pain, as the patient was barely able to move beyond the neutral position. He was able to reach his knees with his fingertips during forward bending, but he had great difficulty returning to an upright position because of sharp right low lumbar pain. Active side bending and rotation of the trunk caused soreness in the low lumbar region and were moderately restricted. Right unilateral pressures on L5 done in sitting position provoked the sharp right low lumbar pain with a spasm end feel. Vertical trunk compression (downward pressure applied to the shoulders with the patient sitting) produced a slight increase in the patient's throbbing pain. Passive vertebral segmental testing done in sitting demonstrated general hypomobility throughout the lumbar spine.

Assessment and Outcome

The referring physician was aware of the patient's previous history of cancer but wanted to avoid medical testing such as radiologic testing if possible. Owing to the patient's 30-year history of low back pain episodes and the fact that this episode was precipitated by a specific event (a lift), the physician considered a trial of physical therapy to be warranted. The physician requested physical therapy for 2 weeks with weekly correspondence scheduled between the therapist and physician.

Because cancer had not been ruled out, joint mobilization for the hypomobile segments was not used. Soft tissue mobilization for the areas of muscle guarding and gentle manual traction for the lumbar spine in sitting were carried out. Hot packs were also used for the lumbar spine. A soft lumbar corset was tried but provided no relief of symptoms. After the third visit, he reported that the sharp pain was virtually gone but that the throbbing and aching pain across the lumbosacral junction still prevented him from lying down. During the fourth visit, significant edema was noted in the lower legs and feet; the patient stated that he had noted the development of swelling over the past 24 hours. He also reported having a very difficult time with a bowel movement. The physician was contacted regarding these new developments, and medical tests were ordered. The test showed numerous metastatic lesions and pathologic fractures in the rib cage, thoracic spine, and lumbar spine, including L5.

This case demonstrates some of the inherent difficulties of differentiating between disease of the musculoskeletal system and mechanical musculoskeletal system dysfunction as the source of symptoms. Generally the onset of symptoms from mechanical musculoskeletal dysfunction is associated with an incident, accident, or repetitive overuse-type of insult to a body region, while symptoms from a disease process are thought to begin insidiously. This patient's history included a very specific precipitating incident, the lift and pull of a fence post. In addition, the behavior of symptoms from mechanical musculoskeletal system dysfunction is generally thought to include a change of body/limb position or movements altering the symptoms, while symptoms from a disease process are thought to vary little with movement or changes in posture. This patient reported very specific positions (recumbent) and movements (sit to stand and bed mobility) that would cause sharp right low back pain. In addition, backward bending caused the same right low back pain, as did right unilateral pressures on L5, but he did state that the deep throbbing pain varied little initially, regardless of posture. Diseases of the musculoskeletal system, such as cancer, that cause a change in the local anatomy and therefore a change in ability to function clinically present differently than diseases of the urogenital or pulmonary systems. As with conditions of mechanical musculoskeletal dysfunction, certain body positions or movements will stress the diseased area (in this case, sites of pathologic fracture), while other postures or movements will not. Therefore, the symptoms of the two clinical entities may have similar behavior. Often other subjective information or objective examination results do not fit the usual pattern of findings associated with mechanical musculoskeletal dysfunction. Such was the case with this patient, who presented with an unusual pattern of symptoms not normally associated with mechanical musculoskeletal dysfunction resulting from a lifting injury. This patient could not lie down in any position because of severe pain. Patients with back pain from mechanical dysfunction may have pain moving from a sitting to recumbent position, but once lying down can get comfortable to some degree.

A good general rule to follow is that if a patient presents with a history of cancer, the symptoms should be assumed to have a pathologic etiology until proved otherwise. In this case, the referring physician was aware of the patient's past medical history and the potential of disease being responsible for the symptoms, hence the physician's request for frequent communication between himself and the therapist, in addition to careful monitoring of the patient's status. If this patient had not been seen by a physician before physical therapy, he would have been referred to one after the initial evaluation.

REFERENCES

1. Mathews JS: Preparation for the twenty-first century: the educational challenge. Phys Ther 69:981, 1989
2. Watts NT: The privilege of choice. Phys Ther 63:1802, 1983
3. WHO: International Classification of Impairments, Disabilities, and Handicaps. World Health Organization, Geneva 1980
4. Sahrmann SA: Diagnosis by the physical therapist: a prerequisite for treatment. Phys Ther 68:1703, 1988
5. Jette AM: Diagnosis and classification by physical therapists. Phys Ther 69:967, 1989
6. Rose SJ: Diagnosis: defining the term. Phys Ther 69:162, 1989
7. Harris BA, Dyrek DA: A model of orthopaedic dysfunction for clinical decision making in physical therapy practice. Phys Ther 69:548, 1989
8. Shenkman M, Butler RB: A model for multisystem evaluation, interpretation, and treatment of individuals with neurologic dysfunction. Phys Ther 69:538, 1989
9. Zohn DA: Crossmatching anatomy with pathology as a means to differential diagnosis. p. 35. In Zohn DA, Mennell JM: Musculoskeletal Pain: Principles of Physical Diagnosis and Physical Treatment. 2nd Ed. Little, Brown, Boston, 1987
10. Salter RB: Neoplasms of the musculoskeletal tissues. p. 304. In: Textbook of Disorders and Injuries of the Musculoskeletal System. Williams & Wilkins, Baltimore, 1970
11. Echternach JL, Rothstein JM: Hypothesis-oriented algorithms. Phys Ther 69:559, 1989
12. Sweet DE, Madewell JE, Ragsdale BD: Radiologic and pathologic analysis of solitary bone lesions III. Radiol Clin North Am 19:785, 1981
13. Spjut HJ: Histologic classification of primary tumors of bone. p. 57. In: Management of Primary Bone and Soft Tissue Tumors. Year Book Medical Publishers, Chicago, 1977
14. Siedal HM, Ball JW, Dains JE, Benedict GW: Examination Techniques and Equipment. p. 21. In: Mosby's Guide to Physical Examination. CV Mosby, St. Louis, 1987
15. Zohn DA: Clinical observations aiding diagnosis. p. 71. In Zohn DA, Mennell JM: Musculoskeletal Pain: Principles of Physical Diagnosis and Physical Treatment. Little, Brown, Boston, 1987

16. Barbera C, Lewis MM: Office evaluation of bone tumors. Orthop Clin North Am 19:821, 1988
17. Cohen J, Bongiflio M, Campbell CJ: Special fractures and injuries. p. 121. In: Orthopedic Pathophysiology in Diagnosis and Treatment. Churchill Livingstone, New York, 1990
18. Siedal HM, Ball JW, Dains JE, Benedict GW: The history and interviewing process. p. 1. In: Mosby's Guide to Physical Examination. CV Mosby, St. Louis, 1987
19. Wilkins RM, Sim FH: Evaluation of bone and soft tissue tumors p. 189. In D'Ambrosia R (ed): Musculoskeletal Disorders: Regional Examination and Differential Diagnosis. 2nd Ed. JB Lippincott, Philadelphia, 1986
20. Madewell JE, Ragsdale BD, Sweet DE: Radiologic and pathologic analyisis of solitary bone lesions I. Radiol Clin North Am 19:715, 1981
21. Jaffe HL: Osteoid osteoma: a benign osteoblastic tumor composed of osteoid and atypical bone. Arch Surg 31:709, 1935
22. Cohen J, Bonfiglio M, Campbell CJ: Musculoskeletal tumors. p. 397. In: Orthopedic Pathophysiology in Diagnosis and Treatment. Churchill Livingstone, New York, 1990
23. Freiberger RH, Loitman BS, Helpern M, Thompson JC: Osteoid osteoma: a report of 80 cases. AJR 82:194, 1959
24. Wuisman P, Harle A, Frohberger U: Parosteal osteosarcoma as a cause of chronic knee pain in an athlete. Sportverletz Sportschaden 3:37, 1989
25. Schajowicz FL, Ackerman LW, Sisson HA: Histologic Typing of Bone Tumors. International Histologic Classification of Tumours No. 6. World Health Organization, Geneva, 1972
26. Healy JH, Ghelman B: Osteoid osteoma and osteoblastoma. Ten most common bone and joint tumors. Clin Orthop 204:76, 1986
27. Turek SL: Tumors of bone. p. 537. In: Orthopaedics Principles and Their Application. 3rd Ed. JB Lippincott, Philadelphia, 1977
28. Klein MJ, Kenan S, Lewis MM: Osteosarcoma, clinical and pathological consideration. Bone tumors: evaluation and treatment. Orthop Clin North Am 20:327, 1989
29. Romsdahl MM, Ayala AG: Surgical management of osteosarcoma. p. 137. In: Management of Primary Bone and Soft Tissue Tumors. Year Book Medical Publishers, Chicago 1977
30. Ragsdale BD, Madewell JE, Sweet DE: Radiologic and pathologic analysis of solitary bone lesions. II. Radiol Clin North Am 19:772, 1981
31. Dahlin DC, Coventry MA: Osteosarcoma: a study of 600 cases. J Bone Joint Surg 49A:101, 1967
32. Sweetnam R: Osteosarcoma. Ann R Coll Surg 44:38, 1969
33. Mankin HJ: Forward. In Lewis MM (ed): Bone Tumor Surgery. JB Lippincott, Philadelphia, 1988
34. Enneking WF: A system of staging musculoskeletal neoplasms. Ten most common bone and joint tumors. Clin Orthop 204:9, 1986
35. McGuire MH, Mankin HJ, Schiller AL: Benign cartilage tumors of bone. p. 4717. In Evarts C (ed): Surgery of the Musculoskeletal System. 2nd Ed. Churchill Livingstone, New York, 1990
36. Barton B, Clifton EJ: Chrondroblastoma in a college athlete. Athletic Training 24:342, 1989
37. Nolan DJ, Middlemiss H: Chondroblastoma of bone. Clin Radiol 26:343, 1975
38. Eckardt JJ, Grogan TJ: Giant cell tumor of bone. Ten most common bone and joint tumors. Clin Orthop 204:45, 1986
39. Chew FS: Skeletal Radiology—The Bare Bones. Aspen Publishers, Rockville, MD, 1989
40. Spjut HJ, Dorfman HD, Fechner RE, Ackerman LV: Tumors of Bone and Cartilage. Armed Forces Institute of Pathology, Washington, DC, 1971
41. Goodman MA: Plasma cell tumors. Ten most common bone and joint tumors. Clin Orthop 204:86, 1986
42. Kapadin S: Multiple myeloma: a clinical pathological study of 62 consecutive autopsied cases. Medicine (Baltimore) 58:380, 1980
43. Durie B, Salmon S: The current status and future prospects of treatment of multiple myeloma. Clin Haematol 11:181, 1982
44. Neff JR: Nonmetastatic Ewing's sarcoma of bone; the role of surgical therapy. Ten most common bone and joint tumors. Clin Orthop 204:111, 1986
45. Roaten S, Lea WA: Dermatology. p. 1111. In Rakel RE (ed): Textbook of Family Practice. 4th Ed. WB Saunders, Philadelphia, 1990
46. Yates D: Indications and contraindications for spinal traction. Physiotherapy 58:55, 1972
47. Galasko CSB: Incidence and distribution of skeletal metastasis. p. 14. In: Skeletal Metastases. Butterworth, Boston, 1986
48. Twycross RG, Fairfield S: Pain in far-advanced cancer. Pain 14:303, 1982
49. Foley KM: The treatment of cancer pain. N Engl J Med 313:84, 1985
50. Glasko CSB: Local complication of skeletal metastasis. p. 125. In: Skeletal Metastases. Butterworth, Boston, 1986
51. Gunn AE, Dickison EM, McBride CM: Physical rehabiliation. p. 23. In Gunn AE (ed): Cancer Rehabilitation. Raven Press, New York, 1984
52. Spratt JS, Donegan WL, Greenberg RA: Epidemiology and etiology. p. 46. In Donegan WL, Spratt JS (eds): Cancer of the Breast. WB Saunders, Philadephia, 1988
53. Giuliano AE, Sparks FE, Morton DI: Breast cancer presenting as renal colic. Am J Surg 135:842, 1978
54. Mettlin C: Breast cancer risk factors. p. 35. In Ariel IM, Cleary JB (eds): Breast Cancer: Diagnosis and Treatment. McGraw-Hill Book Co., New York, 1987

55. Siedal HM, Ball JW, Dains JE, Benedict GW: Breasts and axillae. p. 339. In: Mosby's Guide to Physical Examination. CV Mosby, St. Louis, 1987
56. Haskell CM, Giuliano AE, Thompson RW, Zarem HA: Breast cancer. p. 123. In Haskell CM (ed): Cancer Treatment. WB Saunders, Philadelphia, 1985
57. Ariel IM, Teng Pk, Predente R: Fibrocystic breast disease, diagnosis treatment and association with cancer. p. 60. In: Breast Cancer; Diagnosis and Treatment. McGraw-Hill Book Co., New York, 1987
58. Mammography 1982: A statement of the American Cancer Society. Ca 32:226, 1982
59. Badalament RA, Drago JR: Prostate cancer. Postgrad Med J 87:65, 1990
60. Turek SL: Secondary tumors of bones. p. 587. In: Orthopaedics Principles and their Application. 3rd Ed. JB Lippincott, Philadelphia, 1977
61. Mueller EJ: Cancer of the prostate. Postgrad Med J 86:115, 1989
62. Siedal HM, Ball JW, Dains JE, Benedict GW: Abdomen. p. 363. In: Mosby's Guide to Physical Examination. CV Mosby, St. Louis, 1987
63. Neuwirth H, Figlin RA, deKernion JB: Kidney. p. 769. In Haskell CM (ed): Cancer Treatment. WB Saunders, Philadelphia, 1985
64. Kessel KF, Leslie WT, Rossof AH: Neoplastic diseases. p. 583. In Taylor RB (ed): Family Medicine Principles and Practice. Springer-Verlag, New York, 1988
65. Donald PJ: Thyroid. p. 196. In Head and Neck Cancer. Management of the Difficult Case. WB Saunders, Philadelphia, 1984
66. Salter RB: Reactions of the musculoskeletal tissues to disorders and injuries. p. 17. In: Textbook of Disorders and Injuries of the Musculoskeletal System. Williams & Wilkins, Baltimore, 1970
67. Woolf AD, Dixon AS: The prevention of osteoporosis. p. 146. In: Osteoporosis: A Clinical Guide. JB Lippincott, Phialdelphia, 1988
68. National Research Council (US): Recommended Dietary Allowances. 10th Ed. National Academy Press, Washington, DC, 1989
69. Halioua L, Anderson JJB: Lifetime calcium intake and physical activity habits: independent and combined effects on the radial bone of healthy premenopausal Caucasian women. Am J Clin Nutr 49:534, 1989
70. Nilsson BE, Westlin NE: Bone density in athletes. Clin Orthop 77:179, 1971
71. Genant HK, Block JE, Steiger P et al: Appropriate use of bone densitometry. Radiology 170:817, 1989
72. Halle JS, Smidt GL, O'Dwyer KD, Lin S: Relationship between trunk muscle. Torque and bone mineral content of the lumbar spine and hip in healthy postmenopausal women. Phys Ther 70:690, 1990
73. Smith E, Reddan W, Smith P: Physical activity and calcium modalities for bone mineral increase in aged women. Med Sci Sports Exerc 13:60, 1981
74. Sinaki M, Offord K: Physical activity in postmenopausal women: effect on back muscle strength and bone mineral density of the spine. Arch Phys Med Rehabil 69:277, 1988
75. Dalsky GP: The role of exercise in the prevention of osteoporosis. Comp Ther 15:30, 1989
76. Ettinger B, Genant HK, Cann CE: Postmenopausal bone loss is prevented by treatment with low-dosage estrogen with calcium. Ann Intern Med 106:40, 1987
77. Woolf AD, Dixon AS: Clinical types and associations. p. 73. In: Osteoporosis: A Clinical Guide. JB Lippincott, Philadelphia, 1988
78. Woolf AD, Dixon AS: Differential diagnosis of bone pain and fracture. p. 110. In: Osteoporosis: A Clinical Guide. JB Lippincott, Philadelphia, 1988
79. Waldvogel FA, Medoff G, Swartz MN: Osteomyelitis: a review of clinical features, therapeutic considerations and unusual aspects. N Engl J Med 282:198, 1970
80. Waldvogel FA: Acute osteomyelitis. p. 1. In Schlossberg D (ed): Orthopaedic Infection. Springer-Verlag, New York, 1988
81. Bonakdor-pour A, Gaines VD: The radiology of osteomyelitis. Orthop Clin North Am 14:21, 1983
82. Ho G Jr, Tice AD, Kaplo SR: Septic bursitis in the prepatella and olecranon bursae: an anslysis of 25 cases. Ann Intern Med 89:21, 1978
83. La Cour EG, Schmid FR: Infections of bursae and tendons. p. 92. In Schlossberg D (ed): Orthopaedic Infection. Springer-Verlag, New York, 1988
84. Kanavel AB: Infections of the Hand. A Guide to the Surgical Treatment of Acute and Chronic Suppurative Processes in the Fingers, Hand, and Forearm. 7th Ed. Lea & Febiger, Philadelphia, 1939
85. Neviaser RJ: Closed tendon sheath irrigation for pyogenic flexor tenosynovitis. J Hand Surg 3:464, 1978
86. Rakel RE, Williamson PS: Use of consultants. p. 190. In: Textbook of Family Practice. 3rd Ed. WB Saunders, Philadelphia, 1984
87. Healey PM, Jacobson EJ: Musculoskeletal disorders. p. 186. In: Common Medical Diagnoses: An Algorithm Approach. WB Saunders, Philadelphia, 1990
88. Saunders HD: Evaluation and treatment of musculoskeletal disorders. p. 59. Educ Opportun 1982
89. Boissonnault W, Bass C: Pathological origins of trunk and neck pain: part III–Diseases of the musculoskeletal system. J Orthop Sports Phys Ther 12(5): 219, 1990

SUGGESTED READINGS

American Academy of Orthopaedic Surgeons: Orthopaedic Knowledge Update 3. 1st Ed. Vol. 3, 1990

Avioli LV, Krane SH: Metabolic Bone Disease and Clinically Related Disorders. 2nd Ed. WB Saunders, Philadelphia, 1990

Cohen J, Bonfiglio M, Campbell CJ: Orthopedic Pathophysiology in Diagnosis and Treatment. Churchill Livingstone, New York, 1990

Galasko CSB: Skeletal Metastases. Butterworth, Boston, 1986

Schajowicz F: Tumors and Tumor-like Lesions of Bone and Joints. Springer-Verlag, New York, 1981

Schlossberg D: Orthopaedic Infection. Springer-Verlag, New York, 1988

Woods CG: Diagnostic Orthopaedics—Pathology. Blackwell Scientific, London, 1972

11 Screening for Rheumatic Disease

Paul H. Caldron, D.O., F.A.C.P., F.A.C.R.

The essence of rheumatic disease is inflammation, specifically inflammation that promotes damage to organs in the absence of continuous inciting trauma or an invading pathogenic organism or substance. Such inflammation results from immunologic or metabolic functions intrinsic to the host that have gone awry. The term *inflammation* refers to processes involving cadres of blood and tissue cells and their products that make up a dedicated infantry. This army responds to a great variety of command sources in a rather limited number of ways.

The teleologic missions of these cells are to clean up the aftermath of tissue damage accruing through trauma or an invading organism or substance, to confine the perimeters of the assault, to promote reconstruction and healing, and to formulate recall potential for rapid recognition of recurrent invaders. When the signals for attack continue, or the signals for "cease fire" by the inflammatory process are not heard, despite the lack of an identifiable invader, then further tissue damage is inflicted by chronic inflammatory cells and their products. Intrinsic to the appreciation of this unwanted inflammation is the concept of autoimmunity, wherein our defensive proteins and cells mistake our own cellular elements as foreign in the absence of or following a true invader. When self-tolerance fails, the resulting autoimmune reaction may produce inflammation characteristic of various rheumatic disorders.

Thus, rheumatic disease therapy pivots on controlling unnecessary inflammation. Rheumatologic practice hinges on identifying clinical syndromes of immune dysregulation and metabolic causes of unhelpful inflammation. The challenge of such practice begins with differentiating patients who have primary mechanical or degenerative dysfunction, as well as those with infection or other primary organic disorders, from those who have primary inflammatory diseases, when all these categories may present with similar complaints.

This chapter is intended to aid the physical therapist in recognizing rheumatic disease. Several rheumatologic entities selected because of their likelihood of presenting to independent physical therapy practices are described briefly. Subjective and objective clinical clues to help differentiate primary inflammatory disease from mechanical dysfunction and other medical disease are emphasized. Where appropriate, screening or diagnostic laboratory tests are discussed.

GENERAL SYMPTOMS AND SIGNS OF RHEUMATIC DISEASE

The most fundamental aid to recognizing rheumatic disease in people presenting with musculoskeletal discomfort is a search for systemic components. Such symptoms may be constitutional, including new-onset fatigue, fever, weight change, or loss of appetite, or may include signs of disease in organ systems other than musculoskeletal. Typical manifestations may include mucocutaneous signs, such as rash, mouth sores, hair loss, skin thickening or tightening, or nodules. Joint pain occurring with diarrhea or dysuria, headaches or scalp tenderness, or pleuritic chest pain should also suggest the possibility of systemic rheumatic disorders. Sensitivity to sun exposure, with resultant rash, fever, abdominal, or joint pain, should be noted. Such systemic symptoms are nonspecific, are rarely diagnostic, and often suggest infection. However, the clustering of certain features into groups, in the absence of demonstrable infectious causes, should lead to the suspicion of a rheumatic disorder.

Systemic Lupus Erythematosus

A case in point is that of systemic lupus erythematosus (SLE). This disorder is often considered the prototypical systemic rheumatic disease. As in most inflammatory rheumatic disorders, the incidence is higher in women. Patients with SLE often present with nonspecific arthralgias and myalgias, or polyarthritis. The diagnosis is dependent on the demonstration of abnormalities in several other organs concomitant with the serologic detection of certain autoantibodies (Table 11-1).[1] When suspicion of SLE is raised by the clustering of some of these criterion symptoms, testing for antinuclear antibodies (ANA) is essential. This group of autoantibodies is generally felt to play a substantial role in the pathogenic mechanisms in the various diseased organs. Although no particular antibody test is absolutely diagnostic, these and other autoantibody species can provide strong clues for lupus and a variety of other rheumatic disorders.[2]

Table 11-1. Criteria: Systemic Lupus Erythematosus[a]

Criteria	Further Description
1. Malar rash	Fixed erythema, flat or raised, over the malar eminences, tending to spare the nasolabial folds
2. Discoid rash	Erythematous raised patches with scaling and atrophic scarring
3. Photosensitivity	Skin rash as an unusual reaction to sunlight
4. Oral ulcers	Usually painless, shallow mucosal ulcers
5. Arthritis	Usually nondeforming
6. Serositis	Pleuritis or pericarditis
7. Renal disorder	Proteinuria or cellular casts
8. Neurologic disorder	Seizures or psychosis
9. Hematologic disorder	Hemolytic anemia, leukopenia, lymphopenia, or thrombocytopenia
10. Immunologic disorder	Positive LE cell preparation, anti-DNA, anti-Sm, or false-positive serologic test for syphilis
11. Antinuclear antibody	Screening test for autoantibodies

[a]Four or more of the 11 criteria support a diagnosis of SLE.

Local Tissue Assessment

Another rudimentary task in sorting out rheumatic disease is identifying inflammation in tissues clinically. Localization and demonstration of inflammatory signs guides the evaluation at the bedside. First, the focus of the complaint must be isolated: Does the discomfort arise from muscle, tendon, bursa, or joint?

In general, pain of *joint* origin is characterized by discomfort throughout the range of motion (ROM). Joint pain is usually accompanied by limitation of range either because of mechanical barrier or because of muscle guarding attributable to pain. Pain is felt throughout the articulation. By contrast, *periarticular tendon* or *bursal* pain is usually better isolated with a single pointing finger and more likely to hurt during a definable segment in the ROM. For example, supraspinatus tendon pain is typically located at the subacromial space and occurs most notably between 30 and 60 degrees abduction. By comparison, *muscular* pain may be indicated by local tenderness or by discomfort with a particular isolated motion out of all the available motions of the joint. Muscular pain may be present throughout passive lengthening of an individual muscle or muscle group but is usually worse with active contraction, including isometric contraction. These points on differentiating joint versus tendon or bursa versus muscular origin of pain generally hold true for both inflammatory and mechanical or strain conditions. It is useful to note, however, that the end feel with passive movement testing of inflamed joints is generally more spongy in character than degenerative joint changes because of inflammatory edema.

If the source is indeed articular, the presence of inflammation versus degenerative or mechanical pathology can usually be suggested by historical clues. Typically, patients with noninflammatory conditions will describe "post-rest gel," indicating stiffness in a spine region or peripheral joint after a period of immobility. Post-rest gel loosens momentarily, within a few steps or passages of motion. In contrast, inflamed joints may take 30 minutes to several hours of regular motion, particularly in the morning, to feel freely mobile. In the worse scenario, the patient may feel stiff throughout the day.

Next, the observer must seek the presence of the cardinal signs of inflammation at the joints. These signs include soft tissue (especially synovial) swelling, redness, heat, and tenderness, as well as pain on motion at the site. Bony thickening resulting from noninflammatory-induced cartilage degeneration typifies osteoarthritis, and the cardinal signs of inflammation are generally absent.

In the laboratory, acute-phase reactants such as the erythrocyte sedimentation rate (ESR) and C-reactive protein (CRP) are usually increased when substantial inflammation is present. In the absence of known trauma, plain radiographs are generally helpful only when joint pathology has been present for at least several months. By that time, degenerative changes versus inflammatory effects may be differentiated (Fig. 11-1).

Differentiation of Arthritis

It is imperative for the clinician to distinguish an inflammatory from a noninflammatory (degenerative) chronic arthropathy as early and precisely as possible. Without adequate pharmacologic suppression of inflammation in inflammatory disorders, there is little hope of effective symptom control or joint preservation despite the most meticulous attention to physical therapy. Likewise, early recognition of degenerative osteoarthritis can allow for alteration in the mechanical stresses that hasten cartilage and disc breakdown and may demonstrably retard the rate of further deterioration. In community practice, the distinction of degenerative from inflammatory arthritis is rarely difficult if the observer focuses on the aforementioned historical and examination clues and notes the typical distribution of the involved joints. Distinguishing various subtypes of inflammatory arthritis, again, is aided by the distribution of involved joints and the concomitant extra-articular manifestations.

Osteoarthritis

If osteoarthritis is "wear and tear" induced, intuitively the primary weight-bearing joints (i.e., knees, hips, and

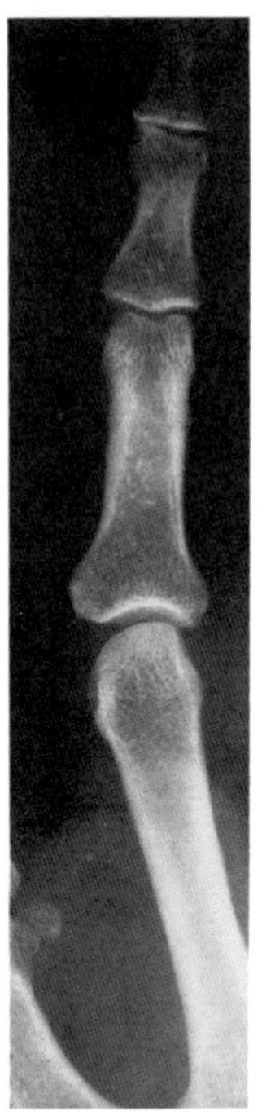

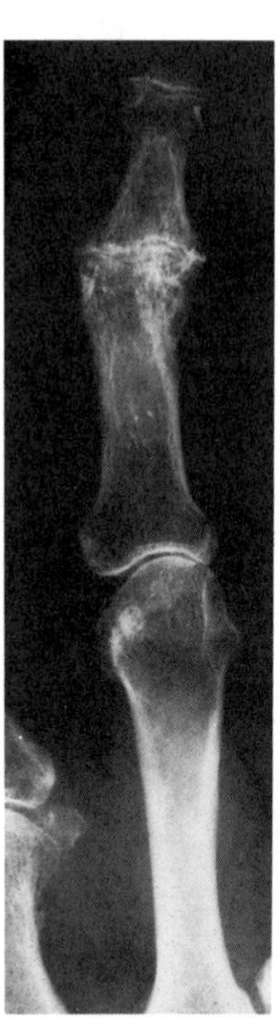

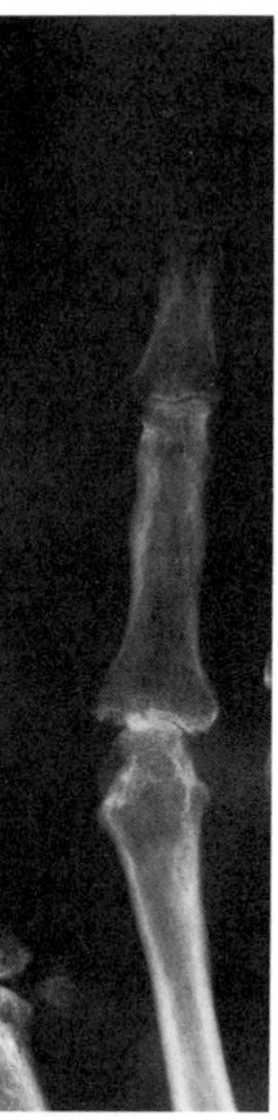

Fig. 11-1. (A) Radiograph of normal index finger. **(B)** Osteoarthritis. Note narrowing of joint cartilage space and periarticular bony thickening of the interphalangeal joints and sparing of the metacarpophalangeal joint. **(C)** Rheumatoid arthritis. Note joint space narrowing with periarticular decrease in bone density and marginal bony erosions. The metacarpophalangeal and proximal interphalangeal joints are involved, while the distal interphalangeal joint is spared. (Courtesy of Healthwest Regional Medical Center, Phoenix, AZ.)

lumbar and cervical spine) should be the most affected. Such is the case. Similarly, small joints, such as the first carpometacarpal articulation, first metatarsal phalangeal joint, and distal and proximal interphalangeal joints, are also commonly involved. In these nonweight-bearing joints, genetic influence and use-intensive accumulated microtrauma lead to narrowing of joint cartilage and bony thickening. Metacarpophalangeal joints, wrists, ankles, elbows, shoulders, and temporomandibular joints are less affected unless there are occupational or athletic influences promoting trauma specifically to these joints (Fig. 11-2). Predictably, the incidence of symptomatic osteoarthritis increases with age equally in the sexes, affecting one-half the population by age 65.[3]

Management of pain and post-rest gel is approached with measures to maintain ROM and muscle tone with the goal of optimizing joint function. Supportive devices, including joint supports, canes, and proper footwear, may be of significant benefit. Simple analgesic medications can be used. Since some degree of inflammatory cell action may be present as deterioration progresses, presumably in an attempt to remove debris, some patients with osteoarthritis have better symptom control with the judicious use of nonsteroidal anti-inflammatory drugs (NSAIDs) than with simple analgesics. Occasional intra-articular corticosteroid injections may have symptomatic benefit. Potent systemic corticosteroids or immunomodulatory drugs have no role.[4] While radiographs help define and grade degenerative joint disease, there are no other laboratory tests of utility in this process. In the near future, however, blood levels of certain cartilage matrix glycoproteins may give an index of the rate of cartilage deterioration.

Rheumatoid Arthritis

The most common form of inflammatory arthritis resulting from chronic immune dysregulation is rheumatoid arthritis (RA). Occurring at any age, the peak incidence is in the 30- to 50-year-old population, with a 3:1 female predominance. All the cardinal signs of inflammatory synovitis become evident in the untreated patient; when present for more than 6 weeks, most infectious or other extrinsic causes of such inflammation can be excluded.

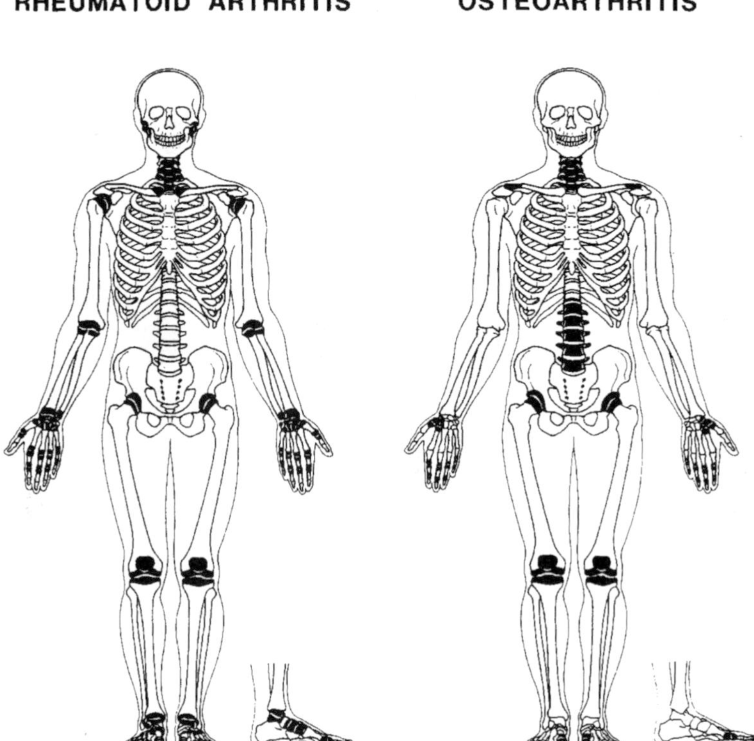

Fig. 11-2. Commonly involved joints in arthritis. (Courtesy of Healthwest Regional Medical Center, Phoenix, AZ.)

Morning stiffness can be very prolonged. The distribution of RA is peculiarly symmetric in most cases or becomes so with the passage of time. The distribution is not influenced by mechanical stresses but by unknown forces that allow the disease to involve virtually any joint variably, typically metacarpal phalangeal (MCP) joints, wrists, elbows, temporomandibular joints, and cervical spine, while inexplicably sparing the distal interphalangeal (DIP) joints and the rest of the spine and sacroiliac joints (Fig. 11-2).

Several extra-articular manifestations can occur, and virtually all organ systems may be affected in particular ways (Fig. 11-3). Sjögren syndrome, a condition involving chronic inflammation in exocrine glands resulting in dryness of eyes, mouth, and vaginal mucosa, often accompanies RA and other autoimmune syndromes. Constitutional symptoms of low-grade fever and fatigue are common, as is the presence of rheumatoid nodules. ESR and CRP usually accord a physiologic numerical value to help follow management of inflammation, and low-grade anemia typically develops. There are no diagnostic laboratory tests. So-called rheumatoid factor is an autoantibody that occurs in about 80 percent of RA patients by 1 year of disease but does not occur exclusively in RA, nor does its absence negate the diagnosis. Physical measures combined with aggressive anti-inflammatory and immunomodulatory drug therapy round out disease management.[5]

Spondyloarthropathies

The term *spondyloarthropathies* is given to a group of inflammatory arthritides that are classed together because of certain shared characteristics. These include asymmetric oligoarthritis, sacroiliitis, dactylitis (inflammation occurring in the DIP joints), enthesitis (inflammation occurring at the site of tendinous and ligamentous insertion into periarticular bone), absence of rheumatoid factor, and an increased prevalence in persons whose genome codes for the cell surface marker HLA-B27.[6] These entities are separated nosologically by the presence of significant inflammatory disease in other organ systems. Psoriatic arthritis, the arthritis of inflammatory bowel disease (enteropathic arthritis), reactive arthritis (Reiter syndrome, post-dysenteric and post-urethritic arthritis), and ankylosing spondylitis are the clinical subtypes. Table 11-2 displays the disease associations and extra-articular manifestations that typically occur with each syndrome. There are often overlapping features, raising the likelihood that each syndrome may represent a set of particular disease expressions for closely linked genes associated with immune dysregulation. The symptoms of ankylosing spondylitis, the prototype of the spondyloarthropathies with inflammatory back pain, are further characterized in the section on rheumatoid back and neck pain.

The spondyloarthropathies may occur in females as commonly as males, though the spinal manifestations are usually much less extensively expressed in women. The outcome in ankylosing spondylitis may be rigid fusion of most or all of the spine with a composite flexion posture. Early radiographic changes are typically seen at the sacroiliac joints, and, with further fusion of vertebral segments, the characteristic "bamboo spine" may become evident (Fig. 11-4). Limitation of spinal motion is measurable, although nonspecific. Inflammatory destruction of root joints (i.e., hips and shoulders) is common in ankylosing spondylitis, and up to one-third of affected persons will have peripheral arthritis in the knees, wrists, hands, ankles, and feet.

While radiographic changes of sacroiliitis and spondylitis are distinctive in well-established disease, no other laboratory tests are diagnostic. ESR may be moderately elevated with the spondyloarthropathies, and rheumatoid factor is characteristically absent. While HLA-B27 and newer genetic markers may define a population at increased risk of these disease expressions, none as yet is diagnostic. HLA-B27 occurs in about 8 percent of the American white population, and only about one in five individuals whose genome codes for this cell surface marker has any correlative signs of disease.

Management of inflammatory back disease and associated extraspinal findings, again, revolves around selected pharmacologic interruption of the inflammatory sequence of events. In the psoriatic and enteropathic variants, the back symptoms may improve with suppression of the associated disease. In addition to the usual physical therapy applications for peripheral joint disease, the therapist is called upon to educate the spondylitic patient in an extension maintenance program so that any eventual axial fusion will occur in the optimally functional position.

Rheumatic Back and Neck Pain

The origins of back pain are myriad and complicated, and the major impact of chronic back pain on health care expenditures and disability has been well recog-

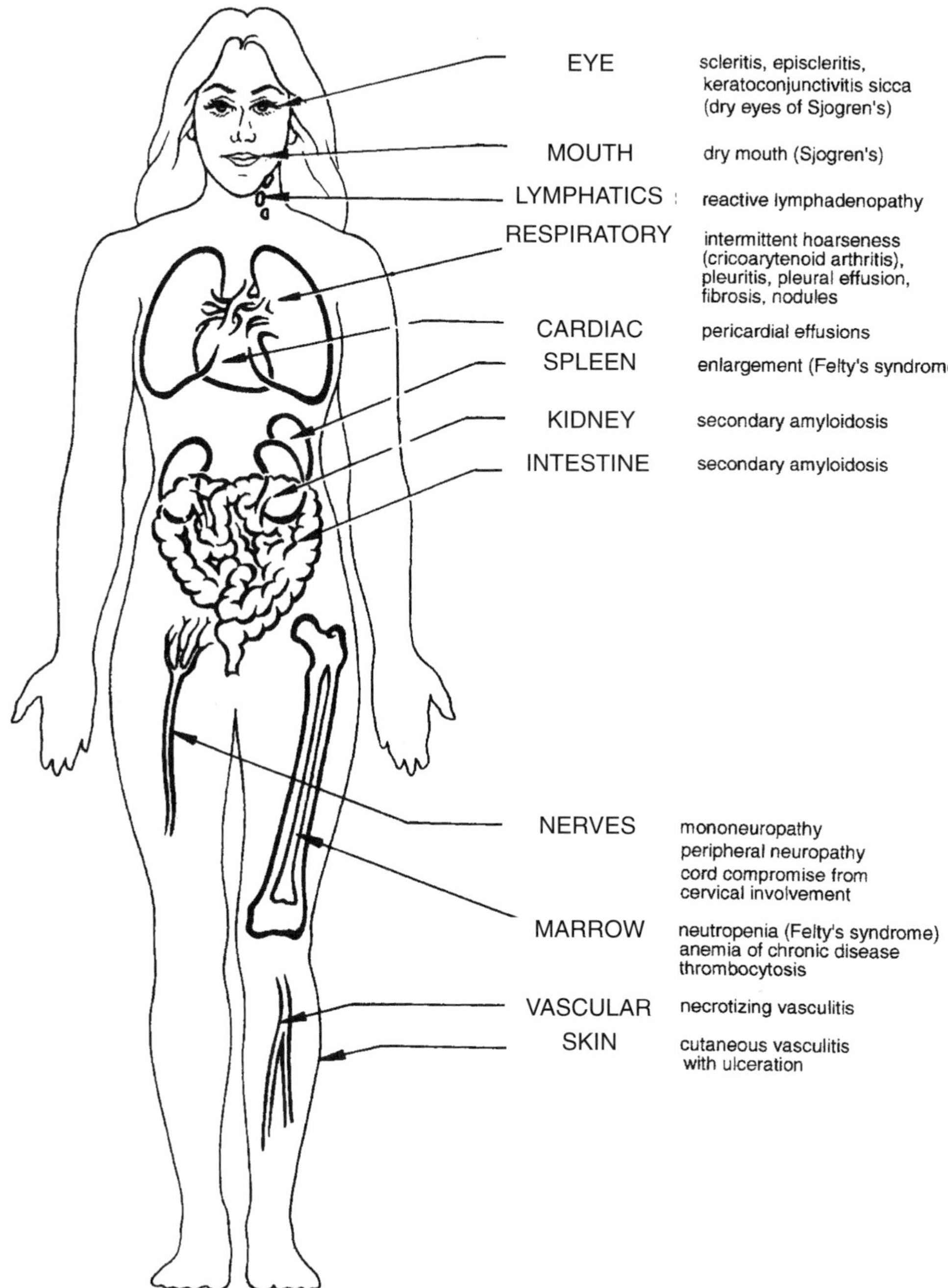

Fig. 11-3. Systemic features that may accompany rheumatoid arthritis. (Courtesy of Healthwest Regional Medical Center, Phoenix, AZ.)

Table 11-2. Differentiation of the Spondyloarthropathies

Spondyloarthropathy	Principal Disease Manifestations	Distribution of Arthritis	Extra-Articular Manifestations
Psoriatic arthritis	Psoriasis	Any small or large joint, including DIP joints (dactylitis), sacroiliitis common	Psoriatic pitting of nails common; eye inflammation
Arthritis of inflammatory bowel disease (enteropathic arthritis)	Crohn's disease; ulcerative colitis	Peripheral oligoarthritis, usually knees, ankles Unilateral sacroiliitis to extensive spondylitis	Eye inflammation, mouth ulcers, skin ulcers (pyoderma gangrenosum)
Reactive arthritis (including Reiter syndrome)	After urethritis or dysentery	Sacroiliitis, peripheral oligoarthritis predominantly of large joints of lower extremities, Achilles tendonitis	Eye inflammation urethritis, mouth ulcers, rash, (keratodermia blenorrhagica), penile rash (circnate balanitis)
Ankylosing spondylitis	Primary spinal arthritis	Spinal and pelvis articulations and entheses, including hips; occasional varying peripheral arthritis	Eye inflammation, aortitis with aortic murmur, lung fibrosis

nized. An exhaustive review of back pain etiologies exceeds the scope of this chapter; however, several key aspects in differentiating some sources of back pain merit particular attention when screening for rheumatic disease. Similarly, clinicians seeing patients with rheumatic disorders must be aware of certain concepts regarding the cervical spine.

Inflammatory Back Pain

Fundamental to discriminating back pain of inflammatory versus degenerative origin or musculoligamentous strain is an understanding of the nature of ankylosing spondylitis (AS). This inflammatory condition, which may affect all of the axial skeleton, tends to have a gradual onset invariably below the age of 40 and is usually dated to the second or third decade. In AS, and in the related spondyloarthropathies, when the sacroiliac or spinal segments are involved, pain and stiffness usually last several minutes to hours after rising and tend to improve with exercise. Since onset is insidious, patients generally are seen after several months of symptoms for which an inciting event cannot be recalled.

Contrast these features with mechanical back pain, which is also quite common in this younger age group who are likely to be engaged in heavy labor or athletic endeavors and at risk for lumbosacral musculoligamentous strain, herniated discs, or stress fractures. These patients would tend to present for evaluations very soon, if not immediately, after an easily recalled task or event that precipitated the back pain. Such conditions would be expected to improve with rest, analgesics, and physical therapy procedures within days to a few weeks. Characteristically, the discomfort associated with such injuries tends to be less after rest and to increase after activity, during the recovery phase. Therefore, the distinguishing clinical features for recognizing inflammatory back pain include (1) pain or stiffness that is worst in the morning and that improves with activity; (2) insidious onset; and (3) pain present for 3 months or more, with an onset of symptoms usually well below the age of 40.[7]

Danger Signs in Back Pain Patients

In relationship to the previous discourse on inflammatory and noninflammatory back pain, a few "red flags" should pique the therapist's attention when interviewing the patient with back pain. Patients should be asked about any known history of cancer. Several solid tumors, such as breast, lung, prostate carcinoma, and sarcomas, often metastasize to bone (see Ch. 10). Leukemias, lymphomas, and multiple myeloma may present with periarticular bone pain or back pain and, by the nature of their cellular origin, may produce various systemic autoimmune symptoms, such as fever, vasculitic rash, weight loss, and fatigue. A known history of malignancy should always raise concern for an association with any new skeletal pain. Undiagnosed malignancy should be suspected in the presence of new atraumatic back or bony pain that is constant and that varies little with position or motion. This red flag must not be clouded over by the presence of other established causes of rheumatic complaints.

Elderly postmenopausal women, and those treated with high doses of corticosteroids for prolonged periods,

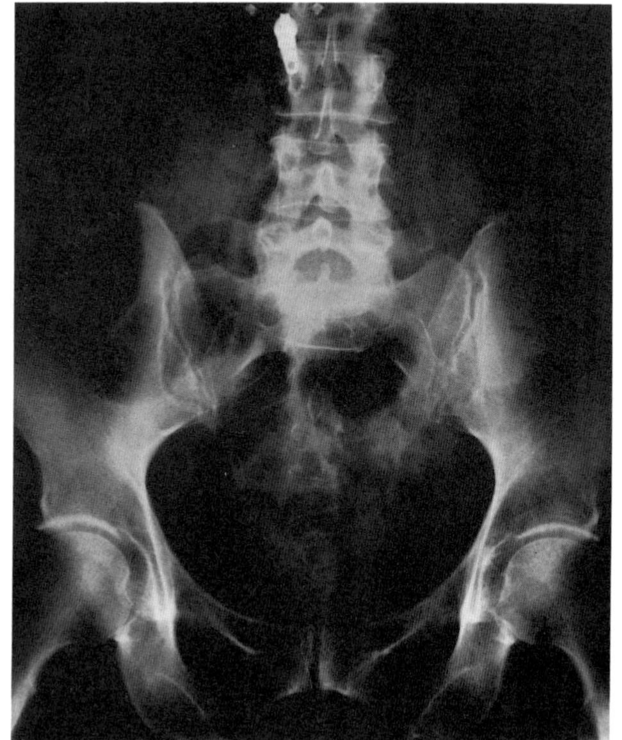

A

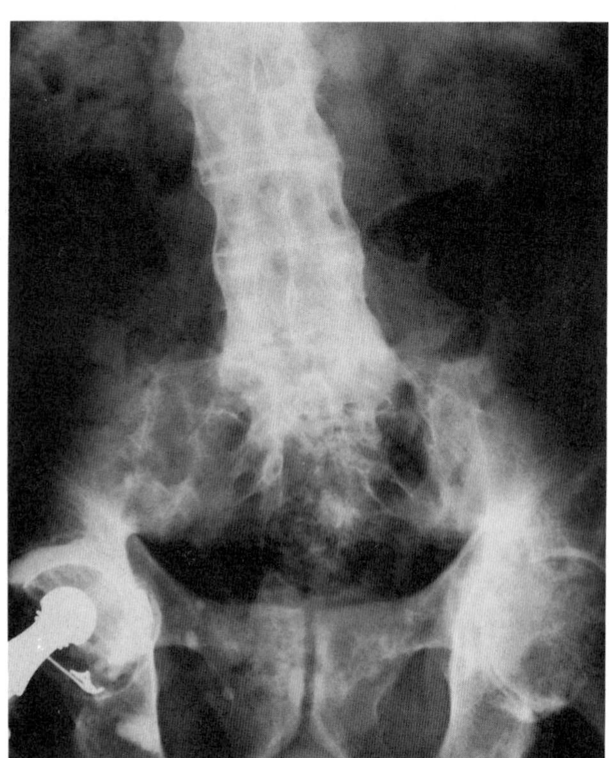

B

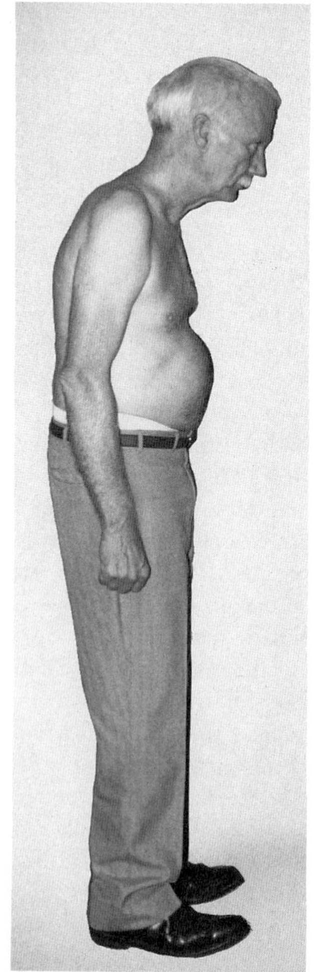

C

Fig. 11-4. (A) Normal pelvis and sacroiliac joints. **(B)** Advanced ankylosing spondylitis with fusion of sacroiliac joints and calcification of spinal ligamentous structures. Hips are affected, the right having undergone total hip arthroplasty. **(C)** Patient with fixed spinous posturing typical of ankylosing spondylitis. Note the increased dorsal kyphosis and cervical flexion. The protuberant abdomen is often found associated with these spinal changes. (Courtesy of Healthwest Regional Medical Center, Phoenix, AZ.)

may be at risk of osteoporosis (i.e., diminished bone density). The probability of hip, wrist, and other appendicular fractures increases with falls or trauma, but such persons may sustain compression fractures of thoracic or lumbar vertebrae with physiologic events, such as coughing, sneezing, squatting, or lifting very little weight. Acute onset of intense spinal pain and paraspinus spasm that worsens with the slightest movement should raise suspicion of compression fracture in these populations. Metastatic pathologic fractures of the spine may be clinically and radiographically identical. In patients not at risk of osteoporosis, further investigation, including computed tomography (CT) scanning, magnetic resonance (MR) imaging, or bone biopsy for carcinoma or infection, must be pursued.

Spinal Stenosis

Narrowing of the caliber of the spinal canal may result from tumor or abscess, inflammatory diseases including RA and ankylosing spondylitis, as well as degenerative changes. Bony facet thickening, disc bulging, posterior longitudinal or ligamentum flavum thickening, and segmental listhesis may compromise the cord or nerve roots (Fig. 11-5). Complaints from the patient of burning, tingling, searing, or aching pain in a radicular distribution will easily prompt an evaluation and diagnosis of neural impingement. However, the symptoms of cord compromise in some patients may be other than neuritic. Several historical clues to neural impingement may be available to the clinician, even when neuritic symptoms are absent and objective changes on sensory, motor, or reflex examination or electrophysiologic testing are not evident.

Symptomatic lumbar canal stenosis secondary to degenerative spondylosis, as opposed to intraspinus abscess or tumor, has a gradual onset. Typical symptoms might include worsening of lumbar pain when standing in one place, such as at the kitchen sink or counter, for which the patient relates having to bend forward at the waist and lean on the arms to get relief. In this circumstance, a sense of weakness or "rubberiness" in the legs or burning ache in the buttocks may accompany the increased low back pain. Sitting or lying further relieves these symptoms. In addition, neurogenic claudication may occur (i.e., buttock pain or leg weakness when walking) with or without increased lumbar pain or neuritic symptoms. Neurogenic claudication must always be distinguished from vascular (ischemic) claudication resulting from peripheral vascular insufficiency. An historical clue is that the pain of vascular claudication tends to arise in the buttocks, thighs, or calves more quickly after a reproducible distance, at the usual walking rate, and

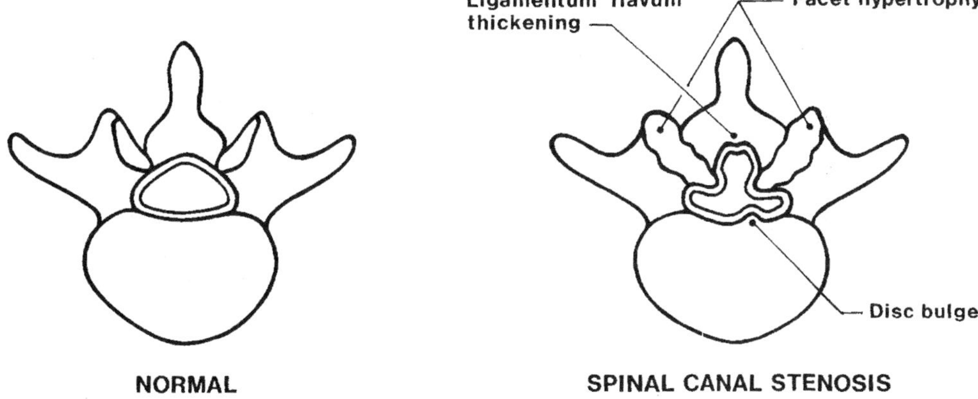

Fig. 11-5. Compromise of the spinal canal in degenerative disease. (Courtesy of Healthwest Regional Medical Center, Phoenix, AZ.)

likewise tends to subside more abruptly with rest and often merely by standing still. Neurogenic symptoms, by contrast, tend to wax and wane more gradually with walking and rest. In either disorder, strength and deep tendon reflexes are usually normal, although in lumbar canal stenosis weakness and transient decrease in reflexes may be detectable if checked immediately after walking. Diminished or absent pedal pulses are a clear indicator of compromised arterial flow. The two conditions, neurogenic claudication from lumbar stenosis and vascular claudication from arterial stenosis, commonly coexist in older persons.

Inflammatory Neck Pain

Nontraumatic cervical stenosis occurs usually as a result of advanced degenerative spondylosis but may result from inflammatory disease, particularly rheumatoid arthritis and ankylosing spondylitis. Symptoms of cord and root compromise may run the gamut from radicular symptoms to weakness, areflexia or spasticity, to drop attacks and loss of bowel or bladder control, and potentially to quadriplegia or respiratory arrest. A progressive presentation of cervical cord compromise may mimic the presentation of multiple sclerosis as a group of focal neurologic deficits, initially intermittent, separated by time of onset and neural pathways.

The rheumatoid cervical spine deserves special comment. Facet and ligamentous disruption with shifting of segments and distortion of the canal and neuroforamina may occur, principally in the midcervical segments (Fig. 11-6). This avenue of change usually occurs indolently. Patients typically complain of weakness, often initially attributed to their peripheral arthritis. By contrast, instability of the atlantoaxial articulation often precipitates more acute complaints. The odontoid process of C2 may become loosened from its ligamentous moorings within the anterior portion of the ring of C1 as a result of inflammation (Fig. 11-7). Similarly, erosive synovitis at this rotatory articulation may lead variably to blunting or disintegration of the odontoid or to whittling of this structure to a fine point. This process may allow the odontoid to move posteriorly into the canal, impinging neural tissue, or migrate upward to impale the brain stem. With unchecked motion, especially with forceful or sustained cervical flexion, the results may be devastating, and sudden paralytic respiratory death is a recognized complication. Harbingers of such life-threatening inflammation include severe neck pain and spasm with intense occipital pain, lightning pains into extremities, drop attacks, incontinence, intermittent paresis of any or all extremities, or complaints from the patient of a sense that his or her head may fall off.[8]

Lateral flexion and extension plain radiographs may give a clue to the amount of motion at the odontoid in the anteroposterior plane. MR imaging best defines the integrity of the relationships of the bony structures and neural components in this area. Management may require neurosurgical intervention with transoral odontoidectomy and fusion of C1 and C2, but this must be

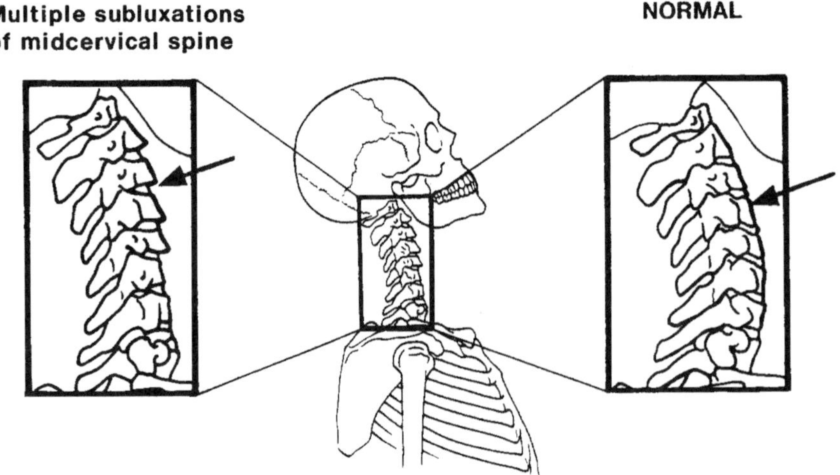

Fig. 11-6. Rheumatoid cervical spine. Multiple segmental subluxations may cause narrowing of the spinal canal and pressure on spinal cord and nerve roots. (Courtesy of Healthwest Regional Medical Center, Phoenix, AZ.)

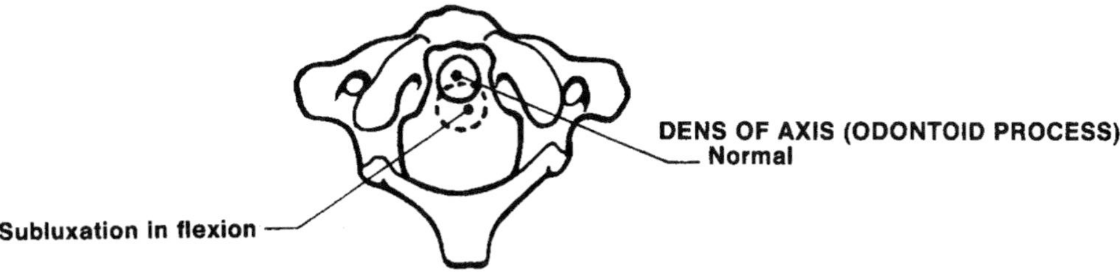

Fig. 11-7. Rheumatoid cervical spine. Remodeling of the dens and loosening of its attachments as a result of inflammation may cause impingement of the spinal cord. (Courtesy of Healthwest Regional Medical Center, Phoenix, AZ.)

weighed against the potentially grave surgical risks. Often the most appropriate management is a rigid cervical collar, strict avoidance of cervical manipulation or inertial injuries, and meticulous care to avoid hypermobilization when intubating or moving the anesthetized rheumatoid patient at surgery.

The cervical spine in ankylosing spondylitis may fuse in its entirety, generally with loss of the normal lordotic curve, to form a single osseus beam. Occasionally, fractures through this fusion mass sustained in a fall will give the patient a sense of regained motion in the neck. Such a history should prompt the clinician to evaluate for potential cervical instability.

Muscular Rheumatism

The approach to differentiating the etiology of muscular disorders in screening for rheumatic disease begins with an attempt to clarify the most prominent aspect of the muscular complaint (i.e., weakness or pain). Overlap of these two principal symptoms is extremely common; however, a careful history and examination will most often discriminate the hallmark feature.

Polymyositis

Inflammation in muscle leads primarily to weakness. Polymyositis is a term applied to conditions of inflammatory cell infiltration in muscle tissue, resulting histopathologically in edema of the interstitial zones, with muscle fiber necrosis and regeneration. The release of elevated levels of creatine phosphokinase and aldolase in the blood is typical, although nonspecific. Characteristic features of inflammation are usually detectable by electromyography (EMG), including insertional irritability, fibrillation potentials, and positive sharp waves.

Polymyositis may occur as a primary disease of unknown etiology. When accompanied by certain skin manifestations, it is called dermatomyositis. A heliotrope rash, appearing as faint erythema and puffiness around the eyes, photosensitive dermatitis of the face and of the neck, papular vasculitic lesions of the extremities and trunk, and Gottron's papules occurring over the dorsum of the MCP and proximal interphalangeal (PIP) joints as thick erythematous lesions that commonly ulcerate, are tip-offs to underlying intense chronic muscular inflammation (see Fig. 11-8). Polymyositis may also occur as a mild or prominent component of other rheumatic diseases, such as SLE, RA, scleroderma, or vasculitis, or represent a paraneoplastic

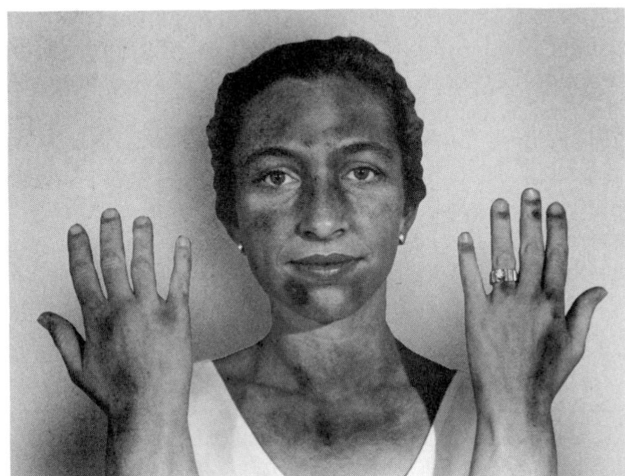

Fig. 11-8. Dermatomyositis. Note heliotrope facial rash, photosensitive dermatitis on neck and hands, and faint Gottron's papules on a few metacarpophalangeal and interphalangeal joints. (Courtesy of Healthwest Regional Medical Center, Phoenix, AZ.)

phenomenon in the presence of recognized or occult malignancy (Table 11-3).[9] Interstitial fibrosis, proximal dysphagia, myocarditis, and arthritis may be clinical features in polymyositis and dermatomyositis.

Muscular inflammation is typified by several common complaints, signaling predominantly proximal limb girdle weakness. Patients develop difficulty arising from chairs without help, climbing stairs, brushing hair or teeth, or similar activities requiring substantial proximal motor power. Muscle pain and tenderness usually pale by comparison to the aspect of weakness in inflamed muscle. Normal sensory findings and reflexes that persist until muscle weakness is advanced help to distinguish polymyositis from neuropathic weakness.

Even on muscle biopsy, differentiating inflammatory muscle disease from primary degenerative muscle disease (muscular dystrophy) may be difficult. Tissue that demonstrates an intense chronic inflammatory cell infiltrate supports the former. Other clinical features with respect to age and the involved muscle distribution may help distinguish the various forms of muscular dystrophy from typical polymyositis. Special stains and electron microscopy can usually sort out inclusion body myopathy, dysgenetic storage myopathies, and parasitic infection of muscle. Inflammatory muscle disease usually requires potent anti-inflammatory and immunomodulatory therapy for extended periods of time.

Myasthenia Gravis

Myasthenia gravis appears to be an autoimmune disorder wherein autoantibodies may destroy the myoneural junction. By both EMG and muscle strength testing, these patients display rapidly ensuing weakness after initial strength following a period of rest and may be present in virtually any muscle. Response to cholinesterase inhibitors may be helpful in diagnosis (Tensilon test),[10] as well as in the primary management. The detection of antibodies to acetylcholine receptors is also supportive. Tumors of the thymus, a primary organ of immune lymphocyte development, may accompany myasthenia gravis and should be sought and potentially resected. Immune modulatory therapy with corticosteroids, immunosuppressive drugs, and plasmapheresis are required in many cases.

Table 11-3. Classification of Polymyositis-Dermatomyositis[a]

Group	Description
I	Primary idiopathic polymyositis
II	Primary idiopathic dermatomyositis
III	Dermatomyositis (or polymyositis) associated with neoplasia
IV	Childhood dermatomyositis (or polymyositis) associated with vasculitis
V	Polymyositis (or dermatomyositis) with associated collagen vascular disease

[a]Classification suggested by Bohan et al.[9]

Polymyalgia Rheumatica and Giant Cell Arteritis (Temporal Arteritis)

Pain, rather than weakness, typifies this nosologic entity. Although a diagnosis of exclusion, the usual clinical features of polymyalgia rheumatica (PMR) cry out for recognition that only comes when the clinician is keenly aware of this clinical syndrome. The pathogenesis is not clear but may relate to subclinical synovitis involving the joints of the shoulder and pelvic girdles. Diffuse but predominantly proximal muscular and joint pain on motion, occurring acutely or subacutely in older people, should suggest PMR. Tenderness of muscles may be present or absent, typically without joint swelling. PMR rarely occurs below the age of 60, and most patients with this syndrome can recall the day, if not the hour, in which the pain began. These older persons can clearly distinguish subjectively their new pain from previous stiffness of degenerative joint disease. There are no diagnostic tests or findings on muscle biopsy, but as a rule of thumb the ESR is elevated numerically to approximate or exceed the patient's age. Low-grade fever and anemia with mild elevation in liver function enzymes are common systemic findings, but muscle enzymes are normal, and no autoantibodies are found. Other pulmonary or gastrointestinal influenzalike symptoms are typically absent. A dramatic, often overnight, response to low doses of corticosteroids is very supportive of the diagnosis of PMR. Bacterial infection should be ruled out with blood cultures. Rarely, a PMR-like presentation may foretell the presence of an occult solid malignancy, and a thorough physical examination is essential.

An important caveat when considering the diagnosis of PMR is the frequent coexistence in such patients of a specific type of vasculitis referred to as temporal arteritis or giant cell arteritis (see Ch. 8). New-onset severe headaches, especially temporal, with eye pain, and visual symptoms such as blurring or double vision suggest temporal arteritis. Other key symptoms may include aching in the masseter, temporalis, or tongue muscles with persistent speaking or chewing, neck pain with swallowing during a meal, scalp tenderness with hair brushing, or bulging and tender temporal arteries. Extremely high ESR is common, and a biopsy of temporal artery is needed for confirmation. Without rapid treatment with high doses of corticosteroids, this idiopathic arterial inflammation may result in blindness, stroke, or other vasculopathic outcomes.

Other forms of vasculitis may present with muscle pain and tenderness but are usually accompanied by cutaneous signs, such as palpable purpura, skin ulcerations, or ischemic digital infarcts.[11]

Fibromyalgia

Fibromyalgia syndrome, also known as fibrositis, must be distinguished from inflammatory muscle disease and synovitis. Patients with this noninflammatory condition complain of tightness and aching in muscles and of joint stiffness, as well as a subjective sense of swelling in the hands and feet and at times variable and fleeting radicular symptoms. Objective signs of joint inflammation are absent, however, and neurologic examination, including motor strength, is normal. Physical examination demonstrates a pattern of tender points (Fig. 11-9) that appears to be reproducible from patient to patient. Several investigators suggest that the symptoms and hypersensitivity of muscles and fibrous tissue are associated with a disturbance of sleep, and a history of nonrestful sleep is usually elicited from such patients.[12] The symptoms may be chronic and ongoing or intermittent in association with stressful times. Laboratory testing, including ESR, should be normal, unless the sleep disturbance is fostered by other medical illness associated with an elevated ESR. Recognition of the syndrome and explanation to the patient are of paramount importance. Instruction in sleep hygiene and use of certain hypnotic drugs may help to restore more physiologic sleep. Regular low-impact exercise also appears to be beneficial when other medical conditions allow. Hypothyroidism is a common clinical entity that mimics fibromyalgia and should be screened (see Ch. 7).

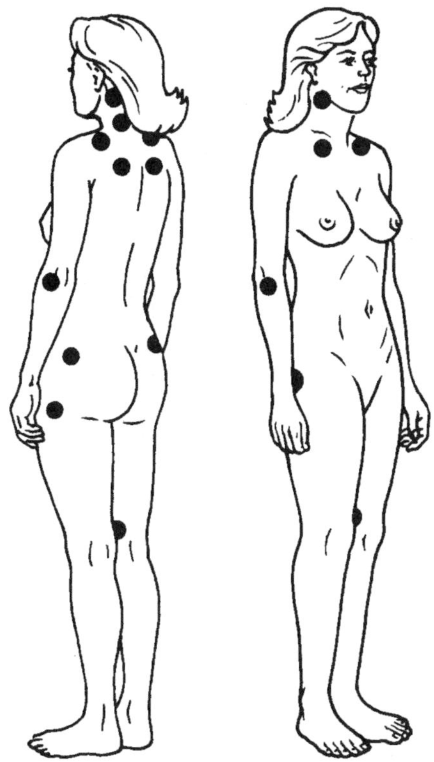

Fig. 11-9. Fibromyalgia, tender points. **Definition:** Pain on digital palpation. **Occiput:** Bilateral, at the suboccipital muscle insertions. **Low cervical:** Bilateral, at the anterior aspects of the intertransverse spaces at C5–C7. **Trapezius:** Bilateral, at the midpoint of the upper border. **Supraspinatus:** Bilateral, at origins, above the scapular spine near the medial border. **Second rib:** Bilateral, at the second costochondral junctions, just lateral to the junctions on upper surfaces. **Lateral epicondyle:** Bilateral, 2 cm distal to the epicondyles. **Gluteal:** Bilateral, in upper outer quadrants of buttocks in anterior fold of muscle. **Greater trochanter:** Bilateral, posterior to the trochanteric prominence. **Knee:** Bilateral, at the medial fat pad proximal to the joint line. (Courtesy of Healthwest Regional Medical Center, Phoenix, AZ.)

Other Noninflammatory Pain Syndromes

Several clinical entities deserve brief note because of their propensity to present to the physical therapist for management, often under a presumed misdiagnosis. A high index of suspicion is required for each of these nosologies.

Benign Hypermobility Syndrome

Patients with lax joints, such as in Ehlers-Danlos type III collagenosis, or other subtle developmental differences in collagen structure, are at risk of premature degenerative joint disease. Commonly, such patients complain in adolescent years of prolonged aching in the joints and tendons after engaging in activities, but no signs of inflammation or degenerative joint disease are evident. A history or demonstration of excessive joint motion is suggestive and may include the ability to extend the fingers passively for close approximation of the wrist, flexing the thumb to the wrist, hyperextension of the elbows or knees to 190 degrees or more, or placing the palms to the floor from a standing position with knees locked in extension. Patients may be able to sit with legs tightly interlocked (so-called lotus position); to lift a foot forward to place it behind the head; or to relate "double-jointedness" with easily subluxed shoulders, hips, or patellae.[13] Maturing collagen begins to lessen such hypermobility. In the meantime, efforts to avoid premature degenerative joint disease by counseling toward low-impact conditioning exercises and the avoidance of sports that embody extension stress (gymnastics, ballet) may be helpful.

Reflex Sympathetic Dystrophy Syndrome

Also known as shoulder-hand syndrome, although it occasionally occurs in the foot, reflex sympathetic dystrophy syndrome represents a poorly understood autonomic response in an extremity to a variety of clinical insults. Progressive causalgic (burning) pain and tenderness, especially in the hand or foot, is accompanied early on by diffuse swelling, coolness, and mottling, and later by atrophy, loss of skin appendages, and contracture. This sequence of events may take weeks or months and must be interrupted by intensive physical therapy. At times corticosteroids and sympathetic blockade are needed to avoid permanent limb dysfunction. Inciting events most commonly include shoulder injury (shoulder-hand syndrome), intrathoracic or intracranial malignancy, stroke, or trauma in the lower extremity.[14]

Aseptic Osteonecrosis

Sudden loss of nutrient arterial flow to subcortical bone may result in flattening of humeral head, femoral head, or femoral condylar bone with acute pain and destruction of these major joints.[15] The typical presentation is that of an adult in the third to sixth decade with atraumatic subacute large joint pain at rest, worsening with motion and weight bearing. Although similar pathology in the wrist or tarsus may follow trauma, the more common settings that should trigger an investigation for osteonecrosis are alcoholism, high-dose corticosteroid use, SLE, and sickle cell disease. Radionuclide bone scanning may suggest osteonecrosis, even before the findings of subcortical lucency or cortical flattening are evident on plain radiographs.

Hypertrophic Osteoarthropathy

Pulmonary, cardiac, or liver disorders may induce this peculiar osseus disease characterized by clubbing of digits, synovitis in distal joints, and aching and tenderness in the shafts of long bones in the extremities (see Ch. 2, Fig. 2-11). Such tenderness correlates with periosteal thickening seen on radiographs, and even earlier on radionuclide bone scanning. Elevation of the extremities often gives temporary dramatic relief of pain, and this complex of findings may resolve rapidly with successful treatment of the underlying visceral pathology.

Referred Pain

Pain referred from intra-abdominal, pelvic, or intrathoracic organs is an important consideration in evaluating atypical musculoskeletal complaints. (This issue is reviewed in Ch. 1.)

Acutely Swollen Joint

Most rheumatologic care is applied to chronic disease entities. While early diagnosis almost universally carries advantages, there is usually time for careful observation of unfolding clinical patterns. By contrast, acute monarthritis with effusion is a clinical presentation that demands urgent clarification and management because of intense pain and the potential for rapid articular destruction.

Acute Septic Arthritis

Bacterial infection in the joint requires prompt and adequate drainage and intensive antibiotic therapy to prevent rapid cartilage destruction and invasion of adjacent bone. The septic joint displays all the signs of inflammation with effusion and is generally accompanied by fever and chills. In addition to immediate aspiration for microbiological studies and joint space decompression, an investigation for the portal of infection is necessary. Even when chronic inflammatory arthritis such as RA is present, joint sepsis must be ruled out when an isolated intensely inflamed joint and fever develop. Indeed, joints with preexisting damage from other disorders are more susceptible to hematogenous seeding of bacterial, fungal, or tubercular organisms.

Acute Crystalline Arthropathy

The term crystalline arthropathy principally encompasses gout and pseudogout. Gout is a disorder of purine metabolism resulting in an accumulation of the byproduct uric acid. Crystals of monosodium urate may develop in various tissues, including synovial lining, and may intermittently shower into the synovial fluid, precipitating an intensely painful inflammatory reaction. Any joint may be involved, but the most commonly susceptible seem to be the first metatarsal phalangeal joint, knee, tarsus, and wrist. Men may be affected as early as the second decade, but women rarely before menopause. The blood uric acid level is usually elevated in gout but is not diagnostic, and gout may clearly be present with normal uric acid levels. Definitive diagnosis depends on microscopic demonstration of monosodium urate crystals in synovial fluid. Acute attacks are managed with anti-inflammatory drugs, and the disease is usually well controlled over the long term with medications to reduce total body load of uric acid (see Ch. 14).

Pseudogout manifests in a very similar clinical fashion as gout, but is not related to monosodium urate handling. Rather, the episodes of acute joint inflammation are induced by calcium pyrophosphate crystals (calcium pyrophosphate deposition). Calcification of joint cartilage may be appreciated on radiographs, and polarized microscopic evaluation of aspirated joint fluid can distinguish the crystal types. Anti-inflammatory drug therapy and analgesics as well as rest are helpful. Some cases of pseudogout are associated with other disorders of metabolism such as thyroid and parathyroid dysregulation or degenerative joint disease.

Hemarthrosis

Hemarthrosis, or bloody joint effusion, must be ruled out in post-traumatic acute effusions of large joints. Spontaneous hemarthrosis can occur in a variety of inherited coagulation disorders, most commonly factor 8 and 9 deficiencies (hemophilia A and B, respectively). Such effusions are usually warm, tense, tender, and painful with motion. Except in the hip, a bluish hue may be appreciated about the joint.

In the absence of evidence of infection, crystals, or blood, joint aspiration of the acutely inflamed joint will still help differentiate a noninflammatory effusion of injury or degenerative joint disease from the onset of new inflammatory arthritis by virtue of the total leukocyte count and differential count in the synovial fluid.

RHEUMATIC SYNDROMES ASSOCIATED WITH INFECTION

Any acutely inflamed joint in the presence of recognized infection in other organ systems is suspect for hematogenous spread of the organism to the joint space. In contrast, as discussed under the spondyloarthropathies, an immunologically mediated reactive arthritis may follow infection with such enteric pathogens as some species of *Salmonella*, *Shigella*, *Yersinia*, *Campylobacter*, and others, or with urinary pathogens such as *Chlamydia* species, without the actual presence of organisms in the joints. Symptoms of intestinal or urogenital infections, therefore, should always be sought in the evaluation of new arthritis (see Chs. 4, 5, and 6).[16]

Similarly, rheumatic fever is an immunoreactive process in susceptible individuals following group A β-hemolytic streptococcal pharyngitis. Along with various cutaneous, cardiac, and neurologic features, acute inflammatory arthritis of one or more joints may occur. Demonstration of high titers of antistreptococcal antibodies (streptozyme test and others) at the peak of joint symptoms is supportive (Table 11-4).[17]

Table 11-4. Jones Criteria for Guidance in the Diagnosis of Rheumatic Fever[a]

Major Manifestations	Minor Manifestations
Carditis	Clinical
Polyarthritis	Fever
Chorea	Arthralgia
Erythema marginatum	Previous rheumatic fever or
Subcutaneous nodules	rheumatic heart disease
Plus	
Supporting evidence of preceding streptococcal infection:	
Increased ASO or other streptococcal antibodies	
Positive throat culture for group A *Streptococcus*	
Recent scarlet fever	

[a]The presence of two major criteria, or of one major and two minor criteria, indicates a high probability of the presence of rheumatic fever if supported by evidence of a preceding streptococcal infection. The absence of the latter should make the diagnosis suspect, except in situations in which rheumatic fever is first discovered after a long latent period after the antecedent infection (e.g., Syndenham's chorea or low-grade carditis). (Based on Stollerman et al.[17])

Infective endocarditis is associated with diffuse myalgias and synovitis of one or more joints. The presence of fever, a new or changing heart murmur, and cutaneous signs of septic emboli are highly suggestive of endovascular infection. Blood cultures will usually readily identify the pathogen (see Ch. 2). In endocarditis, a reactive synovitis or true septic arthritis may occur.[18]

Lyme disease is mediated by the spirochete *Borrelia burgdorferii* and is transmitted by the bite of the *Ixodes dammini* tick. Early manifestations include constitutional symptoms and a violaceous spreading rash, called erythema chronicum migrans. Later manifestations involve a variety of neuropathic and cardiac findings and, weeks to months later, arthritis of one or more joints. Interestingly, some patients are not fully evaluated until seen for arthritis. Because of the increasing incidence and widening endemic areas for this infection, patients with new inflammatory arthritis should be questioned about time spent in wooded areas, tick bites, and the typical rash or antecedent (or concomitant) neurologic or cardiac symptoms. Supportive serology for Lyme antibodies and urine testing for antigens from the spirochete are available. Appropriate antibiotic therapy usually results in cure and appears to be more successful earlier in the disease.[19]

PATIENT CASE STUDY

History

A 17-year-old high school student came to the clinic with a diagnosis of rheumatoid arthritis and a chief complaint of occipital headaches and posterior cervical pain. The headaches and cervical pain were constant, with the intensity increasing with prolonged forward flexed postures such as when studying. Slight relief was noted after the application of ice. These symptoms began 3 years ago insidiously and were intermittent. Approximately 2 months before the evaluation the complaints became constant. The patient could not relate the regression to a particular incident or accident. She noted that her neck would lock up on her at times, making it difficult to move her head. This could happen three to four times per day. She denied any dysthesias, episodes of paralysis, drop attacks, or bowel or bladder incontinence.

The patient was diagnosed with rheumatoid arthritis when she was 15 years old. She noted periodic soreness in both wrists and knees and in the right temporomandibular joint. The patient also noted periods of fatigue, poor appetite, and diarrhea. Her surgical history was negative, and aspirin in high dosages was the only medication she was taking.

Physical Examination

Observation revealed a moderate forward posture with protracted shoulders. Moderate muscle guarding was palpated posteriorly from the occiput to the upper scapular region. Active left rotation of the neck was limited to 10° with a blocked, stuck sensation noted by the patient at end range in the left suboccipital region. She had 95° of right rotation and full forward bending without symptoms. Right sidebending was slightly reduced, with a sharp pulling sensation noted in the left suboccipital region. Backward bending was slightly reduced, with a sharp soreness noted in the left suboccipital area. The complaints noted by the patient during the active movements resolved immediately when the patient returned to neutral position. The patient reported a relief of the headache with manual traction of the head and neck. While maintaining the traction, the patient was asked to rotate to the left. She had 90° of motion without symptoms. This maneuver was repeated three times, after which the patient was asked to rotate to the left without the traction. She was able to rotate full range without symptoms. Passive segmental mobility testing revealed hypermobility at C1–C2 and hypomobility at C7, T1, and T2.

Treatment and Outcome

When the patient returned for the second visit, she had full active left rotation of the neck, but had only 40° of right rotation. She again complained of a blocked sensation at end range in the right suboccipital region. In the sitting position, manual traction was applied to the head and neck and the patient was asked to rotate to the right. She was able to rotate to the right fully, without symptoms. This was the pattern of the initial four to five visits; she would be limited at a certain point in the neck rotation range by a blocked sensation, usually felt on the ipsilateral side of the neck. Her mobility would be restored quickly with the manual traction maneuver or with a muscle energy technique for C1–C2 rotation. As treatment for the dysfunctions continued, the episodes

Review of systems checklist: Rheumatic disease

Item	Yes	No	Comments
1. Constitutional symptoms (fever, weight loss, loss of appetite, fatigue, and malaise) in absence of obvious infection	______	______	______
2. Mucocutaneous signs (i.e., mouth ulcers, rash), especially with sun exposure, or on mid-facial area not explained by infection or allergy	______	______	______
3. Joint pain not explained by strain or injury, especially with swelling, redness, heat, and stiffness	______	______	______
4. Chest pains with deep breathing (pleurisy) or substernal chest pain with lying (pericarditis) in absence of injury or infection	______	______	______
5. Persistent unexplained back or neck pain or stiffness	______	______	______
6. Persistent discomfort with urination, hematuria or cloudy urine, not explained by infection	______	______	______
7. Persistent or recurrent diarrhea not explained by infection	______	______	______
8. Unexplained progressive weakness	______	______	______

Fig. 11-10. Checklist for review of systems in screening for rheumatic disease.

of the patient being stuck during the day steadily decreased and the headaches and neck pain became intermittent and controlled with exercise.

As noted in this chapter joint instability can be a manifestation of rheumatic disease. This patient demonstrates that joint hypermobility may initially present as significant movement restriciton. Therapists need to be cognizant of the presence of diseases that may be manifested by joint instability and, if this history is present, take the necessary precautions regarding treatment techniques until the underlying dysfunction is understood. For this particular patient there were clinical signs that joint hypermobility could be an issue. The fact that her neck would become stuck periodically and that she would be able to restore mobility with some effort and then have full range of motion and that at times her neck would be limited in one direction and then in another support this hypothesis. The segmental mobility testing and the quick, dramatic response to the manual traction confirmed the supposition. The inherent marked range of motion normally available at the C1–C2 segment make it an area that is at risk for instability, and the relationship of the spinal cord to this segment carries potentially serious consequences if the therapist does not take proper precautions. The presence of neurologic signs would warrant a neurosurgical evaluation and avoidance of manipulation.

SUMMARY

Rheumatology is the medical subspecialty dedicated to the investigation and clinical management of rheumatic diseases. The key to screening for rheumatic disease is an appreciation of the observable effects of untoward inflammation in synovium, muscle, skin, and other organ systems (Fig. 11-10; see also Fig. 11-3 and Tables 11-1 and 11-2). Combined with a familiarity with the common syndromes outlined here, such an appreciation of inflammation will allow the physical therapist to guide patients toward appropriate medical management. Excellent comprehensive reviews of rheumatic disease are available in the texts listed under Suggested Readings.

REFERENCES

1. Tan SM, Cohen AS, Fries JF et al: The 1982 revised criteria for the classification of systemic lupus erythematosus. Arthritis Rheum 25:1271, 1982
2. Tan EM: Antinuclear antibodies: diagnostic markers for autoimmune diseases and probes for cell biology. Adv Immunol 44:93, 1989
3. Mankin HJ, Brandt KD, Shulman LE: Workshop on etiopathogenesis of osteoarthritis. J Rheumatol 13:1130, 1986
4. Altman RD: Osteoarthritis: aggravating factors and therapeutic measures. Postgrad Med 80:150, 1986
5. Harris ED Jr: Rheumatoid arthritis. Pathophysiology and implications for therapy. N Engl J Med 322:1277, 1990
6. Healey LA: Manifestations of B27: a hypothesis. Clin Rheumatol Pract Sep/Oct:222, 1984
7. Calin A, Porta J, Fries JF et al: Clinical history as a screening test for ankylosing spondylitis. JAMA 237:2613, 1977
8. Bland JH: Rheumatoid subluxation of the cervical spine. J Rheumatol 17:134, 1990
9. Bohan A et al: A computer-assisted analysis of 153 patients with polymyositis and dermatomyositis. Medicine 56:255, 1977
10. Tether JE: p. 556. In Conn HF (ed): Current Therapy. WB Saunders, Philadelphia, 1965
11. Hunder GG et al: The American College of Rheumatology 1990 criteria for the classification of vasculitis. Arthritis Rheum 33:1065, 1990
12. Campbell SM et al: Clinical characteristics of fibrositis. I. A "blinded," controlled study of symptoms and tender points. Arthritis Rheum 26:817, 1983
13. McKusich VA: Heritable Disorders of Connective Tissue. 4th Ed. Mosby St. Louis, 1972
14. Kozin F et al: The reflex sympathetic dystrophy syndrome. Am J Med 60:321, 1976
15. Ficat P, Arlet J: Baltimore, p. 85. In Hungerford DS (ed): Ischemia and Necrosis of Bone. Williams & Wilkins, 1980
16. Keat A: Reiter's syndrome and reactive arthritis in perspective. N Engl J Med 309:1606, 1983
17. Stollerman GH, Markowitz M, Taranta A et al: Jones criteria (revised) for guidance in the diagnosis of rheumatic fever. Circulation 32:664, 1965
18. Churchill MA, Geraci TE, Hunder GG: Musculoskeletal manifestations of bacterial endocarditis. Ann Intern Med 87:754, 1977
19. Rahn DW: Lyme disease: Clinical manifestations, diagnosis, and treatment. Semin Arthritis Rheum 20:201, 1991

SUGGESTED READINGS

Kelly WM, Harris ED, Ruddy S, Sledge CB (eds): Textbook of Rheumatology. 4th Ed. WB Saunders, Philadelphia, 1993

McCarty DJ, Koopman WT (eds): Arthritis and Allied Conditions. 12th Ed. Lea & Febiger, Philadelphia, 1993

Schumacher HR, Klippel JH, Koopman WT (eds): Primer on Rheumatic Diseases. 19th Ed. Arthritis Foundation, Atlanta, 1993

Sheon RP, Moskowitz RW, Goldberg VM (eds): Soft Tissue Rheumatic Pain: Recognition, Management, Prevention. 2nd Ed. Lea & Febiger, Philadelphia, 1987

12 Screening for Psychological Disorders

Warren J. Bilkey, M.D.
Michael B. Koopmeiners, M.D.

Though poorly understood, the complex interaction between mind and body, psyche and soma, is universally appreciated in health care. Overlapping fields of psychiatry and psychology attempt to describe the process within a diagnostic and treatment framework. The physical therapist is often the first person to confront these issues when dealing with a new patient presenting with complaints of pain and disability.

This poses a seemingly difficult conceptual problem. Physical therapy and psychology are discrete, focused specialties with very different clinical viewpoints and relatively little understanding of each other's methodologies. Many patients are most efficiently addressed by the coordinated input of both disciplines. Early recognition of this need may determine a quick treatment success from a chronic, discomfortingly dependent, seemingly plateaued case that drains the clinician of patience and energy. Such is the subject of this chapter.

This chapter is clinically focused. Rather than presenting a broad academic view of psychology, the discussion is organized around a particularly difficult clinical problem in physical therapy: the pain patient. Orthopaedic, or manual, physical therapy is emphasized.

The psychological aspects of pain are reviewed, beginning with basic definitions and a general review of the effect of pain on the patient and the family. The relationship between pain and human personality is addressed, as is the diagnosis of specific psychiatric disorders and psychoses and their association with pain. Considering the prevalence of depression, this disorder is covered in detail. Related concerns of stress, abuse, and chemical dependency are reviewed. Assessment tools for psychopathology, specifically those appropriate to the practicing therapist, are presented and commented on. Finally, chronic pain syndrome and types of chronic pain rehabilitation are reviewed.

ACUTE AND CHRONIC PAIN

Pain is an unpleasant sensory and emotional experience associated with tissue damage or described in terms of tissue damage.[1] Pain may be acute or chronic, each producing different effects.[2] Acute pain, of recent onset, is typically associated with autonomic activity proportionate to the perceived intensity of the stimulus. Measurable increases occur with cardiac rate, stroke volume, blood pressure, palmar sweating, striated muscle tension, oxygen intake, glycogen release into the circulation, and adrenal release of epinephrine and norepinephrine. There are decreases in gut motility and cutaneous circulation.

The pattern demonstrates the fight-or-flight response. Anxiety reactions are associated with the same pattern of events. Indeed, patients with acute pain normally experience anxiety about the intensity of perceived significance of the pain. Therapeutic reduction of anxiety through medication or counseling usually reduces pain.

Chronic pain is of longer but differentially defined duration. In terms of appropriateness for manual intervention, chronic pain lasts beyond normal soft tissue healing time, ranging from 2 to 12 weeks. In terms of human psychology, chronic pain is of at least 6 months' duration, well beyond the patient's perceived expected time for resolution. A different pattern of normal consequences occurs, including sleep disturbance, change in appetite, decreased libido, irritability, social withdrawal, weakening of relationships, and increased somatic preoccupation. Habituation to the autonomic responses of acute pain may occur if the pain is not intermittent. This pattern of vegetative and other signs is typically seen in depressive reactions.

Psychological testing usually demonstrates depression in chronic pain patients. Depression may be masked by the patient's overwhelming preoccupation with somatic symptoms. Indeed, therapeutic reduction of depression usually results in reduction of pain. Alternatively, treatment of pain will reverse the neurotic depression caused by that pain.

Beyond the normally present depressive response to chronic pain, the afflicted patient is faced by an array of diverse problems.

Problems Facing the Chronic Pain Patient

- Personal issues
  - Loss of mobility
  - Physical change
  - Psychological distress
  - Loss of control of lifestyle
  - Change in body image
  - Diminished coping skills
  - Fear
- Interpersonal issues
  - Increased dependency on spouse and family
  - Sexual dysfunction
  - Diminished role in family functioning
  - Marital discord, separation, divorce
  - Isolation from family and social interaction
  - Impaired interpersonal skills
  - Self-defense of psyche in lieu of organic cause of pain
- Socioeconomic issues
  - Lost income after job loss
  - Confusion about eventual financial settlement
  - Stressful interactions with distrusting employer and agencies
  - Return-to-work issues
  - Monetary and social secondary gain

Persistent pain has a progressive impact on the patient's psychological and social well being.[3] There is confusion about the organic cause of the problem. Frequent humiliating medical examinations, inconvenient or painful tests, and unsuccessful treatment attempts add to the problem by causing psychological distress. The result is depression, anxiety, social isolation, lowered self-esteem, and fear. Fear may be spectacular. In spite of their suffering, these patients may be told, directly or indirectly, that the pain is psychogenic, that it is "all in the head." This approach further harms the therapeutic relationship and forces patients to take on the added burden of defending their psyche.

Secondary gain becomes important as a reinforcement for pain complaints. The more chronic the pain, the more extensive the secondary gain issues, and the more resistant the patient is to treatment. The needed disability compensation provides a financial incentive to hurt. Perhaps more powerful are the social responses to the "sick role," which provide for unmet dependency needs, enhancement of self-esteem, stabilization of weakened or immature personality, and conflict resolution of sexual and aggressive drives.

It is generally regarded that persistence of reinforced chronic pain beyond 2 years' duration is not fully curable. Patients rarely return to work if their pain was sufficient to cause them to be unemployed for more than 1 year.

Pain must be distinguished from nociception, suffering, and disability.[4] Nociception is the stimulus that activates A delta and C fibers, which signal the central nervous system (CNS) that tissue damage is occurring. Pain is the unpleasant sensation arising from perceived nociception. Pain may occur in the absence of nociception, such as with couvade syndrome (abdominal pains in men during their wives' labors or pregnancies). Nociception may occur without pain, as illustrated in Beecher's observations[5] of nonpainful yet severe combat injuries.

Suffering is the emotional response with attendant psychological distress triggered by perceived nociception.[6] Suffering is intimate and personal and is communicated to society by pain behavior. Disability is the social judgment (partially based on medical judgment and law) placed on the patient as a response to collected pain behaviors.

Pain behavior is influenced by culture, personality, and social context. Culture, or ethnic membership, partially determines the expressive style of suffering.[2] For example, Scandinavian Americans and Irish Americans are notably stoic. They tend to inhibit their pain expression. By contrast, Italian Americans and Jewish Americans demonstrate a lower pain tolerance and encourage its expression. Note that pain threshold, and not pain tolerance, remains stable cross-culturally.

Introversion–extroversion is the psychological continuum correlated with expression of suffering. The neurotic introvert will suffer in silence; the extrovert will tend to overcommunicate concerns. All communication and, more importantly, listener bias occurs within the framework of social context. Personality and psychological disorders have additional influence on somatic tolerance, pain threshold, the likelihood to develop chronic pain, resistance to purely mechanical treatment of pain syndromes, and effectiveness of communication with the clinician.

FAMILY DYNAMICS AND PAIN

Family dynamics have a major impact on the development and maintenance of chronic pain.[7] Marital maladjustment may challenge self-esteem and cause depression, with attendant chronic pain. Alternatively, family dysfunction may create dependency needs or leave existing needs unmet. The patient uses pain complaints to help satisfy these needs. Conflict may arise with unsatisfied aggressive drives, with the outlet being chronic pain. Pain may permit denial of unresolved family conflict. Pain is a powerful tool for manipulation of family members to seek attention and to avoid normal family role responsibilities while maintaining a sense of self-esteem. Chronic pain syndrome patients often come from families of chronic pain sufferers.

After a patient develops pain, the family, with benign intent, responds with pain-reinforcing behavior. Providing attention by being constantly present, by assisting with essential activities of daily living (e.g., dressing or bathing the patient, feeding or cutting the food, assisting with transfers or gait), and by being verbally sympathetic to disability and irresponsibility ("since the accident happened, you hurt too much to work") reinforces and perpetuates pain, suffering, and pain behavior. In reducing fear, these inputs further reinforce pain. Perhaps also with benign intent, the family may, in effect, "solve" marital dysfunction by making the sick role of the pain patient the scapegoat. This approach has the effect of stabilizing an unstable dysfunctional family relationship.

In the dysfunctional family, the spouse may become overprotective or may reject the patient. The former tends to fixate on pain behavior rather than on the person. The latter fails to offer sufficient support and participation in pain management.

Family dysfunction can be responsible for the chronic pain syndrome or can perpetuate it. These signs do not preclude mechanical treatment of mechanical dysfunction. Rather, they indicate a need for additional input of competent marital counseling, family therapy, or individual psychological consultation.

Signs of Family Dysfunction That May Have Significant Impact on Chronic Pain

- Current or past history of physical abuse or sexual abuse
- History of alcohol or other drug abuse
- History of criminal activity on the part of children or spouse
- History of extramarital affair of patient or spouse
- Patient says "family problems" exist or describes many family arguments
- Major economic difficulties
- History of suicide attempt by spouse/children
- Family assists with essential activities of daily living of patient (dressing, bathing, feeding)
- Chronic pain for longer than 2 years
- Family speaks for patient and attends all physical therapy sessions
- Family deserts patient at home
- Spouse appears overprotective or over-rejecting of patient
- Unemployed spouse
- Spouse or children living at home have chronic pain

PERSONALITY ISSUES AND PAIN

As with any stress, patients faced with disabling chronic pain employ adaptive defense mechanisms and available social supports to cope. The adaptive mechanisms depend on personality structure. Along the continuum of increasing pathologic behavioral significance, certain personalities, specific and perhaps odd personality traits, personality disorders, neuroses, and psychoses will modify patient suffering, pain behavior, and prognosis for outcome of an entirely manual approach to the presenting pain syndrome.

There is no accepted "unitary theory" of psychiatry that effectively combines normal behavior, thought and emotion, and psychopathology. It is attractive and useful to conceptualize continua of function (e.g., normal, borderline, severe dysfunction/incompetence) or continua of behavior (e.g., normal social interaction, "different," bizarre/threatening). Such is not the case for diagnosis. Psychosis is not simply a more severe neurosis. Indeed, recent trends in taxonomy view psychopathology as a collection of diseases, disorders, syndromes, traits, states, symptoms, and signs based on level of diagnostic certainty.

Realizing that the psychologically disturbed patient can have either mechanical or "psychogenic" pain, or both, puts the clinician in the difficult role of deciding if and when expert psychology consultation is necessary. This concept is never a clinical problem in the absence of diagnosed mechanical dysfunction. Difficulty arises when the mechanical dysfunctions appear not to explain the presented symptoms fully or when appropriate manual treatment fails to resolve symptoms. Should mechanical treatment proceed? Is concurrent referral to the psychology consultant indicated?

PSYCHIATRIC DISORDERS

What follows is a brief review of psychiatric disorders. Three primary references are drawn from two comprehensive textbooks of psychiatry[8,9] and the DSM III-R.[10] The American Psychiatric Association Diagnostic and Statistical Manual of Mental Disorders, 3rd edition, revised (DSM III-R) presents the current universally accepted taxonomy of psychiatric disorders. It lists all disorders and defines their diagnostic criteria. Each disorder is briefly discussed as it pertains to chronic pain. The major psychiatric disorders to be concerned with are the somatoform disorders, personality disorders, and affective disorders.

Somatoform Disorders

Somatoform disorders involve the expression of psychological distress through physical symptoms. Affected patients present physical symptoms that suggest a physical disorder for which there are no demonstrable organic findings or physiologic mechanism and for which there is evidence linking symptoms to psychological issues. These include conversion disorder, somatoform pain disorder, somatization disorder, and hypochondriasis. Factitious disorder and malingering are considered different because, in these cases, the patient presumably has voluntary, conscious control of symptoms. Psychophysiologic conditions are also considered a separate entity because a psychologically induced physiologic mechanism is indeed present to explain the etiology of symptoms (e.g., muscle tension headache).

The clinician must be aware of several major conceptual problems. Absence of a demonstrable etiologic physiologic mechanism for the symptom is the essential feature of somatoform disorders. Because classic medical teaching emphasizes the diagnosis of visceral, bone, joint, and nerve pathology and de-emphasizes the diagnosis and treatment of ligament, muscle, and joint motion dysfunctions, there is a very strong likelihood of misdiagnosis. Indeed, follow-up studies of diagnosed conversion disorder cases demonstrate 13 to 64 percent incidence of subsequent diagnosis of neurologic illness.

The manual clinician presents a significant new technology to medical diagnosis. All patients who present to the manual clinician with a diagnosis of somatoform disorder or malingering should be considered "virgin" and should receive a normal comprehensive, biomechanical assessment of their pain symptoms. Likewise, all medical literature to date on the topic of somatoform disorders must be studied with a pervading concern for blatant inaccuracy.

Psychophysiologic conditions present an equally difficult but more subtle problem because they pretend to provide an answer and may erroneously justify non-indicated treatment methodologies. For example, eager acceptance of muscle tension as an etiology of headache risks ignoring other potentially treatable causes, such as upper cervical spine mechanical dysfunction, regional weakness, cranial dysfunction, and temporomandibular joint dysfunction. Again, all cases require competent biomechanical examination.

Conversion Disorder

According to the DSM III-R, conversion disorder involves a pain-free loss or alteration of physical function that suggests a physical disorder. These are symptoms that the patient is not consciously producing and that cannot be explained by a known physical disorder. Psychological stressors or conflict must be demonstrably related to the onset or exacerbation of symptoms. Pain symptoms are classified under somatoform pain disorder. Autonomically mediated symptoms (e.g., fainting, palpitations, dizziness, tachycardia, dyspnea) are also excluded from the conversion disorder category.

Somatoform Pain Disorder

Somatoform pain disorder is characterized by the presence of severe pain for longer than 6 months either with no explainable pathophysiologic mechanism or in which the severity of complaints or resulting disability is in gross excess of that expected from the demonstrated organic pathology. This wide-ranging disorder tends to be subdivided by pain location (e.g., abdominal, low back, pelvic). Most chronic pain syndrome cases are considered to be somatoform pain disorders. Depression is frequently manifested in these patients.

Many theories have been offered to explain the psychophysiology of somatoform disorder. Unconscious guilt may be expressed as self-punishment with chronic pain, particularly in patients with life histories of abuse and defeat.[11] Another theory proposes effective noninhibition of autonomic activity and afferent stimulation centrally.[12] Behavioral theory implicates positive reinforcement from family members.[13]

Psychological distress, regardless of cause, may be reflected as pain complaint and suffering because somatic symptoms are culturally more acceptable to society, to the patient, and to co-workers. Somatic symptoms usually engender immediate social and professional attention, which unfortunately may reinforce dysfunctional pain behavior. Perhaps most important, pain complaints permit avoidance of the discomfort of direct confrontation with the psychosocial issues causing the psychological distress. Attention to the pain thus delays appropriate care of the psychological disorder.

Somatization Disorder

Somatization disorder is characterized by a history of multiple somatic complaints beginning before the age of 30 and persisting for several years. The clinical presentation tends to be dramatic and flamboyant with obsessively detailed symptoms and past histories of multiple hospitalizations and excessive surgery. Again, no organic pathology is found. Concerns must be significant enough for the patient to see physicians, take prescribed medication, or alter lifestyle. Beyond pain, symptoms complained of range across all organ systems. Somatization disorder has a high frequency of concurrent psychiatric disorder (e.g., depression, chemical dependency, phobia, mania).

Hypochondriasis

Hypochondriasis is characterized by an unrealistic chronic (more than 6 months') preoccupation with fear of having (or belief that one has) a serious disease, based on the patient's interpretation of sensations or physical signs. This fear or belief persists in spite of a negative medical evaluation and reassurance from the physician. The patient with exaggerated somatic awareness, capable of feeling or sensing every minor mechanical dysfunction, may be a borderline or overt hypochondriac. Depression is frequent.

Personality Disorders

Personality disorders are longstanding, inflexible behavior patterns, evident by late adolescence, that cause distress or that impair social and/or occupational functioning. These maladaptive, irrational ways of thinking, feeling, and acting significantly impair human interaction far beyond what is normally regarded as an odd character trait.

Personality disorders are divided into four groups: (1) eccentric (includes the schizotypal, schizoid, and paranoid disorders); (2) dramatic or erratic (includes the histrionic, narcissistic, antisocial, and borderline personality disorders); (3) anxious or fearful (includes the avoidant, dependent, obsessive-compulsive, and passive-aggressive disorders); and (4) self-defeating personality disorder.

Eccentric Personality Disorders

Schizotypal personality disorder typically presents with an eccentric manner of speaking, behavior, and appearance. Patients are nonemotional, paranoid, and socially isolated and have odd beliefs (e.g., superstitiousness: "others can feel my feelings"). By contrast, schizoid personality disorder presents a pervasive indifference to social relationships and a preference for social isolation. These patients are unresponsive to praise or criticism and are aloof and detached. Paranoid personality disorder presents an intense, driven suspiciousness, mistrust, and hypervigilance. A secondary hostility, irritability, and anxiety may occur when stressed.

The eccentric personality disorders are not frequently associated with chronic pain. The symptoms they present should be considered understated. Mechanical dysfunctions causing pain in this group should be approached in a direct, nonemotional, rational, and scientific manner. There is no benefit in attempting to provide emotional support or friendship. After mechanical problems are corrected, there should be prompt resolution of symptoms. If not, one should assume persistent organic pathology and proceed with further diagnostic study.

Dramatic Personality Disorders

Histrionic personality disorder is a pervasive pattern of excessive emotionality and attention seeking. These patients tend to be dramatic, overly gregarious, seductive, manipulative, exhibitionistic, labile, frivolous, aggressive, and demanding. Narcissistic personality disorder is characterized by a grandiose sense of self-importance, conceit, arrogance, low empathy, and hypersensitivity to criticism and compliment (even if not expressed). These patients seek constant attention and admiration and expect favorable treatment. Antisocial personality disorder is a pattern of chronic, socially irresponsible, exploitative, and shameless behavior. Physical fights, illegal acts, unemployment, substance abuse, and inadequate parent and spouse functions are seen. Borderline personality disorder is characterized by instability of mood; chaotic, unstable interpersonal relationships; and self-damaging impulsiveness. Inappropriate emotional outbursts, suicidal threats or gestures, uncertainty of sexual orientation and long-term goals, and frantic efforts to avoid perceived abandonment may be seen.

The dramatic, or erratic, personality disorders have a direct impact on the management of musculoskeletal pain. Symptoms complained of must be assumed to be exaggerated in description of quality, intensity, and resulting disability. The inadequate ego of these patients responds to verbal sympathy and support. There may be real value in specifically treating symptoms before treating cause. This improves patient tolerance for physical procedures that are typically pain provoking. Aggressive pretreatment with short-term analgesic medication or physical therapy modalities may be indicated. Clinicians must be careful to avoid emotional entrapment by the histrionic and narcissistic behavior of their patients. Pain may be an important defense mechanism that stabilizes a weak ego structure in these patients. On rare occasions, successful, or the threat of successful, treatment of the chronic case will result in florid psychopathology—even a psychotic reaction. Such a response should be assumed to be unavoidable by the clinician; competent psychiatric consultation is needed.

Dramatic personality disorder patients may be particularly distressed by pain because it limits their exhibitionism and attractiveness. By contrast, they may be symptomatically unresponsive to appropriate manual intervention, yet persistently seek caring attention. Discharge from treatment may be interpreted as rejection, criticism, or accusation of psychopathology, with a response of angry, threatening emotional outburst. This situation is best approached by being clear with the patient that (1) symptomatic treatment is only transiently effective, since cause is ignored; (2) treatment must terminate when mechanical dysfunction resolves or when disabling dependence on procedures or medication results; and (3) biomechanical dysfunction does not explain all pain, and persistent symptoms require input of other specialists, perhaps even a chronic pain rehabilitation program. The issue is not whether or not the patient truly hurts, or is being understood; rather, it is whether the clinician can provide any further help. Improved mobility and relief of tissue tension may be the only gains—not pain relief.

Anxious or Fearful Personality Disorders

Avoidant personality disorder is characterized by timidity, social discomfort, fear of criticism or disapproval, fear of social embarrassment, low self-esteem, apprehension, mistrust, and exaggerated fear of potential danger in ordinary activities. Dependent personality disorder presents a pervasive pattern of submissive reliance on others for companionship, emotional support, and everyday decision-making. These patients tolerate mistreatment, are hurt by disapproval, and fear abandonment. Obsessive-compulsive personality disorder is the tendency toward disabling perfectionism; preoccupation with rules, organization, and schedule; indecisiveness, inflexibility, and over-intellectualizing. These stubborn, controlling people are disposed toward power struggles. Passive-aggressive personality disorder involves passive, indirect resistance to authority and responsibility. It is vindictive negativism. These patients procrastinate, forget, become sulky and argumentative when asked to perform, and are critical and disgruntled. A "yes, but" response may follow every suggestion.

Somatic and depressive disorders may accompany these anxious or fearful personality disorders. Persistent pain may offer the avoidant personality a convenient "way out," the dependent personality a ready source of needed social support. The inflexible obsessive-compulsive and the resistive passive-aggressive will tend not to carry out recommended therapeutic activities. They will have plenty of excuses. The clinician must remain aloof to power struggles and be simple, direct, and thorough in explanations and directions (e.g., of exercise programs) discussed with the patient. No room should be left for conceptual misinterpretation and argument. The dependent may do exactly as told but still hurt somewhere. The passive-aggressive will not do as told and still hurt. Persistent symptoms must be assumed to follow appropriate manual intervention. As with the dramatic personality disorders, there must be a clear statement to the patient of separation of symptom and cause and of scientific rationale for termination of treatment.

Self-Defeating Personality Disorder

Self-defeating personality disorder is characterized by a pattern of chronic pessimism; resignation to failure, suffering defeat, or exploitation; and tendency to place oneself repetitively in situations that are harmful or painful. These patients reject help or opportunity for pleasure and fail to accomplish crucial tasks they are capable of. Pain patients with self-defeating personality disorder may receive multiple surgeries, setting themselves up for procedures that fail to cure the pain (e.g., by positive symptomatic response to body cast as an indication for surgical fusion). Conversely, they may reject or discontinue effective treatment.

Affective Disorders

Affective disorders include (1) unipolar depression or major depression; (2) unipolar mania or pure mania; (3) bipolar depression; (4) cyclothymia, a mild form of bipolar depression; (5) dysthymia, a mild form of unipolar depression; (6) seasonal affective disorder; and (7) hypomania. The first three entities are the emphasis of this section due to their high incidence levels and potential impact on physical therapy practice.

The primary presentation associated with these disorders is an altered mood state. Depression and mania are primary disorders of mood. Mood, the internal emotional state of the patient, is contrasted to affect, which is the external manifestation of the patient's mood. Affect may not obviously correlate with the patient's mood, making diagnosis difficult. Patients with affective disorder feel a loss of control over their emotions that leads to the distress and functional impairments. These disabling and potentially deadly disorders are difficult to diagnose. Only one-third to one-half of those with major depressive disorder are properly diagnosed.[14]

Depression is remarkably prevalent, both causing chronic pain and resulting from chronic pain.[15] Depression has been described as a normal response in the natural history of all persistent pain.[16]

Epidemiology

Major depression is the most common adult psychiatric disorder, with a lifetime prevalence of one in eight adults. Women have a two to one prevalence over men. In a 6-month period 2.5. to 5 million women meet the diagnostic criteria for depression. In outpatient physical therapy practice there was an 11.4 percent prevalence.[17] Mean onset of diagnosis is 40 years of age, with the majority of diagnoses made between 20 and 50 years of age. Bipolar disease usually presents at a younger age. Major depression occurs in 21 to 43 percent of chronic pain patients.

Etiology

Multiple etiologies have been proposed, but none has been definitively shown to explain all affective disorders. Biogenic amines and a neuroendocrine mechanism such as the limbic–hypothalamic–pituitary adrenal axis have been hypothesized as etiology of depression. Genetics play a strong role in bipolar disorders. Fifty percent of patients with bipolar disorders have one parent with the disease. Conversely, children with one parent with the disorder have a 27 percent chance of developing bipolar disorder. Life events and perceived stress are associated with increased incidence of depression, but no cause and effect has been shown.

Various diseases have depression as an associated condition, (see Table 12-1). Depression is also a side effect of many medications (see Table 12-2), many of which patients seen in a physical therapy practice may be taking.

Table 12-1. Physical Illnesses Commonly Associated With Features of Depression

Central nervous system
Parkinson's disease
Cerebral arteriosclerosis
Stroke
Alzheimer's disease
Temporal lobe epilepsy
Postconcussion injury
Multiple sclerosis
Miscellaneous focal lesions
Endocrine/metabolic
Hyperthyroidism
Hypothyroidism
Addison's disease
Cushing's disease
Hypoglycemia
Hyperglycemia
Hyperparathyroidism
Hyponatremia
Viral
Acquired immunodeficiency syndrome
Hepatitis
Pneumonia
Influenza
Nutritional
Folic acid deficiency
Vitamin B_6 deficiency
Vitamin B_{12} deficiency
Cancer
Pancreatic
Bronchogenic
Renal
Ovarian
Miscellaneous
Systemic lupus erythematosus
Pancreatitis
Sarcoidosis
Syphilis
Porphyria

(From Tollefson,[18] with permission.)

Table 12-2. Drugs Commonly Associated With Depressive Syndromes

Psychoactive agents
Amphetamines
Cocaine
Benzodiazepines
Barbiturates
Neuroleptics
Antihypertensive drugs
Beta blockers, especially propranolol (Inderal)
$Alpha_2$-adrenergic antagonists
Reserpine (Serpalan, Serpasil)
Methyldopa (Aldomet, Amodopa)
Hydralazine (Alazine, Apresoline)
Analgesics
Salicylates
Propoxyphene (Darvon, Dolene)
Pentazocine (Talwin)
Morphine
Meperidine (Demerol)
Cardiovascular drugs
Digitalis/digoxin (Lanoxin)
Procainamide (Pronestyl)
Disopyramide (Norpace)
Anticonvulsants
Phenytoin (Dilantin)
Phenobarbital
Hormonal agents
Corticosteroids
Oral contraceptives
Miscellaneous
H_2 antagonists, especially cimetidine (Tagamet)
Metoclopramide (Reglan)
Levodopa (Dopar, Larodopa)
Griseofulvin (Fulvicin, Grifulvin, Grisactin)
Nonsteroidal anti-inflammatory drugs
Antineoplastic agents
Disulfiram (Antabuse)

(From Tollefson,[18] with permission.)

Boissonnault and Koopmeiner's study[17] of outpatient physical therapy practices showed that 26 percent of patients were on prescription NSAIDs, while 44 percent were taking over-the-counter NSAIDs; narcotics were used by 8 percent; and β-blockers by 5 percent. All of these medications have the potential side effect of depression. The natural history of depression shows that untreated depression will last 6 to 12 months, with a suicide risk of 10 percent. Treated depression lasts on average 3 months. Untreated depression will relapse 50 percent of the time, with each subsequent episode lasting longer. Relapses occur approximately every 4 to 6 years, but the frequency increases with age, especially if left untreated.

Diagnosis

The criteria for diagnosis of major depression are outlined in Table 12-3. Part A, listing symptoms, is the most relevant for the therapist regarding the screening process. Interestingly, the down-in-the-dumps, depressed affect is only one of the potential symptoms and is not necessary for depression to be diagnosed. Decreased energy is reported in up to 95 percent of patients, sleep disorders in 80 percent, impaired cognition in 65 percent, and poor concentration in 90 percent. The symptoms are typically worse in the morning and improve as the day progresses. Ninety percent of the patients will

Table 12-3. DSM III-R Criteria for Major Depressive Episode

A. At least five of the following symptoms have been present during the same two-week period and represent a change from previous functioning; at least one of the symptoms is depressed mood or loss of interest or pleasure. (Do not include symptoms that are clearly due to a physical condition, mood-incongruent delusions or hallucinations, incoherence or marked loosening of associations.)

1. Depressed mood (or irritable mood in children and adolescents) most of the day, nearly every day, as indicated by subjective account or observation by others
2. Markedly diminished interest or pleasure in all, or almost all, activities most of the day, nearly every day (as indicated by subjective account or observation by others of apathy most of the time)
3. Significant weight loss or weight gain when not dieting (e.g., more than 5 percent of body weight in one month) or decrease or increase in appetite nearly every day (in children, consider failure to make expected weight gains)
4. Insomnia or hypersomnia nearly every day
5. Psychomotor agitation or retardation nearly every day (observable by others, not merely subjective feelings of restlessness or being slowed down)
6. Fatigue or loss of energy nearly every day
7. Feelings of worthlessness or excessive or inappropriate guilt (which may be delusional) nearly every day (not merely self-reproach or guilt about being sick)
8. Diminished ability to think or concentrate or indecisiveness nearly every day (as indicated by subjective account or observation by others)
9. Recurrent thoughts of death (not just fear of dying), recurrent suicidal ideation without a specific plan or a suicide attempt or a specific plan for committing suicide

B. It cannot be established that an organic factor initiated and maintained the disturbance. In addition, the disturbance is not a normal reaction to the death of a loved one (uncomplicated bereavement). Note: Morbid preoccupation with worthlessness, suicidal ideation, marked functional impairment or psychomotor retardation or prolonged duration suggest bereavement complicated by major depression.

C. At no time during the disturbance have there been delusions or hallucinations for as long as two weeks in the absence of prominent mood symptoms (i.e., before the mood symptoms developed or after they have remitted).

D. The disturbance is not superimposed on schizophrenia, schizophreniform disorder, delusional disorder or psychotic disorder not otherwise specified.

(From American Psychiatric Association,[10] with permission.)

experience anxiety, making differentiation from panic attack difficult at times.

Various tools have been promoted to assist in the diagnosis of depression, such as Beck's depression inventory, Hamilton rating scale for depression, and Zung self-rating depression scale. All of these tools, though, are associated with high numbers of false-positive findings. The diagnosis is ultimately based on the correlation of history and mental status examination findings.

Clinical Presentation

The initial sign of depression is frequently psychomotor retardation or agitation. Only 5 percent of patients volunteer depressed mood. The history is complicated by the patient having difficulty answering questions and giving short, delayed responses. The self-directed negativism may make it hard to assess the treatment the patient is receiving. Pre-occupation with pain and loss make the therapy assessment that much harder. Depression can also initially present as a pain syndrome for which physical therapy is sought. Any combination of the symptoms noted in Table 12-3 may present themselves to the therapist, warranting communication with a physician.

Physical therapy treatment of mechanical dysfunction can be an important part of the rehabilitation program for a depressed patient. Restoration of function, including the ability to participate in an active exercise program, initially impeded by the presence of mechanical dysfunction, may be paramount for recovery to occur. A dilemma facing therapists is how long to treat the mechanical dysfunction without other intervention (i.e., counseling) being instituted. Scenarios that would direct the therapist toward putting therapy on hold until other treatment has been initiated are (1) the mechanical dysfunction resolves or improves yet the patient notes no functional or symptomatic improvement, (2) the mechanical dysfunction does not change, or (3) the patient notes a significant worsening of symptoms yet no observable or palpable regression can be noted by the therapist.

Lastly, suicide is a potential risk among patients who are depressed. Seventy percent of depressed patients admit to suicidal ideation, and 10 percent will commit suicide. The patients also potentially harm themselves through less risky behavior such as starting smoking, not wearing seat belts, not taking their medication, and not following their rehabilitation program. Therapists may have concerns regarding asking patients if they are considering suicide. "What if I ask a patient if they are considering suicide and they say yes? Now what do I do?" "Maybe the patient is not considering suicide, and by asking I plant the idea." There is no evidence to support the last concern. In fact, recognition of the intent and discussing it with someone is often the initial step toward appropriate treatment being instituted.

After learning of the suicide ideation, the therapist needs to question the patient regarding a specific plan and what resources are available to carry out the plan. If the patient has suicide ideation, plans to use a gun, has a gun at home, and has recently bought ammunition, a medical emergency exists much as if the therapist took a history consistent with unstable angina or found a symptomatic abdominal aortic aneurysm on abdominal examination. The patient's physician must be consulted and arrangements made to see and probably hospitalize the patient. While suicidal intent without a plan and a plan without identifiable resources to carry it out are less worrisome, therapists in doubt should contact the attending physician. See Table 12-4 for a list of factors associated with increased risk of suicide.

Bipolar Disease

Bipolar disease usually starts with a depressive episode, and the first mania episode is diagnosed 6 to 8 years after the first depression. See Table 12-5 for the criteria for diagnosis of a manic disorder. A manic episode starts abruptly over hours or days, with a full-blown episode developing in weeks. Left untreated, the symptoms will subside over several months. Creativity and productivity are initially increased with the mania episode, but over time the episodes occur more frequent and the dysfunction becomes more obvious. Between episodes 50 percent of the patients do well, but up to 33 percent show a steady down hill course. To diagnose a mania episode, one needs to know the patient's baseline behavior. Mania symptoms include euphoria, irritable mood, grandiosity, and distractibility. Maneuvers such as long, sustained stretches are difficult to do with these patients. The patient's behavior must also result in some impairment that may be difficult to appreciate. Jobs and relationships are frequently chosen to complement the mania, but sooner or later the mania episode becomes intolerable and job performance is negatively affected. The diagnosis may not become obvious until the patient has exhausted all support mechanisms. Drug states can be confused with mania and need to be ruled out.

Table 12-4. Features Associated With an Increased Risk of Suicide

Psychiatric diagnosis (especially alcoholism, depression, panic disorder, acute psychosis)
Concurrent medical disease
Previous suicide attempts
Any significant recent loss (e.g., death of a spouse, divorce)
Self-blame, guilt, or hopelessness
Family history of suicide; often, early loss of parent through suicide, fatal illness, desertion, etc.
Age over 45 or younger age with concurrent drug use
Male gender
Unmarried (especially with recent change in marital status)
Protestant religion
Education through college or higher
Unemployment/recent job loss
Living alone
Living in urban area

(From Tollefson,[18] with permission.)

Table 12-5. DSM III-R Criteria for Manic Episode

A manic syndrome is defined as including criteria A, B, and C. A hypomanic syndrome is defined as including criteria A and B but not C (i.e., no marked impairment).

A. A distinct period is marked by an abnormally and persistently elevated, expansive, or irritable mood.
B. During the period of mood disturbance, at least three of the following symptoms have persisted (four if the mood is only irritable) and have been present to a significant degree:
   1. Inflated self-esteem or grandiosity
   2. Decreased need for sleep (e.g., feels rested after only three hours of sleep)
   3. More talkative than usual or pressure to keep talking
   4. Flight of ideas or subjective experience that thoughts are racing
   5. Distractibility (i.e., attention too easily drawn to unimportant or irrelevant external stimuli)
   6. Increase in goal-directed activity (socially, at work, at school, or sexually) or psychomotor agitation
   7. Excessive involvement in pleasurable activities that have a high potential for painful consequences (e.g., engages in unrestrained buying sprees, sexual indiscretions, or foolish business investments)
C. The mood disturbance is sufficiently severe to cause marked impairment in occupational functioning or usual social activities or relationships with others or to necessitate hospitalization to prevent harm to self or others.
D. At no time during the disturbance have there been delusions or hallucinations for as long as two weeks in the absence of prominent mood symptoms (i.e., before the mood symptoms developed or after they have remitted).
E. The disturbance is not superimposed on schizophrenia, schizophreniform disorder, delusional disorder, or psychotic disorder not otherwise specified.
F. It cannot be established that an organic factor initiated and maintained the disturbance. Note: Somatic antidepressant treatment (e.g., drugs, electroconvulsive therapy) that apparently precipitates a mood disturbance should not be considered an etiologic organic factor.

(From American Psychiatric Association,[10] with permission.)

Lastly, seasonal affective disorder is an affective disorder that has a seasonal pattern to it, as the name implies. The symptoms of depression, including dysfunction, are present for at least 2 months, but are followed by a period of no symptoms. Typically the summers are the asymptomatic periods, and the winters are the symptomatic periods, possibly due to decreased melatonin. Dysthymia is a chronic mild form of unipolar depression, while cyclothymia is a chronic mild form of bipolar depression. Hypomania is diagnosed when the patient has the symptoms of mania without the impairments. All of these conditions have symptoms lasting longer than 2 years and do not have the degree of impairment noted in the other more severe diseases.

Generalized Anxiety Disorders

Generalized anxiety disorder involves persistent (more than 6 months) unnecessary worrying about life circumstances. Four types of symptoms are seen: (1) motor tension (shakiness; muscle tension, ache, or soreness; easy fatiguability; and restlessness); (2) autonomic hyperactivity (increased perspiration, dry mouth, lightheadedness, nausea, shortness of breath, palpitations, urinary frequency, diarrhea, hot flashes or chills); (3) apprehensive expectation; and (4) vigilance and scanning (irritability, sleep disorder, difficulty concentrating). Complaints of pain are frequent as part of the motor tension symptoms of anxiety. The anxious patient may or may not relax enough to be examined or therapeutically handled. These patients tend to be overly fearful, presenting a verbal nuisance, but also inadvertently preventing their own appropriate treatment.

Malingering

Malingering is fraudulent, intentional production of physical or psychological symptoms, motivated by a specific goal. Goals include money, avoiding work, avoiding criminal prosecution, and obtaining medication. Malingering is not a psychological disorder. Opportunistic malingering has been described as taking advantage of an accident or injury by exaggerating symptoms or disability for financial gain.[19]

Several physical examination findings may be indicative of malingering or psychological disturbance. With muscle strength testing, there is poor pain-free effort, a jerky on–off agonist contraction, or co-contraction of antagonist muscle. "Touch-me-not" syndrome exists when diffuse tenderness prevents accomplishment of even a rudimentary biomechanical examination. Provision of analgesia through medication, accupuncture, or physical therapy modalities does not enhance the ability to carry out the examination. Obviously contradictory findings are demonstrated. An example is a painful spring test of a lumbar spinous process and a non-painful spring test of simultaneous bilateral transverse processes at the same level. Another example is painful bilateral knee-to-chest posture at less than 90-degree hip flexion, in contrast to comfort sitting. Many relatively controversial findings are used by experienced clinicians. For example, it is rare to see a case of purely organic or mechanical low back pain in which radiation of pain into the leg causes the patient to have falls. I have never seen a patient with organic or mechanical low back pain tolerate less than 15-degree straight leg raise.

To minimize conflict from misdiagnosis of malingering, no attempt should be made by the manual clinician to diagnose the patient on a psychosocial basis. The clinical question is not whether malingering or psychogenic pain is present. Rather, can symptoms be explained by organic pathology or mechanical dysfunction? If so, diagnosed problems should be treated. If not, the clinician cannot help, and the patient is discharged or referred to alternative specialist consultation. If signs indicative of a significant psychosocial problem are found, the patient should receive concurrent psychological evaluation and treatment along with whatever mechanical treatment is needed. Some patients will require separate treatment of pain and of mechanical dysfunction.

Clinical Markers of Malingering

- Symptoms not explainable by examination findings
- Symptoms persist after successful treatment of diagnosed problem
- Symptoms are severe but vague; pain behaviors overdramatized
- Poor cooperation with diagnostic evaluation
- History of recurrent accident or injury
- Injury presents opportunity for financial gain, work avoidance, or evasion of legal proceedings
- Patient requests addictive medication
- Antisocial traits demonstrated

OTHER PSYCHIATRIC DISORDERS

Pain is usually not associated with the remaining major psychiatric disorders: schizophrenic disorders, organic mental disorders (dementia), delusional (paranoid) disorders, and dissociative disorders. Schizophrenia is notable for relative insensitivity to pain, which may obscure the presentation of serious organic disease. Rarely, delusional pain will be present in schizophrenia. In these cases, the complaints are highly bizarre and ill defined. For the sake of completeness, the diagnostic features of these disorders are reviewed.

Schizophrenic Disorders

Schizophrenic disorders are a group of disorders characterized by major psychiatric disturbance and severely disordered behavior. Bizarre delusions, prominent hallucinations, incoherence or marked loosening of associations, grossly inappropriate affect, and/or catatonic, paranoid, undifferentiated, and residual (burned-out psychosis but still functionallly disabled).

Delusional (Paranoid) Disorders

Delusional disorders are characterized by nonbizarre delusions, such as involving real-life situations. Delusions are unrealistic, fixed ideas that persist in spite of logic or objective contradictory evidence. Patients with other psychotic disorders and dementia will commonly have delusions. The specific delusional disorder will not have prominent hallucinations or otherwise bizarre behavior and will not meet the criteria for schizophrenia. Types of delusional disorders include erotomanic (believes to be loved by another), grandiose (inflated worth, power, identity), jealous (infidelity), persecutory (belief of malevolent treatment), somatic (believes has defect or disease), and others not fitting these categories.

Dissociative Disorders

Dissociative disorders are a group of syndromes characterized by a sudden, temporary disruption in identity, consciousness, or motor behavior. These include psychogenic amnesia, multiple personality disorder, psychogenic fugue (sudden travel, new identity, inability to recall one's past), depersonalization disorder (sense of dreamlike automation and detachment from self), and possession/trance disorder (psychogenic altered state of consciousness or possession).

PSYCHOPHYSIOLOGY OF PAIN

An alluring question is whether a psychiatric disorder can cause a segmental or regional mechanical dysfunction that requires psychiatric treatment for the mechanical dysfunction to resolve. Psychophysiologic pain syndromes refer to pain resulting from involuntary psychogenic musculoskeletal dysfunction. The classic example of muscle tension headache presumes stress-induced chronic muscle contraction causing local pain. Undoubtedly, cases do occur even in the absence of cranial dysfunction. Bruxism and chronic tension of masseters and temporalis muscles are considered part of the cause of temporomandibular joint syndrome.

Some patients demonstrate a tendency to contract their cervical paraspinal extensors and trapezii when stressed or inappropriately so when performing light work with the distal upper limbs. Theoretically, these cases would respond to relaxation training or biofeedback therapy. However, electromyographic (EMG) biofeedback muscle relaxation has been shown, in a large number of cases, to aggravate pain.

Alternative psychophysiologic pain states may be induced by regional fascial restriction, perhaps autonomically mediated. Distant segmental mechanical dysfunction may result and confuse the diagnosis. Finally, a general tension state may exacerbate existing mechanically induced painful muscle spasm or may augment the autonomic effects of mechanical dysfunction. The case history at the end of this chapter suggests a pathophysiologic etiology through fascial restriction.

Whether there is significant psychopathology or not, if mechanical dysfunctions are diagnosed they should be treated mechanically. Anyone can develop mechanical pain syndromes, even the psychologically disturbed. The medical literature fails to describe the behavior of patients with psychiatric disorders in whom an organic pain problem develops. There are several suggestions.

Psychopathology is characterized by weak ego structure, poor social support network, insecurity, and immaturity. Thus, pain is perceived as a greater personal threat (there is a limited reserve). Pain more easily disables the psychologically disturbed from an already barely functional level of interpersonal and social relationships.

With organic pain, psychologically disturbed patients have a greater likelihood of being depressed, anxious, or highly fearful. These patients are less likely to decline the relief of addicting analgesic medication or to understand and carry out self-help methodologies (e.g., exercise programs). They may have unrealistically optimistic expectations of success of outcome of therapeutic procedures and may be overly pessimistic about a neutral or negative response. They will tend to challenge the patient–clinician relationship through socially aversive behavior, including bizarre descriptions of pain (heightened or disturbed perceptions), excessive dependency behavior (insecurity, immaturity, and fear), naive attempts to manipulate people and situations (insecurity, immaturity, and fear), "touch-me-not" intolerance to necessary physical handling of the patient in the therapeutic situation (decreased pain threshold of anxiety), and generally increased emotionality of speech and behavior (fear and immaturity).

The medical literature presents confusing data. Waring et al.[20] showed that the mere presence of significant psychopathology fails to predict surgical therapeutic success. However, several retrospective studies demonstrate an association between hypochondriasis, hysteria, anxiety, and depression with poor surgical outcome.[21–23] None of these attempted to rule out mechanical dysfunctions as part of the cause of the symptom complex. As is feasible, the clinician must wade through these issues in attempting to correct mechanical dysfunction.

STRESS AND PAIN

The initial understanding of stress is attributed to the work of Hans Selye. He noted that all human maladies, illnesses, and injuries produced certain common changes within the body or the "syndrome of just being sick." These observed changes were primarily endocrine and visceral, including enlargement of the adrenal cortex, shrinkage of the spleen, and gastrointestinal ulcers, termed the *general adaptation syndrome*.[24]

Allowance is made for specific variations in response to specific stressors. Allowance is also made for individual differences in conditioning factors that selectively enhance or inhibit a particular stress effect. Thus, normally tolerable stress will induce a "disease of adaptation" in a patient predisposed to such. Stressors that produce the stress response include infection, toxin, social environment, physical environment, emotional stimuli, and nervous stimuli.

Stress is divided into eustress and distress. Eustress is the positive successful adaptation to a stressor or challenge, which is helpful and enjoyable. Distress is the negative adaptation to a threat, as well as loss of control, aggression, or failure to cope within the environment. Subsequent to Selye's work, investigators have tended to confuse stress with distress, which is more in line with the generally accepted socially contexted view of the stress response as a purely negative experience.

Sequelae to stress have been described as including medical and psychiatric illness, mood disorders, autonomic dysfunctions, self-defeating behaviors, and pain syndromes.[25] Stress participates in causing illness, possibly delays healing, and complicates coping with the resulting disability. Thus, there is much value to recognizing significant stress and then providing appropriate clinical management to care for the pain patient.

Several associated factors help to define stress. Cognition is a powerful mediator of stress, including recognition of the stressor and appraisal of its relative associated harm (threat) or gain (challenge). Response is shaped by personality attributes: motives, beliefs, and emotional life of the person and relative confidence in one's wealth of coping resources (or self-esteem).[26] The psychological significance of the threat may be more important than the injury itself in effecting a stress response. Indeed, coping is largely anticipatory of the injury.

There are several specific stress–response syndromes[9]: (1) fearful or anxious states of mind associated with perception of the threat and sense of vulnerability; (2) conditioned emotional response generalized from past danger experience and repeatedly evoked by a memory of that experience (responses may be exaggerated in relationship to the current or potential danger); and (3) signal anxiety or other affect (e.g., guilt, shame, disgust, pride, joy) arising consciously or unconsciously to signal arrival of a stress event.

Stress emotions are complex and troublesome. The person subject to stress may typically fear repetition of the stress, have shame over being helpless against the stressor, be angry toward a symbol of the stress source, and then have shame or fear over aggressive ideations.

Coping with stress may include the typical mechanisms of defense: denial, repression (unconscious unawareness of the stress), suppression (conscious expulsion of distasteful thoughts), displacement (or transfer of concern to another person, situation, or object), projection (of emotion/impulse to others), regression (turning back maturational clock), turning against self, intellectual detachment, rationalization, and acting out. Other defenses include sublimation (replacing an unacceptable thought with one that is socially appropriate), undoing (opposite behaviors), and reaction formation. Reaction formation is the unconscious replacement of a "bad" feeling/thought with a conscious, emphasized opposite thought or activity.

Coping represents an effort to postpone or prevent the harm, overcome the injury, or palliate the consequent affective distress. Coping mechanisms may be beneficial, inadequate, or overtly harmful. Examples of the latter would be worsening a problem by ignoring it or adding a new problem to the original stressor, such as chemical dependency added to chronic pain. Success with coping determines the ability to control the effect of a stressor on a person's life. Coping controls whether the stressor is essentially a positive (eustress) or negative (distress) experience in life. The essence of stress is control. Stress is thus best defined as the unpleasant consequence, with attendant emotions, of loss of control over significant aspects of one's life.

Factors that enhance control over stress include strong self-esteem, a positive typical reactive emotion to stress, strong social support network, benevolence of chosen defense mechanism, and perhaps physical fitness and strength. An appropriate assessment of the impact of stress on pain must include these stress-mitigating factors.

In the neurologic rehabilitation setting, the stress-coping process is often referred to as the process of *adjusting to disability*. This frequent complicating factor limits the efficiency and outcome of rehabilitation efforts. In the presence of biomechanical dysfunction, stress should not be considered the sole cause of pain. Stress may delay or limit therapeutic efficacy or may be part of a broader chronic pain disability.

If there is evidence of inadequate control over stress, referral to a psychology consultant is indicated. This would yield a better assessment of control issues, stress emotion, and coping skills. Treatment would enhance coping skills and limit secondary anxiety and depression. This should not be done in lieu of appropriate physical management of mechanical dysfunction associated with the pain complaint. Both treatments should proceed concurrently as feasible.

There are two stress-relevant psychiatric diagnoses: adjustment disorder and post-traumatic stress disorder. Adjustment disorder is a common reactive psychiatric disorder to an identifiable significant stress. This disorder is sufficient to impair occupational or social functioning. Symptoms are in excess of the normal or expected reaction to the stress event. While exclusive of other psychiatric diagnoses, symptom patterns commonly include depressed or anxious mood, disturbed emotion and conduct, work inhibition, physical complaints, and withdrawal.

By contrast, post-traumatic stress disorder is comparatively severe. It occurs from a stress event outside the normal range of human experience that would be considered markedly distressing to almost anyone. The traumatic event is persistently re-experienced through memory, dreams, and experiential and emotional flashbacks. There is intense psychological distress with exposure to symbols or aspects of the stress event (e.g., anniversaries). There are signs of avoidance of stimuli associated with the stress, numbing of general responsiveness, and symptoms of increased arousal (e.g., difficult sleep, irritability, hypervigilance, exaggerated startle response).

A history of physical, emotional, or sexual abuse is an important stress event with potential for long-term maladaptive consequences, including intensification of pain and subsequent disability. In the physical therapy setting, past abuse may yield a "touch-me-not" intolerance to the necessary physical handling of the patient. Dysfunctional posture may exist. For example, one such patient had a persistently elevated shoulder, having been constantly struck there. An involuted, kyphotic, slumped posture has been associated with recurrent sexual abuse. There may be an unexplainable, particularly midline or bilateral, undue soft tissue tension resistant to treatment. Thus, a component of psychophysiologic pain syndrome would be present. A passive, fragile (weak ego) personality may be noted. Most pain psychologists consider an abuse history sufficient grounds for referral for further assessment and treatment. This need is enhanced when the patient admits that issues related to the abuse have not been fully "processed" by subsequent counseling.

CHEMICAL DEPENDENCY

Substance abuse is one of our major public health problems and has a direct impact on the practice of physical therapy. The chemically dependent pain patient will not be able to cooperate fully with therapy procedures, particularly offsite self-treatment techniques. This makes the patient more dependent on procedures administered by the therapist and prolongs recovery. Capacity to cope with pain stress issues is impaired. Psychophysiologic pain syndromes may appear. Some abused substances are biologically toxic and impair tissue healing, notably alcohol and dirty intravenously administered agents.

Pain intensity is often increased by substance abuse (even narcotics) and is diminished by detoxification and withdrawal. Failure to recognize chemical dependency and refer for appropriate treatment endangers patients and the people they interact with. Coexisting treatment of chemical dependency and mechanical dysfunction can be most efficient and useful in addressing the "whole" patient.

Several screening procedures have been designed to help identify chemical dependency. A particularly useful test is the CAGE questionnaire.27 An adaptation of this test would be to expand the four questions to all illicit drugs. A single "yes" response would suggest that a complete chemical dependency evaluation be undertaken. Two or three "yes" answers strongly suggest chemical dependency.

The CAGE Questionnaire

1. Have you ever felt you should cut down on your drinking or drug use?
2. Have people annoyed you by criticizing your drinking or drug use?
3. Have you ever felt bad or guilty about your drinking or drug use?
4. Have you ever used a drug or had a drink first thing in the morning to steady your nerves or get rid of a hangover (eye-opener)?

Additional evidence indicating chemical dependency would arise with

1. Any confirmation by the patient to questioned use of illicit drugs
2. Current or even minimal use of alcohol or an illicit drug when there has been past chemical dependency treatment or in spite of having been advised by a physician against use
3. Heavy caffeine use (12+ cups caffeinated beverage per day)
4. Undue anger, evasiveness, rationalization or defensiveness when asked about drug and alcohol use
5. Undue fidgeting or shakiness on repeated clinical visits
6. Frequently late to or missing appointments
7. Multiple mood-altering drug prescriptions from different physicians
8. Chemical use resulting in the trauma that brought the patient to the physical therapist
9. Driving while intoxicated

Several guidelines are useful to improve information gathering about chemical dependency. The clinician should begin with questions about the least socially threatening agents (caffeine, tobacco, over-the-counter analgesics) and then proceed with questions about alcohol, narcotic analgesics, and street drugs. Questions that require a "yes" or "no" response should be avoided. Also to be avoided is offering educational or advisory responses before the information-gathering process is finished and certainly any value judgments to response statements, such as surprise, disgust, or disapproval.

The overt toxicity and consequent defenseless use of certain agents, such as cocaine and amphetamines, should be kept in mind. If asked, the clinician should state that his or her personal chemical use is not at issue. Vague answers (e.g., "I drink socially," or "rarely") should not be accepted as valid.

PSYCHOLOGICAL TESTING

This discussion reviews the currently useful validated tests of psychological functioning in the pain patient. Owing to the multidimensional nature of pain, psychological testing is organized according to three essential components: measurement of overt behaviors; measurement of cognitive, sensory, affective, and coping responses; and measurement of physiologic variables. Most existing tests were developed by psychologists for interpretation by psychologists. The Pain Distress Scale presented at the end of this section is a quickly administered tool, designed to assist the physical therapist in deciding when to bring in a psychology consultant.

The reader is alerted to some important limitations of psychological testing. There is no objective test to prove that the pain complaint is psychogenic and not organic or mechanical in nature. The value of these tests is improved definition of the psychological aspects of patient functioning and the standardization and formalization of the normal psychological assessment process. There also is no test for psychiatric diagnosis. The diagnosis depends on a detailed interview, on neurologic and mental status examinations, on knowledge of DSM III-R diagnostic criteria, and often on recurrent assessments during psychiatric treatment.

Behavioral Assessment

Perhaps most useful to the clinician is an accurate and meaningful interpretation of pain behavior in the clinical setting. Indeed, this is routinely performed, in every social interaction, including that between patient and clinician. This informal everyday process is subject to the bias, prejudice, evoked emotion, and naivete of the observer. Accuracy requires formalized consistency in clinical activities and observation methodology.

Display of excessive or prominent pain behavior is thought to be an important prognostic indicator of invasive diagnostic and therapeutic procedures. The following methods are designed to measure behavioral dimensions of pain.[28]

Self-observation: The patient monitors and records such activities as medication use, physical activity, pain behaviors, and pain experience. Significant discrepancies among these measures, as well as between self-reported behavior data and direct observation, have been reported.

Automated recording: This method is relatively complex and involves the use of such devices as pedometer, "uptime" clocks, and ambulatory recording of heart rate and skeletal muscle activity.

Direct observation: This method involves a trained observer staff and, preferably, a relatively standardized clinical environment or sequence of patient behaviors (the latter is classically present in the physical therapy setting). The occurrence and frequency of pain behavior (e.g., rubbing, bracing, guarding, grimacing, sighing) are monitored. Studies have shown moderate correlations with patient self-report measures of pain experience. Interrater and test–retest reliabilities are as high as .89 to .96.

The Pain Behavior Scale[29] is a direct observation technique that has been validated for outpatient use. Ten items are observed for frequency, and each is graded numerically and then added up for a final score of 0 to 10.

Formal pain behavior protocols have been correlated with measures of pain-related functional disability, depression, and self-reports of pain intensity.[30] Although statistically significant, correlation coefficients (.25 to .58) show poor predictability of one measure by another. Although valid, assessed pain behavior must be viewed as valuable patient data in its own right that helps describe the overall clinical picture. Each clinician must ultimately determine the significance of these data to practice procedures and prognosis.

Pain Behavior Scale

1. Vocal verbal complaints
   none = 0; occasional = ½; frequent = 1
2. Vocal nonverbal complaints, including moans, groans, and gasps
   none = 0; occasional = ½; frequent = 1
3. Time spent lying down during the day because of pain
   none = 0; 0–60 min = ½; >60 min = 1
4. Facial grimaces
   none = 0; mild/infrequent = ½;
   severe/frequent = 1
5. Standing posture
   normal = 0; mildly impaired = ½ distorted = 1
6. Gait
   normal = 0; mild limp or impairment = ½;
   severe limp or impairment = 1
7. "Body language" indicative of pain, including clutching and rubbing pain site
   none = 0; occasional = ½; frequent = 1
8. Visible equipment use, including crutches, cane, brace, TENS, leaning on furniture
   none = 0; occasional = ½; constant or dependent = 1
9. Stationary motion
   can stand/sit still = 0; occasional position shifts = ½; constant moving to shift posture or position = 1
10. Analgesic medication
    none = 0; non-narcotic nonpsychogenic = ½; medication abuse or demanding increased narcotic dosage = 1

Somewhat different from assessment of pain behavior, yet within the domain of self-report measures, is the Sickness Impact Profile (SIP).[31] The SIP provides a profile of patient functional disability in several areas, including gross mobility, gait, and self-care activities. This 136-item scale and a 24-item modification[32] of the SIP are well validated and have demonstrated sensitivity to change as patients progress.

Cognitive, Affective, Sensory, and Coping Responses

Minnesota Multiphasic Personality Inventory

The Minnesota Multiphasic Personality Inventory (MMPI) is the most frequently used instrument to assess general aspects of personality. Developed during the late

1930s and recently updated as the MMPI-2, there is voluminous literature applying this test to the scope of psychopathologies, stress syndromes, medical illnesses, and chronic pain. Included are many attempts to differentiate "psychogenic" from "organic" pain effectively by the use of MMPI. The reader is referred to alternative sources for a review of this controversial literature.[33]

The MMPI is a 566-item questionnaire scored and interpreted either by computer or by a specifically trained psychology consultant. Output scoring is by scales: scale 1, hypochondriasis; scale 2, depression; scale 3, conversion hysteria; scale 4, psychopathic deviate subscales: familial discord, authority problems, social imperturbability, social alienation, self-alienation; scale 5, masculinity–femininity; scale 6, paranoia; scale 7, psychasthenia (constructed on patients showing obsessive worries, compulsive rituals, or exaggerated fears); scale 8, schizophrenia; scale 9, hypomania (early manic stage of bipolar disorder); and scale 10, social introversion.

Additional scales are used to ensure validity and truthfulness. Beyond these basic scales, many subscales have been developed to assess specific, otherwise unaddressed concerns. Combination scores have been proposed as significant. *Functional* pain has been claimed to be associated with the MMPI conversion V configuration (high scores on scales 1 and 3, low score on 2). Elevation of all three scales is referred to as the *neurotic triad*.

Although the MMPI cannot diagnose the source of pain, to the psychologist there is immense value in defining personality variables important to pain-coping skills and chronic pain rehabilitation. Furthermore, in confirming a clinical diagnosis, the MMPI may justify the prescription of psychoactive medication.

Illness Behavior Questionnaire

The Illness Behavior Questionnaire (IBQ)[34] is a 62-item questionnaire that assesses abnormal illness behavior. Seven independent dimensions are produced: general hypochondriasis, conviction of disease, psychological versus somatic focus of disease, affective inhibition, affective disturbance, denial of life problems unrelated to pain, and irritability. Three normal and three abnormal score patterns are described.[35] In spite of design intent, it is unclear whether abnormal illness behavior or anxiety or distress features of chronic pain are actually being measured.

Millon Behavioral Health Inventory

The Millon Behavioral Health Inventory (MBHI)[36] is a 150-item questionnaire that must be purchased and computer scored. It was originally developed to evaluate psychological functioning in a wide variety of medical, specifically not psychiatric, patients. The generated interpretive report attempts to provide information regarding the patient's likely style of relating to health care personnel, problematic psychosocial attitudes and stressors, and similarity to patient with psychosomatic complications or poor response to medical intervention. Again, output is by specific scales of basic coping styles (introvertive, inhibited, cooperative, sociable, confident, forceful, respectful, or sensitive), psychogenic attitude (chronic tension, recent stress, premorbid pessimism, future despair, social alienation, and somatic anxiety), psychosomatic correlates, and prognostic index.

Symptom Checklist

The Symptom Checklist-90 (SCL)[37] is a 90-item questionnaire that is easily administered and scored. It measures nine major psychological disturbances: somatization, obsessive-compulsive, interpersonal sensitivity, depression, anxiety, hostility, phobic anxiety, paranoid ideation, and psychoticism. Three global measures of psychic distress are derived: somatic distress, cognitive distress, and distrust.

Beck Depression Inventory

The Beck Depression Inventory (BDI) is a single-page, easily administered questionnaire that must be purchased.* Questions pertaining to depression are answered according to a hierarchy of severity. Answer numbers are then totaled to a numerical score, with significant depression, in our experience, having a score greater than 13. This is a very useful test to help diagnose a complicating depression or significant pain distress.

Visual Analogue Scale

Measurement of pain intensity is easily accomplished by the visual analogue scale, a straight line with "no pain" on one end and "unbearable pain" on the other. The patient indicates perceived pain intensity by placing a mark appropriately within that continuum. Numerical categorization may be added by dividing the continuum into 5 or 10 equal spaces. In my experience, patient insistence on scoring their pain intensity beyond the scope of the visual analogue scale has universally led to eventual admission to a chronic pain rehabilitation program. Pain categories (faint, mild, moderate, strong, very strong) may be added. Generally these scales strongly intercorrelate.

McGill Pain Questionnaire

The McGill Pain Questionnaire (MPQ)[38] was developed to assess separately three interrelated but conceptually distinct components of pain: sensory-discriminative, motivational-affective, and cognitive-evaluative. This is done by arranging 20 categories of intensity-ranked, pain-descriptive words. The patient is told simply to circle no more than one appropriate word from each category. Scoring is based on number of words chosen, or according to the sum of the rank values of chosen words from each of the pain dimensions. Good reliability, validity, and sensitivity to change have been demonstrated for the MPQ. In addition to providing a deeper understanding of the pain experience, the data indicate the tendency to overdramatize or minimize pain perception and suffering.

Coping Strategies Questionnaire

The Coping Strategies Questionnaire (CSQ)[39] is a recently developed instrument that assesses the extent to which pain patients use six different cognitive coping strategies (e.g., diverting attention, reinterpreting pain sensations, praying or hoping), and two behavioral coping strategies (e.g., increasing activity level, increasing pain behavior) in response to pain. Because this test is recent, supportive literature is limited. Fortunately, the CSQ provides valuable insight into a critical aspect of pain rehabilitation.

West Haven-Yale Multidimensional Pain

The West Haven-Yale Multidimensional Pain Inventory (WHYMPI)[40] is a 52-item test that is easily administered and scored. This comprehensive inventory of several aspects of the subjective experience of chronic pain is theoretically based on a cognitive-behavioral perspective. It was designed to fill an existing void in the assessment of pain by examining the subjective, behavioral, and psychophysiologic components of pain. It has demonstrated good validity, reliability, and sensitivity to change. Part one of the WHYMPI evaluates five dimensions of the pain experience: perceived interference of pain in various areas of patient functioning, support and concern of significant others, pain severity, self-control, and negative mood. Part two assesses the response of significant others to communications of pain: perceived frequency of punishing, solicitous (enabling) responses, and distracting responses. Part three evaluates patient capacity to function in common daily activities: household chores, outdoor work, usual activities outside the home, and social activities.

Measurement of Physiologic Variables

Physiologic variables include assessments of EMG activity as a measure of existing states of local muscle spasm, of generalized muscle tension associated with stress (typically frontalis), and of reactivity of paraspinal musculature to stress induction. As yet, no specific valid diagnostic information is raised by this assessment measure. EMG biofeedback for treatment depends on such information.

Another physiologic variable is the measurement of myofascial trigger-point pressure sensitivity. A spring-loaded plunger, pressure algometer, is used. Reliable and valid measures of trigger-point sensitivity result, but there is poor correlation with patient reports of pain intensity.

PAIN DISTRESS SCALE

In an effort to assist the busy clinician, a questionnaire is presented that summarizes essential questions to ascertain a need for psychology consultation for the pain patient.

This questionnaire asks basic, close-ended questions concerning depression (#3, 4), chemical dependency (#5, 6, 7), anxiety (#12, 17), adequacy of stress and pain-coping skills (#8, 10, 11, 14, 20), past or present abuse (#15, 16), perceived prognosis (#1, 2, 9, 13), and family functioning (#18, 19). There is good indication to obtain psychology consultation if at least two answers fall on the right margin. Indeed, one such answer may be enough (e.g., recent suicide ideation). Answers in the center must be interpreted within the clinical context. Obviously, they have an impact on prognosis (e.g., perceived inadequate medical evaluation; perceived inevitable persistence of pain), but the need for further referral may rest on the patient's clinical progress or on answers to further questions evoked by test results.

CHRONIC PAIN SYNDROME AND CHRONIC PAIN REHABILITATION

Chronic pain syndrome is defined as disabling pain lasting longer than 6 months, for which there is no associated progressive or treatable abnormality found upon medical or

Pain Distress Scale

1. Do you think you will ever get over your pain?
   yes no
2. Do you feel you have had an adequate medical evaluation?
   yes no
3. Do you feel depressed, or have you lost interest in most of your daily activities?
   no yes
4. During the past 6 months, have you considered suicide?
   no yes
5. How much caffeinated coffee do you drink per day?
   0–12 cups 12+ cups
6. Does alcohol relieve your pain or help you sleep?
   no yes
7. Has anyone ever told you they were annoyed with your use of alcohol, pain killers, or street drugs?
   no yes
8. Do you feel that your life is out of control?
   no yes
9. Do you think you will ever be able to work again?
   yes no
10. Has your pain made you excessively angry, irritable, or violent?
    no yes
11. Do you think you are coping well enough with your pain?
    yes no
12. Does worrying about pain and what you are going through keep you awake at night?
    no yes
13. Do you fear your pain will inevitably get worse?
    no yes
14. What best describes how much you have limited your activities because of pain? (circle one)
    little change, can do work around the house | some bad days of bedrest | stopped all activities
15. Do you think you are being victimized by your employer or by the insurance company?
    no yes
16. Are you being abused now, or have you ever been abused in the past (physical, sexual, or emotional abuse)?
    no yes
17. Have you experienced panic attacks or periods of desperation?
    no yes
18. Do you need help from family members or others for dressing, bathing, or pain treatments?
    no yes
19. Are you having difficulties getting along with spouse, family, or friends?
    no yes
20. Have you ever been hospitalized for a mental illness?
    no yes

biomechanical evaluation. Chronic pain syndrome is thus untreatable by medical, surgical, or physical therapy methods. To avoid confusion with problems of cancer pain, medical stability is deemed an integral component of chronic pain syndrome. Equally important is the secondary disability; this pain impairs normal family life, social interaction, vocation, and future planning. The syndrome may or may not be associated with significant psychopathology.

Identification of chronic pain syndrome is obviously enhanced by competent biomechanical assessment and treatment. Accurate diagnosis and prompt treatment are critical to this disabled population. Failure or delay exacerbates the severity and complexity of the syndrome and worsens the prognosis for success. Treatment of chronic pain syndrome is an evolving field yet in its infancy. Distinct methodologies have been developed, but all center on multidisciplinary input. These include procedural pain clinics and behavioral and cognitive pain rehabilitation programs.

Procedural Pain Clinics

To avoid confusion, procedural pain clinics are distinguished from behavioral and cognitive pain rehabilitation programs. Typically, procedural clinics are anesthesiology, neurology, surgery specialty, and psychiatry based. They emphasize injection procedures, medication (including psychotropics), acupuncture, transcutaneous electrical nerve stimulation (TENS), physical therapy modalities, exercise and educational activities, and surgical evaluation and treatment. Technically they are contraindicated for chronic pain syndrome because their focus is the treatment of causative organic pathology or mechanical dysfunction, which is not present in chronic pain syndrome as defined. Patients who fail the procedural approach are theoretically eligible for behavioral or cognitive pain rehabilitation programs.

Behavioral Rehabilitation Programs

Behavioral rehabilitation programs view chronic pain as a set of behaviors positively reinforced over time by multiple rewards. Rewards include money (disability income) and relief from responsibility at home and at work. Family members inadvertently reinforce the "sick role" by a variety of activities, termed enabling behaviors, which are appropriate only to acute illness and are antithetical to the rehabilitation of chronic disability.

The health care system adds to the problem. Professionals subtly reinforce pain behavior by being verbally attentive to pain complaints, physically handling the complaining patient, ordering dramatic tests, and providing socially acceptable rationalization for the pain (e.g., diagnoses of fibrositis and myofascial pain syndrome). Items are prescribed, such as canes and neck collars, that reinforce the medical rationale of pain behavior. Whether helpful or not, they are socially obvious indicators and justifiers of the "sick role." The ring of credibility that comes from degrees and certifications further convinces the patient that a genuine disability, and perhaps severe medical problem, exists. Manual clinicians may add to the problem by attempting to address pain instead of mechanical dysfunction.

The behavioral approach to chronic pain rehabilitation views pain as a conditioned behavioral response.[41] Treatment seeks first to identify the specific pain behaviors and the specific reinforcers. The patient is then placed in a milieu in which pain behavior is purposely not reinforced and pain-free behavior is positively reinforced. Counseling educates the patient and family members about the nature of chronic pain behavior, avoidance of enabling, and reinforcement of pain-free behavior. Also during this time, the patient is typically engaged in general physical exercise and reactivation. Nonessential medications are withdrawn.

Behavioral rehabilitation is a powerful, proven therapeutic methodology that has no regard for source of pain and by default assumes the absence of disease and mechanical dysfunction. Typically, behavioral programs are expensive 4- to 8-week inpatient programs that require a sophisticated staff capable of recognizing specific behaviors and reinforcers. Consistency of response to patient complaints is essential. Follow-up outpatient counseling is critical to assist the behavioral transition back to home and community.

Cognitive Pain Rehabilitation Clinics

In an effort to improve generalization of the behavior modification to home and community environment, the cognitive approach to chronic pain rehabilitation was developed to supplement or replace behavioral methods.[42] The cognitive approach attempts to teach the patient that pain as an entity is separate from organic disease and can be successfully managed through rational means. The patient is taught about the physiology of pain. For example, the gate control theory of pain directly supports the concept that alternative neurologic input may block neural transmission of pain sense. The patient is then taught self-treatment methods of blocking pain. These include self-hypnosis training, relaxation therapy, accupressure, self-applied deep muscle (fibrocytic) massage, and appropriate biofeedback for pain control or relaxation.

Education cuts the pain–fear relationship by convincing the patient that the pain is not an indication of serious progressive disease. Counseling procedures accomplish several goals. Behavioral patterns are looked for that may add to the suffering and disability of chronic pain. Self-defeating behaviors are identified that both impair coping and further stress relationships. Pacing problems are seen as consistent attempts to overwork physically in spite of chronic pain, ensuring failure and adding to anxiety and stress when the body cannot keep up with self-imposed excessive demands. The impact of pain on specific, nontolerated components of vocational and social activities is assessed. Subtle changes may be recommended, as feasible, that permit the general activity without affecting goal attainment. This includes training in a focused goal setting.

Some of the cognitive techniques that a patient is taught to address pain include intensity reduction by visualizing the turning down of a "gain control" on their body. The patient may "reinterpret" the pain sensation as a neutral (not negative) perception, shift the location of the pain, or visualize reduction of the total area that hurts. Alternatively, the pain may be dissociated or displaced by imaging being someplace else that is pleasant. The patient may change the focus of attention to a specific thought or a specific muscle contraction. Ultimately, instructed techniques may be made "automatic" by practice or suggestion.

Counseling is also involved with assessment of significant psychosocial stressors that amplify suffering and disability. Family dysfunction is evaluated and treated. Stress management skills are taught. The long-term effects of physical or sexual abuse during childhood or of parental chemical dependency are evaluated and treated. Substance abuse and chemical dependency are evaluated and treated.

Depression, which is very common in the chronic pain population, is assessed and treated. Usually antidepressant medication is used to ensure the immediate benefit of improved sleep. Nonessential medications are withdrawn. Physical reactivation occurs through a general exercise program, along with instruction in posture control and proper lifting biomechanics.

As with the behavioral approach to chronic pain management, caution is taken to avoid enabling attentiveness to pain complaints and behaviors. Pain-free behavior is encouraged, including cessation of reliance on a cane or other nonessential orthotic device. From the time of admission, the expectation is clearly communicated that pain can be effectively and independently managed by the patient. With the cognitive approach, concomitant treatment of mechanical dysfunction is not automatically viewed as enabling of pain and disability. Rather, mechanical normalization is viewed as a useful treatment objective to improve physical capabilities, whether or not any effect on pain symptoms is achieved. In contrast to the behavioral approach, behavior is not the clinical focus. Rather, rehabilitation and reactivation in spite of the existing pain become the focus.

An observation raised by review of the chronic pain rehabilitation process concerns the importance of nurturance. Short of significant psychopathology, ego weakness, poor self-esteem, and fear of reinjury seriously lessen the patient's resiliance to the diverse effects of injury. Mounting stresses that result from significant pain are incompletely and inefficiently resolved by the weak, immature, insecure personality. A parental function is thus applied by the chronic pain rehabilitation program. Expression of grief is facilitated. Anger is creatively directed. Fear is soothed by training in goal setting and reasoned problem solving. Effective life management is encouraged and reinforced. A healthy lifestyle is taught. The patient grows in strength and endurance by the exercise component of the pain program. This simple nurturance appears to be invaluable for certain injured patients.

The cognitive approach to rehabilitation is eclectic, involving a diversity of professionals. Such programs are often provided over a 2- to 4-week period, in an outpatient or residential setting. In distinct contrast to the behavioral approach, outpatients may do better than inpatients through easier generalization of learned concepts to the "real world." The less confining the program, however, the greater the need to monitor substance abuse. Postgraduate aftercare sessions facilitate the struggling patient's integration back to the social and familial norm.

Competence in manual technique offers unique and potent resources to chronic pain rehabilitation programs. Primary is the ability to diagnose biomechanical dysfunction efficiently and accurately as the cause of the pain syndrome. Diagnosis is the key to health care. Subsequent "hands-on" conservative and potentially enabling therapy is thus assigned specific, quantifiable outcome goals, independent of mere pain reduction. Also, at least partially resolved is the relationship of pain and physical work capacity of the injured worker.

Concomitant treatment of manual therapy and chronic pain rehabilitation introduces a contradiction that has the potential to sabotage or diminish the effect of either. This problem is avoided in three ways: (1) completing manual treatment before chronic pain rehabilitation, (2) distinguishing separate goals for manual treatment (mechanical normalization for improved work capacity) and chronic pain rehabilitation program (learning to cope with pain), and (3) applying limited components of the chronic pain rehabilitation program during manual treatment. For example, specific family counseling, chemical dependency treatment, medication for depression, and so forth, are provided during manual treatment. The choices depend on the needs of the individual.

Pain patients with chronic, untreated mechanical dysfunction may have acquired sufficient psychosocial stressors to require pretreatment by a chronic pain rehabilitation program before successful manual intervention. Such cases are refractory to medication; these patients are often too irritable (or "touch-me-not") to tolerate the positioning and handling of manual techniques or to carry out recommended exercises. The benefit of the sequential treatment is a realistic, calm patient who is tolerant of the minor physical discomfort of manual treatment and whose expectation of outcome mirrors the clinician's therapeutic goals. The difficult patient is thus made an ideal patient.

EVALUATIVE ALGORITHM

Figure 12-1 presents an algorithm that summarizes the evaluative process in screening for psychological disorders. It is recommended that, at a minimum, several questions be asked from the Pain Distress Scale or on the basis of the problems listed earlier regarding the chronic pain patient, the signs of family dysfunction, and the clinical markers of malingering. As previously stressed, biomechanical dysfunction supporting the symptom spectrum should be appropriately treated. However, if treatment is hampered by, or if the clinical history indicates significant concern for, psychopathology, there is a need for further, more formalized, assessment. This assessment better defines the "whole" of the situation and provides a formal rationale for subsequent specialty referral.

SUMMARY

The preceding sections have reviewed screening for psychological disorders, with a specific focus on the pain patient. This has included a discussion of definitions of pain and how pain affects the patient and the family. Psychiatric disorders, personality disorders, and affective disorders, as well as their interaction with pain, were covered. Issues of stress, abuse, and chemical dependency were reviewed. Useful psychological testing tools were introduced, particularly the Pain Distress Scale. Chronic pain syndrome and its rehabilitation were discussed to provide a framework for how physical symptoms are therapeutically addressed from a psychological perspective.

PATIENT CASE STUDY

History

A. S. is a 36-year-old healthy female nurse who developed work-related, immediate-onset low back pain while lifting a patient. She sought immediate medical attention that diagnosed sacroiliac joint mechanical dysfunction. The problem was treated by manipulation, with good results. However, the problem reoccurred frequently from resumption of lifting activity. She quit work to pursue further education directed toward a more sedentary occupation.

Several months later, she presented in moderate distress. Without trauma, she had experienced exacerbation of severe, sharp pain in the sacroiliac region, with pain spreading into the entire left side of her body, including the hemicranium. There was associated lightheadedness, dizziness, visual blurring, and photophobia.

Objective Examination

Physical examination revealed a sweeping functional scoliosis throughout the spine, severe pubic and sacral torsion, marked tightness of regional abdominal fascia, and tightness of the chest wall, neck, and cranium. Segmental mechanical restrictions were limited to the upper cervical spine, T7 and L3.

Assessment and Outcome

Muscle energy manipulation, deep slow stretch techniques, and high-velocity thrust were administered with good results. Subsequent evaluation and treatment occurred every 2 weeks over the next 8 months. Typically, she would have the expected 1 to 2 days of symptom aggravation, followed by only a few days of significant relief. Severe pain would then recur, varying in location and attendant disability. The fascial restrictions of the abdomen and chest wall, the cranial restrictions, and the pelvic dysfunctions continued to recur in spite of detailed reassessments and competent manipulative intervention, as demonstrated by short-term normalization of biomechanics.

Eventually, significant psychosocial stressors were uncovered. At age 13, she had experienced a near-drowning. She revealed that she was a single mother of two, divorced from an alcoholic spouse who had physi-

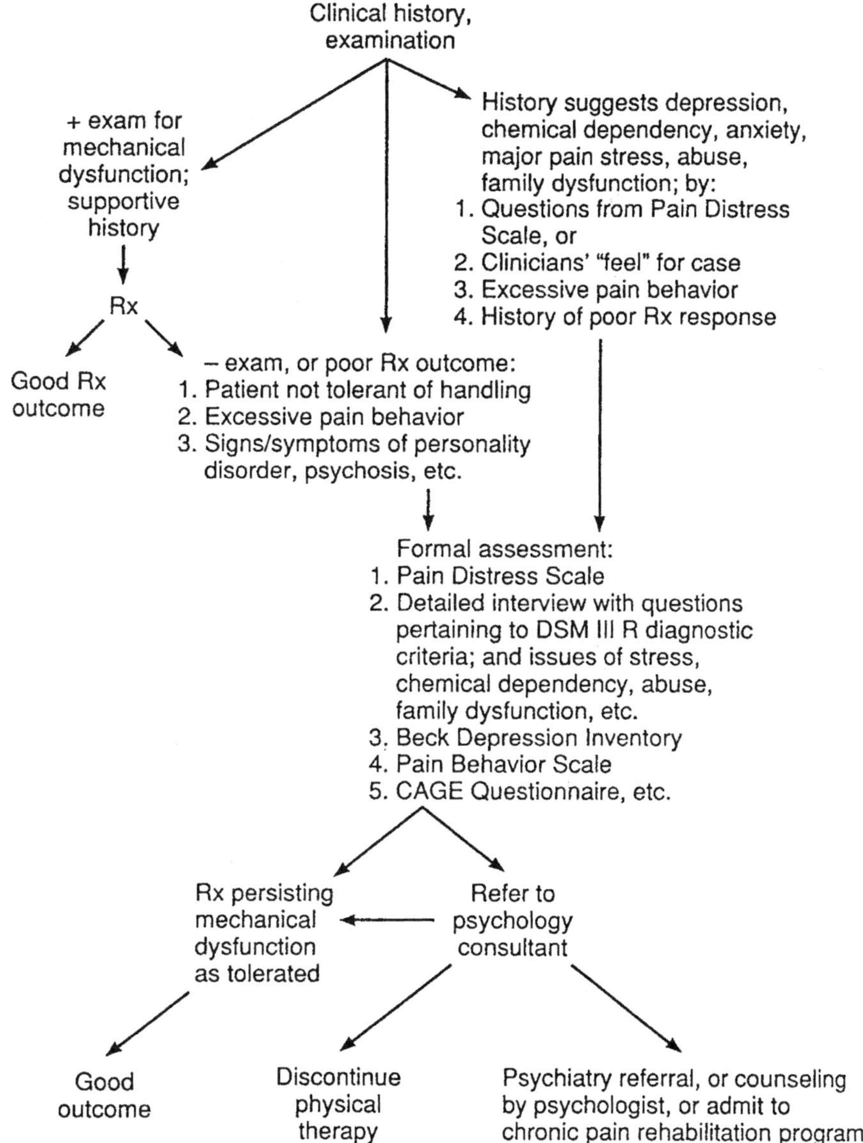

Fig. 12-1. Evaluative algorithm in screening for psychological disorders.

cally abused her. Her 13-year-old daughter had recently attempted suicide. In stoic fashion, no efforts had ever been made to discuss these issues with others or to resolve psychological effects through competent counseling. The next two clinic visits led to further introspection and progressive openness to expression of feelings; eventually, she was able to weep. She was referred to, and indeed read, several books on near-death experiences and family dysfunction.

Dramatic improvement was seen during subsequent biomechanical examinations. Manipulative techniques were now more easily accomplished. The fascia loosened up. She was finally able to advance to strengthening and conditioning exercise. Over the following year, there were infrequent recurrences associated with changes in physical demand and with the psychological stress of her academic activities. One suggestion from this case history is that significant psychosocial stress may mediate mechanical dysfunction through regional fascial restriction.

REFERENCES

1. Fields HL, Abram SE, Budd K et al: Core curriculum for professional education in pain. p. 8. International Association for the Study of Pain. Publications, Seattle, 1991
2. Sternbach RA: Psychologist's role in the diagnosis and treatment of pain patients. In Barber J, Adrian C (eds): Psychological Approaches to the Management of Pain. Brunner Mazel, New York, 1982
3. France RD, Krishnan KR, Houpt JL et al: Personality and chronic pain. p. 76. In France RD, Krishnan KR (eds): Chronic Pain. American Psychiatric Press, Washington, DC, 1988
4. Loeser JD: Perspectives on pain. In Proceedings from the First World Conference on Clinical Pharmacology and Therapeutics. Macmillan, London, 1980
5. Beecher HK: Measurement of Subjective Responses. Oxford University Press, London, 1959
6. Fordyce WE: Pain and suffering. A reappraisal. Psychology 43:276, 1988
7. Roy R: A problem centered family systems approach in treating chronic pain. p. 113. In Holzman AD, Turk DC (eds): Pain Management. Pergamon Press, New York, 1986
8. Talbott JA, Hales RE, Yudofsky SC et al: American Psychiatric Press Textbook of Psychiatry. p. 357. American Psychiatric Press, Washington, DC, 1988
9. Horowitz MJ: Stress and the mechanisms of defense. p. 39. In Goldman HH (ed): General Psychiatry. 2nd Ed. Appleton & Lange, E. Norwalk, CT, 1987
10. American Psychiatric Association: Diagnostic and Statistical Manual of Mental Disorders. 3rd Ed. Rev. Ed. American Psychiatric Press, Washington, DC, 1987
11. Engel GE: "Psychogenic" pain and the pain prone patient. Am J Med 16:899, 1959
12. Miller L: Neuropsychologic concepts of somatoform disorders. Int J Psychiatry Med 14:31, 1984
13. Katon W, Kleinman A, Rosen G: Depression and somatization: a review. Parts 1 and 2. Am J Med 72:127, 241, 1982
14. U.S. Department of Health and Human Services: Depression in Primary Care. Vol 1. Detection and Diagnosis. Publication No. 93-0550. US DHHS, Rockville, MD, 1993
15. Krishnan KR, France RD, Davidson J: Depression as a psychopathological disorder in chronic pain. p. 196. In France RD, Krishnan KR (eds): Chronic Pain. American Psychiatric Press, Washington, DC, 1988
16. Hendler N: Depression caused by chronic pain. J Clin Psychiatry 45:30, 1984
17. Boissonnault WG, Koopmeiners MB: Medical history profile: orthopaedic physical therapy outpatients. J Orthop Sports Phys Ther 20:2, 1994
18. Tollefson GD: Recognition and treatment of major depression. Am Fam Physician 42(5 suppl):559, 1990
19. Yudofsky SC: Conditions not attributable to a mental disorder. p. 1862. In Kaplan HI, Sadock BJ (eds): Comprehensive Textbook of Psychiatry. 4th Ed. Williams & Wilkins, Baltimore, 1985
20. Waring EM, Weisz GM, Bailey SI et al: Predictive factors in the treatment of low back pain by surgical intervention. p. 939. In Bonica JJ, Albe-Fessard D (eds): Advances in Pain Research and Therapy. Raven Press, New York, 1976
21. Blumetti AE, Luciano MM: Psychological predictors of success or failure of surgical intervention for intractable back pain. p. 323. In Bonica JJ, Albe-Fessard D (eds): Advances in Pain Research and Therapy. Raven Press, New York, 1976
22. Caldwell AB, Chase C: Diagnosis and treatment of personality factors in chronic low back pain. Clin Orthop 129:141, 1977
23. Frymoyer JW, Rosen JC, Clements J et al: Psychological factors in low back pain disability. Clin Orthop 195:178, 1985
24. Selye H: Stress without distress. p. 11. In Garfield CA (ed): Stress and Survival. CV Mosby, St. Louis, 1979
25. Appelbaum SH: Stress Management for Health Care Professionals. Aspen Press, Rockville, MD, 1981
26. Lazarus RS: A cognitive analysis of biofeedback control. p. 69. In Prokop CK, Bradley LA (eds): Medical Psychology. Academic Press, San Diego, 1981
27. Mayfield D, Mcleod G, Hall P et al: The CAGE questionnaire: validation of a new alcoholism screening instrument. Am J Psychiatry 131:1121, 1974
28. Feuerstein M, Greenwald M, Gamache MP et al: The Pain Behavior Scale: modification and validation for outpatient use. J Psychopathol Behav Assess 7:301, 1985
29. Richards JS, Nepomuceno C, Riles M, et al: Assessing pain behavior: the UAB Pain Behavior Scale. Pain 14:393, 1982
30. Romano JM, Syrjala KL, Levy RL, et al: Overt pain behaviors: relationship to patient functioning and treatment outcome. Behav Ther 19:191, 1988
31. Bergner M, Bobbitt RA, Carter WB, et al: The Sickness Impact Profile. Med Care 19:787, 1981
32. Deyo RA: Comparative validity of the sickness impact profile and shorter scales for functional assessment in low back pain. Spine 11:951, 1986
33. Bradley LA, Anderson KO, Young LD, et al: Psychological testing. p. 573. In Tollison CD (ed): Handbook of Chronic Pain Management. Williams & Wilkins, Baltimore, 1989

34. Pilowsky I, Spence ND: Patterns of illness behavior in patients with intractable pain. J Psychosom Res 19:279, 1975
35. Pilowsky I, Spence ND: Illness behavior syndromes associated with intractable pain. Pain 2:61, 1976
36. Millon T, Green C, Meagher R: Millon Behavioral Health Inventory Manual. 3rd Ed. National Computer Systems, Minneapolis, 1982
37. Shutty MS, DeGood DE, Schwartz DP: Psychological dimensions of distress in chronic pain patients: a factor analytic study of symptom checklist—90 responses. J Consult Clin Psychol 54:836, 1986
38. Melzak R: The McGill pain questionnaire: major properties and scoring methods. Pain 1:277, 1975
39. Rosenstiel AK, Keefe FJ: The use of coping strategies in chronic low back pain patients. Pain 17:33, 1983
40. Kerns RD, Turk DC, Rudy TE: The West Haven–Yale Multidimensional Pain Inventory. Pain 23:345, 1985
41. Roberts AH: The operant approach to the management of pain and excess disability. p. 10. In Holzman AD, Turk DC (eds): Pain Management. Pergamon Press, New York, 1986
42. Holzman AD, Turk DC, Kerns RD: The cognitive behavioral approach to the management of chronic pain. p. 31. In Holzman AD, Turk DC (eds): Pain Management. Pergamon Press, New York, 1986

SUGGESTED READINGS

Bradley LA, Anderson KO, Young LD et al: Psychological testing. In Tollison CD (ed): Handbook of Chronic Pain Management. Williams & Wilkins, Baltimore, 1989

Goldman HH (ed): Review of General Psychiatry. 2nd Ed. Appleton & Lange, E. Norwalk, CT, 1987

Merskey H: Psychiatry and chronic pain. Can J Psychiatry 34:329, 1989

Turk DC, Rudy TE: Assessment of cognitive factors in chronic pain: A worthwhile enterprise? J Consult Clin Psychol 54:760, 1986

U.S. Department of Health and Human Services: Depression in Primary Care. Vol 2. Treatment of Major Depression. Publication No. 93-0551. US DHHS, Rockville, MD, 1993

13 Screening for Skin Disorders

Charles Shapiro, M.Ed., P.T.
Stanley Skopit, D.O.

Diseases and pathologies of the skin affect millions of Americans every year. These problems can range from minor cosmetic problems to deadly skin cancer. In many cases, the key to treatment and management is early detection before extensive tissue damage or disease progression has occurred. It does not always take the trained eye of a physician specializing in dermatology to screen for skin disorders. The American Cancer Society has long encouraged self-examination and examination by a significant other to help pick up questionable moles that may become problematic. In addition, millions of Americans are seen daily by health care practitioners other than physicians, but it is not routine for those practitioners to give screening of the skin the attention that is warranted.

Physical therapists, in particular, are in a position to conduct a good dermatologic screening as part of their routine assessment of their patients. The physical therapy assessment often involves a thorough family and medical history, a visual inspection, and soft tissue palpation as part of the examination of the patient. Obviously, it would take little effort to expand the physical therapy examination to include dermatologic screening targeted at early detection of specific disorders.

The discussion in this chapter includes an overview of structures and functions of the skin and a straightforward approach to examination. The reader will better understand how to screen for common skin conditions that may require further medical diagnosis or intervention.

One method of approaching differential assessment of skin disorders has been developed by Dr. Stanley Skopit. *Skopit's Ring of Diagnosis of the Skin* (Fig. 13-1) is a straightforward approach to data gathering that leads the clinician through the examination of the skin using a differential diagnostic approach. Skopit's Ring is formed by six interdependent aspects of examination of the skin, including patient *history*, *classification* of skin lesion, *configuration* of skin lesion, *location* of skin lesion, *season* (chronology, or time of onset), and *laboratory findings*. Skopit's Ring has been used successfully for years to train dermatology residents and is used in this chapter as the basis for teaching physical therapists assessment of the skin.

STRUCTURE AND FUNCTION OF THE SKIN

Much of the literature refers to the skin as one of the largest and most important organs of the body. Physical therapists often recognize the integumentary system as including the skin, hair, and nails. Also included in the integumentary system are the eccrine (sweat) glands, apocrine (scent) glands, sebaceous glands, arrectores pilorum muscles, and mammary glands (Fig. 13-2).

Layers of the Skin

A cross section of the skin reveals three layers. The outermost layer, the epidermis, is further divided into the basal layer, prickle layer, granular layer, lucid layer, and horny layer.[1] Cells from the basal layer, which is closest

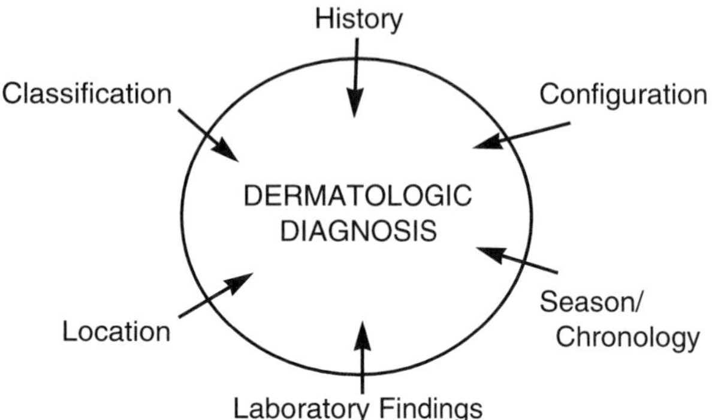

Fig. 13-1. Skopit's ring of diagnosis.

to the underlying dermis, migrate to the superficial horny layer in a 28-day period.[2] The first four layers of the epidermis is referred to as the living epidermis, whereas the outer layer represents the dead end-product.[1] The outermost horny cell layer consists of a nuclear cells containing keratin. The thickness of the keratin layer varies greatly in different body sites, and is found to be very thick over the palm and fingers and thin over the skin of the forearm.

The second layer of the skin, the dermis, consists of fibrous collagen mixed with elastic elastin fibers that support the epidermis. The fibers of the dermis give the property of pliability to the skin as an organ and enables the skin to return to a normal resting state following mechanical deformation. A gel-like ground substance found in the dermis accounts for the skin's ability to accommodate to changes in body weight. Blood vessels, eccrine glands, apocrine glands, sensory nerves, and autonomic nerves are also found in the dermis layer of the skin.

Beneath the dermis lies the subcutis layer, or subcutaneous tissue. This layer is composed primarily of adipose cells and functions as mechanical and thermal protection.

Hair

The hair covers the entire body except for specific areas including the palms of the hands, soles of the feet, and portions of the genitalia. Hair originates in the hair follicle located deep in the dermal layer of the skin. The hair receives its nourishment through a vascular network in the bulb of the follicle. In this bulb is contained the melanin that gives the hair its color. A recurring cycle of hair production occurs by cell division within the lining

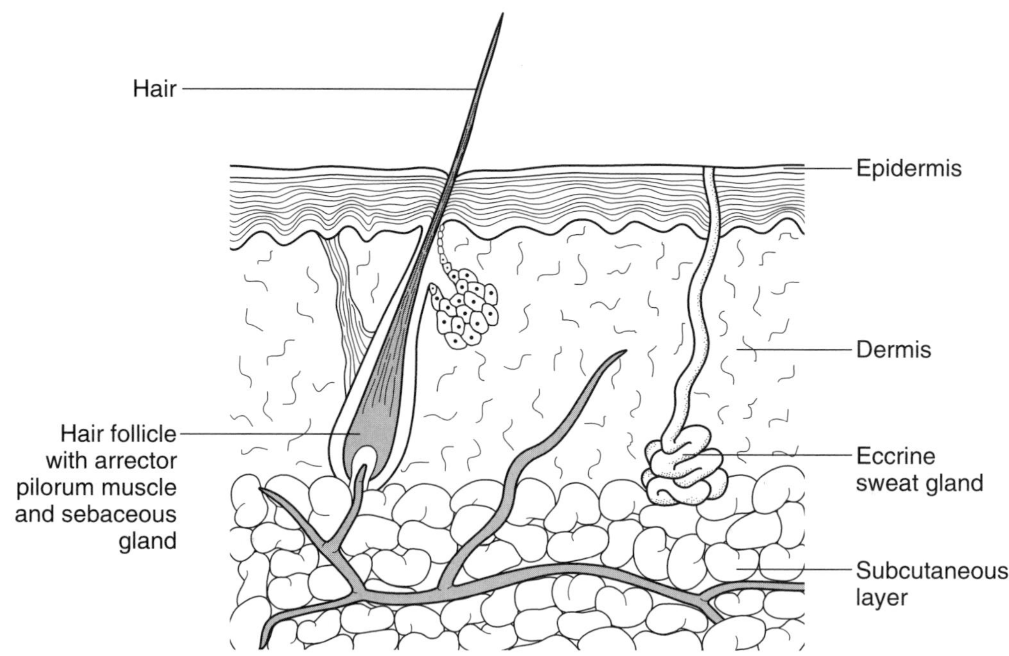

Fig. 13-2. Schematic of normal human skin showing the layers and the interrelationships of the various structures.

of the hair follicle. A sebaceous gland is attached to each hair follicle, which secretes a yellow lipid substance called sebum. Hair goes through three cycles during growth, including a growth phase, an atrophy phase, and a resting stage. Internal diseases may be manifested through changes in the hair.

Nails

The nails are the hard plates covering the ends of the fingers and toes. The fingernails and toenails continue to grow unless irreparably damaged through injury, disease, or amputation. Normal nail growth is approximately 1 mm per week. Changes in the nails may be early indicators of internal disease (Fig. 13-3).

Sweat Glands

There are two types of sweat glands, eccrine glands and apocrine glands. Eccrine glands open directly to the skin surface and are responsible for the regulation of body temperature. Apocrine glands are found in the axillary and genital regions and open into hair follicles. The apocrine glands are stimulated by emotional stress and are responsible for body odor.

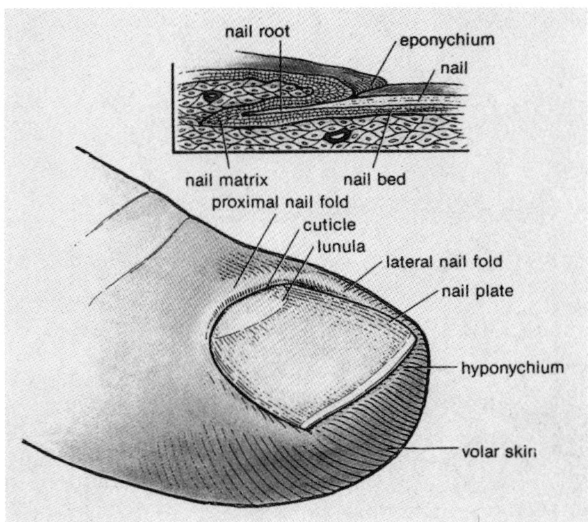

Fig. 13-3. Nail. The nail plate is formed by contributions both from the proximal matrix, lying deep to the proximal nail fold, and from that portion of the matrix extending out into the area identified as the lunula. (From Sams,[2] with permission.)

Color of the Skin

The color of the skin comes from basically four sources. Scattered throughout the deep basal layer of the epidermis are larger pale cells that may contain brown granules. These brown granules, melanocytes, produce a substance called melanin that contributes to skin color and helps protect the skin from damage by the sun. Carotene is a substance found in the subcutaneous fat, especially on the palms and soles, and contributes a yellow color in those areas. Hemoglobin also contributes to coloration of the skin. Oxygenated hemoglobin as carried in the arteries and capillaries will give a bright red color to the skin. Following the loss of oxygen to the tissues, hemoglobin becomes deoxygenated as it is carried through the superficial blood vessels, giving the skin a bluish cast called cyanosis. Any change in the blood's ability to carry oxygen can result in cyanosis.

MANIFESTATIONS OF SKIN DISORDERS

Skin goes through changes due to factors including the normal aging process, environmental conditions, disease, and trauma. Skin disorders can be manifested in several different ways, including color changes, skin lesions, and pruritus (itching).

Color Changes of the Skin

An individual's normal color of skin is determined by the amount of pigment contained within the skin, as well as the quantity and quality of blood flowing to the skin. All individuals have a skin color that is normal for them. Certain changes in skin color are expected with exposure to the elements, as with suntanning. However, in certain abnormal states the skin undergoes a change from the normal color. There are several color changes that the physical therapist should be familiar with as indicators of possible problems. White (pallor), blue (cyanosis), red (erythema), yellow (jaundice), and brown (darkening, hyperpigmentation) are common general color changes of the skin that may be indicators of disease (Table 13-1).

Table 13-1. Abnormal Color Changes of the Skin

Color Change	Physiologic Change	Common Causes
White, pale (pallor)	Absence of pigment or pigment changes	Albinism (albinos), lack of sunlight
	Blood abnormality	Anemia, lead poisoning
	Temporary interuption or diversion of blood flow	Vasospasm, syncope, stress, internal bleeding
	Internal disease	Chronic gastrointestinal disease, cancer, parasitic disease, tuberculosis
Blue (cyanosis)	Decreased oxygen in blood (deoxyhemoglobin)	Methemoglobinemia (oxidation of hemoglobin), high blood iron level, cold exposure, vasomotor instability, cerebrospinal disease
Yellow	Jaundice, excess billirubin in blood, excess bile pigment	Liver disease, gallstone blockage of bile duct, hepatitis (conjunctiva eyes are also yellow)
	High levels of carotene in blood (carotenmia)	Ingestion of food high in carotene and vitamin A
Gray	High level of metals in body	Increased iron, bronze/gray; increased silver, blue/gray
Brown (hyperpigmentation)	Disturbances of adrenocortical hormones	Adrenal or pituitary glands, Addison's disease

Skin Lesions

A skin *lesion* is any single, small area of skin pathology.[2] The term *lesion* refers to the loss of tissue continuity, structure, or function secondary to trauma, disease, illness, or pathology. No one, even a newborn, has perfectly flawless skin. Average adults have as many as 20 to 100 moles (nevi) on their body.

Classification of Skin Lesions

Skin lesions will be classified according to primary, secondary, and special lesions (Figs 13-4 to 13-14; Appendix 13-1). *Primary* lesions are those resulting in the loss of tissue continuity structure or function as a direct result of trauma, disease, illness, or pathology. *Secondary* lesions are those that result secondarily to an existing primary lesion. Secondary trauma such as scratching, rubbing, or bumping of an existing lesion, infection, and inadequate or inappropriate care of a primary lesion can result in secondary lesions more serious than the primary one. *Special* lesions are those that do not quite fit into the category of primary or secondary lesions and present unique properties of their own.

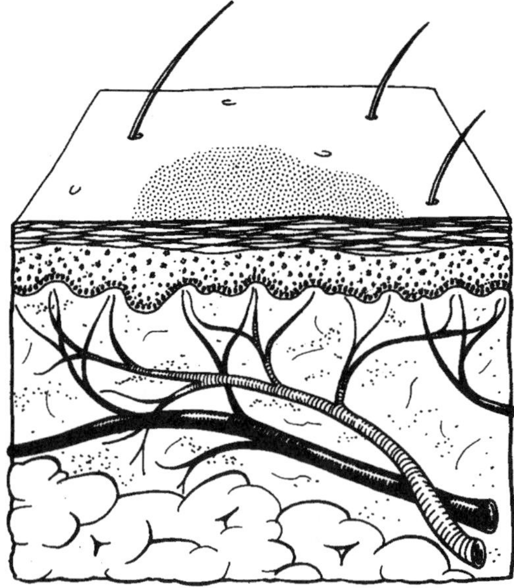

Fig. 13-4. A macule. The only visible abnormality is the color change on the surface of the skin. (From Lynch,[4] with permission.)

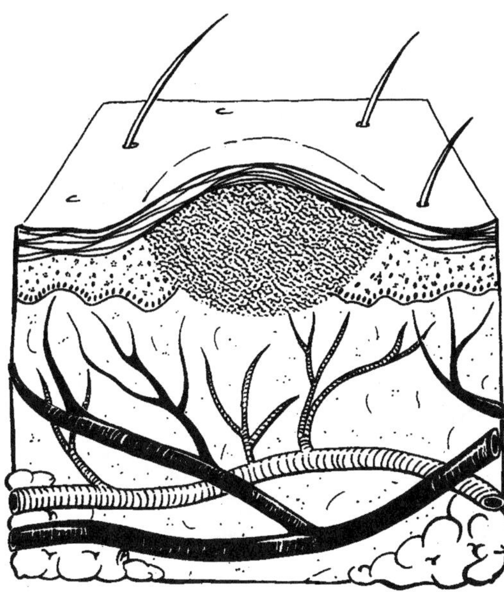

Fig. 13-5. A papule. This figure shows pathology in the epidermis but the histologic abnormality can be located anywhere in the skin. (From Lynch,[4] with permission.)

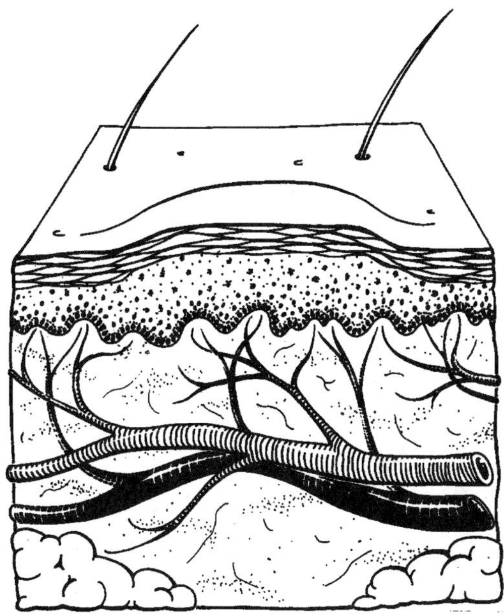

Fig. 13-6. A wheal. The wider spacing of the stippled dots represents fluid that is increasing the space among the nuclei of epidermal cells. However, in many instances the fluid is contained only in the upper dermis. (From Lynch,[4] with permission.)

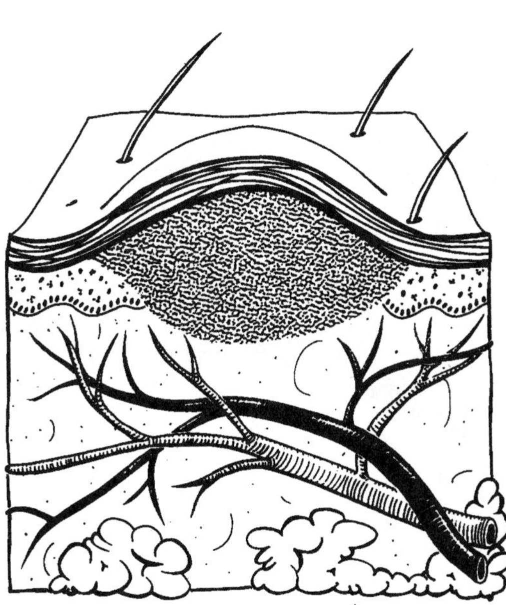

Fig. 13-7. A nodule. Although shown here involving mostly the epidermis, the histopathology of a nodule is more often found in the deeper layers of skin. (From Lynch,[4] with permission.)

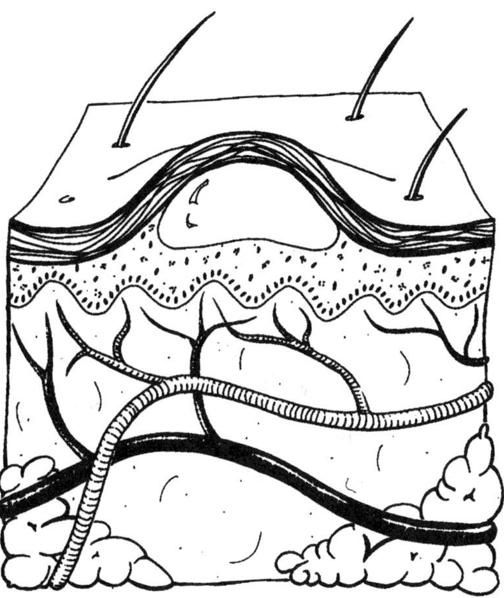

Fig. 13-8. A vesicle. A subcorneal vesicle is shown in this figure. Vesicles can also be located deeper in the epidermis or at the junction of the epidermis and dermis. (From Lynch,[4] with permission.)

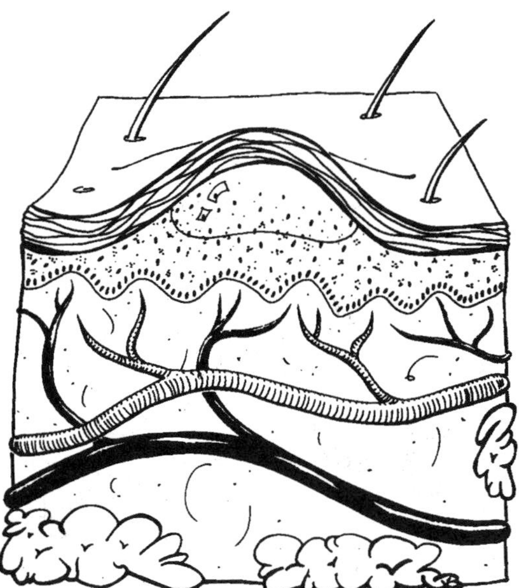

Fig. 13-9. A pustule. The dots in the subcorneal loculation represent the nuclei of neutrophils. As for vesicles, pustules may also be located within the epidermis or at the dermal epidermal junction. (From Lynch,[4] with permission.)

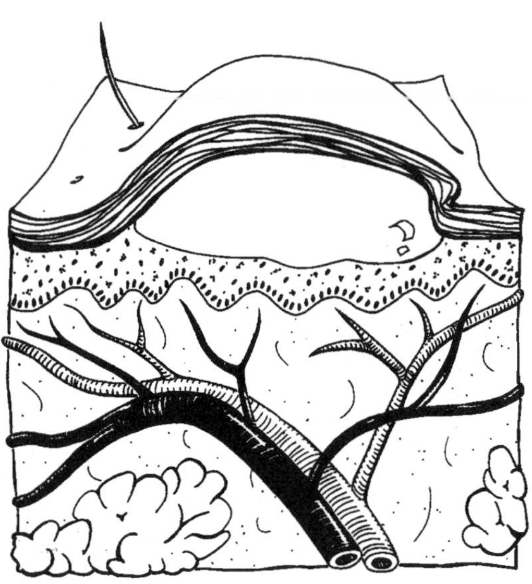

Fig. 13-10. A bulla. The lesion is drawn at the subcorneal level, but most bullae are found at the dermal epidermal junction. (From Lynch,[4] with permission.)

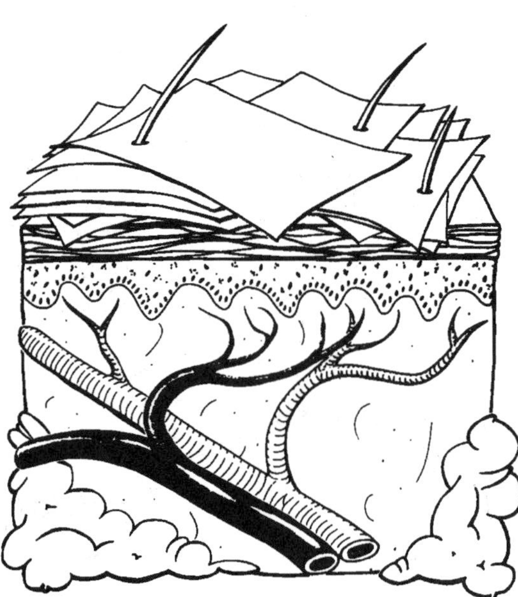

Fig. 13-11. Scale. The square flakes shown would, in actuality, be irregular in shape and would be made up of a mosaic of stratum corneum cells. (From Lynch,[4] with permission.)

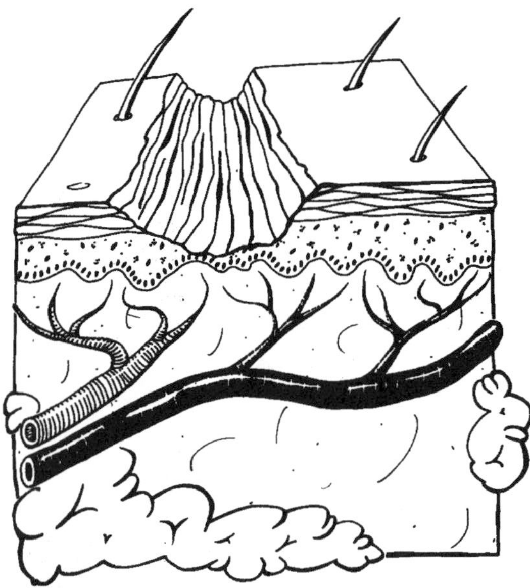

Fig. 13-12. An erosion. The linear furrow shown would probably be due to scratching. (From Lynch,[4] with permission.)

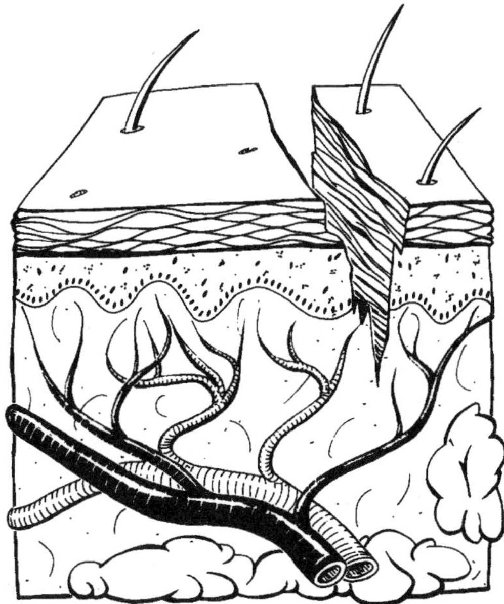

Fig. 13-13. A fissure. This very narrow linear erosion would appear clinically as a red line; the defect itself is often not visible. (From Lynch,[4] with permission.)

Configuration of Skin Lesions

Grouped lesions are a conjugation of lesions usually within a fairly small area. Annular lesions represent a circular, or round, configuration. Linear configurations are basically in a straight line. Linear lesions are an unusual configuration for naturally occurring skin lesions. Linear lesions usually are the result of an outside irritant such as brushing up against poison ivy or a mechanical spreading or manipulation by the individual causing the linear distribution pattern. Serpiginous configuration gives the impression of the lesion creeping from one part to another, possibly multiple lesions joining together.

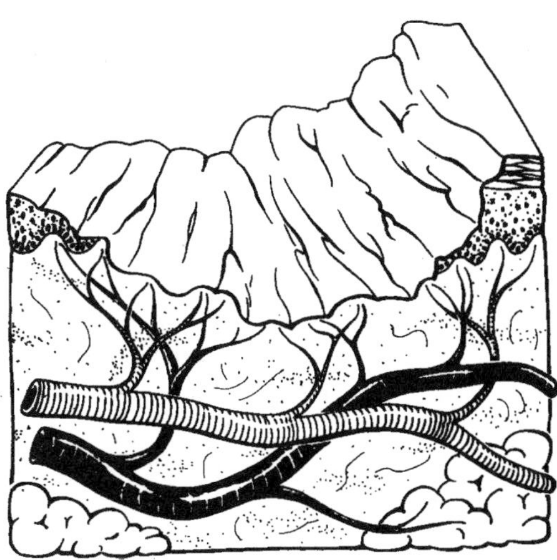

Fig. 13-14. An ulcer. The defect of an ulcer extends into, or through, the dermis. (From Lynch,[4] with permission.)

In addition to the configuration of skin growths, the examiner should consider size, shape, characteristics of the borders, color, and symptomatology. The size of a lesion is important in differentiating one skin growth from another. Vesicle versus bulla, macule versus patch, and papule versus plaque are separated only by their size. A diameter of 1.5 cm is the separation point for each of these pairs.[1]

Lesions can be shaped round, oval, symmetric, or asymmetric. Growths can be flat, depressed, raised above the skin, or raised below the skin. Irregular and ill-defined borders of an isolated lesion are indicative of possible melanoma.

The configuration of the color in some cases is more of a definitive sign of concern than the actual color itself. For example, a growth of multiple shades of brown would raise more suspicion than a growth of solid dark brown color. It is important to recognize whether the color of a lesion is due to pigmentation (growths) or vascularization (rashes, venus pooling). Pigmented lesions are not blanchable, whereas vascular lesions many times are blanchable. A recent change in color of any growth is a red flag for referral.

Location of Skin Lesions

The location of the skin lesion often leads the clinician to the suspected cause of the problem. For example, contact dermatitis is the result of direct contact with the irritant causing the rash. The therapist should examine the lesion to see if there is a pattern associated with exposure of the body part to physical contact with an irritant. Areas of the body that are exposed to the elements of nature may be indicators of contact with tree and plant secretions or poisonous plants such as poison ivy. Exposure to the sun and wind can cause burning and drying of the skin.

Rashes on sun-exposed areas may be the result of a photosensitive reaction in a patient taking photosensitive medications. Individuals can have reactions to contact with clothing, bedding, cosmetics, lotions, or even airborne irritants that may show up on specific locations of the body.

Chronology (Season or Time of Onset)

Rashes associated with allergies may well be associated with spring and fall seasons. Pruritus (itching) is quite common during the winter because artificial heating systems deplete the humidity in the air, causing a drying of the skin.

Rashes associated with periodic exacerbations may also relate to the activities being performed by the patient during certain hours of the day. Exacerbations of the patient's condition during work hours may indicate some exposure to skin irritants at work. Patients who work with chemicals, especially photographic processing chemicals, inks and dyes, cleaning chemicals, and pesticides may be vulnerable to skin lesions.

The length of time since onset is also a very important factor in diagnosing skin lesions. Skin lesions that have existed since birth or for more than 5 years include birthmarks, freckles, moles (nevi), skin tags, and seborrheic keratosis. These represent benign common skin lesions that are rarely problematic. Skin lesions that have existed less than 2 years should be brought to the attention of a physician, and they should be observed regularly by the patient or a significant other. Skin lesions appearing spontaneously in adulthood should be considered a potential problem until proven otherwise. Lesions less than 5 years but greater than 2 years in duration should also be seen by a physician, as a precaution, so that the physician can make an initial diagnosis and establish a baseline for future reference and ongoing evaluation of changes in the lesions.

Causes of Lesions

Most common skin disorders can be classified as either growths or rashes. Growths are permanent eruptions of the skin resulting from a defined mass of tissue. A growth may be benign or malignant. A growth may be a result of the proliferation of cells, a conglomeration of blood vessels, or a foreign body being engulfed by one of the layers of the skin. Rashes are temporary eruptions of the skin frequently associated with childhood diseases and allergic reactions as in heat rash, diaper rash, reaction to foods, and/or drug-induced eruptions. Both growths and rashes present themselves with associated clinical signs and symptoms. Symptoms associated with skin lesions are pruritus (itching), color changes, and sometimes pain. Abnormal skin conditions arise from various causes.

Mechanical Processes

Blisters, calluses, corns, and ulcers can result from abnormal mechanical stresses on the skin. Blisters and calluses develop as a result of abnormal frictional forces, whereas corns and ulcers are pressure related.

Inflammatory Conditions

Inflammation of the skin results in a reddening of the skin and is referred to as erythema. Increased skin temperature can accompany inflammatory skin disorders. Acne, lichen planus, psoriasis, and pityriasis rosea are common inflammatory skin disorders.[3] These conditions are usually localized and are rarely associated with specific internal disease.[3] Exposure to sun, heat, cold, and wind can also cause inflammatory skin conditions.

Infections

Infections of the skin include viral infections, fungal infections, and bacterial infections. Fungal infections include various forms of tinea (athlete's foot, ring worm, fungal infections of the nails). Viral infections include verrucae (common warts, genital warts), herpes simplex (cold sores, fever blisters), and herpes zoster (shingles). Bacterial infections can be a secondary complication of many skin conditions when bacteria invade previously damaged skin. Impetigo, usually occurring in infants and young children, is the most common primary bacterial infection of the skin and is associated with staphylococci. Impetigo can be highly contagious.

Allergies

Allergic skin responses result because of the body's hypersensitivity to a variety of irritants. Contact dermatitis results from direct physical contact with the irritant. Certain types of fibers, dyes, rubbers, and elastics used in clothing can cause skin irritation. Plants such as poison ivy, poison sumac, and poison oak are common irritants. Exposure to metals, metal salts, chemicals, and gases are frequent occupation-related irritants. Cosmetics, perfumes, deodorants, personal hygiene products, and laundry detergents are common causes of contact dermatitis.

Drug reactions and food reactions are two additional causes for allergic skin reactions. Skin lesions are directly related to the administration of the medication (injections, oral medications) or ingestion of food. The skin reaction may appear hours or days after the initial exposure and may resolve spontaneously upon elimination of the drug or food.

Eczema is an allergic skin disorder sometimes associated with a patient history or family history of asthma and hay fever. Eczema can present itself with severe skin lesions, change in pigmentation, and change in texture and elasticity of the skin.

Individuals can also experience an allergic reaction to insect and bug bites. A normal reaction to an insect bite produces a common localized reaction often accompanied by mild pruritus. In an allergic reaction, the patient may experience a severe localized inflammatory response or severe systemic reaction including nausea, vomiting, and fever. A thorough skin examination may be the only way to reveal an insect bite as the cause of such an allergic reaction.

Parasitic Infestation

Certain types of bugs will infiltrate the skin and can be problematic if not detected and treated early. Mites, lice, and ticks are the three most common parasites of human skin. These parasites are transmittable by close contact with other individuals who carry the parasite or, in the case of ticks, with trees, plants, or underbrush such as in heavily wooded areas. Parasitic lesions present themselves as linear burrows and are accompanied by severe itching or a feeling of creeping or crawling under the skin.

Tumors

The skin can develop a variety of growths or tumors. Most tumors are benign, and include common moles called nevi. Nevi can be flat or raised, pigmented or nonpigmented, and hairy or hairless. Dark pigmented nevi can take on a bluish cast due to the translucence of the overlying skin. This is called a blue nevus and is sometimes mistaken for a malignant melanoma. Not all nevi are potential malignancies, but any mole that undergoes a change in size, shape, color, symptoms (itching or pain), or integrity (bleeding) is reason for immediate referral for further medical diagnosis.

The three most common forms of skin cancer are basal cell carcinoma, squamous cell carcinoma, and malignant melanoma. Basal cell carcinoma is the most common form of skin cancer followed by squamous cell carcinoma. Both forms of carcinoma appear to be related to exposure to the sun and are most frequently found on sun-exposed areas of the body. Malignant melanoma is the most deadly form of skin cancer. The occurrence of melanoma is on the rise and is the leading cause of death of all skin disorders.[3]

EXAMINATION OF THE SKIN

History

The initial history includes questions related to the patient's primary physical therapy diagnosis, family and social history, and work history. In most cases the history regarding the skin condition is taken after the initial observation of the skin during the musculoskeletal examination. A more detailed dermatologic history is performed by the physical therapist if the patient has a complaint regarding the skin or if the therapist identifies a questionable lesion. Important questions to include are: Have you noted this spot on your skin? How long has it been there? Has the spot changed size, shape, color, or symptoms (pain, itching, bleeding)? Have you noticed any other spots like this anywhere else on your body? Has a physician looked at this spot? If the questionable lesion is located in an area not easily observed by the patient, (i.e. interscapular region), the questions should be directed as follows: Has anyone noticed and told you about this spot on your back?, and so forth. Physical therapists may want to consider expanding their intake questionnaire to include specific questions about history of cancer (personal or family members), skin cancers, melanoma, and existing skin problems. A history of prior episodes of the same or similar skin condition may quickly lead to an understanding of the current skin condition.

Physical Examination

Examination of the skin is best performed in a room with good lighting and adequate privacy for the patient. The patient should be undressed at least to the underwear to give the examiner the benefit of observing as much surface area of skin as possible. This will give the examiner the opportunity to observe asymmetry and unilateral differences.

Examination of the skin is initially performed by the physical therapist during the observation and palpation portions of the physical therapy examination. Routinely the therapist performs observation for the purpose of identifying postural problems, muscular imbalances, and surgical scars. Palpation is performed to assess muscle tone, spasm, and possible painful trigger points. Physical therapists are encouraged to expand their observation and palpation skills to include assessment of skin lesions and detection of skin manifestations of internal disease.

An initial observation and palpation examination is performed focusing on the primary physical therapy referral diagnosis. If an overt skin problem is detected immediately, the therapist should make a note and complete the rest of the physical therapy examination. Giving immediate attention to the problem may alarm the patient and create anxiety that may influence the rest of the physical examination. Questionable skin lesions should be examined in detail after the therapist has completed all testing pertinent to the patient's primary complaints. As always, universal precautions should be used, as there are many skin conditions that are transmittable by physical contact.

Observation

Good observation of the patient's skin is essential in screening the skin. Close visual inspection will enable the therapist to assess changes in overall coloration of the skin as well as identify questionable lesions that require further inspection and assessment.

Criteria that should be considered when assessing a skin lesion include size, color, shape, and borders. Moles larger than 6 mm in diameter and asymmetrically shaped should raise concern on the therapist's part. Moles that are black, blue-black, or multicolored should also alert the therapist that a pathologic lesion may be present. Ill-defined and irregular borders are not typically associated with benign moles. An ulcerated lesion should also be noted and examined by a physician.

In addition, the therapist should inspect the fingernails, toenails, and hair. The examiner should inspect the nails for color, shape, brittleness, hemorrhages or spots under the nail, abnormal lines or grooves, and an increase of the white area of the nail. Changes in color, shape, and integrity of nails could be indicators of internal diseases (Fig. 13-15). Loss of hair, color changes, and changes of texture of the hair may also indicate underlying problems.

Palpation

Palpation of the skin is used to determine temperature, mobility and turgor, and texture. Palpations for these qualities can be done at the same time the therapist is palpating for muscle tone and spasm.

Temperature

The therapist should compare several areas of the body in assessing skin temperature, keeping in mind areas that are covered by clothing or in contact with furniture or equipment immediately prior to the examination. Localized warmth is associated with inflammation, while a literally hot and swollen joint may indicate infection or hemarthrosis. Generalized warmth of the skin can be indicative of hyperthyroidism, whereas hypothyroidism produces generalized coolness.

Raynaud's disease is a temperature-dependent dermatosis resulting in vasospasm of the digital arteries following exposure to cold temperatures. The condition is referred to as Raynaud's disease when there is no apparent underlying condition and as Raynaud's phenomenon when the condition is associated with an underlying condition such as systemic lupus, rheumatoid arthritis, Buerger's disease, thoracic outlet syndrome, carpal tunnel, drug reactions, following frostbite, or primary pulmonary hypertension.[2]

Mobility and Turgor

Mobility and turgor refer to the ability of the skin to be moved and subsequently return to its resting state. The therapist should lift the skin by pinching it between the thumb and index fingers, assess the mobility, then release it and observe how quickly it returns to its resting state. Decreased mobility of the skin may be indicative of scleroderma or other collagen diseases; however, it is more often associated with common edema.

If decreased mobility of a mole and the adjacent skin is noted when moving the skin in different directions, suspicion should be raised. This may be indicative of a lesion that is growing into deeper layers of the skin.

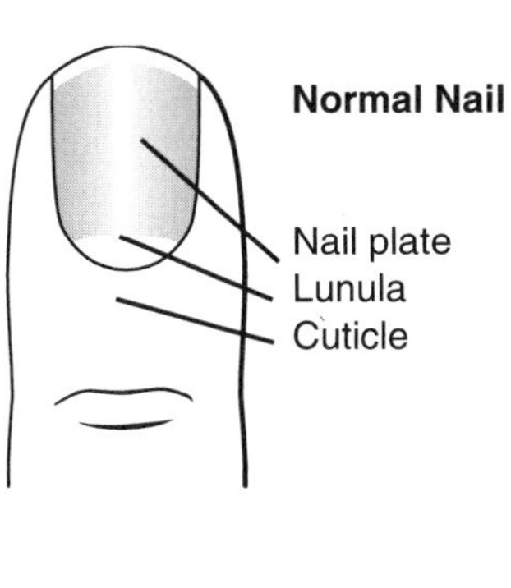

Normal Nail

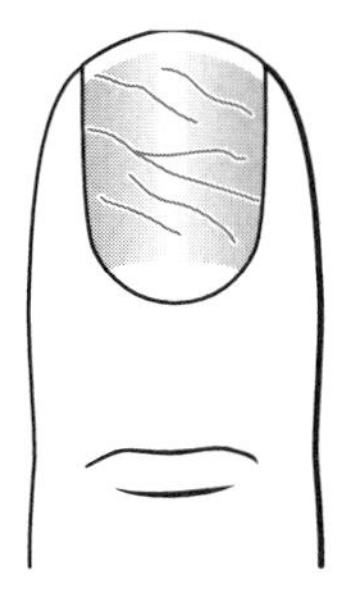

Beau's Lines

Transverse depressions found in any patient who has had a severe systemic insult such as a high fever, infection, renal disease, or hepatic disease

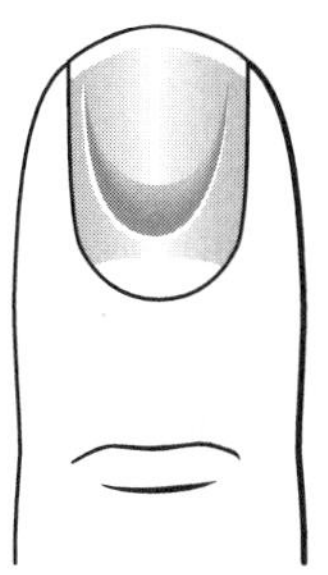

Spoon Nail

Found in patients with iron deficiency

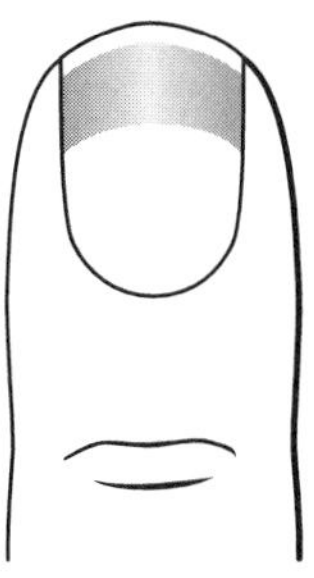

Terry's Nails

The nail bed appears white for more than two-thirds of its length. Found in patients with cirrhosis of the liver and hypoalbuminemia

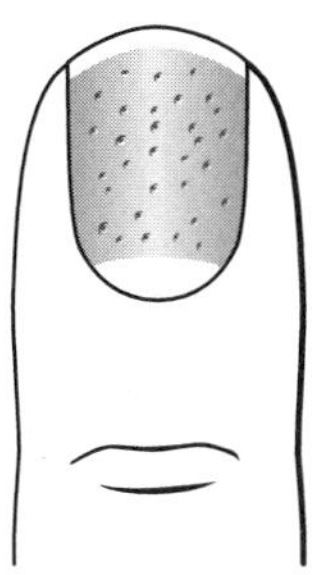

Psoriasis

Pitting of the nail bed is found in 50% of patients with psoriasis

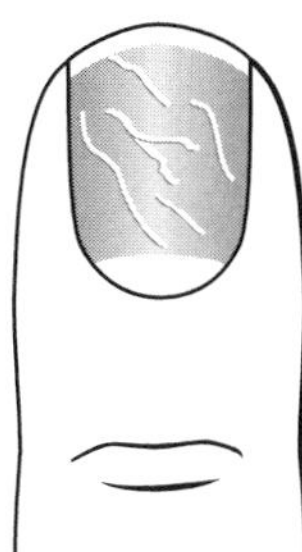

Mee's Lines

A white discoloration of the nail plate that form transverse lines across the nail. The lines usually do not extend across the entire nail. Found in patients following arsenic poisoning, but also found in renal failure, heart disease, and pneumonia.[1]

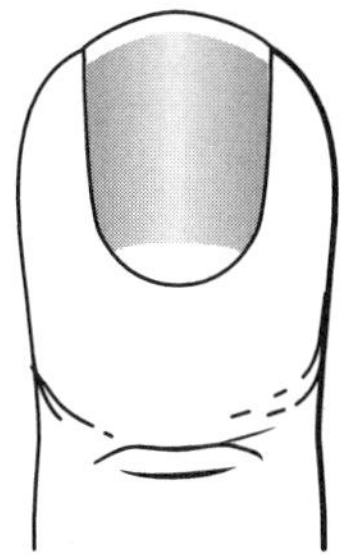

Clubbing

A broadening of the distal appendage with an increased Lovibond's angles as viewed from the lateral side

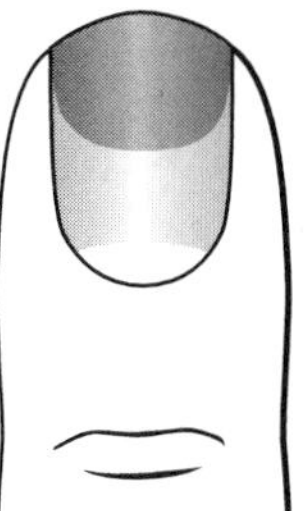

Half-and-Half Nails

A normal white proximal portion of the nail with a distinct brownish distal portion, the latter being over one-third of the nail plate. Indicates chronic renal failure

Fig. 13-15. Common systemic diseases manifested in changes in the nail.

Decreased turgor is associated with dehydration, which should be frequently assessed by therapists working with infants and the elderly. Keep in mind that decreased turgor comes with the aging process, but the therapist should be familiar with norms for all age groups.

Texture

Rough, dry skin can be the result of over exposure to wind and sun and is also common in the winter months associated with heating systems that dehumidify the air. Generalized extreme roughness or cracking of the skin can also be a sign of hypothyroidism. Roughness of the skin over specific body areas may indicate an underlying scale or crust.[2]

Laboratory Tests

The physical therapist is usually not in a position to conduct or order laboratory tests, so details of this aspect are not included in this chapter. Keep in mind, however, that the goals of the physical therapist in screening the skin is not to come up with a definitive diagnosis, but to educate the patient regarding a questionable area and to refer the patient who presents with a skin condition that will require further medical evaluation. Laboratory tests are most appropriately left to the discretion of the physician.

SUMMARY

Since the late 1980s the practice of physical therapy has rapidly been changing to include direct access of patients and the inclusion of physical therapists in wellness programs. Physical therapists are positioned to become an integral part of the health care team, and with this comes the responsibility of expanding our scope of practice. Physical therapists should be encouraged to expand their knowledge of dermatologic conditions and to include a thorough screening as part of their clinical assessments. See Table 13-2 for a summary of clinical findings that should raise concern on the therapist's part.

The systematic approach to screening the skin presented in this chapter will help the therapist understand the underlying cause of most skin conditions presented in the clinic. Taking time to ask the patient more questions about questionable skin conditions will provide many answers. Since dermatologic laboratory testing and prescription of medication are both outside the scope of practice of physical therapists, it will be necessary for the therapist to refer many patients to a physician for definitive diagnosis and treatment. However, the importance of skin screening by physical therapists should not be minimized. The physical therapist who routinely screens for skin disorders may be the catalyst to get the patient appropriate medical treatment before the condition worsens. This will prevent disability and disfigurement and can save lives.

Table 13-2. Summary of Clinical Findings Suggesting a Pathologic Skin Lesion

Linear shape
Asymmetric shape
Irregular borders
Ill-defined borders
Multiple shades of color
Black, blue-black color
Friable/ulcerated
Greater than 6 mm in diameter
Decreased mobility
Firm to hard consistency
Pain
Pruritus
Recent change in color, shape, size
Recent appearance (within 5 years)

PATIENT CASE STUDY 1

History

The patient is a 42-year-old male who was referred to the clinic with left-sided shoulder pain. He reported a gradual onset of pain over 2 weeks, but related no particular incident or trauma to the onset of the shoulder pain. The Patient reported a long history of pain and instability of the left shoulder following a sports injury in high school. The family history includes a father who died of liver cancer at age 87 and a brother who died at age 42 of cancer (primary lesion unknown).

Objective Examination

The patient exhibited limited capsular range of motion specifically in the posterior direction, excessive capsular range anteriorly, limited glenohumeral abduction, and limited glenohumeral flexion. Active range of motion was limited in combined shoulder flexion and shoulder abduction, as well as internal rotation. The patient exhibited a painful arc during active abduction of the shoulder.

Assessment

Acute inflammatory process secondary to subacromial bursitis and possible acute arthritis was diagnosed. The prescribed treatment included modality treatment for the active inflammatory process, passive range of motion, joint mobilization to re-establish normal capsular motion, and instruction in home exercise program.

While completing the initial treatment the therapist noticed a small amount of dried blood adjacent to a small mole on the tip of the patient's left shoulder immediately above the acromion process. When the patient was questioned about the bleeding, he responded "oh, that happens every couple of weeks when I dry off with a towel after a shower, but it always heals and I never thought anything of it."

The therapist examined the mole closer and measured it to be approximately 6 mm in diameter, reddish-brown in color, with regular borders. The mole was slightly raised and at this point appeared to have a soft center due to the bleeding caused by wiping the patient's shoulder. Because of the bleeding, the patient was referred back to his physician, who subsequently sent him to a dermatologic specialist who performed a biopsy of the mole. Laboratory results 1 week later revealed a level IV malignant melanoma.

The patient underwent surgery for a wide resection of the melanoma and removal of left axillary lymph nodes. Laboratory tests of the surgically removed tissue revealed clear borders of the tissue surrounding the tumor and clear lymph node biopsy, a positive prognosis for this diagnosis.

This case demonstrates the importance of physical therapists screening the skin. Although it was obvious from the onset that the apparently minor skin lesion was not contributing to the painful left shoulder condition for which the patient was referred, the therapist's actions and ultimate referral resulted in the positive outcome of what could have been a fatal disease.

PATIENT CASE STUDY 2

History

The patient is a 27-year-old female who came to the physical therapy clinic with complaints of constant, bilateral lower extremity pain. She reported onset of pain 6 weeks ago after beginning an exercise program that included the use of weight machines and running. The patient reported that she used to be a long distance runner until approximately 1 year ago, when she had her first child. She recently began running to get in shape and lose about 10 pounds, but had to stop due to constant pain in the shins.

Objective Examination

A postural evaluation revealed a slight forward head position and a slight decrease of normal lumbar lordosis. Range of motion, strength testing, mobility testing, and special tests were all within normal limits for lumbar spine and bilateral lower extremities.

Physical inspection of the lower extremities revealed large patches of increased pigmentation on the front of the lower legs. With further questioning about this the patient stated that she had noticed the discoloration of the areas of the lower extremities. She had attributed it to irritation of her skin on the exercise equipment and to an increased exposure to the sun, which she'd had little of since giving up running 2 years ago. Further skin inspection was performed that revealed recurrent skin irritation in the axillae bilaterally.

Assessment

The patient exhibited no positive signs of orthopaedic or musculoskeletal pathology that warranted treatment. Signs and symptoms pointed toward a peripheral neuropathy of unknown cause.

Further inquiry into the patient's lifestyle revealed that she had significantly changed her diet and had increased her carbohydrate intake to help her running. Questioning also revealed that she experienced occasional dizziness and blurred vision, which she again attributed to being out of shape. Questions regarding her family history revealed that there is a long history of diabetes, but she has never had a problem with it. Her last complete examination including blood work was approximately 9 months ago.

Due to the skin conditions noted on the patient's legs and axillae, the family history of diabetes, recent changes in diet, and dizziness/blurred vision, the patient was referred back to her family doctor for a complete physical and blood work prior to continuing any exercise program or continuing with a physical therapy program.

One week later the patient phoned and stated that her blood work did reveal that she was diabetic and that at this time she was being managed with oral medications. The same day the patient's physician called the therapist and confirmed the results of the blood work and discussed that his goal was eventually to manage patient's diabetes with diet and exercise.

PATIENT CASE STUDY 3

History

The patient is a 65-year-old female who was referred to physical therapy with a diagnosis of rheumatoid arthritis and bilateral upper extremity weakness. The patient reported that she was diagnosed with rheumatoid arthritis approximately 13 years ago but that she has managed quite well over the years, in spite of her arthritis. She was currently working full-time as an office manager in a computer business. Two weeks ago, she experienced neck pain and arm pain bilaterally. She also complained of generalized weakness and having difficulty in the past 2 weeks carrying out her housework because of weakness in both arms and general fatigue.

Objective Examination

The patient exhibited postural deformities consistent with the diagnosis of rheumatoid arthritis. She showed limitations of range of motion at the shoulder, elbow, wrist, and hand bilaterally. Limitations at all joints were noted to be in noncapsular patterns. Cervical range of motion is limited in all directions, with no increase in pain. Manual muscle strength was bilaterally symmetric and 4/5 range throughout. Gait was slow and guarded, atypical of patient's tested strength and balance. A shallow breathing pattern was noted, but chest sounds were clear.

During the examination, several dozen dark wartlike growths were noted on the patient's middle and upper back. When questioned about these, she reported that she has had "a dozen or so" of these growths for many years; she had been to a dermatologist several times over the years and was always told that these growths were nothing to worry about. She has noticed many more of these in the past month and was waiting until she felt better before going back to the dermatologist.

Assessment

Limited range of motion consistent with long-standing rheumatoid arthritis was diagnosed. There was also generalized weakness and fatigue inconsistent with patient history and activity level.

The treatment plan included a review of medications, use of resting hand splints, and home exercises for strength and range of motion. In addition, the patient was referred back to her family physician for a closer inspection of the skin condition identified during the physical therapy examination. The physician was notified by the therapist of what appeared to be seborrheic keratosis and of the therapist's concern of the appearance of several dozen additional lesions over the past month. The physician was aware of the prior existence of the keratoses, but was not aware of their increase and immediately scheduled the patient for an appointment.

The increase in the number of seborrheic keratoses over a short period alerted the dermatologist that the patient was exhibiting an important warning sign called the sign of Leser-Trélat. This sign suggested a completed work-up for a possible internal malignancy.

The patient was ultimately diagnosed with internal malignancy of the pituitary gland and subsequently underwent surgery and chemotherapy. Both surgery and chemotherapy went well, and the patient has survived 18 months with no recurrence of malignancy.

REFERENCES

1. Sauer GC: Manual of skin disease. 4th Ed. JB Lippincott, Philadelphia, 1980
2. Sams WM Jr: Structure and function of the skin. p. 3. In Sams WM, Lynch PJ (eds): Principles and Practice of Dermatology. Churchill Livingstone, New York, 1990
3. Simandl G: Alteration in skin function and integrity. In Porth CM: Pathophysiology concepts of altered health states. 4th Ed. JB Lippincott, Philadelphia, 1994
4. Lynch PJ: Principles of diagnosis. p. 15. In Sams WM Jr, Lynch PJ (eds): Principles and Practice of Dermatology. Churchill Livingstone, New York, 1990

SUGGESTED READINGS

Arndt AA: Manual of Dermatologic Therapeutics With Essentials of Diagnosis. 4th Ed. Little Brown and Co, Boston, 1991

Bluefarb SM: Dermatology. The Upjohn Company, Kalamazoo, 1984

Callen JP, Jorizzo J Greer KE et al: Dermatological Signs of Internal Disease. WB Saunders, Philadelphia, 1988

Jacobs PH, Anhalt TS: Handbook of Skin Clues of Systemic Disease. 2nd Ed. Lea & Febiger, Philadelphia, 1992

Kusch SL: Clinical Dermatology: A Manual of Differential Diagnosis. Rev Edition. Westwood-Squibb Pharmaceuticals Inc., Buffalo, 1991

Lamberg SI: Dermatology in Primary Care: A Problem Oriented Guide. WB Saunders, Philadelphia, 1986

Lawrence CM, Cox NH: Physical Signs in Dermatology Color Atlas and Text. Wolfe Publishing, London, 1993

Lazarus GS, Goldsmith LA, Tharp MD: Diagnosis of Skin Disease Introduction. FA Davis, Philadelphia, 1980

Levene GM, Calnan CD: A Colour Atlas of Dermatology. Wolfe Publishing, London, 1993

Levene GM, Goolamali SK: Diagnostic Picture Tests in Dermatology. Wolfe Publishing, London, 1986

Lynch PJ: Dermatology for the House Officer. Williams & Wilkins, Baltimore, 1982

Sams WM, Lynch PJ: Principles and Practice of Dermatology. Churchill Livingstone, New York, 1990

Sauer GC: Manual of Skin Disease. 4th Ed. JB Lippincott, Philadelphia, 1980

Simandl G: Alteration in skin function and integrity. In Porth CM (ed): Pathophysiology Concepts of Altered Health States. 4th Ed. JB Lippincott, Philadelphia, 1994

Weston WL, Lane AT: Color Textbook of Pediatric Dermatology. Mosby, St. Louis, 1991

Wilkinson JD, Shaw S, Fenton DA: Dermatology Colour Guide. Churchill Livingstone, London, 1993

APPENDIX 13-1

Glossary

PRIMARY SKIN LESIONS

Bulla: A mass that becomes round by swelling. A large vesicle. A fluid-filled lesion greater than 1.5 cm in diameter.

Macule: An area of perceptible change in color on, in, or of the skin that is not visibly or palpably raised above or depressed below the surrounding general level of the skin. A spot, stain, blemish, or blot. The area of discolored skin is flat and no wider than 1.5 cm.

Nodule: A small node or knobby development in the form of a small mass. A papule that has enlarged in length and width as well as in height or depth.

Papule: A palpable solid lesion no larger than 1.5 cm (pea sized). Papules may be raised above the level of the skin or palpable below the skin, as in a lipoma.

Petechia: A minute hemorrhage resulting in a spot, speck, or freckle on the skin.

Plaque: A papule greater than 1.5 cm. The enlargement of the plaque does not include greater elevation above the skin or greater invasion under the skin.

Purpura: That purplish discoloration that results from hemorrhage into a tissue.

Pustule: A vesicle that has an appreciably purulent content, white or yellow-white in color. Lesions above 1.5 cm diameter are better defined as boils, abscesses, or furuncles.

Rash: An eruption on the skin. Commonly used to describe widespread, red, slightly elevated eruptions.

Tumor: A swelling or growth in the form of a mass. There is no inherent meaning of malignancy or cancer in the word. Many tumors are nonmalignant or benign.

Vesicle: A small blister. A fluid-filled lesion of up to 1.5 cm in diameter.

Wheal: A raised area of the skin appearing as an edematous papule (e.g., a hive).

SECONDARY LESIONS

Crust: Dried serum or exudate of varied colors on the surface of a skin lesion. Crust often accompanies skin conditions such as impetigo and infected dermatitis. Yellow crust is superficial and overlies an erosion. Red or black crust overlies deeper, ulcerative lesions.[1]

Excoriations: Superficial abrasions of the skin usually caused by trauma to a pre-existing insect bite or skin lesion. The traumas resulting in excoriations are frequently caused by the individual seeking relief from itching by scratching the site of the lesion.

Fissures: Linear breaks in the integrity of the skin. Fissures have sharply defined borders. Fissures can also result from a thickening and/or severe drying of the skin. Fissures are frequently found with athlete's foot.

Growth: Permanent eruption of the skin resulting from a defined mass of tissue. A growth may be benign or malignant, and it may be the result of a proliferation of cells, a conglomeration of blood vessels, or a foreign body engulfed by one of the layers of the skin.

Hypertrophic scar: A complication of wound healing that results in exuberant cicatrization (scarring) that resembles keloid formation. Some authors use the terms hypertrophic scar and keloid interchangeably, while others maintain that hypertrophic scars, unlike keloids, do not extend beyond the limits of the wound and eventually flatten themselves out.

Keloids: Raised scars that result from keloidosis. Keloids can be both disfiguring and painful and can extend beyond the limits of the initial wound.

Lesion: The loss of tissue continuity structure or function secondary to trauma, disease, illness, or pathology.

Lichenification: Diffuse area of thickening of the skin accompanied by scaling with increases in skin lines and markings due to a grouping of papules.

Pruritus: Itching that is common to many skin disorders. Pruritus is a skin manifestation that accompanies many skin disorders involving dry or scaly skin but may also be a manifestation of illness or disease such as diabetes mellitus.

Rash: Temporary eruption of the skin frequently associated with childhood diseases, such as heat rash or diaper rash, and certain medications.

Scab: Formation of a hardened collection of clotted blood and sloughing of a tissue that forms on superficial wounds of the skin. The terms scab and crust are sometimes used interchangeably.

Scale: A condition of the skin that appears to be a separation like a husk caused by dead epidermal cells. Scales may be dry or greasy. Scales are present during skin conditions like dandruff and psoriasis. Sometimes scales can be felt as a roughness, even though they are not visible.

Scar: A skin lesion that develops by the formation of dense fibrous tissue covered by atrophic epidermis. Scars may be raised or recessed (pitting) and may be the result of trauma, surgery, or diseases such as chicken pox.

Ulcers: Sores on the skin resulting in excavation of the skin from the outer surface downward. Ulcers are frequently caused by loss of nutrition and/or blood flow to a specific area of the skin. Examples are stasis ulcers of the legs, pressure sores, and ulceration at the site of a melanoma.

SPECIAL LESIONS

Burrow: A subcutaneous tunnel-like lesion usually caused by the invasion of a parasite such as a mite, tick, or scabies.

Comedones: Discolored, dried sebum plugging the excretory ducts of the skin. Frequently associated with acne and referred to as a blackhead.

Milia: Pinhead-sized papules or keratin-filled cysts. Often found on the face and trunk of newborns.

Telangiectasia: A vascular lesion formed by the dilatation of blood vessels. It may appear at birth (birthmark) or in young children. Frequently found on the face or thighs.

14 Clinical Pharmacology for the Physical Therapist

Stephen D. Cain, Pharm.D.
Steven C. Janos, M.S., P.T.

In almost every health care setting, physical therapists deal with patients who are taking some sort of medication. It may be a prescription drug or something as simple as aspirin. In either case, the medication may have enough of an impact on the patient's condition that it affects the clinical presentation or course of treatment. For example, up to 90 percent of ambulatory elderly patients take at least one medication, and most take two or more. As the role of the physical therapist continues to change and we encounter a greater percentage of patients as the entry point into the health care system, we take on a greater responsibility for a more holistic understanding of our patients.

The purpose of this chapter is to present drug classifications used in physical therapy-related patients, a listing and description of individual medications used for common pathologic processes, and side effects that may occur with their usage. This chapter is also designed to give the therapist clinical information that will be useful during the initial patient examination, treatment, and reassessment process.

Additional information for physical therapists concerning drugs and their actions and possible side effects can be obtained from several sources. The most commonly used is the *Physicians' Desk Reference* (PDR). Copies are usually plentiful but may contain more detailed information than the therapist might need. *Drug Use Education Tips* (DUET) is a package published by the American Academy of Family Physicians. It was designed as an easily readable manual for both the health care practitioner and the patient.

The principle of patient education, particularly in the area of information concerning medications, is no longer a debatable philosophy but has been established as a vital component of medical care. We have turned from the consideration of "the need to know" to the establishment of a "right to know" as an integral part of patient care. The DUET manual is a simple, convenient, yet informative way to assist patients toward a better understanding of the medications they may be taking. Patients who have questions about their prescriptions can be given a photocopy of the appropriate page from the DUET package.

Clinical Examination

The initial examination is when the physical therapist first obtains background information on the nature and state of the patient's condition. During the subjective review of symptoms, the therapist should inquire whether the patient is currently, or has in the past, taken medications for the problem. It can be helpful to have the patient fill out a pre-examination questionnaire relative to the medical history. It is useful to send these questionnaires to patients before they arrive for their first physical therapy visit, to give them time to fill in the specific names and dosages of medications they are taking (Fig. 14-1). The following list of questions can be used to screen for medications during the examination.

PHYSICAL THERAPY

To facilitate the evaluation process during your first visit, please complete this questionnaire and give it to your physical therapist at your first visit. Your cooperation is greatly appreciated.

NAME: ____________________ SOCIAL SECURITY #: ______________

AGE: ______ Presently working? Yes No Date last worked: ____________

Occupation/type of work : ________________________________

Leisure activities: ________________________________

1. List any physician, dentist, osteopath, physical therapist, or chiropractor you have seen for your present condition.
2. List all general medical problems for which you have received treatment.
3. Describe any history of joint/muscle problems and treatment you may have received.
4. List all surgeries and hospitalizations you have had and their dates.
5. List all medications you are currently taking.
6. Have you taken steroids (cortisone, Prednisone)? Yes No

   If so, describe the condition for which they were prescribed.

Fig. 14-1. Physical therapy questionnaire.

This information helps in several ways. It assists in the overall determination of the severity of the patient's problem or pain tolerance level, or both. Are the symptoms so bad that medications are not apparently helping, or does the patient complain of high levels of pain, yet takes no medication, even when it is indicated?

The first question is to check with patients for all medications they are currently taking. Patients often will not volunteer information about drugs they do not believe are related to the physical therapy problem. It is important to be as specific as possible with patients in getting the correct name of each drug. If they are not sure, the therapist may review the names of various common medications given for this type of problem with the patient or ask the patient to bring the medication to therapy at the next visit. The therapist may feel the need to call the physician's office for further information. If it is not obvious, patients should be asked why they have been placed on these particular medications. Patients should know what each drug is used for. Often they are not sure why they are taking the drugs, which can lead to improper usage. This is especially true of patients who have either multiple problems or chronic conditions.

Occasionally patients will not offer correct historical information, even upon direct questioning. In many of these cases, a good basic knowledge of drug classifications and further questioning will help ascertain all the facts. For example, a patient reports initially that she has

Subjective Examination Medication Screening

1. What medications (all) are currently being taken (prescription and nonprescription?)
2. What is the dosage of each medication?
3. How often is each medication being taken? (Include times of day.)
4. When was medication prescribed and by whom?
5. When did the patient begin taking each medication?
6. For what purpose was the medication prescribed?
7. Does the medication appear to be beneficial/helping?
8. Do there appear to be any side effects related to taking the medication?
9. Has the medication been taken in the past? If so, what was the effect?
10. When does the medication prescription run out?

not had any surgical procedures in the past yet, when questioned about medications, reports that she is currently taking an estrogen/progesterone supplement. When asked why, she states that she underwent a hysterectomy several years before.

Another patient denies that he has any current medical problems or had any previous surgeries or hospitalizations. When asked about medication, he relates that he is taking lithium, which is an antidepressant medication. Upon further questioning, he admits to recently having been hospitalized for depression. This could be important information to the treating therapist and may have a bearing on the overall treatment course.

We also need to know, if possible, how much of each medication is being taken, how often, and at what time of day. For example, a patient states that he no longer takes his anti-inflammatory medication because it upsets his stomach, a common side effect. Upon further questioning, it is learned that he takes an 800-mg tablet of ibuprofen daily, on an empty stomach. The physician alters the medication to 200-mg tablets qid and makes sure the patient understands that he is to take it with meals. Soon afterward, the patient reports a marked improvement in his condition.

Upon initial examination, it may be important to ascertain from patients when they first started taking their medication. Many times patients state that their medication is not helping the condition, but upon further questioning, the therapist finds that they have only been taking it for 1 to 2 days. Some medications work immediately, but many take several days or longer.

After finding out what medications are being taken, the physical therapist must determine their effectiveness. More often than not, patients can tell whether it has had a beneficial effect or not. Occasionally, the therapist may have to help patients relate their medications not only to pain levels but to function in order to determine their overall response.

It is often important to find out when medications were prescribed and by what physician(s) and when the prescriptions run out. In today's world of specialized medicine, many times patients are taking several medications prescribed by different physicians for different problems. The therapist's role may also be one of a medication screener. If the patient has seen several physicians for the same problem, it is not uncommon to find that each has prescribed a different medication. For those who claim to be currently taking three different nonsteroidal anti-inflammatory drugs (NSAIDs) at the same time for the same problem, it can probably be correctly assumed that this should not be the case; a call to either the referring or the primary physician, or both, is in order.

It may also be important to determine whether patients have been on the present medication before and what the results were. Did it alleviate symptoms earlier and not now? This may be a sign that either the patient is developing a tolerance to the drug or, if the problem is the same, the condition is now worse.

Most patients, when asked a general question such as "Are you presently taking any medication?," will respond with the names of prescription drugs only. It is then the examiner's task to ask about over-the-counter (OTC) medications. This may run the gamut from aspirin to sedatives, laxatives, tonics, nerve pills, vitamins, or birth control pills. It may also be important to ask the patients whether they are using any other recreational drugs or alcohol and about their caffeine and nicotine use (see Ch. 12 concerning the investigation of substance abuse). All these substances can affect the neuromuscular system and the patient's perception of pain or function.

This would also be the time to check out possible side effects of any of these medications (see Appendix 14-1).

Side effects are most often dose related. Most of this material may have been covered in the review of system questioning, but many times a drug-related side effect is not severe enough for the patient to volunteer information, and it is helpful to ask specific questions, depending on the particular medications being taken and common untoward effects.

About 10 to 20 percent of hospitalized patients and 2 to 5 percent of outpatients in whom adverse effects develop will be taking medications. This frequency varies greatly depending on the drug administered, the patient population treated, and the definitions of adverse effects.

Adverse drug reactions may be classified into those caused by excessive intended pharmacologic effects and those caused by unintended actions. Adverse effects from excessive intended pharmacologic affects are all dose dependent. For example, hypoglycemia may be caused by excessive doses of insulin and hypotension by excessive doses of antihypertensive agents.

Adverse effects caused by unintended actions of the drug may be categorized into those attributable to the physical and chemical properties of the drug, the direct cytotoxic effect of the drug, the induction of an abnormal immune response, and inherited enzyme defects. Most adverse drug reactions occur soon after administration and are dose related. The potential side effects of the different medications commonly prescribed are covered in more detail later in this chapter.

Again, most of this information is collected during the initial interview of the patient. Certain questions need to be asked of the patient concerning medications later during the course of treatment. If symptoms are changing, the therapist needs to check subjectively whether or not the patient is continuing on the medication. Is it more or less frequent? Is the dosage the same, or has it been changed? In some cases, one of the first signs of improvement may be a decreasing need for medication during the day. If medications do not seem to be helping the condition after a period of treatment, it may be important for the referring/primary physician to have this information. It is also more likely that patients will develop side effects to certain medications the longer they take them, and this should be followed by questioning at subsequent visits.

As physical therapists, we quite often deal with patients whose primary complaint is one of pain. Although they are hurting, people may not like the connotation of a pain killer, and this may lead to refusal to take the prescribed medication. This can sometimes interfere with the overall management of the patient's condition. For example, it is not unusual for patients given a prescription for an anti-inflammatory medication not to take it because their understanding is that it has been prescribed for pain only. Many times a simple explanation of the role of the prescribed medication will alleviate patients' fears, improve their understanding of treatment, and allow for a better treatment course.

Patients will also at times alter their medication as it relates to their pain before coming to therapy. If their prescribed medication has a profound beneficial effect on their condition, they may decide on their own either to take it just before physical therapy (for better tolerance of the therapy) or not to take it just before therapy (so that the therapist can really see what their condition is like at its worst). These do not necessarily have to be good or bad events, but either way the therapist should be aware of the situation for further insight into the nature of the patient's condition.

Certain medications and conditions should be brought to the physical therapist's attention, such as conditions of angina and diabetes mellitus and their usual prescribed medications.

The therapist should ask patients about medical conditions as well as medications that are being taken. If a patient is taking nitroglycerin for his heart problem and attacks of angina, the drug should be close at hand during the evaluation and/or treatment session. This is also true for the diabetic patient who may be taking insulin or oral supplementation for his condition. In this situation, some type of quick sugar replacement should be readily available for the patient.

PAIN AND INFLAMMATION

Drugs are widely used to treat pain and inflammation in physical therapy patients. NSAIDs, including salicylates, and certain corticosteroids are useful for treating both pain and inflammation. Opiate-like drugs are useful for treating pain, and skeletal muscle relaxants are useful for treating pain as a result of muscle spasm.

Salicylates

Salicylates are the most widely used nonsteroidal anti-inflammatory agents (NSAIA) employed. In the United States, consumption of the salicylate aspirin is on the order of 100 tablets for every man, woman, and child per year. Salicylates can be divided into two groups: those that are acetylated (aspirin) and those that are not. The acetylated portion of the molecule accounts for the differing properties between aspirin and other salicylates (Table 14-1). Both the acetyl and salicylate portions of the molecule account for the pain-relieving, anti-inflammatory, and fever-reducing properties of aspirin. In addition, the acetyl portion of the aspirin molecule confers antiplatelet clotting properties. The pain-relieving, anti-inflammatory, and fever-reducing properties of the nonacetylated salicylate are due only to the salicylate portion of the molecule, and there is no acetyl portion to confer antiplatelet clotting activity. Thus, aspirin has an additional mechanism of action not found on the nonacetylated salicylates.

Mechanism of Action

Precise mechanisms of action for the salicylates have not been clearly established. Aspirin has been found to acetylate irreversibly (and thereby inhibit) the enzyme responsible for prostaglandin synthesis in various tissues. The nonacetylated salicylates do not, but still cause a reduction in prostaglandin synthesis. Inhibition of the enzyme may be reversible for the nonacetylated salicylates.

Salicylates provide mild to moderate pain relief by inhibiting synthesis of prostaglandins that sensitize peripheral pain receptors to various stimuli. Salicylates may act centrally as well by decreasing production of prostaglandins at the level of the hypothalamus.

In much larger doses, salicylates produce an anti-inflammatory effect, useful in treating rheumatoid and nonrheumatoid inflammatory conditions. Although additional mechanisms of action for anti-inflammatory activity have been proposed, prostaglandin inhibition appears to play a major role. The fever-reducing properties of salicylates appear to result from prostaglandin inhibition in the portion of the hypothalamus that controls body temperature. Other mechanisms of action may be involved, however.

Aspirin inhibits platelet aggregation by inhibiting the enzyme responsible for converting arachidonic acid to thromboxane, a substance that promotes platelet aggregation. Nonacetylated salicylates do not inhibit this enzyme and hence are not useful in preventing the formation of thrombi on patients at risk of stroke or myocardial infarct.

Aspirin appears to be somewhat more potent than nonacetylated salicylates in relieving pain and reducing fever. By contrast, the nonacetylated salicylates are equivalent to aspirin in anti-inflammatory potency and thus are useful in treating inflammatory conditions that cannot be treated with aspirin (i.e., patients who are allergic or intolerant to aspirin). The equivalent anti-inflammatory efficacy of the nonacetylated salicylates with aspirin suggests that irreversible inhibition of prostaglandin synthesis is not as important or merely one of many mechanisms producing an anti-inflammatory effect.

Side Effects

Adverse side effects of the salicylates (especially aspirin) mainly involve the gastrointestinal (GI) tract. Two to 10 percent of those taking analgesic doses (less than 3 to 6 g/day) and 10 to 30 percent of those taking larger doses suffer symptomatic disturbances (e.g., dyspepsia, heartburn, epigastric distress, nausea, occasional vomiting, abdominal pain). GI effects can be minimized by taking salicylates with food, antacids, or a large glass of water (240 ml).

Table 14-1. Salicylates

Formulation	Example	Advantage	Disadvantage
Acetylated (Aspirin)			
Effervescent	Alka-Seltzer	Fast acting	1 g sodium per 640 mg
Buffered	Bufferin	Fast acting	
Uncoated	Generic	Fast-acting analgesic effect; onset within 30 min; peak effect 1–3 h; duration of effect 3–6	GI side effects
Enteric-coated	Ecotrin	Prolonged onset of action	GI side effects
Nonacetylated			
Sodium salicylate	Generic		4.0 MEQ sodium
Magnesium salicylate[a]	Doan's pills		Contains magnesium
Magnesium-choline salicylate[a]	Trilisate	Liquid, tablet available	Contains magnesium
Salsalate[a]	Disalcid	bid dosing	

[a]Prescription drug.

About 70 percent of patients taking analgesic doses of uncoated aspirin lose 2 to 8 ml of blood daily as a result of a direct irritant effect on the gastric mucosa. As many as 15 percent lose 10 ml or more. There appears to be no correlation between such occult (usually painless) bleeding and symptomatic GI distress. In a few patients, blood loss can be substantial (e.g., 500 ml); in other patients (those on long-term therapy), iron deficiency can result. Such blood loss is not reduced by taking aspirin with food or commercially available buffered preparations. Enteric-coated aspirin tablets, nonacetylated salicylates that usually produce little or no blood loss, may be a useful alternative in such cases.

A third major GI side effect of salicylates (especially aspirin) is damage to the GI mucosa, ranging from mild inflammation to major ulceration. A direct effect has been implicated but can also occur with rectal or intravenous administration. Such damage can occur with or without either symptoms or bleeding. Enteric-coated tablets have been shown to reduce the incidence of such aspirin-induced erosions; buffered tablets have not.

Since salicylates may aggravate GI bleeding, those with a history of GI bleeding or erosions should avoid them. Patients should avoid combining aspirin with alcohol, since the combination increases the risk of GI bleeding and ulceration. Patients should probably avoid using aspirin within 8 to 10 hours of heavy alcohol ingestion.

Other adverse reactions associated with the salicylates are a sensitivity reaction characterized chiefly by bronchospasm in predisposed patients, as well as tinnitus. Although extremely rare, death has occurred within minutes after ingestion of as little as one or two 5-gr tablets. Patients with the aspirin triad of asthma, nasal polyps, and aspirin allergy appear to be especially susceptible. No prostaglandin synthesis inhibitor such as NSAIAs or the preservative sodium benzoate or tartrazine dye should be administered to these patients. By contrast, it appears that the nonacetylated salicylates may be given cautiously (Table 14-2).

Tinnitus is a ringing or high-pitched buzzing sensation in the head. This side effect is usually observed with either large dosages or long-term use of salicylates, or both. It usually occurs only at dosages employed to treat rheumatoid conditions and in fact is occasionally used by clinicians as a therapeutic end point. Tinnitus and hearing loss that can also occur at higher dosages of salicylates are usually completely reversible. Permanent hearing loss has rarely been reported.

Table 14-2. Comparison of Acetylated Salicylates (Aspirin) and Nonacetylated Salicylates

Aspirin	Nonacetylated Salicylates
Blocks platelet aggregation	No effect on platelet aggregation
High incidence of occult gastrointestinal bleeding	Little or no gastrointestinal blood loss
Can induce bronchospasm	Little cross-sensitivity in aspirin-sensitive patients

Contraindications

Patients whose kidneys are highly dependent on vasodilator prostaglandins should avoid aspirin and NSAIDs. These patients include those with congestive heart failure and liver or renal disease.

Salicylates should be avoided in the last trimester of pregnancy because of an increased risk of adverse hematologic effects in both the mother and neonate, as well as complications in delivery.

Nonsteroidal Anti-Inflammatory Drugs

Eighteen NSAIAs are available in the United States that are not salicylates (Table 14-3). Some agents have

Table 14-3. Nonsteroidal Anti-Inflammatory Drugs

Drug[a]	Usual Dosage (mg)	Indications
Diflunisal (Dolobid)	250–500 8–12 h	R (I)
Fenoprofen (Nalfon)	300–600 tid–qid	RIP
Flurbiprofen (Ansaid)	50–100 bid–tid	R (I)
Diclofenac (Voltaren)	24–40 bid–qid	R (I)
Etodolac (Lodine)	200–400 bid–tid	RP
Ibuprofen (Motrin)	400–800 tid–qid	RIP
Indomethacin (Indocin)	250–500 bid–qid	R (I)
Ketoprofen (Orudis)	50–75 tid–qid	RIP
Ketorolac (Toradol)	10 qid	P
Meclofenamate (Meclomen)	50–100 tid–qid	R (I)
Mefenamic acid (Ponstel)	250 q6h PRN	PI
Nabumetone (Relafen)	1,000–2,000 qd	R
Naproxen (naproxen sodium) (Naprosyn; Anaprox)	250–500 bid (275–550)	RIP
Oxaprozin (Daypro)	1,200 qd	R
Phenylbutazone (Butazolidin)	100 qid	R
Piroxicam (Feldene)	10–20 qd-bid	R
Sulindac (Clinoril)	150–200 bid	R (I)
Tolmetin (Tolectin)	200–400 tid–qid	R (I)

Abbreviations: P, pain; R, rheumatoid osteoarthritis, arthritis; I, nonrheumatic inflammation; ( ), unapproved indications.

[a]Brand names are given in parentheses.

Food and Drug Administration (FDA)-approved indications for treatment of rheumatic diseases, such as rheumatoid arthritis and osteoarthritis. Other agents have approved indications for treatment of pain or nonrheumatic inflammatory conditions, such as bursitis and tendinitis. Other approved indications for these agents are gout, vascular headache, and dysmenorrhea. One agent, naproxen (Naprosyn, Anaprox), has FDA-approved indications for the treatment of all these conditions. In other cases, although FDA approval may be lacking, many of these agents are used to treat one or more of these conditions.

Despite the diversity of approved and unapproved indications for these agents, all agents are considered equally efficacious in treating pain and inflammation. Selection of an agent, then, depends on such considerations as cost, convenience, side effect profile, patient tolerance, and the clinical experience of the physician. Some agents are considered too toxic to be used as a first-time agent (e.g., phenylbutazone, indomethacin). Other agents offer the advantage of once-a-day or twice-a-day dosing (e.g., piroxicam, naproxen). Several agents are available as inexpensive generic compounds (e.g., ibuprofen, indomethacin).

Mechanism of Action

The NSAIDs have a mechanism of action that resembles that of the salicylates. Both block the enzyme responsible for converting arachidonic acid to various prostaglandins and thromboxanes (Fig. 14-2). Such a mechanism of action may account for the similar analgesic, anti-inflammatory, and antipyretic properties of these two classes of drugs, as well as their similar side effect profiles. Unlike aspirin, however, the effect of NSAIDs on platelet aggregation is reversible upon discontinuation of the agent. Other mechanisms of action may be responsible for the anti-inflammatory and analgesic activities of NSAIDs, although inhibition of prostaglandin synthesis appears to play a major role.

Indications

Fifteen of the 18 NSAIDs available in the United States are approved by the FDA for treatment of rheumatic diseases, and rheumatoid disorders account for the primary use of these agents. These agents are generally used as an alternative for patients who cannot tolerate the large doses of salicylates required to treat rheumatoid conditions, although NSAIDs can cause similar side effects.

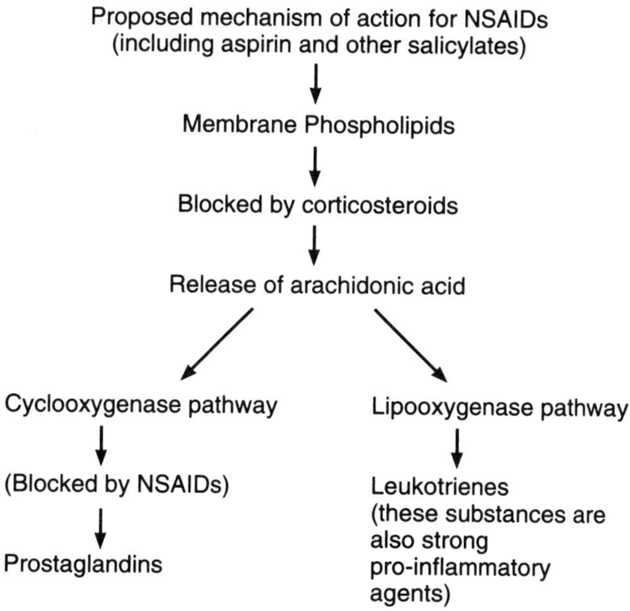

Fig. 14-2. NSAIDs block the cyclo-oxygenase pathway for membrane arachidonic acid. Potent mediators of pain and inflammation are not produced or are antagonized, accounting for their analgesic and anti-inflammatory effect. Corticosteroids that block production of mediators from both pathways are consequently more potent and inflammatory agents.

Rheumatoid conditions for which NSAIDs are employed include rheumatoid arthritis, osteoarthritis, and ankylosing spondylitis.

Eight NSAIDs have FDA approval for treating mild to moderate pain (e.g., musculoskeletal, postoperative, postpartum, visceral pain associated with cancer). Other agents may work just as well. All are believed to act by inhibiting the synthesis of prostaglandins that sensitize peripheral pain receptors. These agents may act centrally as well. Furthermore, their anti-inflammatory effect may also contribute to their analgesic effect.

Although only six NSAIDs have FDA approval for treating nonrheumatic inflammation, almost all agents have been employed to treat these conditions, which include bursitis, tendinitis, athletic injuries, pericarditis, and synovitis. Both the analgesic and the anti-inflammatory activities of the agents account for the clinical value in treating these conditions.

Side Effects

Like the salicylates, the major side effects of NSAIDs involve the GI tract. GI pain, heartburn, and nausea are particularly common, with estimates as high as 30 percent in some cases. Constipation, diarrhea, and vomiting are other side effects that often occur with these agents. To minimize these side effects, it is recommended that NSAIDs be taken with meals, milk, or antacids, but it should also be noted that such administration reduces both the rate and extent of drug absorption, possibly diminishing their therapeutic efficacy. The onset of analgesic action of these agents occurs sooner if taken 30 minutes before, or 2 hours after, meals with at least 8 ounces of water.

Gastrointestinal irritation leading to bleeding, hemorrhage, and perforation of ulcers has been associated with these agents. Patients with a history of upper GI disease should be monitored closely if given these agents, since fatalities have resulted in such cases.

A second major class of side effects associated with NSAIDs involve the central nervous system (CNS). Dizziness and drowsiness often occur with these agents with a reported frequency of 3 to 9 percent. Mild to moderate headache also often occurs, with a reported frequency of 3 to 9 percent.

Indomethacin is particularly significant in causing headaches, with estimates of 25 to 50 percent in some cases. Headaches are often severe and occur especially in the morning.

Another frequent adverse reaction to these agents is skin rash or itching, with a reported frequency of 3 to 9 percent with many agents. Although this allergic reaction is rarely anaphylactic, it warrants medical attention. Patients allergic to aspirin or other NSAIDs should not be administered any NSAID, since cross-sensitivity occurs among these agents. Precautions regarding use of salicylates apply to NSAIDs as well.

Contraindications

Patients should be advised not to combine NSAIDs with alcohol, since the combination increases the risk of GI bleeding or ulceration. Nor should NSAIDs be combined with salicylates or other NSAIDs, as the combination does not offer any increase in therapeutic benefit but does increase the risk of GI irritation and bleeding. Prolonged used of acetominophen (e.g., Tylenol) and NSAIDs increases the risk of adverse renal effects and should be avoided. Caution should be exercised if confusion, diarrhea, dizziness, drowsiness, ocular disturbances, or signs and symptoms of an allergic reaction occur in a patient taking these agents.

Acetaminophen

Acetaminophen is widely employed as both an analgesic and antipyretic by itself and in combination with other agents. It is devoid of anti-inflammatory activity and cannot suppress inflammation in sprains, strains, or rheumatoid conditions. Acetaminophen appears to block prostaglandin synthesis in the CNS with only minimal activity peripherally, in contrast to the salicylates and other NSAIDs. Like the latter two classes of drugs, acetominophen is useful in treating mild and moderate pain and for reducing fever. In normal doses, acetaminophen is safe and relatively free of side effects and accounts in part for its widespread popularity in both over-the-counter and prescription drug products. In an overdose situation, acetaminophen is extremely toxic and can cause rapidly fatal liver failure.

Corticosteroids

Another class of drugs occasionally used to treat inflammatory conditions unresponsive to NSAIDs are the corticosteroids, so named because many are synthetized in the adrenal cortex in humans. (Corticosteroids are to be distinguished from anabolic steroids that are occasionally abused by some athletes in order to increase muscle mass and to enhance their athletic performance.) Corticosteroids are usually divided into two types, on the basis of their predominant activity. Mineralocorticoids have primary effects on sodium retention and potassium excretion and are primarily used in physiologic doses as replacement therapy in certain disorders, such as Addison's disease. These agents have no value in treating inflammatory conditions. Glucocorticoids are the second major type of corticosteroids; in pharmacologic (i.e., large) doses, they have powerful anti-inflammatory effects (Table 14-4). These agents are generally the ones referred to when discussing corticosteroids and are the ones discussed here. Nevertheless, it should be kept in mind that the distinction between these two types of corticosteroids is not complete; some glucocorticoids have mineralocorticoid (sodium-retaining) activity as well (e.g., hydrocortisone, prednisone).

Mechanism of Action

Corticosteroids work through several mechanisms to achieve an anti-inflammatory responses.

By inhibiting the inflammatory process at the cellular level, these agents suppress the symptoms of inflammation (e.g., heat, redness, tenderness). These agents do not treat the cause of the inflammation and are not considered curative agents. When these agents are used for short periods of time, even massive dosages are unlikely to produce adverse effects. By contrast, long-term use of these agents is associated with a number of adverse effects.

Mechanisms of Anti-Inflammatory Activity of Glucocorticoids

1. Stabilizing leukocyte lysosomal membranes
2. Preventing release of destructive acid hydrolases from leukocytes
3. Inhibiting macrophage accumulation in inflamed areas
4. Reducing leukocyte adhesion to capillary endothelium
5. Reducing capillary wall permeability and edema formation
6. Decreasing complement components
7. Antagonizing histamine activity and release of kinin from substrates
8. Reducing fibroblast proliferation of collagen deposition
9. Other possible mechanisms as yet unknown

Table 14-4. Equivalent Doses of Glucocorticoids

Action	Dose (mg)
Short acting (8–12 h)	
Cortisone	25
Hydrocortisone	20
Intermediate acting (12–36 h)	
Methylprednisolone	4
Prednisone	5
Prednisolone	5
Triamcinolone	4
Long acting (36–72 h)	
β-Methasone	0.6
Dexamethasone	0.75

Side Effects

Prolonged use of large doses of glucocorticosteroids may cause decreased secretion of endogenous corticosteroids through negative feedback on the pituitary. These patients may not secrete sufficient corticosteroids in response to stress and, if they are withdrawn abruptly, may show signs and symptoms of adrenal insufficiency (as little as 15 mg prednisone daily beyond 1 or 2 months can cause such suppression). In order to avoid such problems, glucocorticoids should be slowly withdrawn in patients who are discontinuing long-term use of large dosages of these agents.

Another adverse effect of prolonged use of these agents (e.g., prednisone 10 mg/day for years) is the development of osteoporosis, especially in geriatric or debilitated patients. The osteoporosis occurs mainly in the vertebral column and pelvic girdle. Often such osteoporotic changes are asymptomatic until a bone is fractured.

Steroid diabetes is another potential adverse effect of prolonged use of these agents. Glucocorticoids can either precipitate diabetes mellitus in predisposed patients or aggravate the condition in patients who already have it. Hypercortism, a cushingoid state, may also result from long-term use of these agents, manifesting as moon facies with a buffalo hump.

Other adverse effects associated with the use of glucocorticoids are increased susceptibility to, and masking of, infection, sodium retention, and potassium loss; GI side effects (e.g., nausea, vomiting, diarrhea, constipation, peptic ulcer formation); and mind-altering effects ranging from mild euphoria to frank psychosis.

Despite these side effects, short-term use of these agents (e.g., Medrol dospak) is unlikely to produce harmful effects. To minimize adverse effects, these agents should be taken immediately before, during, or immediately after meals or with food or milk. If prolonged use of glucocorticoids is required, they should be administered every other day in the morning and eventually reduced and (preferably) discontinued.

Opioids

For more severe pain, a second class of analgesics are used in place of the salicylates and NSAIAs: the opioids (Table 14-5). The opioids include naturally occurring compounds from the opium poppy, such as morphine and codeine, as well as semisynthetic modifications of these substances, such as hydromorphone (Dilaudid) and oxycodone (Percodan, Percocet). A third class of opioids include completely synthetic substances that resemble morphine in activity, such as meperidine (Demorol), methadone, and, to a lesser extent, propoxyphene (Darvon) and pentacozine (Talwin). All these opioids owe their analgesic (and other pharmacologic) activity to an interaction with opioid receptors existing in different areas throughout the CNS.

Mechanism of Action

Several different kinds of opioid receptors have been discovered. Actions at these receptors account for the analgesic and other effects of the opioids (Table 14-6). Morphine has strong affinity for MU-1 and MU-2 receptors, accounting for its analgesic, euphoric, and other effects. Pentazocine has an affinity for κ- and σ-receptors, thus accounting for its analgesic and "psychotomimetic" effects. Codeine has a weaker affinity for MU-1 and MU-2 receptors than does morphine and thus has weaker analgesic efficacy.

It is proposed that analgesia is achieved when either endogenous opioids (endorphins) or exogenous opioids (e.g., morphine) bind to receptors that block the transmission of pain impulses within the CNS. Both the perception and the emotional response to pain are altered with this binding. Other neurotransmitters believed to be involved in modulating the transmission of pain impulses are serotonin and norepinephrine. Antidepressants that increase the concentration of these two neurotransmitters have been used as adjunctive analgesics in postherpetic neuralgia and vascular headaches (e.g., amitriptyline).

Indications

Opioids such as morphine are indicated for the treatment of severe painn For moderate to severe pain, all other opioid analgesics, with the exception of codeine and propoxyphene, are indicated. For mild to moderate pain, codeine and propoxyphene are indicated.

Oral Opioids

Codeine is the most commonly prescribed oral opioid analgesic in a formulation with either acetominophen or aspirin (e.g., Tylenol #3, Empirin #3). Formulations designated #4 contain 1 gr or 60 mg of codeine, #3 a half-

Table 14-5. Oral Opioid Analgesics

Class	Usual Dosage (mg)	Side Effects
Codeine	15–60 q3–6h (usually prescribed in combination formulation Tylenol #3)	Constipation, drowsiness
Hydrocodone	5–10 q4–6h	Drowsiness, dizziness, increased sweating, flushing of the face
Hydromorphone (Dilaudid)	2 q3–6h	Drowsiness, dizziness, loss of appetite
Meperidine	50–150 q3–4h	Constipation, dizziness, drowsiness, increased sweating, flushing of the face, nausea, vomiting
Morphine	10–30 q4h (initial); dose must be individualized	As with meperidine
Oxycodone	5q3–6h (usually prescribed in combination formulation (e.g., Percodan, Percocet)	Dizziness, drowsiness, nausea, vomiting
Pentazocine (Talwin)	50 q3–4h	Drowsiness, false sense of well-being, nausea, vomiting
Propoxyphene (often prescribed in combination formulation, e.g., Darvocet)	65 q4h	Dizziness, drowsiness, nausea, vomiting

Table 14-6. Characteristics of Opioid Receptors

Receptors	Agonist	Effect
μ_1	Morphine	Analgesia
μ_2	Morphine	Euphoria, respiratory depression, physical dependence, constipation
κ	Nalbuphine	Analgesia, sedation
σ	Pentazocine	Dysphoria, hallucinations, tachycardia, hypertension

grain or 30 mg, and #2 a quarter-grain or 15 mg; #1 formulations are rarely prescribed. The combination of a peripherally acting analgesic (e.g., aspirin) with an opioid analgesic makes therapeutic sense. Pain relief is achieved with two mechanisms of action instead of one. The results of controlled studies have shown that the analgesic effects of each component are additive.

In the doses usually prescribed for the treatment of mild to moderate pain, the side effects of codeine are minor; constipation and drowsiness occur most frequently. When larger doses are employed (e.g., treatment of severe pain), codeine produces side effects similar to those associated with morphine, including respiratory depression. Increasing the oral dose beyond the therapeutic limit of 200 mg increases the incidence of side effects without an increase in analgesia.

Two semisynthetic analogues of codeine are hydrocodone and oxycodone. Both are usually prescribed in combination with a nonopioid analgesic for the same reason as codeine. Hydrocodone is combined with acetaminophen in Vicodin and oxycodone is combined with aspirin or acetaminophen in Percodan or Percocet, respectively. Oxycodone has a slightly greater dependence liability than codeine and is included in Schedule 11 of the Controlled Substances Act. Oxycodone is actually equivalent to morphine in analgesic potency. To limit abuse in the United States, it is combined with aspirin or acetaminophen in a very small amount (4.5 to 5 mg). Both hydrocodone and oxycodene share side effects similar to that of codeine.

Although commonly prescribed (especially in combination with acetaminophen or aspirin for the same reason as codeine) propoxyphene 65 mg was shown in one study to be no more effective than 325 to 650 mg of codeine. Propoxyphene on a milligram basis is only one-half as potent as codeine. Although its dependence liability may be less than that of codeine, its potential for causing life-threatening toxicity has led to its inclusion in Schedule IV of the Controlled Substances Act.

Pentazocine is an opioid that has both analgesic and weak narcotic antagonist properties. It blocks activity at receptors to which morphine binds but stimulates activity at κ-receptors (to produce analgesic) and at σ-receptors (to produce psychomimetic and cardiovascular effects). Pentazocine is effective at relieving moderate pain, but its high incidence of side effects limits its clinical value. Approximately 10 percent of patients will experience psychomimetic side effects such as dysphoria, nightmares, feelings of depersonalization, and, most commonly, visual hallucinations. Nausea, vomiting, and dizziness occur as frequently as the other strong opioids. The other formulation of pentazocine contains naloxone to antagonize the euphoric effects of pentazocine when the tablet is illicitly solubilized and injected intravenously. Evidence suggests that abuse of this drug persists. Pentazocine is included in Schedule IV of the Controlled Substances Act.

Skeletal Muscle Relaxants

A second major class of agents often used as an adjunct to physical therapy are the skeletal muscle relaxants. These agents are used to treat muscle spasms that occur as a result of injury at localized regions of the human body. There are two kinds of skeletal muscle relaxants: direct-acting agents, which block the effects of the neurotransmitter at the level of the neuromuscular junction, and centrally acting agents. The direct-acting agents are usually administered intravenously as an adjunct to general anesthesia during surgery and are not discussed here. Centrally acting agents are usually administered orally and probably achieve most of their muscle relaxant effect through their general CNS depressant (sedative) properties. Three other skeletal muscle relaxants used in treating spasticity as a result of spinal cord injuries or other neurologic disorders, such as multiple sclerosis or cerebral palsy, are caclofen, dantrolene, and the anxiolytic diazepam.

Five major centrally acting skeletal muscle relaxants are available in the United States (Table 14-7). Chlorphenesin and metaxalone are also available but are rarely used.

Side Effects

All centrally acting skeletal muscle relaxants have drowsiness as a major side effect, with cyclobenzaprine particularly notable. Cyclobenzaprine is structurally similar to tricyclic antidepressants and may have side effects

Table 14-7. Skeletal Muscle Relaxants (Central Acting)

Drug[a]	Usual Dose (mg)	Adverse Reactions
Carisoprodol (Soma)	350 qid	Dizziness, drowsiness, GI disturbances
Chlorzoxazone (Paraflex; plus acetaminophen, Parafon Forte)	250–750 tid–qid	GI disturbances, drowsiness, dizziness
Cyclobenzaprine (Flexaril)	10 bid–qid	Drowsiness, dry mouth, dizziness
Methocarbamol (Robaxin)	Initially 1–5 qid 2–3 days, then 750 q4h to 1.5 tid	Lightheadedness, dizziness, drowsiness, nausea, uticaria
Orphenadrine (Norflex SR; Disipal)	100 bid, 50 tid	Dry mouth, weakness, dizziness

[a]Brand names are given in parentheses.

similar to those associated with these agents, such as dry mouth, blurred vision, and increased heart rare. A metabolite of carisoprodol includes meprobamate, a once popular antianxiety agent associated with some abuse potential; this agent should be used with caution in patients who have a history of drug abuse. Orphenadrine shares anticholinergic properties with cyclobenzaprine and should not be administered to patients with glaucoma, prostatic hypertrophy, or cardiac arrhythmias. All these agents are metabolized by the liver and excreted by the kidneys and should be used with caution in patients who have any impairment in these organs. Chlorzoxazone may color urine orange or reddish-purple, and methocarbanol black, brown, or green, especially if allowed to stand.

Baclofen, Diazepam, and Dantrolene

Three other drugs used to treat spasms in neurologic disorders such as spinal cord injury, multiple sclerosis, and cerebral palsy are baclofen, diazepam, and dantrolene. Baclofen is structurally related to a neurotransmitter that blocks conduction of impulses in the spinal cord and may act through this mechanism. Transient drowsiness is the most common side effect of this agent, occurring in 20 to 25 percent of patients. Psychiatric disturbances, such as hallucinations, excitation, confusion, depression, and anxiety, can occur, especially in patients with these pre-existing disorders and in the elderly. Abrupt withdrawal of this agent has precipitated hallucinations, seizures, and increased spasticity in some patients.

Diazepam is an antianxiety agent that enhances the activity of the same inhibitory transmitter by which baclofen is believed to act. Diazepam acts on receptors both in the spinal cord and in the brain and, because of its activity at the latter site, is commonly used as an antianxiety agent and as a sedative. Drowsiness is a major side effect of diazepam, as it is with other benzodiazepenes. Nevertheless, it is a useful muscle relaxant both in chronic neurologic disorders and in acute localized self-limited traumatic disorders.

One agent not indicated for muscle spasms that is related to musculoskeletal trauma is dantrolene. Dantrolene is used orally to treat spasms occurring in neurologic disorders such as multiple sclerosis, cerebral palsy, and spinal cord injury. It is believed to act by blocking the intracellular release of calcium needed for contraction of skeletal muscle fibers. Such activity also accounts for its major side effect of muscle weakness, which may result in slurring of speech, drooling, difficulty in swallowing, choking, and enuresis. Since dantrolene may cause severe liver toxicity, liver function should be monitored. Dantrolene is also contraindicated in patients with a history of liver disease.

OTHER MEDICAL CONDITIONS AND DRUG THERAPIES

Physical therapy patients not only receive drugs specific for pain and inflammation but, like the general population, receive drugs specific for other medical conditions as well. Examples include chronic cardiovascular diseases, such as hypertension and congestive heart failure, or certain psychiatric disorders, such as anxiety, depression, or schizophrenia. An understanding of the action and side effects of the drugs used to treat these medical conditions will prepare physical therapists to evaluate the progress of the therapy they are administering, as well as detect any problems associated with such drug therapy. The concluding portion of this chapter presents a discussion of drug therapies employed to treat common cardiovascular disorders, such as hypertension, congestive heart failure, and angina; psychiatric disorders, such as anxiety, depression, and schizophrenia; neurologic disorders, such as epilepsy; and common medical conditions, such as peptic ulcer disease and asthma.

Cardiovascular Diseases

Hypertension

Hypertension is the most common chronic medical condition, with a prevalence rate of 20 percent among whites and 30 percent among blacks in the United States (in the over 65-year-old population, these rates are 40 percent and 50 percent, respectively). Hypertension has been defined as a systolic blood pressure greater than 140 mmHg or a diastolic blood pressure greater than 90 mmHg, or both. Since blood pressure can vary episodically, three measurements and a thorough medical evaluation should be made before the diagnosis of hypertension is made. Once diagnosed, hypertension should be treated, as it is a major cause of heart failure, kidney failure, stroke, and death.

Management of hypertension has undergone considerable change since 1973, when the National Heart, Lung, and Blood Institute issued their first guidelines. Several new agents have since been introduced that have made obsolete the first-time use of some of the earlier agents.

In 1992, the Joint National Committee on Detection, Evaluation, and Treatment of High Blood Pressure issued its latest recommendations on treating hypertension (JNC V). In contrast to JNC IV, only two classes of agents are proposed as first-line therapy for treatment of hypertension: diuretics and β-blockers. Although JNC V conceded that other classes of agents may be equally beneficial, it was their contention that only diuretics and β-blockers alone have been shown to decrease cardiovascular morbidity and mortality in controlled clinical trials. Nonetheless JNC V recommends five classes of agents as initial therapy in treatment of hypertension: diuretics, β-blockers, angiotensin-converting enzyme inhibitors, calcium-channel blockers, and α_1-blockers (see Table 14-8). Selection of one drug over another should be individualized and should take into consideration the special features of that drug that make it useful for that patient. Older patients seem to respond better to diuretics than do younger patients. Whites appear to respond better to β-blockers than blacks. β-Blockers would not be drugs of choice for patients with diabetes, asthma, or peripheral vascular disease.

Table 14-8. First-Line Therapy for Hypertension

Class/Example[a]	Usual Dose for Treating Hypertension
Diuretics	
Thiazide	
Hydrochlorothiazide	25–50 mg qd
Loop	
Furosemide (Lasix)	40 mg qd
Potassium sparing (triamterene combined with hydrochlorothiazide) in Dyazide and Maxzide	bid, qd
β-Blockers	
Acebutolol (Sectral)	200 mg bid
Atenolol (Tenormin)	50 mg qd
Betaxolol (Kerlone)	10 mg qd
Bisoprolol (Zebeta)	5–20 mg qd
Carteolol (Cartrol)	2.5–5 mg qd
Labetalol (Trandate, Normodyne)	200 mg bid
Metoprolol (Lopressor)	50 mg bid
Nadolol (Corgard)	40–80 mg qd
Penbutolol (Levatol)	20 mg qd
Pindolol (Visken)	5 mg bid
Propranolol (Inderal)	120–240 mg/day in individual doses
Timolol (Blocadren)	10 mg bid
ACE inhibitors	
Benazepril (Lotensin)	10–40 mg qd
Captopril (Capoten)	25–50 mg bid, tid
Enalapril (Vasotec)	10–40 mg qd in divided doses
Fosinopril (Monopril)	10–40 mg qd
Lisinopril (Prinivil, Zestril)	10–40 mg qd
Quinapril (Accupril)	10–40 qd–bid
Ramipril (Altace)	2.5–20 mg qd in individual doses
Calcium-channel blockers (useful for treating hypertension)	
Amlodipine	5–10 mg qd
Diltiazem (Cardizem SR)	60–120 mg bid
Felodipine (Plendil)	5–10 mg qd
Isradipine (Dyna Circ)	2.5–5.0, bid
Nifedipine (Procardia XL)	30–60 mg qd
Nicardipine (Cardene)	20–40 mg tid
Verapamil (Isoptin SR)	240 mg qd
α_1-Blockers	
Doxazosin (Cardura)	1–16 mg qd
Prazosin (Minipress)	1–5 mg bid–tid
Terazosin (Hytrin)	1–10 mg qd

[a]Brand names are given in parentheses.

Diuretics

Diuretics reduce blood pressure initially by causing sodium and water loss. In the long run, diuretics reduce peripheral vascular resistance by a still unknown mechanism. Diuretics such as hydrochlorothiazide are inexpensive, convenient (once-a-day dosing), and effective for a large number of patients, especially in the elderly and among blacks; 40 to 70 percent of all hypertensive patients attain adequate control of their blood pressure with diuretics alone.

Diuretics can also cause potassium loss, which may be manifested by symptoms of muscle weakness, fatigue, and muscle cramps. A more serious, but fortunately rare, consequence of diuretic-induced hypokalemia is ventricular irritability, which may lead to ventricular ectopy or sudden death. Attempts to avoid hypokalemia include supplementation of potassium and/or reduction of sodium in the diet and the use of potassium-sparing diuretics along with or in combination with a potassium-depleting diuretic. Dyazide (hydrochlorothiazide/triamterene) and Maxzide are popular combination diuretics.

Other adverse reactions to both thiazide and loop diuretics (e.g., furosemide) include increases in both serum uric acid concentration (which may manifest itself in gouty arthritis) and serum glucose concentration (which may precipitate the onset of diabetes in certain patients).

β-Blockers

An alternative first-line class of drugs useful in treating hypertension are the β-adrenergic blocking agents, or β-blockers. β-Blockers are as effective as diuretics in lowering blood pressure, and most can be given in once-a-day or twice-a-day dosing. Although several mechanisms have been proposed for the activity of these agents, none has been consistently associated with a reduction in blood pressure.

Although 12 oral β-blockers are available in the United States for treatment of hypertension, clinical differences among them appear nonexistent. Several agents are promoted as cardioselective, that is, β-receptors in the heart are blocked, whereas β-receptors in the lungs, kidneys, and arterioles are spared. Such cardioselectivity is not absolute, however, and at higher doses bronchospasm and arteriolar constriction can occur. Other agents are promoted as being less likely to penetrate the CNS, with less likelihood of causing CNS side effects, such as fatigue and insomnia. Good clinical data substantiating these claims have not been forthcoming.

Adverse side effects of β-blockers result from blockade of β-receptors and include bradycardia, bronchospasm, wheezing, fatigue, decreased exercise tolerance, insomnia, sexual dysfunction, shortness of breath, claudication, weakness, and cold extremities. β-Blockers should not be given to patients with pulmonary disease, peripheral vascular disease, diabetes, or congestive heart failure, as these conditions may be exacerbated by these agents. Patients predisposed to ischemic myocardial events should be tapered off β-blockers, as abrupt discontinuation may result in myocardial infarction or death.

ACE Inhibitors

An alternative first-line class of agents useful for treating hypertension are the angiotensin-converting enzyme (ACE) inhibitors. These agents block the enzyme responsible for converting angiotensin I to the extremely potent vasoconstrictive angiotensin II, a substance that also stimulates aldosterone secretion and sodium and water retention. Blockade of this enzyme also prevents the breakdown of the potent vasodilatory substance bradykinin. The end result of ACE inhibition is a reduction in peripheral vascular resistance.

Seven ACE inhibitors are available in the United States. Side effects of these agents are fewer than those of older agents used to treat hypertension. Initially Captopril was marketed at 100 mg qid (vs. 25 mg bid–tid today) and was associated with a higher than usual incidence of side effects such as skin rash, loss of taste, and neutropenia. There are four major side effects associated with ACE inhibitors.

1. Hypotension, especially in volume-depleted patients (1/1,000)
2. Angiodema, a rare hypersensitivity reaction
3. Hyperkalemia, especially in conjunction with potassium-sparing diuretics
4. Cough, the incidence of which has been reported to be as high as 39 percent (vs. 0.5 to 3 percent as reported in product information sheets (15 percent of patients must discontinue ACE inhibitors as a result of this cough.)

Despite these side effects and their relative expense, ACE inhibitors are becoming popular antihypertensive agents. They are also markedly effective and extremely popular in the treatment of congestive heart failure. However, pregnant patients should not take ACE inhibitors, as injury and death to the developing fetus has been reported with their use.

Calcium-Channel Blockers

The fourth class of first-line drugs useful in treating hypertension are the calcium-channel blockers. Calcium-channel blockers block the influx of calcium into the smooth muscle cells lining arteriolar walls, so that these muscle cells are unable to contract and produce vasoconstriction. Calcium-channel blockers also block the influx of calcium into cardiac muscle cells, thereby blocking contraction of cardiac muscle cells. The sites and intensity of action of the nine calcium-channel blockers available in the United States vary. Bepridil is a recently introduced calcium-channel blocker that, because of its toxicity, is reserved for treating angina in patients who are nonresponsive or intolerant to other antianginal agents. Verapamil and diltiazem have a more pronounced effect on cardiac contractility and are often used to treat cardiac disorders such as angina and arrhythmias. Nifedipine and nicardipine are potent peripheral vasodilators that may cause a reflex increase in heart rate and contractility. Nimodipine is a potent peripheral vasodilator with an affinity for cerebral vessels that makes it useful for treating acute stroke victims. Calcium-channel blockers are effective in treating mild to moderate hypertension, and FDA approval is available for verapamil, nicardipine, and sustained-release diltiazem and nifedipine.

The side effects of the various calcium-channel blockers reflect their mechanism of action. Verapamil and diltiazem are more likely to cause cardiac abnormalities, such as bradycardia, atrioventricular (AV) block, and congestive heart failure. Both agents can also cause anorexia, nausea, peripheral edema, and hypotension. Constipation occurs with verapamil, sometimes severe enough to necessitate surgery for fecal impaction.

Side effects related to the peripheral vasodilating properties of the vasodilating calcium-channel blockers include headache, flushing, dizziness, ankle edema, hypotension, nausea, and tachycardia. Reflex tachycardia is usually not a problem with long-term use, except in patients with ischemic heart disease. Other side effects often subside with continued use of these agents.

Despite their high cost, calcium-channel blockers are becoming popular agents for treating hypertension, cardiac arrhythmias, angina, and other medical conditions (e.g., migraines).

A fifth class of agents that JNC V recommends as initial treatment of hypertension are the α_1-blockers. α_1-blockers dilate both arterioles and veins and have a favorable effect on HDL/cholesterol levels. Terazosin (Hytrin) has also been approved for treatment of benign prostatic hypertrophy.

These agents are associated with a "first-dose" effect manifested by marked hypotension and syncope with sudden loss of consciousness after the first few doses. This effect results from impaired venous return and may be minimized by starting with the lowest dose possible at bedtime and slowly increasing doses every 2 weeks. Dizziness and headache have been common side effects of these agents.

Many other agents are available to treat hypertension, although none is considered a first-line choice. If an additional agent is needed (and 70 percent of patients will require one), an alternative first-line agent is usually selected. Other antihypertensive agents include those that act centrally to decrease sympathetic outflow (methyldopa, guanabenz, guanfacine) and/or peripherally (clonidine) and direct-acting arterial vasodilators (hydralazine, minoxidil). All are effective antihypertensive agents, but their noticeable side effect profile has substantially limited their clinical value.

Congestive Heart Failure

Congestive heart failure (CHF) has rapidly become one of the most important health problems in the United States. An estimated 4 million Americans have chronic CHF, and its incidence more than doubles each decade in those aged 45 to 75. CHF is the most common discharge diagnosis for patients over 65 years of age and is the most prevalent cause of death in hospitalized patients.

CHF results from a failure of the heart to pump blood to meet the body's needs. In normal patients, approximately 60 percent of the blood presented to the ventricles is ejected during contraction. In CHF patients, the figure is 10 to 20 percent. Several factors may account for this reduced ejection fraction: (1) too much blood presented to the ventricles (preload); (2) too much pressure working against the ventricles (e.g., hypertension, afterload); or (3) a damaged myocardium, most commonly as a result of coronary artery disease. Hypertension is a major factor in CHF, and cardiac disease is the primary cause.

As a result of decreased perfusion to the kidneys, renin is released, angiotensin is formed, and sodium and water retention occurs. If the right ventricle is failing, fluid backs up in the veins, manifesting symptoms of right-sided failure. If the left ventricle is failing, fluid backs up into the lungs, manifesting symptoms of left-sided failure (Table 14-9). CHF patients often show symptoms of both left-sided and right-sided failure. The goal of therapy in these patients is to abolish their disabling symptoms and improve their quality of life. In spite of aggressive pharmacologic treatment, the outcome for CHF patients is poor. In the Framingham study, 60 percent of men and 40 percent of women died within 5 years of the diagnosis of CHF.

Diuretics

The first class of drugs usually employed after sodium restriction fails to control the volume overload is the diuretics. Thiazide diuretics (e.g., hydrochlorothiazide) are good first choices for mobilizing fluid; if these agents fail, the more potent loop diuretics are employed (fuorsemide, bumetanide). Since the loop diuretics cause significant potassium loss, potassium levels should be followed, particularly because many CHF patients are also on digoxin, and low potassium levels predispose to serious digoxin toxicity. NSAIAs also interact with diuretics and interfere with their effectiveness. The side effects of diuretics are discussed under therapy for hypertension.

Digitalis Preparations

Digitalis preparations are often used when diuretics alone fail to arrest the symptoms of CHF. Digitalis inhibits the enzyme responsible for exchanging intracellular sodium for extracellular potassium, thus freeing up more sodium to be exchanged with calcium. Calcium enhances cardiac contractility, increasing both the force and rate of contraction. Digitalis also slows the ventricular rate of contraction, allowing more time for the ventricles to fill and thus increase cardiac output.

Digoxin is the most commonly prescribed digitalis preparation. It has one of the lowest therapeutic indices of any drug on the market. Its therapeutic serum level is approximately 1 to 2 ng/ml. Toxic symptoms may appear when levels exceed 2.5 ng/ml. It is estimated that approximately 20 percent of patients develop signs of toxicity while on digitalis, that rhythmic disturbances occur in up to 80 to 90 percent of digitalis toxic patients, and that up to 18 percent of these patients may die from these arrhythmias. Almost all known arrhythmias can occur with digoxin toxicity.

Table 14-9. Symptoms Associated with Heart Failure

Left-Sided Failure	Right-Sided Failure
Cardiomegaly	Anorexia
Cough	Abdominal discomfort
Dyspnea on exertion	Hepatojugular reflex
Paroxysmal nocturnal orthopnea	Jugular venous distention
Pleural effusions	Nocturia
Tachypnea	Edema
Wheezing	Weight gain

Noncardiac signs of digitalis toxicity include those relating to the GI tract and CNS. Noncardiac signs do not always precede cardiac signs of digitalis toxicity, and arrhythmias may present as the only toxic sign. For this reason, patients must be closely followed on digitalis preparations. Given the modest benefits attributed to digoxin and its considerable toxicity, some clinicians have elected to use vasodilators instead of digoxin as their second choice of treatment for CHF.

Vasodilators

Vasodilators are generally reserved for treatment if both diuretics and digoxin have failed in managing CHF. Vasodilators can be of three types: those that dilate arterial vessels (reduce afterload), those that dilate venous vessels (decrease preload), and those that do both. Calcium-channel blockers and hydralazine are examples of afterload reducers. Various forms of nitrates are available for preload reduction. ACE inhibitors and prazocin are examples of mixed or "balanced" vasodilators (Table 14-10).

There are certain drugs that are often overlooked causes or exacerbators of CHF. Cardiac drugs such as arrhythmic agents, β-blockers, and several calcium-channel blockers decrease cardiac contractility and cardiac output. Even topically applied β-blocking drugs (Timolol) have been implicated. NSAIAs also cause or exacerbate CHF as a result of sodium and water retention (some agents have increased blood volume by 50 percent in some cases). Salicylates, androgens, estrogens, and medicinals high in sodium also increase volume overload, thus producing the symptoms of CHF.

Angina

Coronary heart disease is the leading cause of death in the United States (30 percent of all deaths). It is often first manifested as symptoms of angina. These symptoms, such as substernal chest pain that sometimes radiates to the left arm, shoulder, or jaw, occur when cardiac work

Table 14-10. Drug Treatment for Congestive Heart Failure

Class	Side Effect
Diuretics	
Thiazide (HCTZ, chlorthalidone) Loop (furosemide, bumetaldine) Potassium-sparing (triamterene, amiloride)	Weakness, fatigue, muscle cramps, GI symptoms, sexual dysfunction
Digoxin	Cardiac (50% of adverse reactions) includes PVCs, ventricular tachycardia, AV dissociation, accelerated nodal rhythm, atrial tachycardia with block, AV block Gastrointestinal system (25% of adverse reactions) includes anorexia, nausea, vomiting Central nerve system (25% of adverse reactions) includes blurred/yellow vision, headaches, weakness, apathy psychosis
Unloading agents	
Preload reducing (venous dilators) Nitrates, topical, oral nitroglycerin, isosorbide	Headache, flushing, dizziness, hypotension
Afterloading reducing (arterial dilators)	Headaches, flushing, nausea, vomiting, fluid retension, lupus-like syndrome
Hydralazine	
Calcium-channel blockers Nifedipine, Nicardipene, Diltiazem, Verapamil	Dizziness, lightheadedness, headache, edema, weakness, constipation with verapamil)
Balanced vasodilators ACE inhibitors	Hypotension, rash, taste disturbances

Abbreviations: AV, atrioventricular; GI, gastrointestinal; PVCs, preventricular contractions.

and myocardial oxygen demand exceed the ability of the coronary arteries to supply adequate oxygen. Myocardial oxygen demand depends on heart rate, myocardial contractility, degree of ventricular filling, and the force against which the ventricles must work to eject blood. Drugs that decrease any of these factors will reduce myocardial oxygen demand.

A major determinant of myocardial oxygen supply is the extent of coronal artery obstruction by atherosclerotic plaques. When obstruction of these arteries exceeds the 70 percent range, symptoms of angina begin to appear. Pharmacologic agents have been introduced on the market in an effort to lower serum cholesterol, a substance that appears to be a major component of these atherosclerotic plaques.

Three classes of drugs are used to correct the imbalance between myocardial oxygen supply and demand in angina patients. Nitrates cause smooth muscle relaxation of both the venous and, to a lesser extent, the arterial systems. By reducing both the amount of blood the ventricle has to eject (because of its venous pooling) and the force against which it has to be ejected (because of its arterial dilation), nitrates reduce oxygen demand, therefore reducing symptoms. Nitrates are available in many forms (Table 14-11). Many are used prophylactically and a few to treat acute episodes.

β-Blockers decrease myocardial oxygen demand by decreasing heart rate, contractility, and blood pressure. β-Blockers complement the activity of nitrates by limiting the latter's reflex increase in heart rate. Nitrates offset the increase in left ventricular size induced by β-blockers. As mentioned under Hypertension, β-blockers should be gradually tapered if they are to be discontinued in patients with myocardial ischemia. Otherwise acute myocardial infarction and sudden cardiac death may result (i.e., β-blocker withdrawal syndrome).

The third class of agents used to treat angina are the calcium-channel blockers. Calcium-channel blockers differ in their ability to produce peripheral vasodilation (and the force against which the ventricles must work), decrease contractibility, or slow conduction across the AV node. The overall effect will depend on which agent is used; the net result will be a reduction in cardiac work and myocardial oxygen demand. Calcium-channel blockers are particularly useful in treating angina resulting from vasospasms of the large coronary arteries. Patients with heart failure or cardiac condition disorders (e.g., bradycardia) should not be given calcium-channel blockers because of the negative effects of these agents on cardiac contractility.

Another attempt at reducing the risk of developing angina has been to combine drugs with diet in an attempt to lower plasma cholesterol. A 15 percent decrease in cholesterol levels has been associated with a 30 percent reduction in the risk of developing coronary heart disease. If diet modification and other nonpharmacologic measures (e.g., weight control, smoking cessation, exercise) fail, drug therapy with one of the cholesterol-lowering drugs may be appropriate (Table 14-12).

Table 14-11. Nitrate Products

Drug	Strength	Example	Initial Dose
Isosorbide nitrate			
Sublingual	2.5, 5, 10 mg	Sorbitrate, Isordil	2.5–5 mg
Chewable	5, 10 mg	Sorbitrate, Isordil	
Oral tablets	5, 10, 20, 30, 40 mg	Sorbitrate, Isordil	5–20 mg qid
Oral (sustained-release capsules, tablets)	40 mg	Sorbitrate SA, Isordil Tembids	40 mg q8–12h
Nitroglycerin			
Sublingual	0.15, 0.3, 0.4, 0.6 mg	Nitrostat	0.3 mg
Translingual spray	0.4 mg/metered dose	Nitrolingual	0.4 mg
Transmucosal buccal controlled-release tablets	1, 2, 3 mg	Nitrogard	1 mg
Sustained-release tablets/capsules	2.5, 2.6, 6.5, 9 mg	Nitrobid	2.5 mg tid
Transdermal patches	2.5, 5., 7.5, 10, 15 mg	NitroDur II, Transderm-nitro	1 patch
Topical	2% in a lanolin-petroleum base	Nitroglycerin	½ inch

Arrhythmias

Antiarrhythmic agents are used to treat and prevent abnormalities in the rate and rhythm of heart contractions that may impair the ability of the heart to function efficiently as a pump. Antiarrhythmic agents have been classified by Vaughn Williams into four types on the basis of their effects on the electrophysiologic properties of cardiac cells. Class I agents are local anesthetics that depress the initial phase of a cardiac cell's generation of an electrical impulse. Class II agents are β-blockers that slow down the sinus rate, depress contractility, and slow down the conduction of impulses between the atria and the ventricles. Class III agents markedly prolong the period during which a cardiac cell cannot be restimulated. Class IV agents are calcium-channel blockers that slow activity calcium-dependent cells on the SA and AV nodes. Selection of an antiarrhythmic agent depends on both the pathology of the arrhythmia and the effects of the drug, both of which are highly variable. Selection of an individual agent is thus largely empirical. See Table 14-13 for a list of these antiarrhythmic agents.

Table 14-12. Drugs Used in Hyperlipidemia

Drug[a]	Dosage	Side Effects
Cholestyramine (Questran)	4 g tid initially, 4 g qid to 6 ×/d maintenance	Constipation, abdominal pain, heartburn, flatulence, nausea
Colestipol (Colestid)	15–30 g qd given bid–qid	Constipation, nausea, flatulence
Niacin	0.25 g tid, increasing to 2.5 g tid with meals	Flushing, uticaria, anorexia, hyperglycemia, peptic ulceration, jaundice, hyperurecemia
Fluvastatin (Lescol)	20–40 mg qd	Dyspepsia, diarrhea, abdominal pain, headache
Pravastatin (Pravachol)	10–40 mg qd	Nausea/vomiting, diarrhea, localized musculoskeletal pain, headache
Simvastatin (Zocor)	5–40 mg qd	Headache
Probucol (Lorelco)	500 mg bid with meals	Diarrhea, flatulence, nausea
Gemfibrozil (Lopid)	600 mg bid	Hyperglycemia, nausea dizziness, skin rash
Lovastatin (Mevacor)	5–40 mg bid with meals	Headache, insomnia

[a]Brand names are given in parentheses.

Table 14-13. Oral Antiarrhythmic Agents

Group	Example[a]	Usage Dosage
IA	Quinidine	200–300 mg tid–qid
	Procalnamide	50 mg/kg/day in divided doses q6h
	Disopyramide (Norpace)	400–800 mg qd in divided doses
IB	Tocainide (Tonocard)	1,200–1,800 mg in divided doses tld
	Mexiletine (Mexitil)	200–300 mg q8h
IC	Encainide (Enkaid)	25–50 mg tid
	Flecainide (Tambocor)	100 mg q12h
	Propafenone (Rythmol)	150–300 mg q8h
II	Propranolol	10–30 mg tid–qid
	Acebutolol (Sectral)	200–600 mg bid
III	Amiodarone (Cordarone)	(Maintenance dose) 400 mg qd
	Sotalol (Betapace)	80–160 mg bid
IV	Verapamil	240–320 mg in divided doses (for arterial fibrillation) 240–480 mg in divided doses (for PSVT)
I	Moricizine (Ethmozine)	200–300 mg tid

[a]Brand names are given in parentheses.

Quinidine is the most widely used oral Class I agent and is used for treating both supraventricular and ventricular arrhythmias. Quinidine is used orally to prevent the progression of ventricular tachycardia into serious ventricular arrhythmias that can lead to sudden cardiac death. GI effects occur often (30 percent) with quinidine (nausea, vomiting, diarrhea), resulting in discontinuation of therapy in up to 10 percent of patients. A sustained-release product taken with meals, as well as substitution of a different salt of quinidine, minimizes these effects. Symptoms of *cinchonism* (e.g., tinnitus, blurred vision, headache), as well as serious arrhythmias and hypotension (quinidine syncope), can occur if blood levels are exceeded.

Procainamide is an alternative oral Class I agent with effects on the heart very similar to those with quinidine. GI effects occur less frequently with procainamide, as does the development of serious arrhythmias. Up to 30 percent of patients treated chronically with procainamide may develop a syndrome resembling systemic lupus erythamatosus (e.g., fever, rash, myalgia, arthritis) that resolves upon discontinuing the agent.

A third oral Class I agent reserved for patients unable to tolerate or respond to quinidine or procainamide is disopyramide. Disopyramide frequently produces anticholinergic symptoms, such as dry mouth (40 percent), blurred vision (28 percent), urinary retention (10 to 20 percent), and constipation (30 percent). Disopyramide has a potent depressant effect on cardiac contractility that can lead to heart failure.

Moricizine is a Class I antiarrhythmic agent that shares properties with all three subclasses of Class I agents. Because of its ability to cause arrhythmias itself (proarrhythmic effect), its use is restricted to treatment of ventricular arrhythmias that are life threatening, such as sustained ventricular tachycardia.

Two oral formulations similar to lidocaine are tocainide and mexiletine. Both are considered equivalent in treating and preventing ventricular arrhythmias. Side effects are similar with each agent and are mainly gastrointestinal (30 to 40 percent) and neurologic (10 to 20 percent).

Encainide, flecainide, and propafenone are Class I agents reserved for serious arrhythmias that are unresponsive to other agents because of their ability to cause serious arrhythmias themselves. Encainide has actually been withdrawn from the market but is available on a limited basis.

β-Blockers block the effects of catecholamine-induced increases in cardiac contractility and heart rate. Patients with increased circulating levels of catecholamines (e.g., myocardial patients) often benefit from β-blockers, and β-blockers alone have been proved to reduce the risk of sudden cardiac death in these patients. For side effects of β-blockers, see the discussion on hypotension.

Amiodarone is an orally available Class III agent useful for treating both supraventricular and ventricular arrhythmias. Its toxicity is such that it is reserved only for life-threatening arrhythmias unresponsive to other agents. Sotalol is another orally available Class III agent useful for treating ventricular arrhythmias unresponsive to other agents. Sotalol also has Class II (β-blocking) properties.

Class IV antiarrhythmic agents include the calcium-channel blockers verapamil (the only FDA-approved antiarrhythmic calcium-channel blocker) and diltiazem. Both are effective in treating supraventricular arrhythmias because of their depressant effect on the SA node. By delaying conduction through the AV node, calcium-channel blockers reduce the fast ventricular rate in atrial fibrillation and flutter and abolish tachyarrhythmias in paroxysmal supraventricular tachycardia. For side effects on calcium-channel blockers, see the discussion of hypotension.

Psychotrophic Drugs

Benzodiazepines

Benzodiazepines are among the most widely used class of drugs in the world. In the United States, 5 percent of all prescriptions filled are for a benzodiazepine. Of the 15 benzodiazepines available in the United States, 8 are approved by the FDA, primarily for the treatment of anxiety; 5 are for insomnia (Table 14-14). Such labeled indications do not reflect pharmacologic differences between these agents, but rather marketing strategies of the manufacturers; the sedative flurazapam has anxiolytic properties, and the anxiolytic diazepam is widely used as a sedative.

Benzodiazepines have anxiolytic, sedative, anticonvulsant, and muscle relaxant properties. These actions occur as a result of an *enhancement of the effects* of a major inhibitory neurotransmitter in the CNS, γ-aminobutyric acid (GABA). GABA is the most important inhibitory neurotransmitter in the CNS and is involved in nerve

Table 14-14. Benzodiazapines

Drug[a]	Usual Daily Dosage (mg)
Agents used in treatment of generalized anxiety disorder	
Alprazolam (Xanax)	0.25–0.5 tid
Chlordiazepoxide (Librium)	5–10 tid–qid
Clorazepate (Tranxene)	15–60 individual dose
Diazepam (Valium)	2–10 bid–qid
Halazepam (Paxipam)	20–40 tid–qid
Lorazepam (Ativan)	1 mg bid–tid
Oxazepam (Serax)	10–15 tid–qid
Prazepam (Centrax)	20–60 individual doses
Agents used in treatment of insomnia	
Estazolam (Pro Som)	1–2 h
Flurazepam (Dalmane)	15–30 h
Quazepam (Doral)	7.5–15 h
Temazepam (Restoril)	15.–30 mg h
Triazolam (Halcion)	0.125–0.25 h

[a]Brand names are given in parentheses.

transmission of nearly one-third of brain impulses. Although pharmacologically similar, benzodiazepines differ in their approved indications and their pharmacokinetic properties. Selection of an agent for anxiety or sedation will depend on the onset and duration of the desired agent.

Zolpidem (Ambien) is only one of three nonbenzodiazepines that bind to benzodiazepine receptors in the brain. Such selectivity is thought to account for its minimal effect on the various stages of sleep in contrast to the benzodiazepines. Its use is restricted to the short-term management of insomnia.

Antidepressants

Depression severe enough to warrant medical attention is fairly common in our society, with a lifetime prevalence estimated to be about 15 percent (10 percent in males, 20 percent in females). Depression is highly amenable to drug treatment (80 to 90 percent success rate with careful monitoring). Unfortunately, one study indicates only 1 in 10 depressed patients receives adequate doses of antidepressants. Conservative estimates associate 16,000 suicides annually in the United States with depressive disorders.

Three classes of drugs are available for treating unipolar depression: traditional tricyclic antidepressants, newer antidepressants such as fluoxetine and trazadone, and monoamine oxidase inhibitors (MAOIs). All three classes are considered efficacious in treating depression; some of the newer agents have a more favorable side effect profile than that of the older agents, and the MAOIs may be more effective in treating depression with atypical symptoms.

Mechanism of Action

The proposed mechanism of action of antidepressants has recently undergone revision. Originally it was proposed that a deficiency of the neurotransmitters norepinephrine and serotonin on the synapses of the CNS accounted for the depressive state. By blocking their uptake, it was proposed that antidepressants increased their concentration, and thus neurotransmission. Since antidepressant activity often lags several weeks after this blockade, and since certain other antidepressants do not produce such blockade, it was subsequently proposed that changes in receptor sensitivity to these neurotransmitters (observed with long-term use of antidepressant therapy) accounted for the antidepressant activity of these agents. The recently proposed dysregulation hypothesis suggests that antidepressants correct the dysregulation of neuronal firing associated with the depressive state by allowing more norepinephrine to be released per impulse, with more effective neurotransmission.

Tricyclic Antidepressants

The tricyclic antidepressants (TCAs) are the oldest and most commonly used antidepressants. These agents commonly produce anticholinergic, neurologic, and cardiovascular adverse reactions. Anticholinergic effects occur most frequently and include dry mouth, blurred vision, constipation, and urinary hesitancy. Occasionally, more severe reactions, such as urinary retention, more severe reactions, such as urinary retention, paralytic ileus, and acute glaucoma, also occur. Elderly patients are susceptible to a central anticholinergic syndrome characterized by confusion, disorientation, delusions, and hallucinations.

Sedation is the most common neurologic effect, with some agents less likely to cause this effect than others (Table 14-15). These agents also lower the seizure threshold. Seizures have occurred in patients started on antidepressants.

The most common serious side effects associated with TCAs are cardiovascular, with a quinidine-like effect on cardiac condition. In patients with pre-existing defects in cardiac conduction and in overdoses, fatal arrhythmias can occur. Postural hypotension is another cardiovascular effect of the TCAs that often occurs early in

Table 14-15. Comparison of Antidepressants

Drug[a]	Daily Dosage Range (mg)	Side Effect Frequency	
		Sedative	Anti-cholinergic
Tricyclic agents			
Amitriptyline (Elavil)	75–300	VH	VH
Clomipramine (Anafranil)	250 maximum	H	H
Doxepin (Sinequan)	75–300	H	M
Desipramine (Norpramin)	75–300	S	S
Imipramine (Tofranil)	75–300	M	M
Nortriptyline (Pamelor)	50–200	M	M
Protriplyline (Vivactil)	15–60	S	H
Trimipramine (Surmontil)	75–300	H	M
Newer agents			
Maprotiline (Ludiomil)	150–300	M	M
Amoxapine (Ascendin)	100–600	M	H
Trazadone (Desyrel)	50–600	M	S
Venlafaxine (Effexor)	75–225	S	S
Bupropion (Weelbutrin)	225–450	M	M
Selective serotonin reuptake inhibitors			
Fluoxetine (Prozac)	20–80	S	S
Paroxetine (Paxil)	20–50	S	S
Sertraline (Zoloft)	50–200	S	S

Abbreviations: VH, very high; H, high; M, moderate; S, slight.
[a]Brand names are given in parentheses.

therapy and especially in the elderly. Certain TCAs are more likely to produce this effect than others.

TCAs are extremely dangerous drugs when taken in overdose. In the United States they follow alcohol, sedatives, and narcotics in causing death due to drug overdosing.

Newer Antidepressants

The newer antidepressants include amoxapine, maprotiline, trazodone, bupropion, venlafaxine, and a new class of agents called the selective serotonin reuptake inhibitors (SSRIs). Overall, their clinical effectiveness is equivalent to that of the TCAs, although their side effect profiles often differ. Amoxapine is a derivative of the antipsychotic loxapine and shares many of the adverse side effects associated with the antipsychotic agents (see under Antipsychotic Agents in this chapter), in addition to those of traditional TCAs. Maprotiline shares side effects similar to those of TCAs, with a greater incidence of seizures in an overdose situation. Trazodone causes less anticholinergic and cardiac conduction side effects than do the TCAs but is similar to several TCAs in causing sedation and postural hypotension. Two newer antidepressants that have minimal anticholinergic and cardiovascular side effects are bupropion and venlafaxine. Both agents are more likely to have a stimulant, rather than a depressant, effect on the CNS, with occasional occurrences of anxiety and insomnia.

SSRIs block the neuronal uptake of serotonin in the CNS. Fluoxetine, paraxetine, and sertraline have quickly established themselves as popular agents for treatment of depression. Minor side effects reported with these agents include nausea, diarrhea or constipation, insomnia or drowsiness, and headache.

Monoamine Oxidase Inhibitors

A third class of antidepressants useful in patients refractory to, or intolerant of, other classes of antidepressants are the MAOIs. These agents are also useful in patients with atypical depression or in those with certain phobic disorders. Postural hypotension, sexual dysfunction (e.g., delayed ejaculation and inhibition of orgasm), and weight gain are common adverse side effects of MAOIs. Weight gain is related to a craving for carbohydrates and is sometimes indicative of a therapeutic response.

A rare but potentially fatal adverse reaction of MAOIs is hypertensive crisis, which occurs when these agents are taken concurrently with certain foods or drugs, especially those high in tyramine (Table 14-16).

Table 14-16. Food and OTC Drugs to Be Avoided by Patients on MAOI

Aged, matured cheeses (e.g., cheddar, camembert)
Smoked or pickled meats, fishes (e.g., herring, sausages)
Yeast extracts (e.g., Brewer's yeast)
Red wines (e.g., Chianti, burgundy, sherry)
Cold, hayfever, or weight-reduction preparations containing
- Phenylpropranolamine
- Ephedrine
- Phenylephrine
- Pseudoephedrine

Abbreviations: MAOI, monoamine oxidase inhibitor; OTC, over-the-counter.

Lithium

An agent useful in treating bipolar disorder (manic-depressive illness) is lithium. Bipolar patients experience periods of mood elevation that alternate with normal mood states. Depression often (but not always) occurs in these patients. Lithium is 60 to 80 percent effective in aborting acute episodes of mania after 1 to 2 weeks of treatment and is 80 percent effective in preventing recurrences of such episodes. According to one theory, lithium acts either by enhancing the uptake or by reducing the release of neurotransmitters in the synaptic cleft throughout the CNS, or by both. Side effects of lithium involve the GI tract, the CNS, and the kidneys. During initial therapy, up to 30 percent of patients will experience GI side effects, such as nausea, vomiting, diarrhea, and anorexia. If these side effects reappear during therapy, excessive lithium levels should be suspected.

Lithium often produces CNS and neuromuscular effects, including muscle weakness (30 percent of patients) and a fine hand tremor (50 percent of patients). These effects occur at therapeutic doses but usually subside with continued use. Four percent of patients continue to have an action tremor that can be managed by lowering the dose of lithium or using β-blockers. Neurologic symptoms, such as coarse tremors, stuttering, myoclonic jerking, and seizures, occur with lithium toxicity.

Fifty percent of patients begun on lithium therapy experience a diabetes insipidus-like syndrome characterized by a mild polyuria and polydipsia caused by an inhibition of antidiuretic hormone in the kidney. Dosage reduction or the use of sustained released tablets diminishes these effects. Other side effects of lithium include hypothyroidism, weight gain, cardiac conduction effects, and dermatologic reactions.

Neuroleptic Agents

A class of drugs taken by physical therapy patients with a diagnosis of schizophrenia are neuroleptic agents, otherwise known as antipsychotic agents or major tranquilizers. Neuroleptic agents diminish the outward symptoms of schizophrenia; they do not cure the disorder, and often patients have to be on these drugs for life. Neuroleptic agents appear to act by inhibiting the neurotransmitter dopamine in various portions of the brain. The agent clozapine (Clozaril), however, appears to act by a different mechanism. Neuroleptic agents can be divided into two types: low potency and high potency (Table 14-17). Low-potency agents such as chlorpromazine (Thorazine) and thioridazine (Mellaril) are associated with a high incidence of sedation, orthostatic hypotension, and anticholinergic side effects (e.g., dry mouth, urinary retention, constipation). High-potency agents such as haloperidol (Haldol) and fluphenazine (Prolixin) generally lack these side effects but, in contrast to the low-potency agents, have a high incidence of extrapyramidal reactions as a result of their dopamine-blocking properties in the substantia nigra of the brain (Table 14-18). Three of these common reactions occur early in therapy (Table 14-19) and are often controlled with anticholinergic agents such as benztropine (Cogentin), antihistamines such as diphenhydramine (Benadryl), or dopamine-enhancing agents such as amantadine (Symmetrel). These reactions are by and large reversible. Tardive dyskinesia, the fourth extrapyramidal reaction, usually occurs months to years after therapy has started and is often irreversible. There is no effective treatment for tardive dyskinesia; thus, it is imperative that neuroleptic agents be used only to treat psychosis in the smallest effective dose for the shortest period of time. Daily use of haloperidol as a minor tranquilizer is not an acceptable use of the drug.

Table 14-17. Comparison of Neuroleptic Agents

Drug	Usual Oral Dosage Range (mg)	Frequency of Side Effects			
		*	**	***	****
Low potency					
Chlorpromazine (Thorazine)	200–1,200	H	H	H	M
Thioridazine (Mellaril)	150–800	H	L	H	VH
Clozapine (Clozaril)	300–450	H	H	M	L
High potency					
Loxapine (Loxitane)	20–250	M	M	M	H
Perphenazine (Trilafon)	16–64	M	M	M	H
Trifluoperazine (Stelazine)	10–60	M	M	M	H
Thiothixene (Navane)	10–80	M	M	M	H
Molindone (Moban)	20–225	M	M	M	H
Fluphenazine (Prolixin)	5–60	M	M	M	VH
Haloperidol (Haldol)	10–100	L	L	L	VH

Abbreviations: *, sedation; **, anticholinergic; ***, orthostatic hypotension; ****, acute extrapyramidal effects. VH, very high; H, high; M, moderate; L, low.

Table 14-18. Side Effects of Neuroleptic Agents

Side effect
Anticholinergic
Dry mouth
Constipation
Nasal dryness
Dry skin
Urinary hesitancy/retention
Blurred vision
Inhibition of ejaculation
Extrapyramidal
Acute dystonias
Oculogyric crisis
Trismus
Opisthotonus
Torticollis
Akathisia
Subjective desire to be in constant motion
Pseudoparkinsonism
Pill-rolling movements of hands
Slowing of body movements
Masklike facies
Cogwheeling of extremities
Stiffness
Stopped, shuffling gait
Postural instability
Festinating gait
Salivary drooling
Tardive dyskinesia
Sedation
Orthostatic hypotension

Medical attention is warranted if patients develop abnormal tongue or finger movements while on neuroleptic agents. Often tardive dyskinesia develops slowly with mild tongue movements. Later, manifestations of the reaction include lip smacking, puckering, sucking lip movements, jaw movements, protrusion of the tongue (fly-catcher tongue), and difficulty swallowing. Blinking, grimacing, and arching of the eyebrows also often occur. In severe cases, these involuntary movements of the reaction can involve the extremities, causing choreiform and other abnormal movements.

Table 14-19. Extrapyramidal Reactions Associated with Neuroleptic Agents

Reaction
Reversible
Acute dystonias (e.g., torticollis, retrocollis, opisthotonos, oculogyric crisis, laryngospasm)
Akathisia (subjective desire to be in constant motion, manifested by patient's constant pacing or inability to sit still
Parkinsonism (e.g., shuffling gait, difficulty with starting-and-stopping movement, bradykinesia, muscular rigidity, masked facies, tremor, postural instability, drooling)
Possibly irreversible
Tardive dyskinesia—manifesting often as abnormal movements of the face (e.g., tremor of upper lip—rabbit syndrome, tongue protrusion, fly-catching syndrome), buccal (pressing of tongue, bon-bon sign), neck (retrocollis, torticollis), trunk (axial hyperkinesia, athetoid movements), extremities (chorea of hands or toes, athetosis, ballistic movements), grunting, vocalizations, and other symptoms

Epilepsy

Epilepsy is estimated to affect 0.05 to 1 percent of the general population. Physical therapists will occasionally encounter these patients in their practice. Although there are more than 30 different types of seizures, four major types predominate in this disorder. Partial seizures, both simple and complex, and generalized tonic-clonic (formerly known as grand mal) respond to four different types of antiepileptic drugs (AEDs). Absence seizures (formerly known as petit mal) respond to an agent that is ineffective for the other seizures, as well as to an agent that is effective for all the others.

AEDs control the manifestations of epilepsy; they do not cure the disorder. Nevertheless, after a seizure-free interval, many patients can be slowly taken off these agents. AEDs act either by increasing the seizure threshold through a decrease in brain cell excitability or by limiting the spread of seizure discharge in the brain (through a slowing down of nerve cell electrical transmission). Some agents appear to stimulate an inhibitory pathway by increasing the brain concentration of GABA, an inhibitory neurotransmitter.

In the United States, five primary AEDs are available to treat these four major seizure disorders. One of them, phenytoin (Dilantin) has been among the top 25 most prescribed drugs for years. Another agent, valproate (Depakene, Depakote) is the most prescribed AED in Europe, partly because of its effectiveness in treating all major seizure disorders. A third agent, carbamazepine (Tegretol), was originally introduced on the market for the treatment of trigeminal neuralgia but is gaining increased popularity because of its effectiveness and relatively low toxicity in treating most major adult seizure disorders. A fourth agent, ethosuximide, is useful only for treating absence seizures that commonly affect children. Phenobarbital and primidone (Mysoline) are the fifth type of AED available and are considered together because primidone is in part metabolized to phenobarbitol (see Table 14-20 for a list of AEDs).

Two new agents have been recently approved for treatment of seizure disorders in the United States. Felbamate was approved for treatment of partial seizures in adults.

Table 14-20. Comparison of AEDs

Drug[a]	Dosage Range (mg)	Type Seizures Useful for	Side Effects
Ethosuximide (Zarontin)	250–500 qd	Absence	GI (e.g., nausea, vomiting) CNS (e.g., ataxia, drowsiness)
Felbamate (Felbatol)	400–600 tid–qid	Simple and complex partial	GI (e.g., nausea, vomiting) CNS (headache, drowsiness)
Gabapentin (Neurontin)	300–600 tid	Simple and complex partial	CNS (drowsiness, dizziness, ataxia)
Phenytoin (Dilantin)	300–400 qd	Generalized tonic-clonic; simple and complex partial	CNS (e.g., nystagmus, ataxia) GI (e.g., nausea, vomiting) Gingival hyperplasia
Phenobarbital	50–100 bid–tid	Generalized tonic-clonic; simple and complex partial	CNS (e.g., drowsiness, lethargy)
Primidone (Mysoline)	125–500 tid–qid	Generalized tonic-clonic; simple and complex partial	CNS (e.g., ataxia, drowsiness) GI (e.g., nausea, vomiting)
Carbamazepine (Tegretol)	400–1,200 qd bid dosing	Generalized tonic-clonic; simple and complex partial	CNS (e.g., dizziness, drowsiness) GI (e.g., nausea, vomiting)
Valproic acid (Depakene, Depacote)	Maximum recommended dosage: 60 mg/kg/day	Absence, generalized tonic-clonic; simple and complex partial	GI (nausea, vomiting) CNS (drowsiness)

Abbreviations: CNS, central nervous system; GI, gastrointestinal.
[a]Brand names are given in parentheses.

However, reports of aplastic anemia associated with its use has led its manufacturer to recommend a suspension of its use. Gabapentin is also approved for treatment of partial seizures in adults. Dizziness and drowsiness are minor side effects associated with its use.

Peptic Ulcer Disease

An estimated 15 to 20 percent of all Americans will develop peptic ulcer disease. The most frequently occurring ulcers are duodenal and gastric, and many physical therapy patients will be taking agents either to treat or to prevent recurrence of these ulcers. Other physical therapy patients will be taking a class of these agents (the H_2 antagonists) as treatment for gastroesophageal reflux disease.

Antacids have traditionally been the mainstay of therapy for the treatment of peptic ulcer disease but, because of their often unacceptable side effects (e.g., 27 percent incidence of diarrhea) and inconvenience (multidose per day regimen), they have been replaced by the H_2 antagonists, a sucralfate, or omeprazole. H_2 antagonists act by binding to H_2 receptors on the parietal cell of the GI tract, blocking the release of gastric acid by these cells. In the United States, four H_2 antagonists are available, most of which have FDA-approved indications for treatment and maintenance of duodenal ulcer, as well as treatment of benign gastric ulcer. Nizatidine does not have FDA approval for treating the latter condition and ranitidine, unlike the other three, has FDA approval for treating gastroesophageal reflux disease (Table 14-21). Nevertheless, all four agents are probably equally efficacious in treating these conditions.

In treating peptic ulcer disease, any of these agents can be administered as a single nighttime dose, when acid secretion is highest. Food does not interfere with the absorption of these agents, so they may be taken without regard to meals. Antacids, however, interfere with absorption and should be taken 30 minutes to 1 hour apart from these agents.

Table 14-21. Dosing Guidelines for H_2 Antagonists

Drug[a]	Active Duodenal Ulcer (mg)	Healed Duodenal Ulcer (mg)	Active Benign Ulcer (mg)	Gastroesophageal Reflux (mg)
Cimetidine (Tagamet)	800 hs or 300 qid	400 hs	800 hs or 300 qid	Not currently indicated
Ranitidine (Zantac)	300 hs or 150 bid	150 hs	150 bid	150 bid
Famotidine (Pepcid)	40 hs or 20 bid	20 hs	40 hs	Not currently indicated
Nizatidine (Axid)	300 hs or 150 bid	150 hs	Not currently indicated	Not currently indicated

[a]Brand names are given in parentheses.

H_2 antagonists are relatively free of adverse side effects. The overall incidence of adverse effects with cimetidine is 4 to 5 percent, mostly affecting the GI tract (2.1 percent) and CNS (1.2 percent). In elderly patients and in patients with kidney and liver dysfunction, more severe CNS adverse effects have occasionally been reported (e.g., confusion, agitation, hallucinations); in patients on high-dose long-term therapy with the agent, gynecomastia has developed.

Ranitidine is similar to cimetidine in its side effect profile but, unlike cimetidine, does not cause gynecomastia. In addition, ranitidine does not appear to interact with the liver metabolism of drugs in the manner exhibited by cimetidine. Famotidine and nizatidine are relatively new H_2 antagonists. Little information is available on the side effect profile of these drugs. There is no reason to believe that their side effect profile will differ remarkably from that of the other agents. Famotidine causes muscle cramps, headaches, and constipation in up to 2 percent of patients.

Sucralfate (carafate)is an aluminum salt of sulfated sucrose that forms a gel when exposed to the acid medium of the stomach. This gel serves to coat the ulcer and prevent backdiffusion of acid. Since sucralfate is not absorbable, side effects are rare (constipation in 2 percent; nausea, metallic taste, dry mouth in less than 1 percent). Drugs should not be coadministered with sucralfate, since binding with the agent may occur.

Omeprazole (Prilosec) is the latest agent approved for the treatment of peptic ulcer disease. It suppresses gastric acid secretion by specifically inhibiting the proton pump of gastric parietal cells. Approved indications include active duodenal ulcer and severe erosive esophagitis or poorly responsive gastroesophageal reflux disease. Dosage for both is 20 mg qd × 4 to 8 weeks. Side effects appear to be minimal.

Oral Contraceptive Agents

Many physical therapy patients are taking oral contraceptive agents (OCAs); thus, it is important for the physical therapist to be familiar with how these agents work and what their minor and major adverse effects are. OCAs are available in two formulations: combination products containing both an estrogen and a progestin and a product containing only a progestin, often known as the *minipill*. Combination products have undergone substantial changes since the first was introduced on the market in the United States in 1960. This product contained 200 mg of the progestin and 3,000 μg of the estrogen. Today's triphasic products contain varying amounts of the progestin, all less than 1 mg, and varying amounts of the estrogens, usually 30 to 40 μg. Reducing the amount of hormones in the agents has not reduced their effectiveness as contraceptive agents but has substantially reduced the incidence of adverse side effects.

Estrogens act as contraceptives by exerting a negative feedback effect in the female monthly cycle. The net result is suppression of ovulation and inhibition of implantation of a fertilized ovum. Progestins also exert a negative feedback effect on the monthly cycle, suppressing ovulation and creating an environment in the uterus that is harmful for implantation. When taken properly, oral contraceptives are extremely effective; the last observed failure rate for combination oral contraceptives is 0.5 percent; for progestin-only products, the lowest observed failure rate is 1 percent.

Side Effects

Most of the side effects of OCAs are dose related. The introduction of lower dose agents has reduced the incidence of these side effects. Nausea is the most common adverse effect of OCAs; it can be minimized by taking the agent at bedtime. Taking the agent at bedtime can also reduce the risk of chloasma or facial hyperpigmentation that develops and can be exacerbated by exposure to sunlight when estrogen levels are high. Such symptoms as headache and breast tenderness are also helped by bedtime dosing. These effects, as well as the improvement in acne, are secondary effects of the estrogen component in combination formulations. Other CNS effects associated with OCAs are dizziness, mental depression, lethargy, and decreased libido.

Cardiovascular effects are the most serious adverse effect of OCAs. Women using OCAs are at two to four times greater risk of the development of superficial or deep venous thrombosis and pulmonary embolism than are nonusers. Myocardial infarctions and strokes have also occurred more often in users than in nonusers, although most studies involved users of the older higher estrogen formulation. The risk of hypertension is also higher in users of older formulations of OCAs. It is infrequently encountered with the newer agents. Lastly, there is an increased risk of subarachnoid hemorrhage in OCA users, particularly those who are hypertensive and who smoke.

Many of the cardiovascular risks associated with the estrogenic component of oral contraceptives can be avoided with the use of the progestin-only agent, the minipill. In addition to being useful for nursing mothers (progestin is usually not present in breast milk), progestin-only pills avoid the estrogen-causing side effects, such as nausea, fluid retention, breast tenderness, headaches, chloasma, hypertension, and corneal edemas. Minipills, however, are less effective than combination products and must be taken every day. Irregular menses occur frequently, with some women having as few as two menstrual periods annually.

Patients on OCAs should memorize the mnemonic ACHES (see box on this page), the five early danger signs for patients on the pill, and should alert their physician if any of these symptoms appear.

Indications

Besides contraception, estrogens and progestins are often used to treat symptoms that some women experience during menopause. Approximately 75 to 85 percent of all women in their climacteric years will experience hot flushes (or hot flashes), characterized by a feeling of warmth in the chest, neck, and facial areas, often with visible red flushing. Other symptoms that may occur include headaches, dizziness, palpitations, nausea, vomiting, diaphoresis, and night sweats. Some women develop changes in the vagina that cause discomfort, especially during and after intercourse (atrophic vaginitis). Both symptoms are associated with declining estrogen levels and are responsive to estrogen therapy.

Estrogen products indicated for these two conditions include oral, transdermal, and topical formulations. Oral products, such as conjugated estrogens (Premarin) and transdermal estradiol (Estradiol), are usually administered cyclically (e.g., 3 out of 4 weeks), to avoid overstimulation of the uterus. Estradiol patches have the convenience of twice-weekly application. For atrophic vaginitis, the topical cream should be applied daily for 1 to 3 months, then intermittently, for relief of symptoms. To prevent overgrowth of the lining of the uterus (endometrium), progestins (e.g., medroxyprogesterone, Provera) are often administered with estrogens for 10 days each month.

Another approved indication of estrogens is in the prevention of osteoporosis in postmenopausal women. Taking estrogens seems to slow down the bone loss that occurs in some postmenopausal women. A common schedule is 0.625 of conjugated estrogens administered daily for 3 out of 4 weeks.

Side Effects

Prolonged postmenopausal use of estrogens has been associated with an increased risk of the development of endometrial cancer. The coadministration of progestins during the last 10 days of the cycle has been shown to reduce the risk; nevertheless, any sign of vaginal bleeding warrants medical attention, as such bleeding could be an early sign of endometrial cancer. Postmenopausal use of estrogens has also been associated with an increased risk of gallbladder disease requiring surgery. These risks are explained more fully in the information sheets that pharmacists are obligated to dispense to patients with their prescriptions for estrogens and progestins.

Other side effects of estrogens include nausea, vomiting, weight gain, breast tenderness, and breast enlargement. The use of estrogens alone is associated with a dose-related risk of uterine bleeding; the addition of a progestin may increase this risk but also normalizes the bleeding pattern and reduces breakthrough bleeding. Progestins themselves may cause breakthrough bleeding, spotting, changes in menstrual flow, edema, weight gain or loss, mental depression, and many other side effects.

ACHES: Early Danger Signs of the Minipill

Abdominal pain (severe): may be sign of gallbladder disease, hepatic adenoma, pancreatitis, or blood clot

Chest pain (severe): may indicate a pulmonary embolism or myocardial infarction

Headache (severe): may be a sign of stroke or migraine headache

Eye problems, including blurred vision, flashing lights, or blindness, may be indications of hypertension or stroke

Severe leg pain, especially in the calves or thighs, may indicate venous thromboembolism

Asthma

Asthma is a chronic inflammatory condition of the airways that affects an estimated 10 million Americans. In contrast to other treatable diseases, the number of deaths caused by asthma appears to be increasing. Previously the focus of therapy for this disease was on its bronchoconstrictive component and on bronchodilating agents. New appreciation for the inflammatory component of the disease has led to an emphasis on the use of anti-inflammatory agents as prophylactic therapy, particularly the (inhaled) topical corticosteroids.

Although the mode of action of the inhaled corticosteroids is uncertain, these agents appear to act at various stages of the inflammatory process in asthma. Several formulations of inhaled corticosteroids are available in the United States (Table 14-22); all appear equally effective and in many cases can be given in twice-daily dosing. Occasionally, patients will require orally administered corticosteroids. The same precautions apply as in their chronic use in other inflammatory conditions (see under Corticosteroids). A somewhat less effective inhaled anti-inflammatory agent is cromolyn sodium. It is particularly useful in children because of its negligible side effects.

For patients experiencing only occasional symptoms of wheezing, coughing, or difficulty in breathing, symptomatic treatment with an inhaled bronchodilator may be sufficient. Patients experiencing these symptoms in response to exercise may also benefit from prophylactic use of these agents. The largest category of inhaled bronchodilators are the β-agonists (antagonists?). All appear equally efficacious, and all are associated with minimal adverse side effects (Table 14-22).

An alternative, somewhat less effective, inhaled bronchodilating agent is the anticholinergic ipatropium bromide. Patients with chronic obstructive pulmonary disease may benefit more from the marginal improvement in bronchodilation provided by ipatropium.

An orally administered bronchodilatory agent that is widely used is theophylline. Theophylline is associated with several adverse side effects and interactions that may regulate its use to a third-line agent in the future. Although the bronchodilating activity of theophylline is weak, some patients benefit from its use. Theophylline is

Table 14-22. Antiasthmatic Agents

	Dosage Range, Prophylaxis	Side Effects
Anti-inflammatory agents		
Corticosteroid aerosols		
Beclomethasone (Beclovent, Vanceril)	2–3 puffs tid–qid	Throat irritation, hoarseness, dysphonia, coughing
Flunisolide (Aerobid)	2 puffs bid	
Triamcinolne (Azmacort)	2 puffs tid–qid	
Cromolyn sodium (Intal)	2 puffs qid	Rare
Bronchodilating agents		
β_2-agonists (inhalers)		
Albuterol (Proventil, Ventolin)	2 puffs q4–6h	Rare with β_2-agonist inhalers
Terbutaline (Brethaire)	2 puffs q4–6h	
Bitolterol (Tornalate)	2 puffs q8h	
Pirbuterol (Maxair)	2 puffs q4–6h	
Salmeterol (Serevent)	2 puffs bid	
β_2-agonists (oral)		
Albuterol (Proventil, Ventolin)	2–4 mg 16–8h	Tremor, tachycardia, palpitations
Terbutaline (Brethine)		
Anticholinergic agents (inhaler)		
Ipatropium (Atrovent)	2 puffs qid	Dryness of oropharynx, cough
Miscellaneous agents		
Xanthines (Oral theophylline)	Dosage must be individualized; maximum 900 mg qd in divided doses	Nausea, vomiting, palpitations, tachycardia, headache
Cromolyn inhaler (Intal)	2 puffs qid	
Nedocromil (Tilade)	2 puffs qid	Unpleasant taste

not effective as an inhalant and must be given by either the oral or the intravenous route.

Diabetes

Of the 12 million Americans with diabetes, 10 percent are insulin dependent. The other 90 percent can usually be managed with diet, exercise, and oral hypoglycemic agents, although many of these patients require insulin as well. Insulin is available in three different strengths in the United States (U40, U100, U500) and in three different forms (short acting, intermediate acting, and long action) (Table 14-23). Human insulin produced through biosynthesis (recombinated DNA) or semisynthesis is probably less immunogenic than that obtained from beef or pork sources.

The goal of insulin therapy is to maintain normal blood glucose concentrations so as to avoid either hypoglycemic reactions (blood glucose less than 50 to 60 mg/dl) or symptoms of hyperglycemia (e.g., polyuria, polydipsia, fatigue). Studies are under way to determine whether insulin therapy will prevent or delay the complications of diabetes.

Insulin reactions occur when blood glucose levels are too low. These reactions usually appear suddenly and are most frequently caused by poor timing or by skipping meals, by extra exercise without additional food, and by the accidental administration of too much insulin. Symptoms include shakiness, nervousness, sweating, dizziness, tingling, irritability, and hunger. Insulin reactions should be treated immediately with a fast-acting carbohydrate (e.g., 5 ounces of regular soda such as Coke, 8 Lifesavers, 6 jelly beans) and by stopping all activity and resting for 10 to 15 minutes. Left untreated, insulin reactions can lead to convulsions and unconsciousness. In these cases, glucagon should be administered or the patient should be taken promptly to the emergency department.

Any stress on the body, such as illness (e.g., common cold, flu), infection, injury, or emotional stress, can cause the release of several hormones that oppose the action of insulin. This state of insulin resistance causes the body to turn to body fat for an energy source. The subsequent formation of ketones combined with high blood glucose levels can lead to ketoacidosis and possibly diabetic coma and death. Diabetic patients must be attentive to any illness or other situation associated with severe stress to the body. Any signs of dehydration or symptoms of ketoacidosis, such as nausea, stomach pain, vomiting, chest pain, rapid shallow breathing, and difficulty staying awake, warrant immediate medical attention, as death would otherwise result.

For noninsulin-dependent diabetics, five oral hypoglycemic agents are available for use after diet and exercise have failed to control high glucose levels (Table 14-24). These agents appear to make tissue cells more responsible to the hypoglycemic activity of the depressed levels of insulin in these patients. Duration of action and side effect profile account for the major differences among these agents. Tolbutamide (Orinase) is the shortest-acting sulfonylurea and must be dosed two or three times a day. Several of the other short-acting agents can be dosed once a day, with the exception of chlorpropamide. Side effects of the sulfonylureas are infrequent and mild. GI, dermatologic, and hypoglycemic reactions account for most of the adverse reactions. GI disturbances can generally be relieved by taking the agent at mealtime. Chlorpropamide causes a facial flushing reaction when alcohol is ingested in

Table 14-23. Comparison of Insulin Preparation

Insulin	Onset (h)	Duration of Activity (h)	Example
Short-acting			
Regular	½–1	5–7	Regular Iletin I, Novolix R, Humulin R
Semilente	1–2	12–16	Senilente
Intermediate-acting			
NPH	1–2	24	NPH, Humulin N, Novolin N
Lente	1–3	24	Lente, Humulin L, Novolin L
Long-acting			
PZ1	6–8	36	PZ1
Ultralente	6	36	Ultralente, Humulin U

Table 14-24. Sulfonylureas Used to Control Blood Glucose

Drug[a]	Daily Dosage Range
Acetohexamide (Dymelor)	250 mg–1.5 g
Chlorpropamide (Diabense)	100 mg–250 mg
Tolazamide (Tolinase)	100 mg–3.0 g divided dose
Glipizide[b] (Glucotrol)	2.5–40 mg
Glyburide[b] (Diabeta, Micronase)	1.25–20 mg

[a]Brand names are given in parentheses.
[b]New agent.

one-third of chlopropamide-treated patients. Other adverse reactions to chlorpropamide include water retention and, because of its long duration of action, occasionally prolonged hypoglycemia.

Conclusion

Drug therapy often plays a role in the conservative care of patients seen by physical therapists. It may be a means to an end, as in an acutely inflamed joint and NSAIDs, or it may be "the cure," as in the case of diabetes mellitus and insulin. Medications may affect patients in many different ways and may therefore influence the therapist's examination findings, as well as the patient's response to treatment. These drugs (prescription and OTC) may resolve some symptoms while precipitating new ones (side effects). They are another variable to be considered in the puzzle of patient examination and treatment. Their roles, actions, and side effects must be understood for all the "pieces" to fit. To be ignorant of the roles played by drugs in the care of patients can only handicap the clinician in being able best to evaluate, treat, and manage patients.

Patient Case Study 1

A 54-year-old woman is seen with the diagnosis of spondylolisthesis and a primary complaint of low back pain. Early in her treatment course, she was placed on Darvocet (opioid) for pain. Within several days, she was noted to have a flare-up of psoriasis on the arms and ankles and, upon questioning, a recent case of diarrhea. This information was passed on to the physician, and the medication was discontinued. She was later placed on Motrin (NSAID). As physical therapy treatment progressed, she improved both subjectively and objectively, with her only complaint being an inability to sleep through the night, waking at about 3:00 A.M. with low back discomfort. She had been taking her evening dose of medication with dinner at approximately 5:00 P.M. When this was moved back to 9:00 P.M. with a snack, her final complaint of pain at night resolved.

Patient Case Study 2

A 48-year-old woman was seen with the primary complaint of right-sided low back and thigh pain and a diagnosis of degenerative disc disease of the lumbar spine. Besides her mechanical lower back problem, it was noted upon initial examination that she was having respiratory problems as well. She stated that she had a history of respiratory infections. After her second physical therapy treatment, she returned several days later for her third visit and stated that all low back and leg symptoms were nearly gone. The initial thought was that this was secondary to therapy, but upon further questioning, she had recently started a course of prednisone (corticosteroid) for her respiratory problems.

Patient Case Study 3

A 42-year-old woman was seen for primary complaint of right shoulder pain. Upon questioning, it is learned from the patient that she has similar pain at the left shoulder, neck, and lower back, as well as a recent insidious onset of left knee pain and swelling. When questioned about medications, she stated that she takes only Tylenol (acetaminophen). The review of systems reveals a history of gastritis, easily irritated by aspirin or NSAIAs. After the initial clinical examination, the patient was referred by the physical therapist to a rheumatologist, who was able to allay the patient's fears about medication for her condition and placed her on a *controlled* trial of NSAIDs. In conjunction with physical therapy, all symptoms were soon alleviated without gastric upset.

SUGGESTED READINGS

American Academy of Family Physicians: Drug Use Education Tips. Kansas City, MO, 1988

Ciccone CD: Pharmacology in Rehabilitation. FA Davis, Philadelphia, 1990

Conn PM, Gebhart GF: Essentials of Pharmacology. FA Davis, Philadelphia, 1989

Deglin JH, Vallerand AH: Davis Drug Guide for Nurses. FA Davis, Philadelphia, 1993

Gilman AG, Goodman LS, Rall TW, Murad F: The Pharmacological Basis of Therapeutics, McGraw, New York, 1990

Physician's Desk Reference (PDR), Medical Economics, Oradell, NJ, 1995

Appendix 14-1

Review of Systems: Side Effects/Subjective Complaints (in Order of Most Common Occurrence)

1. Gastrointestinal distress (dyspepsia, heartburn, nausea, vomiting, abdominal pain, constipation, diarrhea, bleeding)
   A. Salicylates
   B. NSAIDs
   C. Opioids
   D. Corticosteroids
   E. β-Blockers
   F. Calcium-channel blockers
   G. Skeletal muscle relaxants
   H. Diuretics
   I. ACE inhibitors
   J. Digoxin
   K. Nitrates
   L. Cholesterol-lowering agents
   M. Antiarrhythmic agents
   N. Antidepressants (TCAs and MAOIs, lithium)
   O. Neuroleptics
   P. Antiepileptic agents
   Q. OCAs
   R. Estrogens and progestins
   S. Theophylline
2. Pulmonary (bronchospasm, shortness of breath, respiratory depression)
   A. Salicylates
   B. NSAIDs
   C. Opioids
   D. β-Blockers
   E. ACE inhibitors
3. Central nervous system (dizziness, drowsiness, insomnia, headaches, hallucinations, confusion, anxiety, depression, muscle weakness)
   A. NSAIDs
   B. Skeletal muscle relaxants
   C. Opioids
   D. Corticosteroids
   E. β-Blockers
   F. Calcium-channel blockers
   G. Nitrates
   H. ACE inhibitors
   I. Digoxin
   J. Antianxiety agents
   K. Antidepressants (TCAs and MAOIs)
   L. Neuroleptics
   M. Antiepileptic agents
   N. OCAs
   O. Estrogens and progestins
4. Dermatologic (skin rash, itching, flushing of face)
   A. NSAIDs
   B. Corticosteroids

C. β-Blockers
D. Opioids
E. Calcium-channel blockers
F. ACE inhibitors
G. Nitrates
H. Cholesterol-lowering agents
I. Antiarrhythmic agents
J. MAOIs and lithium
K. OCAs
L. Estrogens and progestins
M. Antiepileptics

5. Musculoskeletal (weakness, fatigue, cramps, arthritis, decreased exercise tolerance, osteoporosis)
   A. Corticosteroids
   B. β-Blockers
   C. Calcium-channel blockers
   D. ACE inhibitors
   E. Diuretics
   F. Digoxin
   G. Antianxiety agents
   H. Antiepileptic agents
   I. Antidepressants
   J. Neuroleptic agents
6. Cardiac (bradycardia, ventricular irritability, AV block, CHF, PVCs, ventricular tachycardia)
   A. Opioids
   B. Diuretics
   C. β-Blockers
   D. Calcium-channel blockers
   E. Digoxin
   F. Antiarrhythmic agents
   G. TCAs
   H. Neuroleptics
   I. Oral antiasthmatic agents
7. Vascular (claudication, hypotension, peripheral edema, cold extremities)
   A. NSAIDs
   B. Corticosteroids
   C. Diuretics
   D. β-Blockers
   E. Calcium-channel blockers
   F. ACE inhibitors
   G. Nitrates
   H. Antidepressants (TCAs and MAOIs)
   I. Neuroleptics
   J. OCAs
   K. Estrogens and progestins
8. Genitourinary (sexual dysfunction, urinary retention, urinary incontinence)
   A. Opioids
   B. Diuretics
   C. β-Blockers
   D. Antiarrhythmic agents
   E. Antidepressants (TCAs and MAOIs)
   F. Neuroleptics
   G. OCAs
   H. Estrogens and progestins
9. HEENT (tinnitus, loss of taste, headache, lightheadedness, dizziness)
   A. Salicylates
   B. NSAIDs
   C. Opioids
   D. Skeletal muscle relaxants
   E. β-Blockers
   F. Nitrates
   G. Calcium-channel blockers
   H. ACE inhibitors
   I. Digoxin
   J. Antiarrhythmic agents
   K. Antianxiety agents
   L. Antidepressants (TCAs and MAOIs)
   M. Antiepileptic agents

Abbreviations: ACE, angiotensin-converting enzyme; MAOIs, monoamine oxidase inhibitors; NSAIDs, nonsteroid anti-inflammatory drugs; OCAs, oral contraceptive agents; TCAs, tricyclic antidepressants.

15 Medical Emergencies in Physical Therapy

James Leonard, D.O., P.T.
Tim Harbst, M.D.

The trend in health care is toward outpatient treatment, which is generally felt to be more cost effective. Patients with rehabilitation needs are frequently discharged from the hospital more acutely, with the expectation that they will carry out their therapy program in a clinic setting.

Therapists may be dealing with patients who are prone to acute medical emergencies and need to be prepared for these. This will require

1. Preparation in the following areas of training
   - Basic cardiopulmonary resuscitation
   - Familiarity with signs and symptoms seen in common emergency situations
   - Emergency "plan of action" that is understood by the staff
   - Proper supportive care
2. Proper emergency equipment
   - Oral CPR mask
   - Blood pressure cuff
   - Stethoscope
   - Oral airway
   - Portable oxygen
   - Thermometer
   - Juice (orange, grape, etc.)
   - Spine board
   - Basic first aid kit (band aids, etc.)
3. Ready access to emergency transport, with 911 and other emergency numbers posted at all phones
4. Continued periodic retraining of personnel in proper procedures and a documented preparedness plan
5. Current records on patients'
   - Major medical problems and a brief history of these
   - Allergies
   - Current medications
   - Patients' treatment plans and progress

When the signs and symptoms of a major problem that requires emergent action are recognized, the response should be to alert other personnel and to stabilize the patient while summoning appropriate emergency transport. Major problems to be aware of include

1. Nonresponsiveness
2. Seizures
3. Falls
4. Sudden unexplained severe symptoms, such as pain, shortness of breath, numbness, weakness, and alteration of consciousness

Therapists are more frequently the point of entry of the patient into the health care system. Because of this, the patient may not have had a full medical examination prior to the evaluation. This places more emphasis on the importance of an initial evaluation, including questions relating to the patients past and general health. It also requires therapists to sharpen their evaluative tools and look at not only the peripheral neuromusculoskeletal system but also at the mental status, cranial nerves (see Ch. 9), and possibly the abdomen (see Ch. 4) and vital signs (including heart rate, blood pressure, and temperature) (see Ch. 2).

Remember, if it is not documented, it did not happen. This applies to the therapist's history and physical examination, preparedness issues, and any incident that may occur in the clinic setting.

While a therapy department should be prepared with regards to procedures, equipment, and personnel training, attention should also be given to education regarding specific situations that may be encountered. Awareness of signs and symptoms that point to an emergent situation can hasten the appropriate treatment. For example, if a patient loses consciousness in the therapy gym area while ambulating, one would consider hypotension, a cerebral event, and possibly severe pain as potential causes. If the patient regains consciousness rapidly, then this helps to simplify the list of possibilities. If not, and the cause cannot be well defined, adhering to the basic principles of supportive care and following the training given in basic CPR is the most appropriate path.

One of the most important aspects of training is that it gives the staff an immediate plan of action and helps to reduce the elevated stress level that can occur. This will hopefully streamline the process for staff and improve response time and quality of care.

There are several specific situations that are frequently encountered that merit review. We list the major signs and symptoms encountered, briefly review pathophysiologic mechanisms and major possible diagnostic entities that could be the cause, and discuss appropriate interventions.

AUTONOMIC DYSREFLEXIA

This is most frequently seen in individuals with a complete spinal cord injury at the T6 level or above. Common symptoms include headaches that are sudden in onset and frequently a flushed sensation. Signs include bradycardia or tachycardia, elevated blood pressure, sweating, and flushing of the skin. The mechanism of this is thought to be caused by an uninhibited autonomic nervous system due to lack of supraspinal control or to a hypersensitivity of receptors.

Treatment includes elevating the patient's head and torso to allow for venous pooling in the legs to lower cardiac output. This will reduce the risk of a cerebral hemmorhage or seizures that could result from the elevated blood pressure.

After the patient's head and upper body is elevated, look for possible sources of the dysreflexia, which include bladder distention, bowel impaction, or an edematous leg suggestive of a deep venous thrombosis. Frequently spinal cord–injured patients will be prescribed antihypertensive medications such as Nifedipine, which they are instructed to take sublingually if symptoms of dysreflexia develop.

LOSS OF BOWEL/BLADDER CONTROL

Many patients, especially those with lumbar pain disorders, will experience some alteration of bowel and bladder function. Regarding the bowel, diarrhea, constipation (often due to medications), and increased pain with defecation are frequent complaints. It is rare that a patient will have noticeable stool incontinence.

Bladder symptoms can be more difficult to evaluate. Patients may have some minimal dribbling or urgency with their pain or difficulty initiating urination, possibly due to effects of medications. Of more concern is when a patient has such symptoms as frequent incontinence of small amounts, lack of sensation when urinating, and difficulty emptying the bladder. For instance, patients may say that when they leave the toilet they feel as is they have to urinate again immediately. Incontinence in large amounts would also be a symptom warranting concern.

Sexual dysfunction may occur simultaneously. Symptoms could include difficulty achieving orgasm or inability to achieve or maintain an erection. It is difficult to differentiate these types of symptoms of peripheral nerve dysfunction from those due to pain or emotional stressors.

Signs of cauda equina syndrome include decreased or absent sensation in the perirectal region, usually tested with pinprick or light touch. Also lack of voluntary contraction of the external anal sphincter is a positive sign. It is difficult to grade a contractile force of this muscle, as many patients fail to contract tightly due to the discomfort and the emotional stress of having a rectal examination done.

The etiologies of this disorder are multiple, from pelvic masses affecting the peripheral nerves to lumbar or cervical disc herniations compressing the spinal cord. Cerebral vascular events or mass effects in the brain are also possible causes.

If the patient has a sudden onset of these symptoms, especially in the cases of spinal pain disorders, then it may be a surgical emergency, and physician evaluation is indicated. Contacting the patient's physicians and ensuring that this situation is investigated is the appropriate course of action. The obvious concern is that the patient could have some permanent loss of bowel and bladder or sexual function if this disorder is not recognized and treated promptly.

SUICIDE RISK

When patients allude to suicide, even tangentially, or seem distraught, they may be at risk for self-harm. Asking the patients if they are considering suicide would be an appropriate question. If they respond "yes," then asking them how often the suicidal thoughts cross their mind is necessary. The therapist need not fear that such direct questioning will give the patients suicide ideation or that they will be more likely to carry out the act. This direct line of questioning will help to determine quickly how serious the situation is.

Assess the details regarding their ideation, including the general nature of suicidal thoughts, what is done to dismiss them, and their frequency. Also ask what they would do if the suicidal thoughts became overwhelming and what are their reasons for not committing suicide. Also explore any history of attempts and any plan that was formulated.

A minimal risk would include factors such as infrequent ideation, thoughts that are easily dismissed, several reasons for not killing self, a plan for overwhelming thoughts, no significant history, and no formal plan. A serious risk would include factors that are opposite to a minimal risk as noted. In particular, assess their plan: how formalized and realistic is it, have they written a note, have they recently given away objects, is there preferred method of death?

If the plan is serious, reassure the patient and consult with the patient's physician while the patient is still in the therapy department. Ideally, there will be a plan established to deal with the suicide risk before the patient leaves the therapy session. If the patient is already working with mental health professionals, consult with them also (see Ch. 12 for additional information).

PAIN FOLLOWING A FALL IN THERAPY

If a patient falls during treatment, determine whether the accident is witnessed. Was there any loss of consciousness and, if so, for how long? Is the patient alert, and is there any pain? If there is any spine or extremity pain, carefully assess the patient before moving, as one may want to consider using a spinal board. Note if there is any alteration in mental status, any peripheral symptoms such as numbness or weakness, or any incontinence that occurred during or after the episode.

This setting emphasizes the importance of having a brief medical record easily available during treatment. Other medical problems such as osteoporosis, diabetes, cardiac arrthymias, and history of transient ischemic events could point toward the etiology of the fall and indicate a need to address these medical problems prior to pursuing more agressive therapy approaches.

If the patient has severe pain, then emergent or urgent physician evaluation is indicated. Ensure that the patient is as comfortable as reasonably possible and that the vital signs are stable, and arrange transport for further evaluation. Make sure that adequate personnel are available before attempting to move a patient, especially when a carry type of lift is used for transportation.

If the patient has fallen and is unconsciousness, assume that there is a spinal or potentially an extremity fracture (such as a hip) until proven otherwise.

PAINFUL SWELLING IN AN EXTREMITY

A patient complaining of pain, tenderness, warmth, discoloration, and swelling in an extremity should raise an index of suspicion in the treating therapist. Further questioning would include whether the symptoms are new or old, if there is any history of recent trauma, any coexisting renal or cardiac disease that could be associated with this (i.e., peripheral vascular insufficiency, congestive heart or chronic renal failure). Does the patient have any shortness of breath, chest pain, or lightheadedness? Did the patient have any recent surgery or been on bedrest for any lengthy period of time? Is there a history of blood clots or bleeding disorders? Is the patient on any anticoagulant medications?

Physical examination should include noting any edema distally in the extremities. If there is, is it unilateral or bilateral? Is there pitting, and how proximal in the extremity does it go? Are the distal pulses palpable? Is there any discoloration, pain on palpation, or temperature change?

A major concern would be that of venous thrombosis and the subsequent risk of a pulmonary embolus. Unfortunately, > 50 percent of the time a diagnosis of acute deep venous thrombosis cannot be made on the basis of the physical examination alone. Also, in certain populations such as spinal cord or head injury patients there may be altered sensation or cognitive status that would interfere with their ability to notice or report symptoms. Therefore, a high level of suspicion would necessitate physician consultation.

CHEST PAIN

Few complaints are more alarming in a physical therapy clinic than either gradual or sudden onset of chest pain. All chest pain complaints should be taken seriously. At the onset of symptoms, activity should be discontinued and the vital signs checked. If blood pressure is lower than normal (a difference of 20 mm Hg in either systolic or diastolic is usually considered significant), then the patient should be placed in a position with the head lower than the heart (Trendelenburg position).

If the patient does not stabilize within a few minutes, then emergency transportation for further evaluation is required. If the patient does stabilize quickly, then the patient's physician should be contacted and a medical evaluation performed before engaging in any further strenuous therapy treatment.

When a patient presents with a history of cardiac problems, investigation of the condition is essential (Table 15-1). The patient should describe the symptoms associated with the heart problem (i.e., chest pain, nausea or vomiting, dyspnea, diaphoresis). Are the symptoms associated with a certain amount of physical activity, following meals, or during stressful periods? How does the patient treat himself? Does he lie down and/or take nitroglycerin?

Being familiar with the patient's heart condition allows the therapist to determine if the current chest pain complaint is the patient's typical angina. If so, the initial action should be just as if the patient were at home; lie down and take nitroglycerin. Vital signs should be checked, and if within a few minutes the symptoms have not resolved then the emergency plan should be initiated.

Table 15-1. Differential Diagnosis of Chest Pain

Organ System	Etiology
Cardiac	
Ischemic (see Ch. 2)	Myocardial infarction
	Unstable angina
	Prinzmetal's angina
	Stable angina
	Hypertrophic cardiomyopathy
Valvular	Aortic stenosis and insufficiency
	Mital value prolapse
Inflammatory	Myocarditis
Vascular	Dissecting thoracic aortic aneurysm
Pulmonary (see Ch. 3)	Pulmonary embolism
	Mediastinitis
	Pneumothorax
	Pulmonary hypertension
	Pneumomediastinum
	Pneumonia
	Pleurisy
Skin	Herpes zoster
Neurologic	Spinal nerve root compression
Musculoskeletal	Rib fracture and chest wall contusion
	Costochondritis
	Intercostal muscle strain
	Fractures
	Bursitis
	Cervical spine disease
	Thoracic outlet or scalenus anticus syndrome
	Arthritis
Gastrointestinal (see Ch. 4)	Boerhaave's syndrome
	Biliary disease
	Pancreatitis
	Gastroesophageal reflux
	Esophageal spasm
	Esophagitis
	Achalasia
	Peptic ulcer disease
	Subdiaphragmatic abscess
Psychogenic (see Ch. 12)	Aniexty syndromes
	Hyperventilation syndrome
	Factitious chest pain

LOSS OF CONSCIOUSNESS

This can be differentiated into two types: a brief interruption of consciousness (syncope) or a prolonged interruption (coma). Initial management will be the same for either condition: address and stabilize airway, breathing, and circulation (the ABCs) and initiate immediate physician assessment. The differential diagnosis of loss of consciousness is listed in Table 15-2.

Regardless of the etiology, patients need to be monitored, including their level of alertness, blood pressure, pulse, and respiration rate. If the pressure is low, position the patients with their head below their heart (the Trendelenburg position). If the patients respond and recover quickly, further medical assessment can be done on an urgent basis. However, when patients do not respond quickly (within a few minutes), emergent transportation and assessment is indicated.

HYPOTENSION (SHOCK)

While the causes can be several, hypotension, often known as shock, can be defined as a decrease in perfusion and oxygen delivery to central organ systems and peripheral tissues.

In a clinic setting, two common causes of hypotension are cardiac, such as myocardial infarction, or decrease in intravascular volume, resulting in decreased cardiac output and the development of symptoms of feeling weak or actually losing consciousness.

A common problem occurs in the inpatient setting when patients have been confined to bed for several days. When they first begin to sit, stand, or ambulate, there is peripheral vasodilation, inadequate cardiac output, and, frequently, the onset of symptoms. Other patients with autonomic instability such as those with diabetes or spinal cord injury are also at risk for these symptoms.

Regardless of the cause, patients need to be positioned so that their circulation improves, that is, with their head lower than their heart in the Trendelenburg position. In addition, vital signs need to be monitored, along with the patients level of consciousness. The ABCs of basic cardiac life support should also be followed.

Table 15-2. Differential Diagnosis of Loss of Consciousness

Seizure
Hypoxia
Hypoglycemia
Hyperventilation
Extension of CVA/cerebral hemorrhage
Intoxication/overmedication
Psychogenic causes
Syncope

When patients continue to be symptomatic despite rest and proper positioning, physician consultation is indicated. When patients quickly recover, appropriately adjusting their level of activity to accommodate their symptoms is prudent.

PULSELESS/NONBREATHER

If a patient is nonresponsive and a pulseless/nonbreather, staff should make note if the situation was a witnessed or unwitnessed event to estimate the amount of time the patient was oxygen deprived. The ABCs (airway, breathing, circulation) of basic cardiopulmonary life support need to be followed. Begin CPR (cardiopulmonary resuscitation) while summoning emergency transport. Call for help to assist with CPR.

The key to a successful approach in this situation is preparedness and practice. Having staff continually recertified in basic cardiac life support is essential.

SHORTNESS OF BREATH

Acute shortness of breath (dyspnea) is defined as a patient experiencing an "inappropriate awareness of breathing." The significance of dyspnea may vary according to context. In a sports medicine or reconditioning exercise program, the patients are expected to become "winded." However, the return to baseline respiratory rate and intensity typically occurs within minutes. Those patients who demonstrate dyspnea for longer than expected or for no apparent reason need to be addressed. Common causes for dyspnea are listed in Table 15-3.

Knowing the patients' medical and clinical histories will allow the therapist to place complaints in perspective. The authors know of patients who have been immobilized for relatively short periods of time (car ride, bed confinement, long plane trip) and have developed an undetected deep venous thrombosis. The patients proceeded to develop a pulmonary embolus with the

Table 15-3. Common Causes of Dyspnea

Upper airway obstruction (COPD, angioedema, foreign body)
Cardiac (ischemia, valve insufficiency, pulmonary edema)
Pulmonary (asthma, embolism, pneumothorax, aspiration)
Allergic reaction (anaphylaxis)

only common presenting complaints of shortness of breath and acutely impaired aerobic endurance.

One also must not forget the obvious cause of dyspnea, which is airway obstruction. Patients with impaired cranial nerve function may have difficulty handling and clearing their own secretions. A tracheostomy tube may or may not be in place. In either case, it is imperative to have access to and be able to clear the airway using suction equipment. If the situation is emergent, the airway needs to be maintained and emergent transport facilitated for further care.

SEIZURES

Seizures can be categorized into two types: partial (focal) or generalized. It is not uncommon for a focal seizure to progress into a generalized one.

If a patient is being observed at the time of onset of a seizure, it is important to note how it began. Was there any staring, eye-rolling, or comments on the patient's part to indicate a seizure coming on?

Being aware of the patient's history is important. Previous head injury, diabetes, drug dependence, or recent alcohol withdrawal may predispose to seizure activity. Also check to see if the patient is on antiseizure medication, as a subtherapeutic level may be the cause.

Treatment in the therapy department centers around maintaining the patients' airways, preventing aspiration, and ensuring that they do not harm themselves with the thrashing activity that may be occurring. Lie them on their side to minimize risk of aspiration. Remove dentures if present and, if possible, insert an oral airway. Monitor the patients to ensure that the oral airway stays in place and that they will not harm themselves.

Most seizures will only last a few minutes. Continue to monitor the patient postseizure, including recording vital signs. Be aware that seizures are a symptom, and, if the underlying cause is not treated, then seizure activity may resume. If seizures persist for more that a few minutes, then emergency medical personnel should be summoned and the patient transported for further care. If the activity ceases rapidly, then the patient's physician should be contacted before the patient leaves the department. A patient should not be allowed to drive immediately after a seizure, as another episode could occur while driving.

THE AGITATED/COMBATIVE PATIENT

In our society, violence is an increasing concern and part of our existence. The health care setting is no exception. Assaultive episodes are increasing in health care settings due to cultural, sociologic, and political factors. Educating health care staff about assault is helpful in management of this problem, but has failed to reduce the incidence of confrontation and assaulting behaviors. To reduce risk of injury to patient and staff, one must recognize predictors of violence.

The most commonly recognized and encountered predictors of violent behavior are

1. Drug or alcohol intoxication
2. Drug or alcohol withdrawal
3. Acute organic brain syndrome
4. Traumatic brain injury
5. Acute psychosis (includes schizophrenia and manic mood disorders)
6. Paranoid character disorder
7. Borderline personality disorder (when demands are not being met)
8. Antisocial personality disorder
9. History of violent outburst
10. Temporal lobe epilepsy
11. Passive-aggressive personality disorder

In the clinical setting, the therapist may not have the advantage of a complete behavioral history of the patient at the time of initial contact. One needs to maintain an awareness for potential violent behavior by observing behavioral clues.

1. *Posture*. If the patient is tense, as evidenced by sitting on the edge of the chair or gripping the armrest, be alert as increased tension often precedes violent behavior.
2. *Speech*. Loud, forceful speech indicates increased potential for violence.
3. *Motor activity*. Restless agitation, pacing, and inability to sit still are some of the most important signs of potential violence.

One last important note is that for hospitalized patients with organic brain syndrome and dementia, the highest incidence of assault is associated with activities of daily living (ADLs). It is thought that any activity that involves the invasion of personal space increases the risk of assault in these patients.

The first priority in the management of the combative patient is to protect the patient and other people in the immediate vicinity from harm. The first step in dealing with a potentially violent situation is to speak calmly and reassure the patient. If a particular topic or situation is causing or contributing to the agitation, try to redirect the patient away from the source of aggravation. Try to be nonconfrontional and nonthreatening in dealing with the patient at this time. Maintaining a minimum distance of 18 inches from the patient and positioning oneself at a 45-degree angle to the patient will communicate a nonthreatening attitude. Speaking in a calm, controlled voice with a reassuring tone and respectful attitude will communicate an ability to maintain control of the situation.

The therapy facility should have a prearranged plan for handling a combative patient. Some mechanism for communication among personnel should be available in all treatment and transportation areas where someone may potentially be alone with a patient such as in individual treatment rooms, elevators, and bathrooms. If an incident occurs in a small room, keep the door open, and do not stand between the combative patient and the exit so that the the patient does not feel trapped. A prearranged signal should be utilized to alert staff of the situation. Rather than shouting, "Call security stat," thereby conveying panic, the therapist should notify another staff member with a code work or phrase (i.e., "Page Dr. Goodwill") in order to summon additional personnel to the area. In some cases, all available personnel gathered as a show of force may be enough to diffuse the situation. However, if the patient is head injured or has organic brain syndrome, a show of force may escalate the patient's agitation. A single person introduced into the interaction with a head injured patient will often distract the patient sufficiently to diffuse the confrontation. The patient's diagnosis and probable cause for agitation will dictate the most appropriate action. After personnel arrive, the primary staff member (either the person having the best rapport with the patient or the team leader) should once again calmly insist the patient settle down. The primary care physician should then be consulted (if not already on the scene) for the next step of management.

When "talking a patient down" is not effective and the safety of patients and/or staff is threatened, physical restraint must be utilized. To be effective, at least five staff members are needed—one person each for the patient's extremities and head. Special care should be taken to prevent the patient biting others. Once subdued, medication, physical restraints, or seclusion can be utilized. The treatment of choice will depend on the clinical setting.

If a patient wields a weapon, the recommended policy is to calmly tell the patient of potential harm that could happen and ask the patient to put away the weapon. At no time should the therapist ask for the weapon or try to take the weapon away. In the midst of an exchange, the patient may experience a change of mind potentially resulting in a struggle and serious injury. If the patient refuses to put away the weapon, clear the area of people to the following recommended distances:

Ten feet from unarmed combative person
Twenty-one feet from a person armed with a club or edged weapon
Line of sight of a person armed with a firearm

Staff and other patients should be careful to avoid blocking potential escape routes. Armed persons should be approached only by security personnel. Once apprehended, patients will need to be evaluated for their potential of causing harm to themselves or others. A psychiatric evaluation and placement in protective custody may be necessitated. For those patients whose agitation or combativeness is an anticipated part of recovery from a particular injury (traumatic brain injury), a behavior modification program should be implemented as soon as the patient is able to minimally understand and cooperate. Medications may also be utilized to decrease agitiation. To provide accurate and consistent feedback regarding treatment effectiveness, an agitiation-aggression rating scale can be used (see Table 15-4). Obviously, to implement this system, a team approach must be utilized.

Finally, personnel in a facility that regularly treats agitated/combative patients should consider additional training in handling this problem. Training should include redirection/distraction techniques, techniques to escape from manual holds, and group restraint techniques. The Veterans Administration (VA) system provides these programs. Behavioral medicine specialists and/or self-defense experts may be other potential resources.

Table 15-4. Agitation-Aggression Rating Scale

Patient Attitude	Action
Calm, complacent, cooperative	None
Restless, irritable	Let patient vent; offer options; motivate to complete
Boisterous; angry tone; muscle tensing	Distract; redirect; change focus
Distressed, threatening, clenching fists	Distance self; summon back up; discontinue task
Flees or attacks	Protect self; control patient with assistance

THERAPEUTIC POOL EMERGENCIES

As a treatment modality, a therapeutic pool offers a unique benefit to any program. Before participating, patients must be screened for contraindications (see Table 15-5). These contraindications must be enforced for the patients' and other pool users' own protection. Other conditions require one-to-one staff-to-patient ratios (see Table 15-6).

The most frequent pool injuries occur on the deck and around the pool due to slips and falls. Emergencies actually occurring in the water are rare. The most obvious in-water emergency is drowning. This accident is most unlikely in any supervised setting, as anyone having trouble or difficulty can immediately be assisted out of the pool. If rescue is needed, use of a towel or shepherd's hook is recommended over an in-water rescue. Diving accidents with the potential for spinal injuries can be avoided by prohibiting and enforcing rules against diving. Most therapeutic pools are not designed for diving activities.

Table 15-5. Patient Conditions Contraindicating Pool Use

Cardiac problems (indicated by sharp change in pulse, respirations, and body temperature)
Open and draining wounds and skin infections (athlete's foot, ringworm)
Contagious disease
Incontinence if uncontrolled
Uncooperativeness (unless brought under control, patient will be discharged from pool)
Abnormally high fever
All infections, including ear, sore throat, influenza, and gastrointestinal infections
Water-borne infections: typhoid, cholera, and dysentery
Kidney diseases where participant cannot adjust to fluid loss
Diseases affecting the body's ability to regulate its temperature
Perforated ear drums

An exception to immediate removal from the water is when a patient is having a seizure. In this situation, the patient should be stabilized away from the pool sides. This will prevent any thrashing and striking the side of the pool. Do not attempt to restrain the patient or place any objects in the month. Once the seizure has ended (less than 5 minutes) remove the patient. If the seizure shows no sign of resolving within minutes, then status epilepticus may be occurring. Immediate transport to the nearest emergency room is required.

As in land-based exercise programs, exercise intolerance is a concern with pool use (see Appendix 15-1). Some signs and symptoms of a serious medical problem include labored breathing, mental confusion, decreased coordination, paleness, and rapid pulse. These signs and symptoms may indicate cardiac dysfunctions or hypoglycemia (see Appendix 15-2). If the patient is known to have either of these problems, institute appropriate treatment and action.

A final concern is the possibility of exposure to chlorine gas. When breathed, chlorine gas causes violent lung spasms and may necessitate hospitalization. Significant exposure can cause death. The easiest way to avoid exposure is to perform chlorine tank exchanges when the pool area is vacant. Another staff member should be standing by with a self-contained breathing apparatus. All staff should be trained to recognize and test for chlorine gas.

Emergency procedures must include an alarm system for immediately clearing the pool and premises. If exposure occurs, remove the victim(s) to fresh air and initiate the ABCs of resuscitation as indicated. Keep the victim warm and lying down until assistance arrives and transportation to a local emergency facility is possible. A predetermined procedure for handling chlorine leaks needs to be implemented. The typical procedure includes notification of the local fire/rescue department.

Table 15-6. Patient Conditions Indicating a 1:1 Staff: Patient Ratio

Inability to assume upright position
Cardiac problems
Uncooperativeness
Mentally not alert or constantly falling asleep
Fainting
Dizziness
Fear of water

SUMMARY

The best way to handle an emergency is to anticipate its occurrence. This will help to reduce the anxiety that can occur when a situation suddenly arises. It also prevents wasting precious seconds in an emergent situation and allows the staff to proceed with a prearranged plan of action.

While common sense can help one through many of the above-mentioned situations, it will not help if the therapist is not aware of the condition in the first place. Including a review of common emergency problems in the in-service schedule seems appropriate. Periodically practicing emergency preparedness and continually having staff recertified in basic cardiac life support are essential.

While we have addressed this discussion to the therapists, we must point out that educating the entire department staff is essential to early recognition of problems and implementation of appropriate treatment. It may be advisable to have some of the reference texts similar to the ones we refer to available in the clinic.

SUGGESTED READINGS

Atkinson JH Jr: Managing the violent patient in the general hospital. Postgrad Med 7:193, 1982

Berkow R (ed): The Merck Manual. 16th Ed. Merck Research Labs, West Point, PA 1992

Bloch R (ed): Management of Spinal Cord Injuries. Williams & Wilkins, Baltimore, 1986

Callahan ML (ed): Current Practice of Emergency Medicine. 2nd Ed. BC Decker, 1991

Dubin WR: Evaluating and managing the violent patient. Ann Emerg Med. 10:481, 1981

Goodman C, Snyder T: Differential Diagnosis in Physical Therapy. WB Saunders, Philadelphia, 1990

Marshall S, Ruedy J: On Call: Principles and Protocols. 2nd Ed. WB Saunders, Philadelphia, 1993

Woodley M, Whelan A: The Washington Manual of Medical Therapeutics. 27th Ed. Little Brown, Boston, 1992

Appendix 15-1.

Signs and Symptoms of Exercise Intolerance

Chances are that no emergencies will occur in class, but instructors should be prepared and familiar with the emergency procedure at the facility in where they teach. Continually monitor the class participants for signs of exercise intolerance or difficulty with a particular exercise or movement and modify accordingly.

INSTRUCTOR MUST KNOW:

1. CPR training
2. Emergency procedures
3. Contraindications for each participant
4. Signs of distress

SIGNS OF A HEART ATTACK:

1. Breathlessness
2. Dizziness
3. Fainting
4. Excessive sweating
5. Nausea
6. Pain in arm, chest, jaw, teeth, ear (spreads to shoulders and neck)
7. Uncomfortable pressure, fullness or squeezing or pain in the center of chest lasting two minutes or more

IF THESE SYMPTOMS ARE PRESENT, THE EMERGENCY MEDICAL SYSTEM SHOULD BE ACTIVATED IMMEDIATELY.

DANGER SIGNS OF SERIOUS PHYSICAL PROBLEMS

Determine if medical help is needed by checking for:

1. Facial expression signifying distress
2. Mental confusion
3. Decreased coordination
4. Paleness, rapid pulse
5. Labored breathing

The following are signs that an individual is experiencing discomfort while exercising:

1. Dizziness, fatigue
2. Rubbing a joint
3. Strained facial expression
4. Lack of balance
5. Change in usual behavior

If you see any of these signs, question the person during class about the problem.

(From Lutheran Health System, LaCrosse, WI, 1992, with permission.)

Appendix 15-2.

Recognition and Treatment of Hypoglycemia (Low Blood Sugar)

Hypoglycemia is a common medical emergency you may encounter in the pool environment. **It requires prompt recognition and immediate treatment!**

RECOGNITION

Warning Signs
- Shakiness and tremors
- Pale appearance
- Rapid and strong pulse
- Fingers feeling asleep
- Sudden mood swings or inappropriate behavior
- Drowsiness and sleepiness or inability to concentrate
- Headache, confusion
- Yawning, lethargy

Severe Reactions
- Loss of consciousness
- Convulsions or seizures

TREATMENT

As soon as you recognize symptoms (warning signs), treatment should be initiated at the pool side when possible. Even if in doubt whether the symptoms indicate low blood sugar, it is always best to treat as if it is low blood sugar. Use one of the following:

Four to six ounces of fruit juice or soda (not diet)
One tablespoon of honey or sugar
Glutose, Insta-Glucose, BD Glucose Tabs, or Cake Mate

If symptoms do not subside dramatically within 10 minutes, repeat the treatment, and enact the emergency action plan.

(From Lutheran Health System, LaCrosse, WI, 1992, with permission.)

16

Radiologic Assessment of the Musculoskeletal System

Robert D. Karl, Jr., M.D.
Jill A. Floberg, P.T.

IMAGING ASSESSMENT IN PHYSICAL DIAGNOSIS

Diagnostic imaging supports, clarifies, and acts to confirm the findings from the physical therapist's history and neuromusculoskeletal physical examination. The intent of this chapter is to introduce physical therapists to the various imaging modalities available in current medical practice and to emphasize the use of imaging studies in the diagnosis and evaluation of the conditions more commonly encountered by physical therapists.

Before any imaging studies are considered, the emphasis must be on a complete history and physical and neurologic examinations. In current practice models, most physical therapy patients are seen by other health care practitioners before their referral to the physical therapist. In this practice model, the referring provider is responsible for arriving at the correct diagnosis before requesting physical therapy treatment. Increasingly, therapists receive referrals requesting evaluation and treatment, frequently without diagnostic information. Physical therapists also treat patients who do not have a referral from another health care practitioner. In this evolving practice model, physical therapists must take more complete patient histories, perform more complete physical and neurologic examinations, and decide which laboratory and radiologic tests, if any, are necessary to confirm the working clinical diagnosis before therapy is instituted. Equally important is the necessity to exclude pathologic and traumatic conditions that are not amenable to physical therapy.

This chapter provides an overview of imaging studies normally used to assess the clinical problems encountered in daily practice. The major diagnostic imaging modalities, including their strengths and weaknesses, are highlighted. As often as possible, the latest clinical literature is cited. This discussion is followed by a description of anatomic regions, with suggestions for the most appropriate choices of imaging procedures for various clinical presentations.

Imaging modalities continue to undergo rapid change, and as a result imaging algorithms are constantly being revised. This chapter integrates an appropriate discussion of the cost-effectiveness of the various diagnostic imaging techniques, which is being ever more closely monitored by the various governmental and third-party agencies at all levels. Examples of imaging studies are presented to help the physical therapist put diagnostic imaging into a clinical perspective.

IMAGING MODALITIES AND BASIC CONCEPTS

Conventional Radiography

The production of x-rays occurs when a tungsten target (the anode) is bombarded with a beam of electrons. The resulting interaction of the tungsten and the electrons produces radiant energy that has a wavelength shorter than that of visible light. When Professor Wilhelm Konrad Roentgen, a physicist at the University of Würzburg, first observed the effects of this previously unknown energy, he named them "x-rays" after the mathematical symbol "x" for the unknown. These energy waves, or x-rays, have the ability to penetrate body tissues. In x-ray imaging, differential absorption, known as *attenuation*, of the beam of x-rays by body tissues of different electron densities is the source of the different contrasts identified on an x-ray film. Greater absorption by a tissue results in fewer x-rays reaching and exposing the film, producing a brighter image on the film. The relatively dense bony structures absorb the most x-rays and appear bright or white on the x-ray film. By contrast, the least dense tissue (air) absorbs the fewest number of x-rays and appears black on the x-ray image. Soft tissues are primarily water density, intermediate between bone and air, and appear gray on the film.

Viewing x-ray films, or radiographs, is a mental exercise in three-dimensional image reconstruction. A radiograph is a two-dimensional representation of a three-dimensional structure, much as a landscape painter presents a three-dimensional scene on canvas. Unlike the artist's painting, however, a radiograph represents the superimposed or composite image of internal body structures. Therefore, when viewing an x-ray image, the observer must think in three-dimensional layers.

When the x-ray beam passes through the body from front to back the film is named an *anteroposterior* (AP) film. Conversely, if the x-ray beam passes from back to front, the film is termed a *posteroanterior* (PA) film. To assist in the three-dimensional image thought process, a second radiographic exposure of the body part should be obtained at a 90-degree angle to the first view. This is termed the *lateral view*. Additional views are also frequently obtained to demonstrate anatomic structures to the best advantage. These additional views are described in the appropriate sections below. Just as the artist's skills increase with practice, the ability to recreate an anatomically correct three-dimensional image mentally from radiographs also improves with practice.

Conventional films or radiographs are widely used in the assessment of musculoskeletal problems. Radiographic examinations are readily available, relatively inexpensive, and excellent for the initial screening of primary skeletal pathology. They are the initial imaging study of choice in trauma for detecting fractures. They are also useful for detecting unstable injuries with the use of flexion, extension, and stress views obtained with force applied manually to the joint under evaluation, in order to determine ligamentous or other structural instability. Routine films are the initial screening study for most chronic conditions, readily detecting the range of pathology from congenital abnormalities to degenerative arthritis.

The radiographic examination is limited in its ability to detect subtle fractures in complex joints or in dense body structures and is very limited in its ability to assess soft tissue changes. Static radiographic images of complex and dynamic structures can only indirectly hint at underlying biomechanical abnormalities.

The radiographic examination is also limited in its ability to detect the presence of metastatic tumor in bone. Bone has a limited ability to respond to metastatic disease. The radiographic appearance of bone involved by metastatic tumor reflects the balance between bone production (osteoblastic activity) and bone destruction (osteolysis).[1] When osteoblastic activity predominates, the resulting lesion appears more dense or sclerotic than normal bone, the most common appearance with prostatic cancer. Conversely, when bone destruction is the predominant activity, less bone is present, and the lesion appears less dense than normal bone, or lytic, the most common appearance with lung and breast cancer. Conventional radiographs are relatively insensitive for the detection of metastatic disease in bone because almost 50 percent of the bone must be destroyed before the lesion can be visualized radiographically. Therefore, for the detection of metastatic disease, skeletal imaging with nuclear medicine is the most effective means of detecting early bony involvement, because this modality images metabolic activity.

Finally, with radiographic studies, there is concern about patient exposure to ionizing radiation. Although a minor consideration when filming a foot using proper equipment and technique, it is a more serious concern when the examination is of the lumbar spine or pelvis, where there will be significant gonadal exposure to radiation. Modern techniques and sensitive (high-speed) films have helped reduce gonadal exposure. Judicious decisions about the appropriateness and value of radiographic examinations will serve to reduce radiation exposure further.

Computed Tomography

A computed tomographic (CT) scan is produced through the use of x-rays passing through the body, as are conventional radiographs. In a CT scan, the x-rays are produced by an x-ray tube that rapidly rotates around the patient. Instead of producing a direct image on film, the x-ray beam passing through the body is measured by an electronic detector. A computer uses the data from the detector in order to reconstruct an image of the internal organs of the body, first on a television monitor and then subsequently printed on film.

Each axial image produced is a cross-sectional slice of the body, much like lifting a single slice of bread from a loaf. The entire series of axial images is used to reconstruct a three-dimensional image of the body, similar to repackaging the individual slices of bread to make the whole loaf. The result is an image of the inside of the body with exquisite anatomic detail that cannot be achieved with conventional radiographs.

A CT scan is effective because it images both the muscular and skeletal systems simultaneously. It yields superb cross-sectional anatomy and has excellent tissue contrast resolution. While conventional films have the ability to discriminate tissue density differences of about 5 percent, CT can distinguish density differences of about 1 percent, permitting differentiation of adjacent soft tissues. CT is also particularly valuable in detecting and characterizing skeletal abnormalities, especially in the spine, pelvis, and extremity joints, where complex articular relationships are present.

A CT scanner uses x-rays and exposes the patient to radiation, but the exposure is kept to a minimum through the use of a pencil-thin or collimated x-ray beam. Like a radiographic examination, a CT scan is noninvasive and, for most patients, a comfortable procedure. CT scanning is a valuable tool in assessing the musculoskeletal system, is widely available, and is a cost-effective method for evaluating many of the conditions commonly seen in physical therapy practices.

Magnetic Resonance Imaging

Magnetic resonance (MR) imaging, once an exotic technology, is now a routine part of diagnostic imaging. MR is the imaging method of choice for the central nervous system (CNS) and is widely used in the assessment of the musculoskeletal system.[2–5]

Advances in diagnosis using musculoskeletal MR are possible because of the superb soft tissue contrast available with this technique. Conventional radiographs are superior for visualizing cortical bone and assessing stability after trauma with flexion, extension, or stress views. Whereas CT provides superior cross-sectional anatomic definition, MR with its exquisite soft tissue contrast, permits complete assessment of the surrounding extraosseous structures (cartilage, tendons, ligaments, muscles) and intraosseous marrow.[6] Although MR does not detect direct cortical bony injury, its sensitivity in detecting abnormal amounts of blood and water (edema) in the underlying marrow has led to an evolving role for MR in the detection of occult trauma.

MR has become the study of choice for demonstrating soft tissue tumors,[7–10] tumor infiltration of adjacent vascular and soft tissue structures, the intramedullary extent of tumor,[11] and the detection of recurrent tumor after therapy.[12]

MR requires a new approach in thinking[13] and image interpretation because it is based on physical principles that are different from those of x-rays, γ-rays, or ultrasound. All medical imaging studies depend on physical interactions between energy photons (packets of energy) and body tissues. CT and radiographic images are based on the differential absorption of energy by body tissues of varying electron density and on the detection of the remaining transmitted energy by receptors on the opposite side of the body (the film or CT detector). By contrast, MR produces images by means of magnetic fields and radio waves and depends on the proton (not electron) density of the body tissues.

MR relies on the behavior of protons (the nuclei of hydrogen atoms) to align with the axis of a strong magnetic field when placed within that magnetic field. When these protons absorb an applied radio wave energy from the transmitter of the MR unit, they temporarily lose the initial alignment. As the hydrogen atoms realign, they transmit a faint radio signal. This signal is detected and amplified by the MR unit and fed into a computer that plots the origin and intensity of the signal and presents this information in the form of an image. Different tissues contain varying amounts of water. Water has the highest concentration of hydrogen atoms; therefore, tissues with differing water content absorb and emit radio signal energy at different intensities. The stronger the signal, the brighter the image. It is this varying signal intensity that permits differentiation and characterization of normal and abnormal tissues. In simplest terms, the MR unit can be thought of as a sophisticated radio transmitter and receiver operating in a magnetic field,[14] and the MR can be thought of as an image of water distribution within the body.

Additional terms used in MR are T1 and T2. These tissue-specific time constants refer to the rate of proton realignment with the external magnetic field after excitation by radio wave energy (T1) and the rate of decay of the transverse magnetization over time (T2). These tissue-specific time characteristics are important because they allow contrast differentiation between tissues. For example, fat has a very short T1 and produces a bright signal, whereas tumors have a relatively long T1 and appear dark on the MR. Cortical bone has a relative paucity of free water protons and is represented as a signal void on MR.

MR is generally considered safe according to the National Institutes of Health (NIH).[15] There have been no published reports of harmful effects from the electromagnetic field per se.[16] The most important risk is that from ferromagnetic objects becoming ferromagnetic projectiles in the strong magnetic field and from ferromagnetic objects within the body, such as aneurysm clips, intraocular foreign bodies, or shrapnel, becoming dislodged. Patients with cardiac pacemakers or neurostimulators should not undergo MR examinations because of the risk of damage or deactivation of the device.

The limitations of MR currently appear confined to the inability to visualize cortical bone, the relative length of time required to complete the study (usually 40 minutes for a complete examination of a joint, longer for the spine), patient claustrophobia, and the considerable expense of the examination. However, MR has become more widely available and is routinely used in the diagnosis of musculoskeletal pathology.

Nuclear Skeletal Imaging

Nuclear imaging of the skeletal system, also referred to as skeletal scintigraphy, or more simply as bone scan, involves the use of (safe) trace amounts of radioactive materials to study the physiology and metabolism of the body. Skeletal imaging is successful because bone is a vascular, living, dynamically active tissue and not just a rigid framework supporting the soft tissue structures. A metabolically active lesion in bone, whether caused by tumor, inflammation, or trauma, concentrates the radioactive material to a greater degree than normal bone and appears more "intense" on the nuclear medicine images. It is generally accepted that approximately one-half of the bone must be destroyed before the changes can be noted radiographically. Therefore, because nuclear skeletal imaging is so sensitive, it will frequently reveal the presence of disease before it can be detected clinically and before routine radiographs demonstrate abnormalities. Nuclear medicine procedures are safe, easy to perform, and comfortable for the patient. Except for a single intravenous injection of a very small amount of liquid (about 1 to 2 ml), these procedures are noninvasive.

The traditional role of nuclear skeletal imaging has been in the detection of metastatic disease. However, newer techniques, newer radiopharmaceuticals, and advances in instrumentation (cameras and computers) during the past decade have greatly increased the specificity and anatomic resolution of nuclear imaging studies. These advances have expanded the role of radioisotopic imaging to include the evaluation of traumatic and sports-related injuries.[17,18] As physical therapists have become aware of the expanded capabilities of this imaging modality, it is a more frequently used tool in the evaluation of a wide variety of both traumatic and nontraumatic conditions and for the differentiation of soft tissue from skeletal pathology.

Technetium skeletal imaging (the bone scan) is the most frequently requested nuclear medicine examination for the evaluation of musculoskeletal disorders. Technetium (Tc 99m) is a short-lived radioisotope with a half-life of approximately 6 hours. The carrier compounds to which the technetium radioisotope is tagged are diphosphonates, usually methylene diphosphonate (MDP). These compounds are rapidly cleared from the bloodstream and are concentrated in the skeleton. As the isotope undergoes radioactive decay, it emits a γ-ray with an energy of 140 keV. This energy makes Tc 99m an ideal agent for imaging with the currently available high-resolution gamma cameras.

The bone scan is both a sensitive and an effective method of screening for potential skeletal pathology. However, because bone scanning images metabolism and not anatomy, its high sensitivity, that is, the ability to detect the presence of disease in a symptomatic patient, comes at the expense of lowered specificity, the ability to exclude the presence of disease in a normal patient. Because it is acutely sensitive to the earliest changes in metabolic activity, any process that affects bone, such as changes in blood supply, trauma, tumors, infections, or degenerative changes, will demonstrate an abnormality on the scan. Additional studies will usually be necessary to define the underlying abnormality further.

Routine Tc 99m skeletal images are obtained 3 to 4 hours after the administration of the radiopharmaceutical. The usual views consist of anterior and/or posterior images of the affected part. Oblique and lateral images are also often obtained.

Although less common, the physical therapist may see the results of gallium and indium studies performed to detect inflammatory conditions such as postoperative infections, infections in the intervertebral discs, joint infections, and infections of bone associated with foot ulcers in diabetic patients.

Gallium 67 is a radioisotope that is very sensitive for inflammatory lesions in the skeleton. It is most often used in the evaluation of osteomyelitis and is available in most nuclear medicine laboratories. Indium 111–labeled white blood cells (WBCs) are also very effective in the diagnosis of infection. However, because this test requires a complex technique to prepare the compound for injection, it is a relatively expensive study and is not routinely available.

All the radiopharmaceuticals used, whether technetium, gallium, or indium, are administered in the smallest amounts possible to minimize the radiation dose to the patient. This may amount to a radiation exposure that is less than that of a radiographic examination of the lumbar spine.

Bone scanning is a technique that is widely available and rapidly performed without complex patient preparation. It has a high degree of accuracy and reproducibility. Bone scanning is useful for imaging in all age groups and is almost totally without adverse reactions. It can be readily and safely repeated for serial follow-up of management and response to therapy. Bone scanning with technetium-tagged diphosphonates is readily available in any nuclear medicine department and is relatively low in cost.

Ultrasound

Diagnostic ultrasound is commonly used in modern medical practice to evaluate a wide variety of conditions from heart disease to early pregnancy. Ultrasound is a safe and effective means of visualizing the body's internal structures. Instead of ionizing radiation, like radiography and CT, ultrasound uses very high-frequency sound waves to create images of the internal organs. A transducer sends these high-energy sound waves into the body and "listens" for their return as they are reflected off internal tissues. A computer analyzes the location and intensity of the reflected sound and creates a picture of the interior of the body that is subsequently photographed.

Although diagnostic ultrasound is used frequently in general medical diagnosis, it is used infrequently in the detection of musculoskeletal pathology. Diagnostic ultrasound does have the ability to distinguish solid from cystic soft tissue masses and is used to direct needle aspirations of soft tissue masses. Its usefulness in musculoskeletal imaging is limited because the sound waves are unable to penetrate bone. Still, ultrasound examination is valuable in assessing the popliteal fossa and in differentiating between a Baker's cyst and other causes of popliteal swelling, such as a popliteal artery aneurysm. In skilled hands, it has proved useful in assessing the rotator cuff muscles for evaluation of shoulder impingement syndrome. However, with the current advances in musculoskeletal imaging attained by CT and MR, even these limited uses of ultrasound are being supplanted. Thus, except in characterizing certain soft tissue masses, diagnostic ultrasound is not a major imaging tool for the musculoskeletal system.

CERVICAL SPINE

Because of its complex anatomy, the cervical spine requires a variety of diagnostic studies for assessment, since no one single method may be adequate to answer completely the clinical questions encountered in patient evaluation. Radiographs, CT scans, MR, nuclear medicine studies, and myelography are all applicable imaging studies for the cervical spine.

Trauma

The physical therapist is rarely involved in diagnosing acute trauma, with the exception of athletic events, where the physical therapist may be present but is not ultimately responsible beyond initial first aid for patient management. It is critical that the patient with suspected spine injuries be immobilized until the radiographic study has excluded spinal injury.[19] The determination of the full extent of the injury may require additional evaluation by CT, myelography, or MR.

Routine radiographs are the most effective primary screening method for detecting the presence of significant cervical spine injuries.[20] The lateral film is the most important study and permits visualization of 90 percent of significant injuries.[21] In the traumatized patient, the initial assessment of the cervical spine is with a cross-table lateral film. This view can be obtained with the patient's head and neck stabilized and permits detection of obvious fractures and abnormalities of alignment. The examination is completed with the addition of AP and odontoid views. If no unstable fracture is identified on the initial examination, flexion and extension lateral views may be obtained to assess soft tissue injury and instability. Additional information may be obtained with CT scanning, which is excellent for assessing complex cervical spine fractures and localizing bone fragments.[22–24]

MR has also been evaluated for its usefulness in assessing the extent of injury in cervical spine trauma.[25,26] MR is superior to CT and conventional films in identifying spinal cord injury, acutely herniated intervertebral discs, and epidural hematomas.[27] An additional asset of MR is the ability to perform multiplanar three-dimensional imaging in the axial, sagittal, and coronal planes. The unique insight provided with MR in spinal cord injuries is invaluable for neurologically compromised or high-risk patients.[28,29]

Nontrauma

A more common scenario for the physical therapist is the assessment of the nontraumatized patient with either neck pain or radioculopathy, or both. The standard cervical spine radiographic series consists of an AP film, a lateral film, bilateral oblique views to visualize the neuroforamina, and an odontoid view to assess the atlantoaxial articular relationship.[30]

In addition to the assessment of alignment, routine films are excellent for identifying vertebral anatomy. This includes narrowing of the intervertebral disc (Fig. 16-1), degenerative arthritis of the articulating facets, and neuroforaminal narrowing.

As visualized on the lateral view, there should be a gently curving line connecting the anterior vertebral margins—the prevertebral line of alignment. A parallel curving line connects the posterior margins of the vertebral bodies, the posterior vertebral line of alignment, which defines the anterior margin of the spinal canal. In addition, a gradually curving line should connect the bases of the spinous processes, the spinolaminar line of alignment, which defines the posterior margin of the spinal canal.

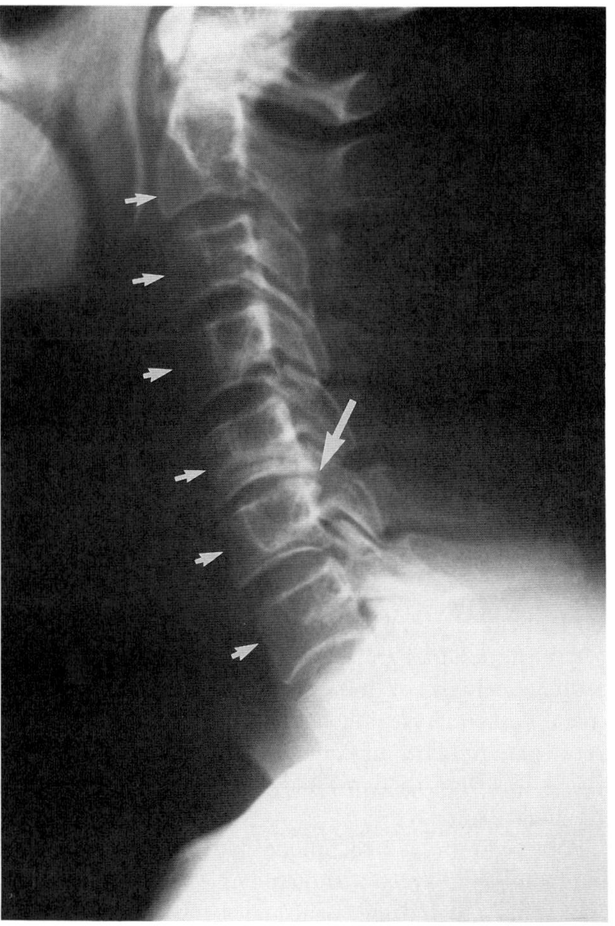

Fig. 16-1. This 41-year-old man complained of chronic cervical and right arm pain. Lateral film from his cervical spine radiographic examination reveals a normal anterior line of alignment (arrowheads). There is narrowing of the C5–C6 intervertebral disc with posterior osteophytes (arrow). An oblique view (not shown) revealed encroachment of the right C5–C6 neuroforamen by the osteophytes.

Further information about alignment and stability can be obtained with flexion and extension views. These are particularly useful for assessing atlantoaxial subluxation. Normally, the transverse ligament maintains the correct anatomic relationship between the odontoid process (dens) of C2 (the axis) and the anterior arch of C1 (the atlas). The normal distance in adults is 1 to 2 mm and up to 5 mm in children, who have greater ligamentous laxity. In trauma or in inflammatory processes, this ligament may be stretched or torn. Atlantoaxial subluxation is the most common abnormal finding in the cervical spine in patients with rheumatoid arthritis.[31] The result is an increased distance between the posterior margin of the anterior arch of C1 and the anterior margin of the odontoid process identified on flexion views. The consequence of atlantoaxial subluxation is compression of the anterior surface of the spinal cord by the posterior margin of the odontoid process with flexion.

Additional imaging of the cervical spine has previously been directed toward assessment of bony anatomic detail with CT scanning and assessment of cord or nerve root impingement with myelography. While CT scans provide superb definition of the bony anatomy of the cervical spine,[32] they fail to delineate neural and soft tissues. In addition, CT scans frequently failed to adequately assess the C6–C7–T1 levels because of beam-hardening artifacts caused by the patients scapulae and humeri.

Although CT during the 1970s significantly increased the ability to assess the bony anatomy of the cervical spine, MR during the 1980s has revolutionized the detection and definitive diagnosis of degenerative diseases of the cervical spine in a noninvasive manner and on an outpatient basis. Routine cervical spine films, including oblique views, are still necessary to assess the bony anatomy of the cervical spine and to detect neuroforaminal encroachment by osteophytes, a relative blind spot for MR.[33] CT scanning is still used to assess complex cervical spine fractures. However, MR has now replaced myelography and CT with myelography (the CT myelogram) as the second study of choice for the evaluation of most cervical spine pathology.

The excellent soft tissue contrast of MR permits exquisite visualization of the contents of the spinal canal (Fig. 16-2), including the epidural space, the cervical cord, the nerve roots, the disc margins, and the cerebrospinal fluid (CSF) without the attendant risks and discomfort of the invasive cervical myelogram. The ability of MR to assess the cord as well as the nerve roots in suspected cases of radiculopathy is considered essential.[34,35] Approximately 12 percent of patients with the clinical diagnosis of cervical spondylolysis will have myelopathy or radiculopathy from another cause.[36] The detection of intramedullary pathology, while present in a minority of cases, will significantly alter the diagnosis and treatment.

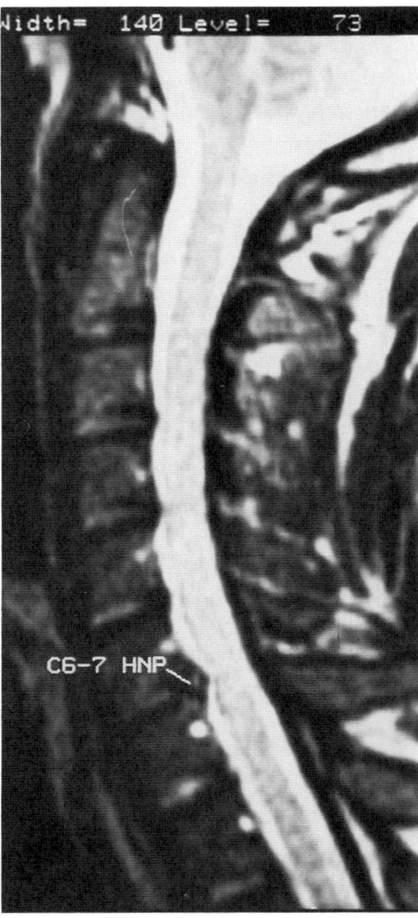

Fig. 16-2. This 29-year-old man sustained a cervical injury in a fall. Initial radiographs of his cervical spine were normal. He continued to complain of pain radiating into the right arm. Physical examination revealed decreased triceps strength on the right. An MRI scan was obtained. The T2-weighted sagittal image reveals a disc herniation at the C6–C7 level with anterior impression on the cervical cord. Axial MR images (not shown) revealed the disc herniation to impinge upon the right C7 nerve root. (Courtesy of Leonard Sisk, MD.)

Although CT myelography with intrathecal contrast still provides the best anatomic assessment of the epidural space, MR is noninvasive, provides almost the same quality of detail of the epidural space, provides more information about the spinal cord, and is more cost-effective. Furthermore, through the development of new imaging techniques with intravenous paramagnetic contrast agents and newer fast scanning techniques, coupled with improvements in both the hardware and software (resulting in improved signal-to-noise ratios), MR has essentially replaced CT and myelography in cervical spine imaging.

THORACIC SPINE

The thoracic spine as such has little individual representation in the literature. Although much less studied from the musculoskeletal perspective, thoracic spine complaints find their way to the physical therapist with regularity if not frequency.

Trauma

The rib cage provides relative stability for the thoracic spine. Thus, most injuries involve the lower thoracic spine, particularly at the thoracolumbar level. Mechanisms of injury include hyperflexion with resultant anterior wedging of the vertebral bodies, axial loading with resultant burst fractures, and, less commonly, hyperextension and shearing injuries. Compression fractures caused by acute flexion are the most common thoracic spine injuries.

Thoracic spine injuries are frequently associated with tracheobronchial and cardiovascular injuries, hemothorax, pneumothorax, and diaphragmatic tears. As with other spinal trauma, the goal is to provide stabilization while other associated life-threatening injuries are being treated.[19]

After the initial assessment of the bony structures with plain-film examination, additional information is obtained with MR imaging. MR detects the soft tissue changes associated with acute trauma such as cord hemorrhage or edema and adjacent musculotendinous hematomas or ruptures.

Traumatic disc herniations occurring in the thoracic spine are best evaluated with MR imaging, which visualizes the relationship of the intervertebral discs with the adjacent spinal cord. MR is also better in evaluating the delayed sequelae of thoracic spine trauma such as a syrinx.[37]

Nontraumatic Thoracic Pain

Scoliosis and compression fractures secondary to osteoporosis are the most common musculoskeletal problems of the thoracic region presenting to the physical therapist. Other abnormalities include congenital anomalies; metastatic disease affecting the vertebral bodies with collapse or destruction of the pedicles; and changes in the intervertebral disc, including degenerative disease, Scheuermann's deformity,[38] and infections.

Radiographic assessment is the first imaging study of choice in the evaluation of patients with thoracic pain. Plain radiographs provide important diagnostic information regarding vertebral alignment, congenital anomalies, skeletal changes caused by tumor and fracture, and the status of the intervertebral disc. The routine radiographic assessment of the thoracic spine consists of AP and lateral views. These views are more valuable for assessing vertebral alignment if performed with the patient in the erect position. The upper thoracic vertebrae are frequently obscured by the superimposition of the shoulder girdles. Additional coned views with the patient very slightly obliqued are necessary to visualize the upper thoracic segments.

Radionuclide imaging is used to determine multiplicity and extent of lesions. CT provides information about tumor matrix and the extent of bone destruction. MR is useful in the evaluation of intracanalicular and paraspinous extension of lesions.

Scoliosis

Scoliosis is defined as one or more lateral abnormalities of the spinal curve, often associated with abnormal rotations and increased kyphosis and lordosis. Although the most common cause of scoliosis is not precisely known and is labeled idiopathic, there is a strong familial association, and most scoliosis probably occurs through genetic transmission. Idiopathic scoliosis accounts for approximately 80 percent of cases of scoliosis and is diagnosed by excluding the other causes of scoliosis.[39] This is in contrast to congenital scoliosis, probably not of genetic origin, which is attributable to the presence of an underlying structural bony abnormality. Scoliosis may also be due to neuromuscular conditions, neurofibromatosis, trauma, and tumors. Radiographic assessment is valuable for assessing the presence of underlying bony abnormalities and for quantitating and following the spinal curve(s).

Evaluation of scoliosis as part of student physical screening has become a common practice in many of the school systems in more than one-half of the states. These screening programs based on physical examination have led to an increased number of radiographic examinations of the spine.[40] After the initial screening examination, subsequent follow-up examinations in scoliotic patients frequently include radiographs with each visit, often at 3- to 6-month intervals, until skeletal maturity is reached.

Females, aged 9 to 14 years comprise approximately two-thirds of the screened population requiring additional evaluation.[41] Developing breast tissue is particularly sensitive to the carcinogenic effects of radiation.[42] In these female patients undergoing multiple examinations, cumulative doses to the breasts of more than 10 cGy have been reported,[43] a potentially significant dose. To protect the breast tissue of adolescent girls from excess exposure to radiation during radiographic examinations additional precautions are necessary. These techniques include fast film and screen combinations known as "rare earth" systems, compensating wedge filters that remove unnecessary radiation from the thoracic area, breast shields, and the PA position. When combined, these methods can reduce exposure to the breast by a factor of 12 or more.[40,41,43]

Osteoporosis

In the elderly population, therapists must be alert to the possibility of patients presenting with back pain caused by collapse of vertebrae weakened by osteoporosis. Osteoporosis is a generalized term referring to a state of decreased mass of normally mineralized bone. Of the many conditions that cause osteoporosis, the most common is postmenopausal bone loss. If the bone density becomes so low that the skeleton cannot support the normal activities of daily life, pathologic fractures occur, most commonly of the vertebral bodies and proximal femurs. Major contributing factors include inadequate nutrition, inadequate hormonal regulation, inactivity, and heredity.

Accurate detection and quantitation of bone mineral content, if readily available, would be integral to the management of osteoporosis and other metabolic bone diseases. Routine radiographs are of little benefit in the early detection of bone loss. Unfortunately, up to 50 percent of the bone mass must be lost by the time radiographic changes can be identified. Therefore, when routine radiographs demonstrate the washed-out appearance characteristic of osteoporosis, the disease is beyond the early stages. Although not beneficial in quantifying osteoporosis, routine radiographs are valuable in assessing the complications of osteoporosis, primarily the collapse of one or more vertebrae.

Several methods for the quantitative assessment of osteoporosis exist, but a persistent lack of precision among these techniques has prevented incorporation of bone mineral analysis into the usual diagnostic armamentarium.[44] Single-photon absorptiometry (SPA), using a single-energy γ-ray, measures bone mineral content of the distal radius and os calcis. However, these measurements do not correlate well with the mineral content of the proximal femur or spine, the most important fracture sites in osteopenic states.[45] Dual-photon absorptiometry (DPA), using two γ-rays of differing energies, measures cortical and trabecular bone in both the hip and spine. However, it has poor spatial resolution, and extensive time is required to complete and analyze the examination.[46] Quantitative computed tomography (QCT) yields high spatial resolution and is the best predictor of vertebral compression fractures. However, it is limited in the assessment of femoral mineral content by software requirements; requires very expensive equipment, which is usually in demand for other studies; and involves high radiation doses.[47] Dual-energy radiographic absorptiometry (DRA), currently limited in availability, offers excellent resolution, greater speed, increased precision, and long-term reproducibility. This technique, using x-ray beams of alternate energies, may become a useful tool for the evaluation and long-term follow-up of patients at risk of osteoporosis.[48]

Neoplasm

Middle-aged and older patients commonly present with complaints of chronic and/or increasing back pain. Degenerative arthritis is a common condition in this age group, as is metastatic disease, which may frequently present before the primary malignancy is diagnosed. Therapists must be cognizant of the concurrent presentation of these two conditions and choose appropriate clinical and imaging assessments to differentiate between them.

Metastases are the most common neoplasms of bone. Lung, breast, genitourinary, and gastrointestinal primary tumors account for approximately 80 percent of skeletal metastases.[49] Seventy percent of skeletal metastases in women are due to cancer of the breast, and in men 60 percent are due to prostate cancer. Dissemination from the primary tumor is usually through the bloodstream to the bone marrow in those skeletal regions engaged in active hematopoiesis (i.e., the spine, pelvis, and ribs).[50] As these skeletal regions have the greatest blood supply, the axial skeleton is the most likely site for metastatic disease. By contrast, it is uncommon for metastases to present distal to the elbow and knee.

Metastases frequently involve the pedicles of the vertebrae and are the major cause of the "missing" pedicle attributable to bone destruction (Fig. 16-3A). These patients frequently present with the clinical complaint of localized pain. Pathologic fractures may be visualized in up to 15 percent of cases.

In most cases, however, routine radiographs are insensitive for the detection of metastatic disease and will usually reveal only arthritic changes or may even be normal.[51] Those patients whose medical history and pain pattern suggest that the symptoms could be due to a systemic process and whose initial radiographs are not diagnostic should have a whole-body radionuclide bone scan to detect occult disease and to measure the extent of the disease (Fig. 16-3B).

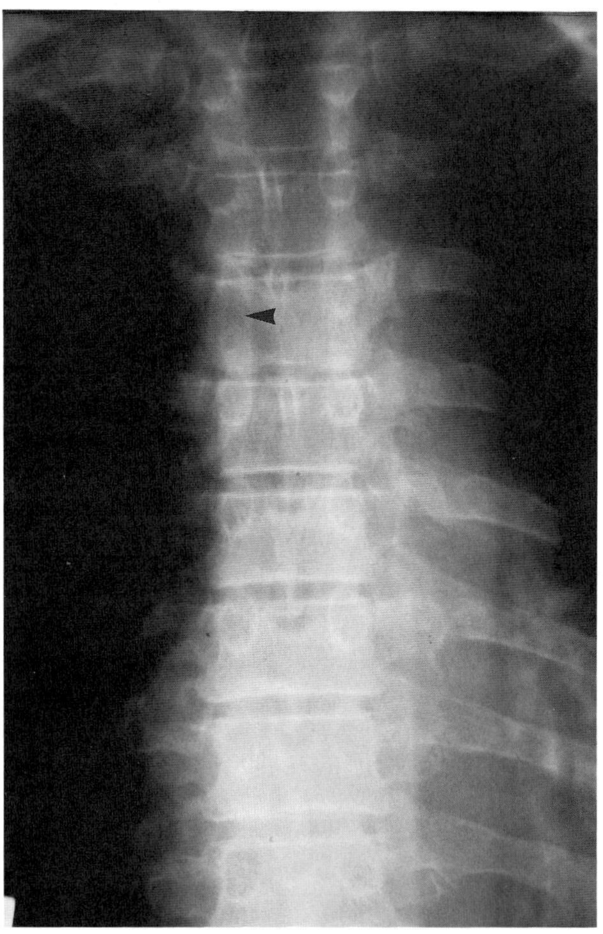

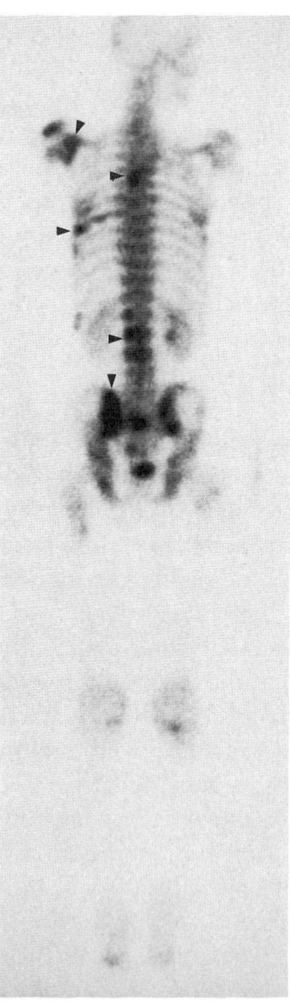

Fig. 16-3. This 42-year-old heavy smoker complained of mid-thoracic pain for 3 months. He was referred for physical therapy. Radiographs of the thoracic spine had not previously been obtained but were requested after the therapist's evaluation. **(A)** The AP film of the thoracic spine reveals absence of the right pedicle of the fourth thoracic vertebra (arrowhead). A chest radiograph (not shown) revealed a mass in the left lung that was subsequently proved to be bronchogenic carcinoma. The patient was referred to an oncologist who ordered a total-body bone scan. **(B)** The posterior image reveals multiple abnormal areas of increased uptake in the spine, ribs, left shoulder, and pelvis (arrowheads) representing metastases.

Detection of metastases on bone scans is frequently the first indication of the presence of an underlying primary tumor. Radionuclide skeletal imaging is the most effective means of detecting skeletal metastases, with a sensitivity of more than 95 percent for localizing skeletal metastases.[52] It is imperative to obtain an early diagnosis of metastatic disease in high-stress or weight-bearing areas. Early diagnosis permits timely intervention with internal stabilization and/or radiation therapy to prevent the development of pathologic fractures.[53] Mechanical back pain caused by disc and facet disease does not usually result in altered bone metabolism, and the radionuclide scans will be negative. A positive scan almost always indicates underlying bone pathology.

LUMBAR SPINE

The presentation of a patient with back pain is a daily occurrence in the physical therapist's practice. To diagnose the etiology of the pain in these patients is a greater clinical challenge[54] than to diagnose the etiology of pain in the peripheral joints, because the spine is much less accessible to direct clinical examination. Before assessing these patients, there must be a solid understanding of the common pathologies and abnormalities that present as low back pain. As a result of the difficulty in clinically determining the etiology of a patient's back pain, a variety of radiographic studies have become available to assist in the evaluation of these patients. These studies include conventional radiography, CT scanning, MR, myelography, and discography. The selection of the most appropriate imaging study is best determined after assessing the results from a thorough history and physical and neurologic examinations.

Trauma

CT, plain radiographs, and, rarely, myelography are currently used in the diagnosis of acute spinal trauma. Conventional radiographs are frequently adequate for the assessment of lumbar spine injuries.[55] After the initial radiographic assessment, if additional anatomic information is necessary, CT is more definitive[23] in assessing the extent of the fractures and the potential complications of bony fragments compromising the spinal canal.

MR has recently been added to the armamentarium available to assess the spine in the traumatized patient. After the patient is stable, MR can be used to assess the status of the spinal canal visualizing retropulsed fragments, acute disc herniations, and cord edema.

Acute Lumbar Pain

In evaluating the patient with acute nontraumatic lumbar or lumbosacral pain, there are significant medicolegal concerns about what, if any, imaging tests to order.[56] In most cases, radiographs are not needed unless symptoms fail to improve within 6 weeks after a trial of conservative therapy, particularly in patients under the age of 40. However inappropriate,[57] many clinicians and even many patients insist on obtaining lumbar spine radiographs at the initial evaluation for back pain. Daffner[58] reviewed Nachemson's study[59] and estimated that 7 million lumbar spine radiographic examinations are performed yearly, at a cost of $500 million (1986). Routine lumbar spine radiographs have a relatively low yield in the detection of significant disease in the patient with acute nontraumatic back pain[60] and represent a significant radiation dose to the gonads.

It has been common practice to obtain a radiograph in patients with acute back pain to exclude major pathology such as neoplasm, infection, trauma, or spondyloarthropathy. However, by obtaining a careful history, the therapist will usually identify the presence of chronic or progressive symptoms in patients with these pathologic conditions. This group of patients should actually be classified as having chronic, not acute, back pain.

Therefore, lumbar spine films should be obtained only rarely in the acutely symptomatic patient with no history of acute external trauma. Most of these patients have ligamentous or muscle strain caused by overuse or misuse, which will respond to conservative treatment.

When nontraumatic back pain does not respond to conservative measures, radiographic studies are appropriate. Routine radiographs of the lumbar spine consist of an AP film and a lateral film. Frequently the examination will also include a spot film centered at the L5–S1 junction, for greater anatomic detail at this level. This examination is frequently performed with the patient erect, to emphasize vertebral alignment in the weight-bearing position. Although not recommended because of the low diagnostic yield and greatly increased gonadal radiation exposure,[61] both oblique views of the lumbar spine are often considered part of the routine radiographic examination.

Routine radiographs, particularly if obtained with the patient erect, are excellent for the detection of alignment abnormalities. These include scoliosis, spondylolisthesis (forward slippage) (Fig. 16-4), and retrolisthesis (reverse slippage). Underlying conditions detectable on plain radiographs that can produce these alignment abnormalities include congenital vertebral anomalies, transitional lumbosacral vertebrae with unilateral sacralization, degenerative disc disease, and spondylolysis (a defect in the posterior supporting elements of the vertebrae). Routine radiographs are also useful in detecting the presence of compression or other types of fractures, of lytic or destructive lesions of the spine, and of osteoarthritis of the facet joints and in assessing the presence and extent of spondyloarthropathies such as ankylosing spondylitis.

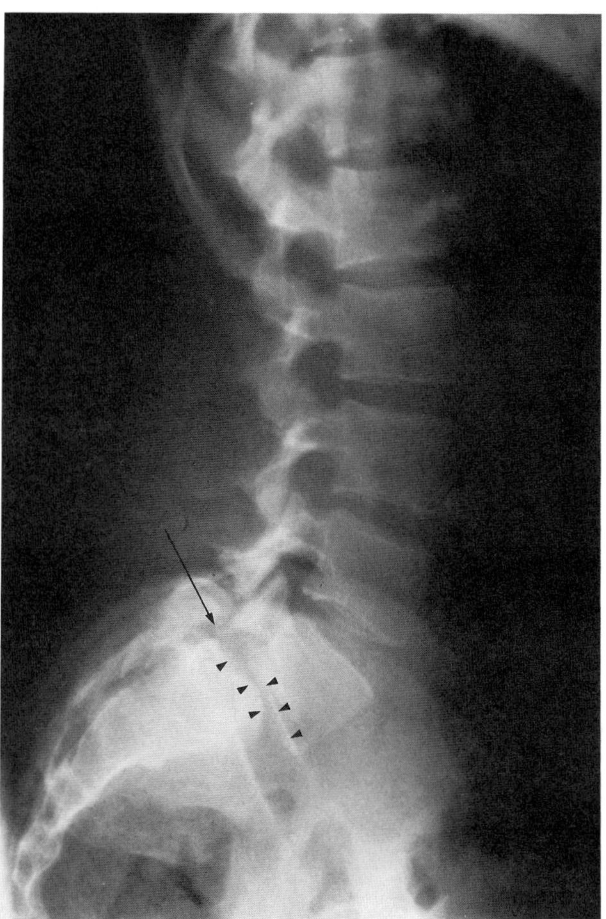

Fig. 16-4. This 25-year-old soccer player complained of chronic and increasing back pain made worse with running or prolonged standing. A standing lateral radiograph of the lumbar spine reveals a grade II spondylolisthesis of L5 on S1 (arrowheads) caused by a bilateral L5 spondylolysis (arrow).

Flexion and extension views may also be obtained to determine the presence of abnormal mobility of the vertebrae. The most common cause of abnormal movement of the vertebrae is a defect in the posterior bony neural arch (the pars interarticularis), termed *spondylolysis*. Although this defect may be visualized on AP or lateral radiographs, oblique projections are sometimes necessary to confirm its presence.

The second most common cause of instability is a combination of degenerative changes of the articulating facets[62] and narrowing of the intervertebral disc, known as *spondylosis*.[63] These abnormalities can produce not only abnormal movement of the vertebrae but may also result in abnormalities of alignment known as *spondylolisthesis* and *retrolisthesis*. Either with or without associated neurologic defects, lumbar spondylosis, spondylolisthesis, and retrolisthesis are significant causes of low back pain.

Chronic Pain, Neurologic Deficits, the HNP, and Spinal Stenosis

Before a discussion of appropriate secondary imaging techniques for the lumbar spine is presented, a brief review of common causes of protracted low back pain is integral to understanding the principles of imaging selection.[54,64]

In patients presenting with chronic low back pain, with or without radicular symptoms, muscle weakness, and sensory loss, the frequent clinical diagnosis is either disc herniation or spinal stenosis, or both. Disc herniation can occur either suddenly as the result of acute overload or gradually as the result of aging. With the normal aging process, there is a gradual loss of the water content of the nucleus pulposus and a concomitant gradual loss of height of the disc.[65] This process is accompanied by weakening and stretching of the outer fibers of the annulus fibrosis. This diffuse circumferential widening of the disc is termed a *bulging annulus fibrosis*. This is a normal process of aging and is usually not symptomatic. The weakened annulus may permit focal herniation of the central nucleus pulposus into the spinal canal (HNP).[65,66] If the herniated nuclear material is still contained within the annulus, the condition is termed *disc prolapse*. If there is a tear in the outer annular fibers permitting escape of nuclear material, it is termed *disc extrusion*. The herniated disc material may further extend through the posterior longitudinal ligament and migrate within the spinal canal.

Clinically, it is impossible to differentiate between a symptomatic diffusely bulging disc and a symptomatic focal herniation (HNP), whether attributable to prolapse or extrusion.[66] If a nerve root is not impinged, the patient will usually remain asymptomatic. Disc herniation occurs most commonly at the L4–L5 and L5–S1 levels, because these are the levels of maximum lumbar movement.

Spinal stenosis, also a frequent cause of back pain, is a general term that includes both congenital and acquired (degenerative) conditions that lead to narrowing of the spinal canal, the lateral recesses, and the neuroforamen.[67] This encroachment results in nerve root entrapment and compression. Patients present with low back pain or buttock pain, frequently exacerbated with standing or walking, and often relieved by lying down or sitting and bending forward.[68] The clinical diagnosis is not obvious, and adjacent disc disease may occur concurrently, further confusing the clinical assessment.

Acquired stenosis is more common than congenital stenosis. Acquired spinal stenosis is narrowing of the spinal canal as a consequence of bony or soft tissue changes. These include degenerative changes of the posterior articulating facets with secondary osteophyte formation, inward buckling of the ligamentum flavum, commonly and incorrectly referred to as "hypertrophy" of the ligamentum flavum, and impingement on the canal by the bulging annulus fibrosis of a degenerated disc.[69,70]

Congenital stenosis can occur in conditions such as achondroplasia, in which the spinal canal is narrowed as a result of anatomic abnormalities. Usually, however, there is no known underlying cause and no specific hereditary pattern, and it occurs equally in both sexes.

Routine radiographs are not useful for the detection of HNP and are of only very limited value for the detection and evaluation of spinal stenosis. They are useful only to exclude other causes of back pain, such as obvious tumor, spondylolisthesis, and deformities associated with compression fracture.

The screening study of choice for the evaluation of the patient with back pain and a suspected HNP or spinal stenosis remains the CT scan (Fig. 16-5). CT provides an anatomic visualization of the spine that cannot be achieved with conventional radiographs. Before the advent of CT, myelography was the diagnostic tool of choice for the assessment of lumbar disc disease. CT can evaluate the more common posterolateral and posterior disc herniations with accuracy equal to myelography.[71,72] In addition, CT is superior to myelography because of its ability to assess true lateral disc herniations (disc material protruding lateral to the neuroforamen), which are not visualized with myelography.[73] CT is valuable in detecting free disc fragments in the spinal canal, which can migrate from the level of origin and present symptoms referable to another level.[74] CT can also visualize stenosis involving the neuroforamen and lateral recesses. The accuracy of CT imaging for HNP is superior to myelography, and its assessment of the bony structures of the spine is superior to that which can be obtained with MR.

If there is discordance between the clinical symptoms and the CT findings, additional imaging with MR is indicated. An MR scan offers a slight increase in sensitivity for disc herniations and may serve to exclude other pathology, such as an epidural metastasis or a cauda

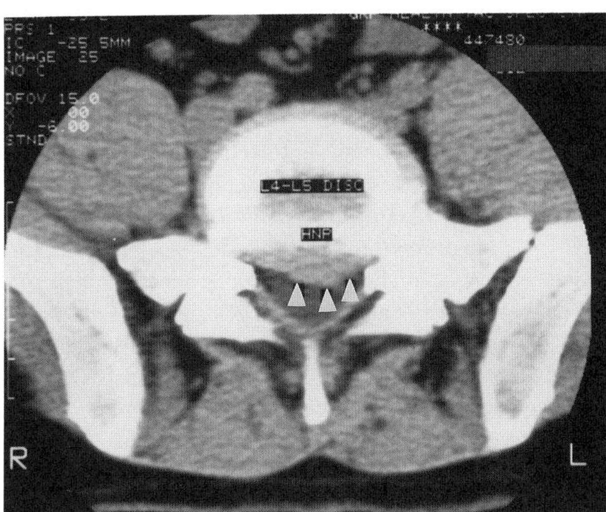

Fig. 16-5. This 28-year-old man was stacking heavy boxes when he experienced acute severe back pain radiating into his left leg. Neurologic examination suggested compression of the left L5 nerve root. A CT scan of the lumbar spine was requested. An axial CT image through the L4–L5 intervertebral disc level reveals a large posterior disc herniation (arrowheads) compressing the thecal sac and left L5 nerve root.

equina tumor. MR can clearly demonstrate the neural elements and any impingement on the thecal sac or nerve roots. Its sensitivity and noninvasiveness make it the preferred alternative to myelography.[75] With the availability of MR for spinal imaging, there are now few indications for performing myelography.

Discography, the injection of iodinated contrast material into an intervertebral disc under fluoroscopic guidance, was once highly regarded as a major tool in the assessment of the patient with back pain and suspected herniated disc. Today, the role of discography is controversial. Opinions range from it being a very useful tool to having no role whatsoever in the assessment of the symptomatic patient.[76]

Discography is an invasive technique that often requires a second or control level disc be evaluated at a nonsymptomatic level if a positive response is elicited at suspicious levels. MR imaging, however, also correctly identifies herniated discs, and the results between CT discography and MR are comparable. Discography has been described as an expensive, outmoded technique that contributes nothing of value.[77,78] The North American Spine Society Executive Committee[79] has issued a statement recommending that discography be reserved only for equivocal cases where the choice of therapeutic interventions is unclear, after other imaging modalities have been used. Therefore, MR is recommended as the screening test of choice for the evaluation of patients with back pain and/or radiculopathy.

The key to the best management of the patient with low back pain is the correlation of the history; physical and neurologic findings; the anatomic information available from radiographic, CT, and MR studies; and the metabolic information available from the bone scan. Even with the advent of MR, CT remains the most cost-effective method of correlating clinical symptoms and arriving at the diagnosis of HNP or spinal stenosis.

HIP AND PELVIS

Although often difficult to assess clinically as to the underlying etiology and site of pain, the hip and pelvis are regions that lend themselves well to evaluation with the multiple available imaging modalities. Particularly with the advent of MRI, evaluation of the hip can be relatively quickly and accurately completed.

The routine radiographic assessment of the pelvis consists of an AP film. This radiograph includes the iliac crests, the hips, and the proximal femurs to the level of the lesser trochanters, with the femurs in a neutral position. If the hips are of specific interest, a second AP radiograph of the pelvis with the hips flexed approximately 45 degrees and the femurs in abduction and external rotation ("frog leg lateral") is also obtained. Oblique views of the pelvis are necessary to assess the sacroiliac joints. A lateral radiograph of the pelvis is seldom obtained because overlapping skeletal structures obscure bony detail. Gonadal shielding should be used to minimize radiation exposure.

Plain radiographs are excellent for the detection of osteoarthritis, fractures,[80] and other mechanical or structural abnormalities. However, for the detection of common pathologic conditions including metastatic disease and Paget's disease, nuclear medicine imaging, with its superior sensitivity, is the preferred study. Skeletal scintigraphy can easily detect the early metabolic changes associated with metastatic disease or Paget's disease,[81] an inflammatory disease of bone probably caused by a slow viral infection,[82,83] well before the radiographs become positive.

Osteoarthritis

Plain radiographs are excellent for the detection of osteoarthritis. Changes in the hip occur in the stressed or weight-bearing superolateral surfaces of the hip joint. Osteoarthritis is characterized radiographically by asymmetric joint space narrowing, irregularities of the adjacent articular surfaces, subchondral and juxta-articular cysts or erosions, increased density of adjacent articular surfaces (sclerosis), and marginal osteophytes.[84]

Osteonecrosis

Osteonecrosis (formerly termed avascular necrosis, ischemic necrosis, or aseptic necrosis) is a complex syndrome of clinical, radiographic, and histopathologic findings. The etiology is thought to be due to repeated trauma resulting in disruption of the blood supply, leading to death of bone cells and subsequent fragmentation.

Osteonecrosis of the hip, also known as Legg-Calvé Perthes disease in children, is a not uncommon clinical problem involving the hip. In post-traumatic osteonecrosis of the hip, the initial event is usually the result of a femoral head dislocation or fracture. True idiopathic osteonecrosis of the femoral head occurs in children, usually under the age of 10, and in men between the ages of 30 and 50.

The early clinical symptoms are nonspecific, usually consisting of focal pain, often increased with motion or weight bearing. Although early clinical signs and symptoms of osteonecrosis of the femoral head are not specific, early diagnosis is important. Treatment during the initial stages of the disease with surgical intervention may prevent or minimize subsequent deformities.

The initial diagnostic study of choice is a radiograph to exclude an obvious infection, tumor, or fracture. However, initial radiographs are usually normal and may remain so for many weeks. A radionuclide bone scan may be positive and has previously been the second study of choice in the detection of the metabolic changes associated with early osteonecrosis. Currently, MR, with its high sensitivity for the detection of tissue changes and better spatial resolution, has superseded bone scanning as the method of choice for evaluating suspected osteonecrosis of the radiographically normal hip[85,86] (Fig. 16-6).

With MR, osteonecrosis appears as focal regions of low signal intensity in the marrow, indicating replacement of the marrow by edema, hemorrhage, and fibrous tissue.[87,88] The subchondral sclerosis, articular surface flattening, and collapse and bony fragmentation identified on conventional radiographs or CT scans are late changes that occur after the disease is well advanced and frequently beyond successful treatment.[89]

Trauma

Falls, particularly with a rotational component, are a frequent occurrence in the older population and represent a large percentage of inpatient physical therapy clients. In the outpatient population, the mechanism of the fall may be insufficient to produce a visible fracture or dislocation, but occult fractures of the femur or fractures of the acetabular rim are common. The patient presents with persistent hip pain or pain referred to the knee. The initial diagnostic evaluation is the plain radiograph. If the patient remains symptomatic, a bone scan may be performed to detect the increased metabolic activity associated with an occult fracture, or a CT scan may be performed to assess the bony anatomy.[90] CT delineates the precise extent of fractures, particularly acetabular fractures and complex fractures involving the articular surfaces. CT also detects associated joint abnormalities, such as osteochondral fractures and intra-articular loose bodies (Fig. 16-7). In patients with hip dislocations, MR may be used to detect marrow edema associated with acetabular or femoral head compression fractures.

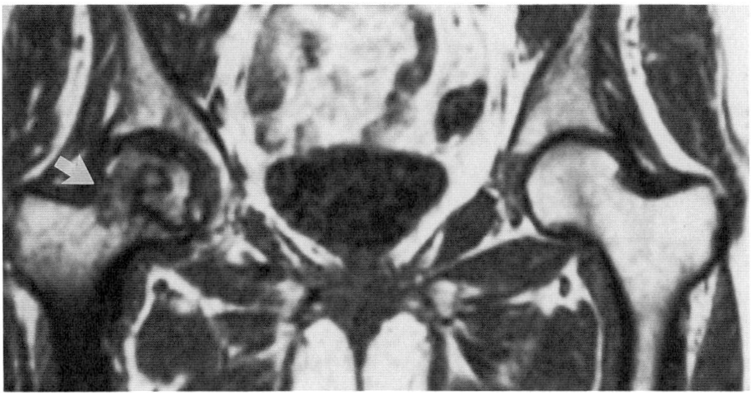

Fig. 16-6. This 65-year-old woman has been receiving high doses of steroids. She has been complaining of increasing right hip pain for the past 6 weeks. Routine radiographs of the hips were not conclusive, and an MR scan was ordered. A coronal T1-weighted image of the hips reveals a large zone of decreased signal intensity in the right femoral head (arrowhead), consistent with marrow edema secondary to osteonecrosis. (Courtesy of Leonard Sisk, MD.)

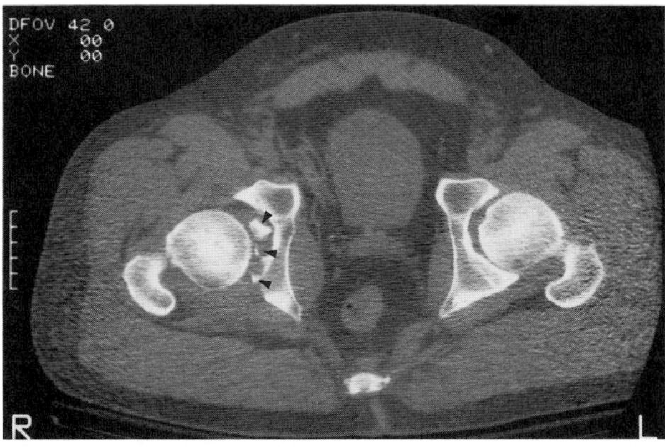

Fig. 16-7. This 30-year-old woman suffered a posterior dislocation of her right hip during a motor vehicle accident. After reduction, a CT scan was obtained revealing multiple intra-articular fragments (arrowheads). Surgery was necessary to remove the fragments before successful rehabilitation could be started.

Stress Fractures

Patients engaging in vigorous physical activities may present with pain in the groin, hip, buttock, or thigh, all symptoms suggesting the clinical diagnosis of stress fracture. Stress fractures of the pubic rami are common in runners, particularly women, who overstride when matched with a taller running partner. Stress fractures of the femoral neck are also common. It is particularly critical to diagnose these femoral neck stress fractures early, in order to prevent the potentially catastrophic complications of a completed fracture.

Routine radiographs are the initial study of choice and may permit the diagnosis of stress fracture. Because these are very subtle fractures, however, the initial radiographs are frequently normal. If the initial examination is negative or nondiagnostic and the patient's symptoms persist, nuclear medicine imaging should be the next diagnostic examination.[17,18,91] While MR may also visualize stress fractures before plain radiographs become positive,[5] nuclear medicine imaging, because of its sensitivity in detecting the early bony metabolic changes associated with overuse injuries, is still the second imaging modality of choice to detect early stress fractures in the hip and pelvis.

KNEE

The knee is one of the most frequently injured joints and often presents a diagnostic dilemma for the physical therapist. The knee is a vulnerable joint because it is exposed to both direct trauma and torsional stresses. Increasing participation in sports and fitness-related activities has resulted in greater numbers of knee injuries with both acute and chronic presentations that require evaluation. The clinical differentiation among bony, cartilaginous, and soft tissue injuries frequently cannot be specific. The application of correct rehabilitation strategies depends on accurate identification of the involved structures.

Current diagnostic imaging modalities for the knee include plain radiographs, bone scans, arthrography, CT, ultrasound, and MR. The routine radiographic study is the most appropriate initial study of the knee. It can determine displaced cortical fractures, foreign bodies, and intra-articular and tendinous calcifications.

The routine radiographic examination of the knee consists of AP, lateral, tangential patellar (sunrise), and open-joint projection (tunnel or notch) views. If the AP and lateral radiographs are performed with the patient in the erect weight-bearing position, valuable information is obtained regarding the degree of degenerative thinning of the articular cartilage, described as joint space narrowing. Additional oblique projections are occasionally useful in acute trauma for the clarification of possible fractures. Stress views are helpful to determine the presence of collateral ligament injuries. Occasionally, a repeat radiograph obtained after a delay of 10 to 14 days may be useful in demonstrating periosteal reaction and/or bone resorption at the margins of previously undetected fractures.

The next study of choice is an MR examination, which can demonstrate all of the surrounding and supporting soft tissues as well as subcortical (marrow) bone injuries not seen on conventional x-ray films. MR has a significant role in the diagnosis of acute injury when the physical examination is difficult due to pain and swelling.[92]

Diagnostic ultrasound is a rapid and less expensive means of evaluating the popliteal fossa for soft tissue masses and of evaluating the suprapatellar bursa. Radionuclide skeletal imaging is of value in detecting occult fractures, correlating clinical symptoms with radiographic changes in degenerative joint disease, identifying metastatic disease, and detecting the metabolic changes associated with osteonecrosis and osteochondritis dissecans. CT is useful for assessing the relationships of bony fragments in complex articular fractures. With sagittal and coronal reconstructions, CT is particularly useful for the pre-operative assessment of depressed tibial plateau fractures.

Meniscal and Ligamentous Injuries

Everyone, regardless of fitness level or lifestyle, is at risk of meniscal injuries. The diagnosis is usually suggested by the clinical examination. Arthrography and arthroscopy were formerly used for further evaluation in patients with confusing clinical symptoms or when spasm and guarding made the clinical examination difficult.

While arthrography (Fig. 16-8), CT-arthrography,[93] and arthroscopy have all achieved an accuracy of 90 percent or greater in the evaluation of meniscal and ligamentous injuries, all are invasive studies. MR is noninvasive and is able to produce high-quality images with high contrast and high resolution, without exposing the patient to ionizing radiation or surgery.[94,95] As a result, MR has virtually replaced conventional contrast arthrography in the assessment of the knee.

Tissue characterization with MR is superior to other imaging modalities. The ability of MR to image ligaments, marrow, subchondral bone, and cartilage makes it ideal for assessing the knee because so many of the abnormalities involve a soft tissue component. With MR, early soft tissue changes in patients with trauma, arthritis, and infection can be detected.[96,97]

The hallmark of meniscal abnormality on MR is increased signal intensity within the meniscus. This increased signal intensity in meniscal tears is due to synovial fluid leaking into the torn meniscus. Within the meniscus, any signal intensity that communicates with an articular surface indicates a torn meniscus. This finding corresponds with meniscal tears with both a sensitivity and a specificity of greater than 90 percent (Fig. 16-9).[98–100] Multiplanar MR imaging[101] has also demonstrated increasing usefulness in the evaluation of the articular cartilage, particularly when coupled with gadolinium contrast enhancement.[102,103]

MR is excellent in determining the presence, extent, and severity of injuries involving the collateral and cruciate ligaments of the knee.[104,105] Both the lateral collateral ligament and superficial fibers of the medial collateral ligament are extracapsular and therefore cannot be completely evaluated by either arthrography or arthroscopy.[106] In addition, the posterior cruciate ligament is not well seen on either arthroscopy or arthrography.

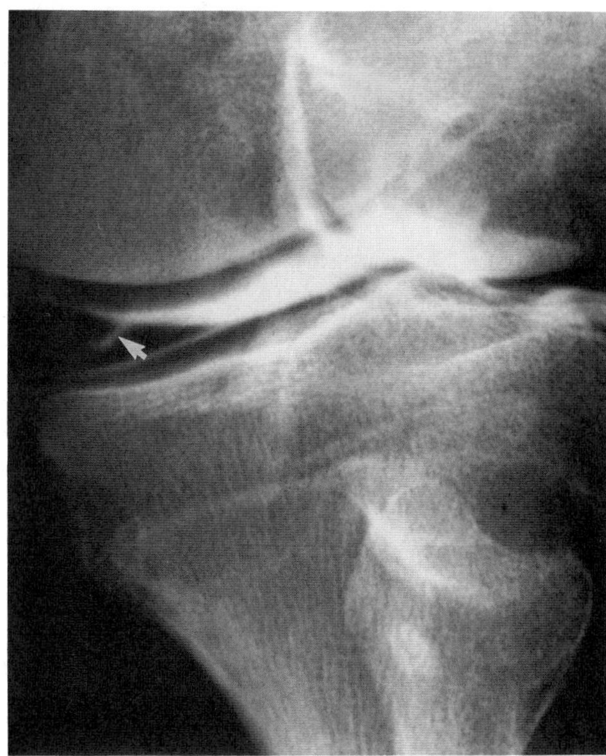

Fig. 16-8. This 24-year-old softball player "twisted his knee" sliding into second base. A conventional single-contrast arthrogram of the right knee reveals a tear of the superior surface of the medial meniscus (arrowhead).

The anterior cruciate ligament (ACL) is the most frequently injured ligament. It may be difficult to assess clinically when acutely swollen and painful. Furthermore, the clinical presentation of an ACL injury may often be confused with meniscal and other ligamentous injuries. MR has become the study of choice for the evaluation of the ACL and other ligaments. Multiplanar imaging can demonstrate not only the ligamentous injuries themselves but also meniscal, other ligamentous, and bony injuries that frequently accompany the primary injury.[107–110]

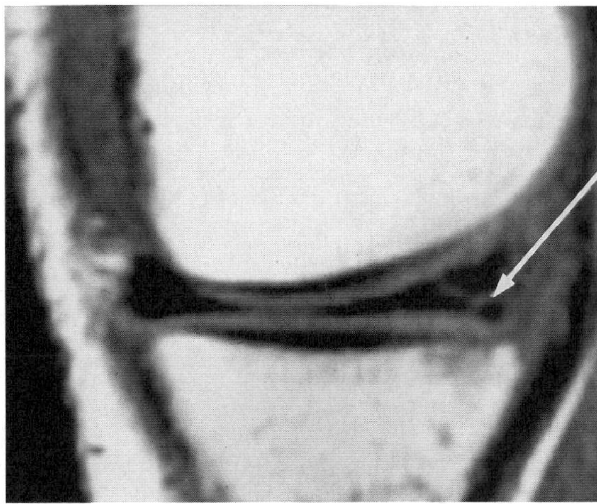

Fig. 16-9. This 30-year-old runner tripped and injured his right knee. A T2-weighted MR scan revealed a tear of the anterior horn of the medial meniscus demonstrated by a linear zone of increased signal intensity (arrow) extending to both the superior and inferior articular surfaces. (Courtesy of Leonard Sisk, MD.)

Physical examination is usually sufficient in patients with chronic injuries and instability. There has not been good correlation of clinical findings of instability with MR identification of medial and lateral collateral ligament tears.

Osteochondral Fractures, Osteochondritis Dissecans, and Osteonecrosis

Osteochondritis dissecans, commonly of the medial femoral condyle, but also occurring in the lateral femoral condyle, patella, tibial plateaus, and talar dome of the ankle, may occur as the result of an undiagnosed osteochondral fracture or may be related to an overuse or stress syndrome. These injuries are a not uncommon sequelae of severe "sprains." The initial radiographs are normal. In the symptomatic patient with normal radiographs, radionuclide imaging can be of benefit in differentiating skeletal from associated soft tissue injuries and can localize the abnormality to the affected condyle. Subsequent conventional or CT images or arthrography may be necessary to confirm the diagnosis, identify bony fragments, and confirm the extent of cartilaginous fragmentation.

MR has also proved especially useful in the detection of early osteonecrosis in the femoral condyle or tibial plateau and may be of value in the detection of early osteochondritis dissecans, bone infarcts, meniscal and Baker's cysts, and occult fractures.[111]

Osgood-Schlatter Lesion

The Osgood-Schlatter lesion occurs as a result of repeated avulsions of the hyaline columnar cartilage of the apophyseal ossification center of the tibial tubercle.[112] It occurs predominantly in boys between the ages of 11 and 15 years, when the tibial tubercle is in the apophyseal stage.[113] There is frequently a history of increasing physical activity but seldom a history of a specific traumatic event. The diagnosis is made clinically. These patients present with painful swelling over the tibial tubercle. The tibial apophysis normally undergoes ossification from multiple centers. Since it is normally asymmetric, radiographs of the affected knee or comparison with the opposite knee seldom add to the clinical evaluation.[114]

Baker's Cyst

First described by Dr. William Baker, a nineteenth century surgeon, these "cysts" are a common cause of pain and swelling in the popliteal fossa. These popliteal "cysts" are not true cysts, but represent a communication between the knee joint and the gastrocnemiosemimembranosus bursa. There is usually an intra-articular abnormality, often traumatic internal derangement or a synovial inflammatory condition, such as rheumatoid arthritis, which produces an effusion. Fluid from the knee joint enters the bursa through a one-way check-valve mechanism.

Rupture of a popliteal cyst or inflammation of or hemorrhage into the cyst can present with clinical symptoms that suggest deep venous thrombophlebitis. An enlarged cyst can also compress the popliteal vein, again producing the symptoms of thrombophlebitis.

Although arthrography and MR can identify Baker's cysts, a noninvasive diagnostic ultrasound examination is the study of choice to evaluate swellings in the popliteal region. Ultrasound can identify a Baker's cyst and differentiate among other causes of popliteal swelling such as a popliteal artery aneurysm, venous thrombosis, a soft tissue tumor, or abscess. If indicated, percutaneous aspiration of the cyst can also be performed using ultrasonic guidance.

Plicae

Plicae are abnormal folds of the synovial membrane that may produce symptoms of pain and palpable soft tissue thickening if they become trapped between adjacent articular surfaces. They usually present along the medial aspect of the knee and occasionally along the lateral aspect of the patellofemoral articulation.[115,116] MR imaging is able to visualize these plicae and differentiate among other entities that may present with similar symptoms such as chondromalacia patellae or ligamentous injuries.

In the imaging assessment of the knee, routine radiographs remain the initial study of choice. Radionuclide bone scanning is currently the supplemental study of choice for the detection of occult fractures; CT scanning is the study of choice for the anatomic assessment of identified fractures. Arthrography is useful for evaluating cartilaginous fragments in the joint; arthroscopy is the modality of choice for evaluating chondromalacia of the patella. Ultrasound is the imaging modality of choice for popliteal masses; MR is the imaging study of choice after the initial plain radiograph examination is completed. It is a noninvasive study with no morbidity that reveals the pathologic detail of meniscal and ligamentous injuries. Although MR is not the procedure of choice for evaluating fractures, either acute or occult, this may change as experience is gained with MR of trauma.[117–119]

FOOT AND ANKLE

Although anatomically distinct structures, each susceptible to specific injuries and pathologic conditions, the foot and ankle are grouped together for imaging purposes, because the same principles apply in their evaluation. The initial approach, as always, is a careful history and physical examination. After the initial examination, plain films remain the first imaging study of choice.[18] CT and MR have enhanced the ability to assess and diagnose ligamentous and bony injuries. CT allows accurate assessment of complex fractures and articular relationships, while MR imaging is useful in the evaluation of subcortical (marrow) bony, cartilaginous, and soft tissue injuries.[120]

Routine views of the ankle include AP, oblique, and lateral radiographs. Routine views of the foot also consist of three views: AP, oblique, and lateral. Routine radiographs are excellent for the detection of arthritis, calcaneal spurs, advanced stress fractures, and traumatic fractures and dislocations. They are occasionally useful for the detection of osteochondritis dissecans and tarsal coalitions. They are relatively insensitive for the detection of early stress fractures and for the more serious underlying pathology that would preclude treatment with physical therapy (e.g., osteomyelitis).

If the initial radiographic examination is abnormal, a CT examination may be necessary to define further the anatomic abnormality identified, such as a suspected tarsal coalition.[121] Normally, however, if the initial radiographic examination is not diagnostic and the patient remains symptomatic, a nuclear medicine bone scan is the next diagnostic imaging study of choice.[17,122]

Radionuclide skeletal imaging is superb in the early detection of occult or suspected fractures (Fig. 16-10A), early stress fractures, and early osteomyelitis.[123] A bone scan also aids in the differentiation of anatomic variants, such as accessory ossicles[124] from avulsion fractures when the initial radiographs are normal, or nondiagnostic, or raise additional questions. Fractures can be detected by bone scanning within 24 to 48 hours of the traumatic event.[125] These fractures will demonstrate abnormally increased uptake of the radiopharmaceutical, in contrast to the normal uptake that occurs with anatomic variants. If the bone scan is normal, treatment can proceed with confidence, with the knowledge that a significant bony lesion is not present.[126] If, however, the bone scan is abnormal, further imaging is necessary, with either repeat radiographs or a CT scan (Fig. 16-10B), for a specific anatomic diagnosis.

CT has been applied to a broad range of diagnostic problems of the foot and ankle, including trauma, overuse injuries, tarsal coalitions, arthritis, and osteomyelitis. CT provides cross-sectional imaging of the foot and ankle to diagnose calcaneal fractures, subtalar coalitions, tarsal-metatarsal fractures, and dislocations and even primary soft tissue pathology and impingement syndromes.

New techniques have given MR an enhanced role in the assessment and diagnosis of musculoskeletal conditions in the foot and ankle. MR of the foot and ankle is best performed with a dedicated extremity coil that permits high resolution. It is useful for diagnosing the myriad of foot and ankle symptom complexes producing pain and instability due to ligamentous and other soft tissue pathology.[127]

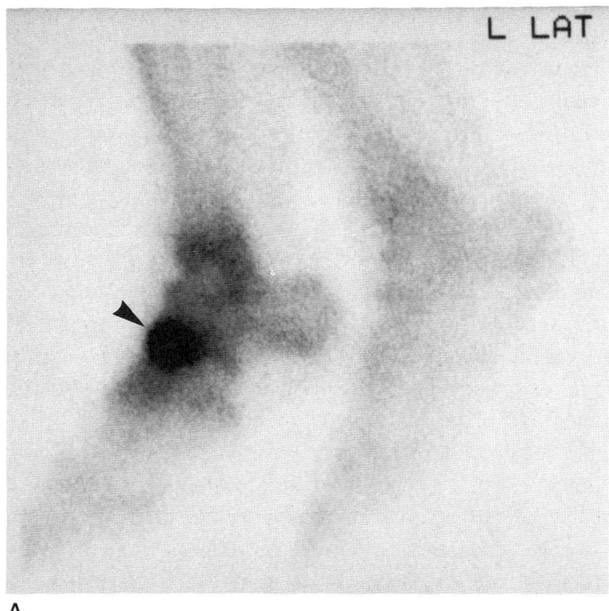

A

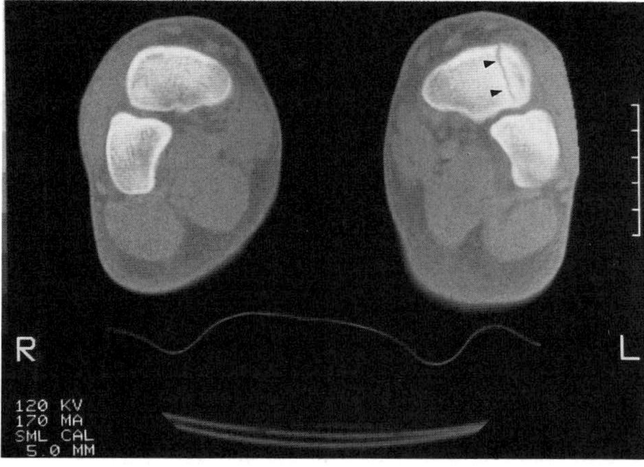

B

Fig. 16-10. This 19-year-old basketball player complained of persistent left foot pain since suffering a severe "sprain" during the final game of the season. Three sets of routine foot radiographs were normal. His symptoms did not improve with physical therapy. **(A)** A radionuclide bone scan requested after the third negative radiographic examination demonstrated intense abnormal uptake in the left tarsal navicular bone (arrowhead). **(B)** A CT scan was then obtained, revealing a fracture of the navicular (arrowheads), which subsequently progressed to nonunion and required internal fixation to achieve healing.

Stress Fractures

Stress fractures, usually occurring with unaccustomed or accelerated physical activity, develop gradually over a period of days to weeks. Persistent physical activity results in continuing bone resorption,[128] which in turn can led to a completed fracture and unnecessarily prolonged healing. The diagnosis of stress fractures is usually made clinically on the basis of the history and physical examination of a patient who is involved in increasing physical activity. Included in the differential diagnosis is tendinitis, arthritis, and other musculoskeletal disorders. The radiographic detectibility of a stress fracture at initial presentation is well below 50 percent.[129]

Skeletal scintigraphy has the ability to identify stress fractures weeks before the appearance of radiographic changes[130] and has a sensitivity approaching 100 percent.[131] The early detection of stress fractures permits prompt treatment, preventing progression of the fractures and the associated complications.[132,133] This is especially true with stress fractures of the midfoot,[134,135] which are particularly difficult to diagnose radiographically because of the complex and overlapping anatomy. Because isotopic scanning is so sensitive, multiple stress fractures will often be identified, even though only one site is symptomatic.

Osteonecrosis

When it occurs in the foot, osteonecrosis[136] usually involves the navicular bone and is referred to as Kohler's disease,[137] or the distal ends of the second and third metatarsals, known as Freiberg's infractions.[138] The initial clinical symptoms are nonspecific, usually consisting of focal pain that increases with motion or weight bearing. Early diagnosis and appropriate treatment are important to minimizing subsequent deformities. The initial radiographs are usually normal and remain so for up to 8 weeks. The radionuclide scan will usually be positive and will permit the correct diagnosis. Delayed radiographs may demonstrate increased sclerosis, fragmentation, or flattening of the involved articular surfaces.

MR is excellent for the diagnosis of osteomyelitis. Although radionuclide scintigraphy remains the most commonly used imaging modality for detection because of its wide availability and documented sensitivity, MR is equally sensitive and even more specific for the diagnosis of osteomyelitis.[139]

Tarsal Coalition

Tarsal coalitions are frequent congenital abnormalities of the feet in which various bony, cartilaginous or fibrous unions between the tarsal bones may occur.[123] They are an important cause of foot and calf pain and of peroneal spastic flatfoot. The most common tarsal coalition is the calcaneonavicular, with the talocalcaneal or subtalar coalitions the second most common. Clinical symptoms often present after strenuous physical activity and are frequently thought to be due to stress fractures.[140] The first imaging study, after the clinical evaluation, should be the routine radiograph. While routine radiographs may reveal a bony calcaneonavicular coalition, they will often fail to visualize fibrous or cartilaginous unions. If these initial films are not diagnostic, radionuclide bone scanning will demonstrate focally increased uptake in the region of the coalition,[140] even if the coalition is fibrous or cartilaginous. With the abnormal radionuclide skeletal images as a guide, precise anatomic imaging with CT can complete the assessment of the painful foot condition. It is important to note that because of the complexity of the anatomic relationships, the imaging assessment of the foot and ankle commonly includes more than a single diagnostic modality.

Soft Tissue Abnormalities

MR has demonstrated a clear superiority in imaging tendinous abnormalities. Tendinitis in the foot most commonly involves the flexor tendons.[141] Tenosynovitis is detected by fluid in the tendon sheath on MR. Complete ruptures of the Achilles tendon are usually diagnosed with physical examination. MR is useful in the assessment of other Achilles tendon injuries and can differentiate between partial tears (Fig. 16-11) and inflammation of the Achilles tendon. It is particularly useful in differentiating tears of the Achilles tendon

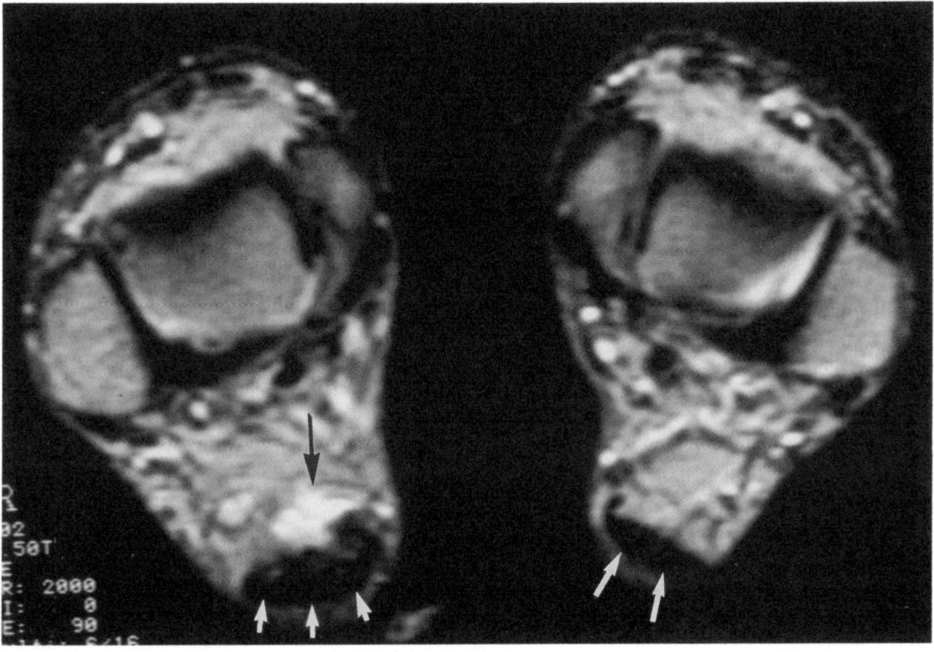

Fig. 16-11. This 53-year-old former Olympic competitor injured his right ankle while running barefoot on the beach without prior warm up or stretching. Clinical examination suggested an Achilles tendon injury. An MR image was requested for confirmation and surgical planning. A selected axial T2-weighted MR image at the level of the ankle joint revealed diffuse thickening of the right Achilles tendon (arrowheads). The adjacent high-signal edema (arrow) extending into the tendon revealed the disruption of the normally smooth contour of the tendon, indicating a partial tear. The left Achilles tendon (short arrows) is normal. Surgical debridement and repair was recommended, but he instead elected nonoperative treatment with physical therapy. Recovery was complete, and he has resumed competitive running.

from tears of the posterior tibial tendon. MR may also be useful in defining the extent of separation of the tendon ends in an Achilles rupture prior to deciding whether surgery or casting would be appropriate.[142]

Tarsal tunnel syndrome is an entrapment neuropathy, usually caused by a soft tissue mass (lipoma, ganglion cyst, nerve sheath neoplasm, fibrosis secondary to adjacent trauma) in the region of the tarsal tunnel resulting in compression of the posterior tibial nerve. Patients present with burning plantar foot pain. The diagnosis is usually readily apparent with MR imaging.[143]

MR is useful in the diagnosis of the sinus tarsi syndrome, which is due to instability of the subtalar joint of the hindfoot resulting from tears of the ligaments uniting the talus and calcaneus.[144] MR has also been used to study Morton's neuromas, the result of fibrosis and enlargement of the nerve sheaths of the interdigital nerves.

Physical examination remains the evaluation tool of choice in detecting the laxity of ankle ligaments and is usually straightforward. MR can clarify equivocal cases.[145] The diagnosis of plantar fascitis is also normally made by clinical examination. Therefore MR, though useful, is not normally needed in the diagnostic process.[146]

SHOULDER

Shoulder pain and dysfunction are frequently encountered problems in the daily practice of the physical therapist. The mobility of this joint is critical to daily function; thus, dysfunction may be particularly disabling. Patients typically present with an inability to meet their work-required performance standards or to perform their daily activities.

The shoulder joint poses a unique challenge for imaging. This complex, highly mobile joint consists of the glenohumeral, acromioclavicular, scapulothoracic, and sternoclavicular joints. Radiographic evaluation with plain radiographs is an important initial diagnostic step after the clinical history and physical examination. Routine radiographs consist of two AP images with the humerus in external and internal rotation. Additional tangential, transthoracic, oblique, and axillary views are often performed after traumatic injuries. These plain radiographs are excellent for fractures and dislocations, are usually adequate for degenerative changes, and may demonstrate calcific deposits. Owing to the complex anatomy, plain radiographs are not generally sensitive or specific for other shoulder pathology. They are only occasionally diagnostic in the chronic impingement syndrome. Plain radiographs not adequate for the common clinical problems of rotator cuff tears, injuries to the glenoid labrum, and other complications of trauma, biceps tendinitis, and rupture or intra-articular deposits.

Rotator Cuff Disease and the Shoulder Impingement Syndrome

Abnormalities of the rotator cuff are common, ranging from tendinitis to partial and complete tears. There are multiple etiologies[147] for rotator cuff pathology: age-related degeneration, failure from overuse, irritation from the chronic trauma of bony impingement, and acute trauma. It has been suggested that up to 95 percent of all rotator cuff lesions result from chronic impingement of the supraspinatus tendon against the undersurface of the coracoacromial arch.[148] This area of injury is called the critical zone, a poorly vascularized portion of the rotator cuff through which tears occur. Neer[148] classified the rotator cuff impingement injuries into three progressive stages. The initial stage, resulting from overuse, consists of reversible edema and hemorrhage of the supraspinatus tendon. Untreated, this progresses to the second stage of progressive inflammation leading to chronic fibrosis, finally progressing to the third stage of complete disruption. Early diagnosis and treatment are critical to prevent further progression of symptoms and improvement of function.

Clinically, the shoulder impingement syndrome consists of pain at the lateral margin of the shoulder. It is also referred to as rotator cuff tendinitis, subacromial bursitis, and supraspinatus tendinitis. The history and physical examination are frequently inadequate to pinpoint the cause of shoulder joint pain.[147,148]

Plain radiographs,[149] arthrography,[150] and occasionally MR[151] can be used to grade the acromial shape and can demonstrate a low-lying anterior acromion process that narrows the space between the anterior acromion and the humeral head. Early correct diagnosis is necessary because identification of the precise etiology leads to appropriate conservative treatment or surgical intervention. The plain radiographic findings of narrowing of the acromiohumeral distance occur late in the course of the disease. Therefore, because of the relative insensitivity of plain radiographs, additional imaging is frequently performed early in the evaluation of the painful shoulder.

Formerly, positive contrast arthrography was the study of choice for the detection of complete and partial rotator cuff tears. The anatomy and mobility of the shoulder made MR examination difficult. The early lack of appropriate surface coils coupled with poor signal-to-noise ratios led to suboptimal images. However, advances in MR imaging hardware, including specialized surface coils, and software during the past several years have given MR imaging diagnostic capabilities that have surpassed those of arthrography. Therefore, MR imaging has now replaced contrast arthrography as the imaging study of choice after the plain-film examination.

Tears of the supraspinatus tendon are directly visualized as a "gap" or discontinuity of the tendon, often with retraction of the supraspinatus muscle (Fig. 16-12A).[152,153] Other findings include fluid in the subacromial-subdeltoid bursa.

MR can also reveal the conditions of the ends of the tendon in a complete tear and the degree of associated muscle atrophy. Cystic erosions of the humeral head and acromion, a frequent component of rotator cuff disease, are also well visualized with MR imaging (Fig. 16-12B).

MR is helpful in assessing the postoperative shoulder with recurrent symptoms. MR can reveal recurrent tears and can reassess the undersurface of the acromion following acromioplasty.

Ultrasound imaging of the supraspinatus tendon has met with some success.[154] Although noninvasive, it requires a very high degree of skill from both the sonographer and the sonologist that is not widely available. Until this technique is more readily available, it cannot be recommended as a routine imaging modality.

Trauma

Although the glenohumeral joint is one of the most mobile, it is also one of the most unstable joints. After the initial evaluation and reduction of an apparently uncomplicated shoulder dislocation, it is common that patients will remain symptomatic or will suffer recurrent dislocations. Plain radiographic evaluation may reveal normal bony structures but is inadequate to evaluate the glenoid labrum. Double-contrast CT arthrotomography (Fig. 16-13) is currently the study of choice for evaluating glenohumeral instability because of its ability to visualize the glenoid labrum and image capsular abnormalities.[155–158] However, advances in MR imaging have also demonstrated an improved ability to visualize labral injuries with an accuracy that is approaching CT arthrotomography.

Calcific Tendinitis

In calcific tendonitis, calcific deposits form within the substance of the tendon and may remain clinically silent or be associated with chronic low-grade symptoms. These calcific deposits are usually detected with routine radiographs.

THE ELBOW

The elbow is a complex hinged joint that allows for multiple planes of movement. It is commonly injured, frequently involved with overuse injuries, and is a frequent source of chronic impairment.

The usefulness of MR in the evaluation of the elbow has been demonstrated for several years, but is only now gaining wider acceptance in the medical community.[159,160] MR permits imaging of the osseous structures, especially the bone marrow, articular cartilage, and the soft tissues of the elbow. The ligaments, muscles, tendons, and neurovascular structures are all well visualized. MR also offers multiplanar imaging capabilities that exceed those of CT and plain-film tomography.

Previously it was difficult to image the elbow with MR because, with the patient's arm at the side, the elbow was not in the center of the magnetic field where the image resolution is greatest. The alternative position, with the arm outstretched overhead, was often difficult to accomplish with a painful elbow. However, the introduction of surface coils with small fields of view now allow a patient to lie with the arm at the side. Improvements in computer software allow off-center imaging in the magnetic field and produce thin section images with high resolution.

Trauma

As in the other extremity joints, routine radiographs are the initial imaging study. The initial examination consists of an AP film with the elbow in extension and a lateral film with the elbow flexed to 90 degrees. Additional oblique views are often obtained in trauma cases to bet-

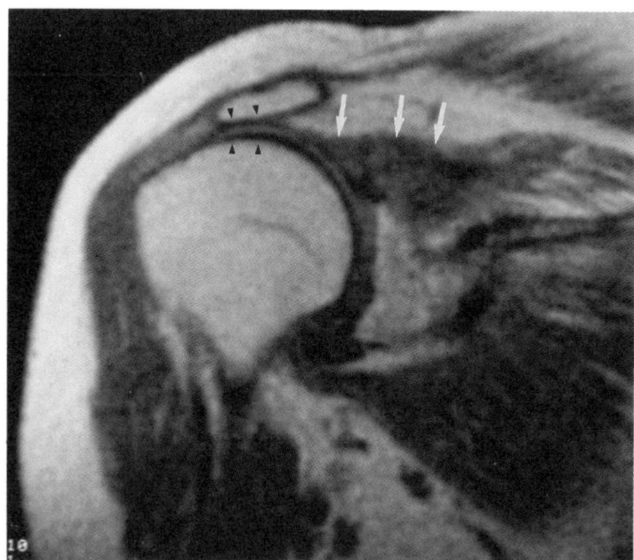

A

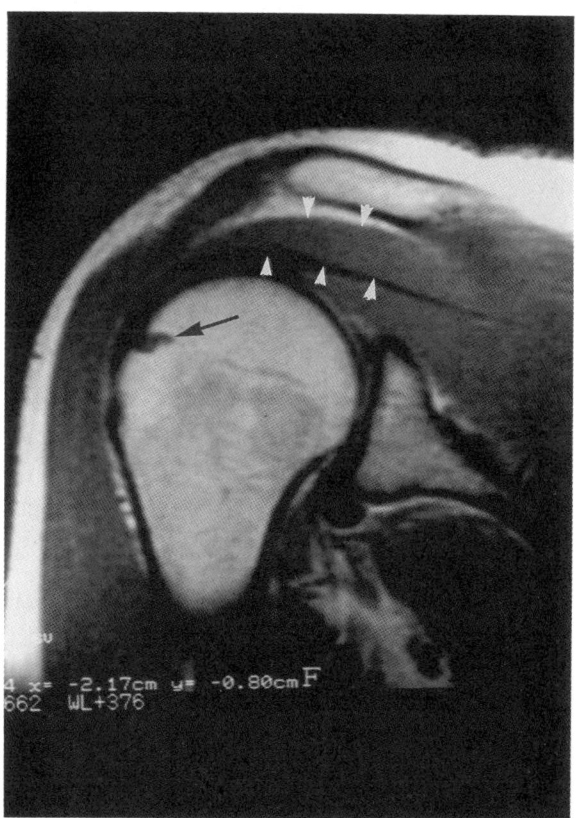

B

Fig. 16-12. (A) This 82-year-old woman experienced onset of right shoulder pain while lifting a heavy flower pot onto a fence post. She did not seek treatment at the time, hoping that the pain would resolve. Over the next 6 months, increasing right shoulder pain and progressive inability to do keyboarding or to lift her coffee cup led her to seek treatment. Clinical examination suggested a rotator cuff tear. An MR examination was requested prior to planned surgery. A coronal T1-weighted image revealed a complete disruption of the supraspinatus muscle (arrows) and obliteration of the normal acromial-humeral space (arrowheads) (cf Fig. 16-12B.) She decided that the recommended surgery and subsequent rehabilitation were not worth the risks and time at her age and chose treatment with physical therapy instead. **(B)** While trying to keep up with his 22-year-old son in weight lifting, this 47-year-old man experienced sudden right shoulder pain that was unresponsive to conservative measures and anti-inflammatory medications. A coronal T1-weighted image revealed an intact supraspinatus muscle and tendon (arrowheads). However, a cystic erosion in the head of the humerus was seen (arrow), and other images (not shown) demonstrated additional cystic erosions, possibly associated with microavulsions at the tendinous insertions. He is responding to physical therapy.

ter visualize the articular surfaces, especially the radial head. These routine views are excellent for the detection of most fractures and dislocations and may also identify intra-articular loose bodies. Frequently, and especially with radial head fractures, the initial examination may reveal only a joint effusion and will not reveal the fracture. Follow-up films in 10 to 14 days may then reveal the fracture.

Further evaluation of the elbow has most commonly been performed with arthrography using either air or iodinated contrast, often in conjunction with conventional tomography or CT imaging. These studies, with a relatively limited degree of invasion, are very useful for the detection of articular abnormalities such as osteochondral fractures or osteochondritis dissecans, or for the localization of intra-articular loose bodies.

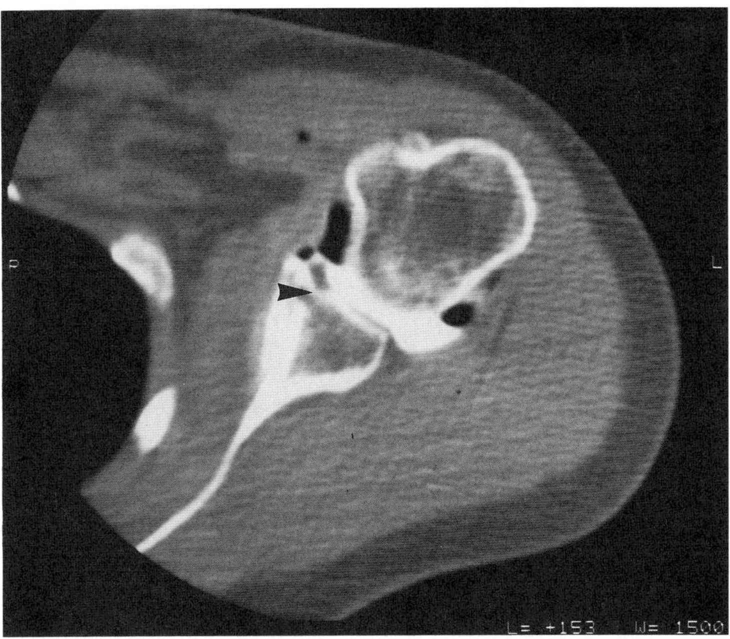

Fig. 16-13. This 32-year-old softball player suffered an anterior dislocation of her left shoulder in a collision with an opposing player. Successful reduction was accomplished, and postreduction radiographs revealed no fractures. She was referred to physical therapy for evaluation and treatment of persistent shoulder pain. When her symptoms did not improve, the consulting orthopaedist requested further evaluation with a CT-arthrotomogram. Axial CT imaging revealed a depressed fracture of the anteroinferior glenoid rim (Bankart fracture) and disruption of the anterior margin of the labrum (arrowhead). After arthroscopic surgery, rehabilitation was successful.

MR imaging has been frequently used in the evaluation of the athletic injury, where early diagnosis permits earlier surgical intervention and a more rapid recovery. MR is valuable in the diagnosis of tendon injuries and ligamentous injuries, especially the ulnar collateral ligament, allowing the differentiation from other injuries that produce similar symptoms.[161] It can differentiate between a complete or partial tear or tenosynovitis and can aid in treatment planning decisions regarding surgical interventions or nonoperative management.

Myositis ossificans is a frequent sequelae of elbow trauma seen by therapists. Skilled clinical evaluation of the recovering injury is required for early detection. Bone scanning as early as 3 weeks post-trauma reveals increased metabolic activity in the soft tissues well before radiographs indicate the presence of bony bridging. Bone scanning can also determine the maturation of the process as an aid to planning prior to excision.

Nontrauma

Lateral epicondylitis (tennis elbow) is a clinical syndrome associated with inflammation of the extensor carpi radialis brevis tendon. Patients often present with no history of acute trauma. Clinically, the diagnosis is usually made by careful physical examination. MR imaging may be useful in patients who do not respond to conservative therapy or when surgery is being considered so that the extent of inflammation and any tendon abnormalities may be documented.[162]

Synovial and bursal abnormalities are much better visualized with MR than with other imaging modalities. Effusions, synovial hyperplasia, and intra-articular loose bodies may be easily detected with MR.

WRIST AND HAND

The hand and wrist are discussed together in this chapter as they form a complex anatomic unit, interrelated by function and subjected to many common traumatic and pathologic disorders.

Trauma

Although advances in diagnostic imaging have led to more complex methods of evaluating hand and wrist conditions, most abnormalities are still visualized on conventional plain films. Therefore, after obtaining an appropriate clinical history and performing a physical examination, the plain-film examination remains the initial radiographic study of choice.[163]

The standard radiographic examination of the wrist consists of at least two views, a posteroanterior (PA) and a true (90-degree) lateral. Additional films are frequently obtained and may include oblique views, an ulnar-deviated PA film for scaphoid assessment, clenched fist views for ligamentous stability, and a carpal tunnel view to visualize the hook of the hamate.[164–166] The scaphoid view is particularly important as more than 40% of all wrist fractures may involve the scaphoid bone.

The standard radiographic examination of the hand includes at least three views, a PA, a PA oblique, and a lateral view. Additional views of the hand are not normally necessary unless to clarify a specific anatomic question.

If the initial radiographic examination of either the hand or the wrist is not definitive, follow-up films in 10 to 14 days may reveal a fracture that was initially radiographically occult. Follow-up films are of particular importance in suspected scaphoid fractures because the consequences of a missed fracture, such as osteonecrosis or nonunion, may have significant, long-term, adverse effects.[167] Radionuclide scintigraphy is also frequently used to evaluate for radiographically occult but clinically suspected fractures. A negative bone scan virtually excludes the possibility of an occult fracture.[168,169]

CT, although not part of the initial diagnostic evaluation, is a mainstay in the assessment of complex wrist fractures.[170] True, direct multiplanar imaging (axial, sagittal, coronal) of the wrist is possible. The advantage of direct multiplanar imaging (as opposed to computerized reconstructions) is that high resolution imaging of complex articular relationships and multiple fracture planes is possible. Another indication for CT of the wrist is the confirmation of suspected fractures when the plain radiographs are negative and the bone scan is positive. Finally, CT is helpful in assessing fracture healing and the postoperative wrist.

MR imaging of the wrist is not frequently used in the assessment of acute trauma of the wrist, although it does have a role in the assessment of post-traumatic sequelae such as osteonecrosis of the scaphoid.

Nontrauma

Conventional films remain the first imaging modality of choice in the assessment of nontraumatic conditions of the hand and wrist. They are readily available, relatively inexpensive, and can satisfactorily demonstrate many of the nontraumatic conditions affecting the hand and wrist. CT is not frequently used, although it may help to clarify the skeletal abnormality indicated by a positive bone scan when the plain radiographs are not diagnostic. Arthrography of the wrist is frequently used to diagnose ligamentous tears and perforations, as well as degeneration of the triangular fibrocartilage, all of which can lead to instability of the wrist, chronic pain, and dysfunction.[171–174]

MR imaging is now assuming a significant role in the assessment of soft tissue pathology of the hand and wrist.[175] In contrast to wrist arthrography, which often requires injection into three separate compartments, MR is a noninvasive study that allows for simultaneous visualization of osseous abnormalities and direct visualization of ligaments and tendons, as well as articular cartilage and the synovium.

Ligamentous Abnormalities

Many of the intrinsic and extrinsic ligaments of the wrist are visualized with MR imaging. Tears of the triangular fibrocartilage are detected with a high degree of accuracy, as are those of the scapholunate and lunotriquetral ligaments.[176,177] Identification of tears in these particular structures is important because they result in functional disability and are amenable to surgical repair.[178] With an accuracy as good as or better than arthrography, MR is becoming the preferred study for the identification of ligamentous abnormalities.[179]

Carpal Tunnel Syndrome

Carpal tunnel syndrome is a common neuropathic condition caused by compression of the median nerve in the carpal canal.[180] The diagnosis of carpal tunnel syndrome relies on a multifaceted approach, including clinical examination with findings of impairment, EMG results, and imaging assessment. MR is useful in the assessment of the carpal tunnel syndrome, particularly in patients with positive clinical findings and negative EMG studies. MR may demonstrate fluid in the tendon sheaths (tenosynovitis) secondary to overuse or arthritis, infiltration and thickening of the tendon in patients with rheumatoid arthritis, complete tears of the flexor tendons, benign tumors such as a ganglion cyst or neuroma, or bony changes secondary to an injury to the hook of the hamate.[180]

Osteonecrosis

The most common location of osteonecrosis in the wrist is the proximal scaphoid following a fracture.[181] The next most common site is the lunate bone, occurring spontaneously and known as Kienbock's disease (Fig. 16-14). These are difficult diagnoses to make clinically, and usually the plain radiographs are normal, especially early in the course of the disease before bony collapse and fragmentation has occurred. Bone scintigraphy is sensitive for the detection of the metabolic changes associated with avascular necrosis. However, MR has demonstrated equal or greater sensitivity and greater specificity for the detection of osteonecrosis[182,183] and is the preferred imaging modality.

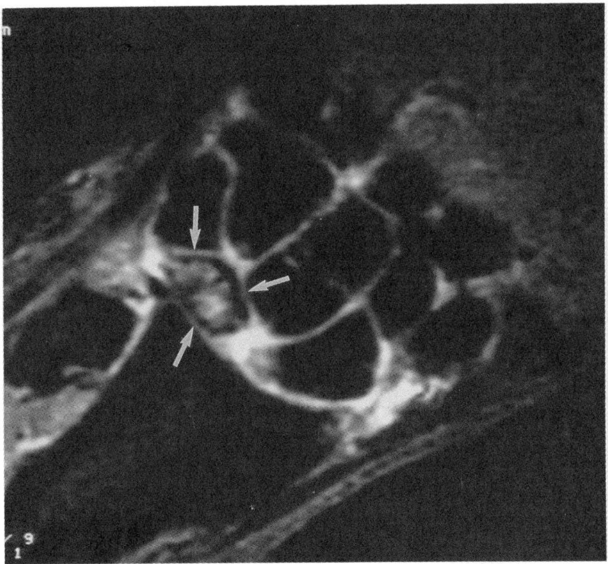

Fig. 16-14. Following a hyperextension injury of his left wrist, this 51-year-old man experienced increasing pain and disability over a 6-month period. Routine radiographs were normal. A radionuclide bone scan (not shown) revealed increased uptake in the lunate. A STIR coronal MR image of the left wrist revealed increased signal intensity (arrows) indicating edema associated with osteonecrosis. He has been offered an ulnar lengthening surgical procedure.

Arthritis

The role of MR imaging in the assessment of rheumatoid diseases is still being refined.[184] In patients with rheumatoid arthritis, studies have demonstrated a greater sensitivity of MR to detect early erosions[185,186] and cystic changes.[187] Other studies report that MR can detect synovial inflammation following the intravenous administration of paramagnetic contrast agents such as gadolinium.[188] The greatest potential of MR may be to assess objectively the response to therapy in patients with rheumatoid arthritis.[184]

Reflex Sympathetic Dystrophy

Radionuclide skeletal imaging may contribute significantly to the evaluation of patients with symptoms suggestive of reflex sympathetic dystrophy syndrome. The clinical presentation consists of poorly localized pain and tenderness, diffuse swelling, and dystrophic skin changes. The etiologic factors are diverse and poorly understood, but are thought to induce a complex of neurologic reflexes associated with vasomotor instability.[189]

Three-phase scintigraphy reveals increased blood flow in the initial and second phases (arterial and capillary perfusion), and the third phase demonstrates increased skeletal labeling, particularly in the periarticular regions of the affected extremity.[190] Radionuclide skeletal imaging, with its high sensitivity and specificity, not only aids in the diagnosis of reflex sympathetic dystrophy but is beneficial in predicting which patients are most likely to respond to systemic steroid therapy.[190–192] Follow-up scans after successful therapy will demonstrate a return to a normal pattern.

CONCLUSION

This chapter emphasizes an approach to diagnostic imaging for the physical therapist. Rather than analyze all possible traumatic, degenerative, or pathologic conditions of the musculoskeletal system, this chapter emphasizes an approach to the diagnosis and evaluation of the more common conditions encountered in daily practice.

Information is provided to help physical therapy clinicians make appropriate decisions about diagnostic imaging studies. While the typical practice model does not rely on the therapist to make the primary request for imaging studies, the therapist should review the patient's imaging studies and the reports that accompany them. Furthermore, the therapist is in an excellent position to collaborate with the referral source to select studies that aid in the accurate assessment of the patients' problems.

It cannot be stated strongly enough that before any imaging studies are considered, the emphasis must be on a complete history, physical assessment, and neurologic examination. Therapists must be constantly alert to patterns of findings that suggest problems not amenable to physical therapy treatment and make appropriate referrals. There is no need for "fishing expeditions" in diagnostic imaging. The physical therapist has a responsibility to collaborate with the imaging specialist before obtaining imaging studies. It is the radiologist's role to recommend the imaging modality that will answer the clinical question with the greatest degree of sensitivity and specificity. Greater communication of information among health care providers will ultimately lead to more accurate diagnoses, better patient care, and more focused therapy.

REFERENCES

1. Galasko CSB: Mechanisms of lytic and blastic metastatic disease of bone. Clin Orthop 169:20, 1982
2. Burk DL Jr, Dalinka MK, Scheibler ML et al: Strategies for musculoskeletal magnetic resonance imaging. Radiol Clin North Am 26:653, 1988
3. Stoller DW: Musculoskeletal applications of magnetic resonance imaging. Appl Radiol 17:39, 1988
4. Edelman RR, Siegel JB: Advances in musculoskeletal MRI. MRI Decisions 5:27, 1988
5. Mandelbaum B: Optimizing sports medicine care with MRI. Diagn Imag 10:124, 1988
6. Moon KL Jr, Genant HK, Helms CA et al: Musculoskeletal applications of nuclear magnetic resonance. Radiology 147:161, 1983
7. Wetzel LH, Levine E, Murphey MD: Comparison of MR imaging and CT in the evaluation of musculoskeletal masses. Radiographics 7:851, 1987
8. Kransdorf MJ, Jelinek JS, Moser RP Jr et al: Soft-tissue masses: diagnosis using MR imaging. AJR 153:541, 1989
9. Totty WG, Murphy WA, Lee JKT: Soft-tissue tumors: MR imaging. Radiology 160:135, 1986
10. Pettersson H, Gillespy T III, Hamlin DJ et al: Primary musculoskeletal tumors: examination with MR imaging compared with conventional modalities. Radiology 164:237, 1987
11. Vogler JB III, Murphy WA: Bone marrow imaging. Radiology 168:679, 1988
12. Vanel D, Lacombe MJ, Couanet D et al: Musculoskeletal tumors: follow-up with MR imaging after treatment with surgery and radiation therapy. Radiology 164:243, 1987
13. Sochurek H: Medicine's New Visions. Mack, Easton, PA, 1988
14. Winkler ML: The fundamentals of MRI: a primer for the referring physician. Curr Concept Magn Reson Imag 1:3, 1988
15. National Institutes of Health Consensus Development Conference Statement on Magnetic Resonance Imaging, October, 1987
16. Shellock FG: Biological effects of MRI: a clean safety record so far. Diagn Imag 9:96, 1987
17. Holder LE, Matthews LS: The nuclear medicine physician and sports medicine. In Freeman LM, Weissman JS (eds): Nuclear Medicine Annual—1984. Raven Press, New York, 1984
18. Pavlov H: Modern Imaging of the Athletic Injury. Postgrad Radiol 8:3, 1988
19. McCort JJ: Radiology's role in trauma evaluation. Postgrad Radiol 10:159, 1990
20. Harris JH, Edeiken J, Monroe B: The Radiology of Acute Cervical Spine Trauma. 2nd Ed. Williams & Wilkins, Baltimore, 1987
21. Berquist TH: Imaging of adult cervical spine trauma. Radiographics 8:667, 1988
22. Post MJ, Green BA, Quencer RM et al: The value of computed tomography in spinal trauma. Spine 7:417, 1982
23. Pech P, Kilgore DP, Pojunas KW, Haughton VM: Cervical spinal fractures: CT detection. Radiology 157:117, 1985
24. Acheson MB, Livingston RR, Richardson ML, Stimac GK: High-resolution CT scanning in the evaluation of cervical spine fractures: comparison with plain film examinations. AJR 148:1179, 1987
25. Hackney DB, Asato R, Joseph P et al: Hemorrhage and edema in acute spinal cord compression. Demonstration by MR imaging. Radiology 161:387, 1986
26. Kulkarni MV, McArdle CB, Kopanicky D et al: Acute spinal cord injury: MR imaging at 1.5T. Radiology 164:837, 1987
27. Chakeres DW, Flickinger F, Bresnahan JC et al: MR imaging of acute spinal cord trauma. AJNR 8:5, 1987

28. Mirvis SE, Geisler FH, Jelinek JJ et al: Acute cervical spine trauma: evaluation with 1.5T MR imaging. Radiology 166:807, 1988
29. Kulkarni MV, Bondurant FJ, Rose SL, Narayana PA: 1.5 Tesla magnetic resonance imaging of acute spinal trauma. Radiographics 8:1059, 1988
30. Christensen PC: Radiographic study of the normal spine. Radiol Clin North Am 15:133, 1977
31. Park WM, O'Neill M, McCall IW: The radiology of rheumatoid involvement of the cervical spine. Skel Radiol 4:1, 1979
32. Dorwart RH, LaMasters DL: Applications of computed tomographic scanning of the cervical spine. Orthop Clin North Am 16:381, 1985
33. Simon JE, Lukin RR: Diskogenic disease of the cervical spine. Semin Roentgenol 23:118, 1988
34. Masaryk TJ, Modic MT, Geisinger MA et al: Cervical myelopathy: a comparison of magnetic resonance and myelography. J Comput Assist Tomogr 10:184, 1986
35. Teresi LM, Lufkin RB, Reicher MA et al: Asymptomatic degenerative disc disease and spondylosis of the cervical spine: MR imaging. Radiology 164:83, 1987
36. Crandell PH, Batzolorf U: Cervical spondylotic myelopathy. J Neurosurg 25:57, 1966
37. Myer S: Thoracic spine trauma. Semin Roentgenol 27:254, 1992
38. Alexander DJ: Scheuermann's disease. A traumatic spondylodystrophy? Skel Radiol 1:209, 1977
39. McAlister WH, Shackelford GD: Classification of spinal curvatures. Radiol Clin North Am 13:113, 1975
40. Educational program on exposure reduction in scoliosis radiography in full swing. Radiol Health Bull 19:1, 1985
41. Downey EF Jr, Butler P: Less radiation and better images: a new scoliosis radiography system. Milit Med 149:526, 1984
42. Howe GR: Epidemiology of radiogenic breast cancer. p.63. In Boice JD Jr, Fraumeni JF Jr (eds): Radiation Carcinogenesis: Epidemiology and Biological Significance. Raven Press, New York, 1984
43. Protecting the breast during scoliosis radiography. FDA Drug Bull 5:1, 1985
44. Reinbold WD, Genant HK, Reiser UJ et al: Bone mineral content in early-postmenopausal osteoporotic women: comparison of measurements methods. Radiology 160:469, 1986
45. Riggs BL, Wahner HW, Dunn WL et al: Differential changes in bone mineral density of the appendicular and axial skeleton with aging: relationship to spinal osteoporosis. J Clin Invest 2:328, 1981
46. LeBlanc AD, Evans HJ, Marsh C et al: Precision of dual photon absorptiometry measurements. J Nucl Med 27:1362, 1986
47. Firooznia H, Golimbu C, Farii M, Schwartz MS: Rate of spinal trabecular bone loss in normal perimenopausal women: CTR measurement. Radiology 161:735, 1986
48. Sartoris DJ, Resnick D: Dual-energy radiographic absorptiometry for bone densitometry: current status and perspective. AJR 152:241, 1989
49. Resnick D, Sartoris DJ (eds): Bone Disease. 4th Ser. Test and Syllabus. American College of Radiology, Reston, VA, 1989
50. Springfield DS: Mechanisms of metastasis. Clin Orthop 169:15, 1982
51. Pagani JJ, Libshitz HI: Imaging bone metastases. Radiol Clin North Am 20:545, 1982
52. McNeil BJ: Value of bone scanning in neoplastic disease. Semin Nucl Med 14:277, 1984
53. Gainor BJ, Buchert P: Fracture healing in metastatic bone disease. Clin Orthop 178:297, 1983
54. Mooney V: The syndromes of low back disease. Orthop Clin North Am 14:505, 1983
55. Rogers LF: Radiology of Skeletal Trauma. 2nd Ed. Churchill Livingstone, New York, 1982
56. Gehweiler JA Jr, Daffner RH: Low back pain: the controversy of radiologic evaluation. AJR 140:109, 1983
57. Hall FM: Overutilization of radiological examinations. Radiology 120:443, 1980
58. Daffner RH: Radiographic evaluation of low back pain. Contemp Diagn Radiol 9:7:1, 1986
59. Nachemson AL: The lumbar spine: an orthopaedic challenge. Spine 1:59, 1976
60. Scavone JG, Latshaw RF, Rohrer GV: Use of lumbar spine films. Statistical evaluation at a university teaching hospital. JAMA 246:1105, 1981
61. DeLuca SA, Rhea JT: Are routine oblique roentgenograms of the lumbar spine of value? J Bone Joint Surg 63A:846, 1981
62. Helbig T, Lee C: The lumbar facet syndrome. Spine 13:61, 1988
63. Epstein BS, Epstein JA, Jones MD: Degenerative spondylolisthesis with an intact neural arch. Radiology 15:275, 1977
64. Resnick D: Annual oration: degenerative diseases of the vertebral column. Radiology 156:3, 1985
65. Lukin RR, Gaskill MF, Wiot JG: Lumbar herniated disk and related topics. Semin Roentgenol 23:100, 1988
66. Heiss JD, Tew JM Jr: Diskogenic diseases of the spine: clinical aspects. Semin Roentgenol 23:93, 1988
67. Dorwart RH, Vogler JB III, Helms CA: Spinal stenosis. Radiol Clin North Am 21:301, 1983
68. Paine K: Clinical features of lumbar spinal stenosis. Clin Orthop 118:77, 1976
69. Pleatman CW, Lukin RR: Lumbar spinal stenosis. Semin Roentgenol 23:106, 1988

70. Weisz GM, Lee P: Spinal canal stenosis. Concept of spinal reserve capacity: radiologic measurements and clinical applications. Clin Orthop 179:134, 1983
71. Raskin SP, Keating JW: Recognition of lumbar disc disease: comparison of myelography and computed tomography. AJR 139:349, 1982
72. Haughton VM, Eldevik OP, Magnaes B, Amundsen P: A prospective comparison of computed tomography and myelography in the diagnosis of herniated lumbar disks. Radiology 142:103, 1982
73. Williams AL, Haughton VM, Daniels DL, Thornton RS: CT recognition of lateral lumbar disk herniation. AJR 139:345, 1982
74. Schipper J, Kardaun JWPF, Braakman R: Lumbar disk herniation: diagnosis with CT or myelography? Radiology 165:227, 1987
75. Modic MT, Masaryk T, Boumphrey F et al: Lumbar herniated disc disease and canal stenosis: Prospective evaluation by surface coil MR, CT, and myelography. AJR 147:757, 1986
76. Schellhas KP, Pollei SR: The role of discography in the evaluation of patients with spinal deformity. Orthop Clin North Am 25:265, 1994
77. Greenspan A: CT-diskography vs MRI in intervertebral disk herniation. Appl Radiol 3:34, 1993
78. Scullin DR: Lumbar diskography (letter). Radiology 162:284, 1987
79. Executive Committee of the North American Spine Society: Position statement on diskography. Spine 13:1343, 1988
80. Fernbach SK, Wilkinson RH: Avulsion injuries of the pelvis and proximal femur. AJR 137:581, 1981
81. Vellenga C, Pauwels EK, Bijvoet OL et al: Untreated Paget disease of bone studied by scintigraphy. Radiology 153:799, 1984
82. Frame B, Marel GM: Paget disease: a review of current knowledge. Radiology 141:21, 1981
83. Singer FR, Mills BG: Evidence of a viral etiology of Paget's disease of bone. Clin Orthop 178:245, 1983
84. Forrester DM, Brown JC, Nesson JW: The Radiology of Joint Disease. WB Saunders, Philadelphia, 1978
85. Patten R, Shuman WP: MRI of Osteonecrosis. MRI Decisions 4:2, 1990
86. Glickstein MF, Burk DL Jr, Schiebler ML et al: Avascular necrosis versus other diseases of the hip: sensitivity of MR imaging. Radiology 169:213, 1988
87. Mitchell MD, Dundel HL, Steinberg ME et al: Avascular necrosis of the hip: comparison of MR, CT and scintigraphy. AJR 146:67, 1986
88. Mitchell RG, Rao VM, Dalinka MK et al: Femoral head avascular necrosis: correlation of MR imaging, radiographic staging, radionuclide imaging, and clinical finding. Radiology 162:709, 1987
89. Stansberry SD, Swischuck LE, Barr LL: Legg-Perthes disease: incidence of the subchondral fracture. Appl Radiol 19:30, 1990
90. Ho C, Sartoris D: Modern assessment of hip fractures. Postgrad Rad 10:85, 1990
91. Zwas ST, Elkanovitch R, Frank G: Interpretation and classification of bone scintigraphic findings in stress fractures. J Nucl Med 28:452, 1987
92. Spenser BG: Knee MRI. Postgrad Radiology 11:198, 1991
93. Ghelman B: Meniscal tears of the knee: evaluation by high-resolution CT combined with arthrography. Radiology 157:23, 1985
94. Tyrrell RL, Gluckert K, Pathrial M et al: Fast three-dimensional MR imaging of the knee: comparison with arthroscopy. Radiology 166:865, 1988
95. Reicher MA, Hartzman S, Duckwiler GR et al: Meniscal injuries: detection using MR imaging. Radiology 159:753, 1986
96. Crues JV, Morgan FW: Magnetic resonance imaging of the knee. Contemp Diagn Radiol 11:28;1, 1989
97. Bellon EM, Keith MW, Coleman PE: Magnetic resonance imaging of internal derangements of the knee. Radiographics 8:95, 1988
98. Crues JV, Mink J, Levy TL et al: The accuracy of magnetic resonance imaging in the evaluation of meniscal tears of the knee: the first 144 cases. Radiology 164:445, 1987
99. Jackson DW, Jennings LD, Maywood RM et al: Magnetic resonance imaging of the knee. Am J Sports Med 16:29, 1987
100. Stroller DW, Martin C, Crues JV et al: MR imaging: pathologic correlation of meniscal tears. Radiology 163:731, 1987
101. Quinn SF, Brown TR, Szumowski J: Meniscii of the knee: radial MR imaging correlated with arthroscopy in 259 patients. Radiology 185:577, 1992
102. Hayes CW, Conway WF: Evaluation of articular cartilage: radiographic and cross-sectional imaging techniques. Radiographics 12:409, 1992
103. Winalski CS, Weissman BN, Aliabadi P et al: Intravenous Gd-DTPA enhancement of joint fluid: a less invasive alternative for MR arthrography, abstracted. Radiology 181 (P):304, 1991
104. Li DKB, Adams ME, McConkey S: Magnetic resonance imaging of the ligaments and menisci of the knee. Radiol Clin North Am 24:209, 1986
105. Mink JH, Levy TL, Crues JV: Tears of the anterior cruciate ligament and menisci of the knee: MRI imaging evaluation. Radiology 167:769, 1988
106. Lee JK, Yao L, Phelps CT et al: Anterior cruciate ligament tears: MR imaging compared with arthroscopy and clinical tests. Radiology 166:861, 1988

107. Vahey TN, Broome DR, Kayes KJ et al: Acute and chronic tears of the anterior cruciate ligament: differential features at MR imaging. Radiology 181:251, 1991
108. Ruwe PA, Wright J, Randall RL et al: Can MR imaging effectively replace diagnostic arthroscopy? Radiology 183:335, 1992
109. Remer EM, Fitzgerald SW, Friedman H: Anterior cruciate ligament injury: MR imaging diagnosis and patterns of injury. RadioGraphics 12:901, 1992
110. Mink JH, Deutsch AL: MRI of the Musculoskeletal System. p. 251–385. Raven, New York, 1990
111. Lee KR, Cos GG, Neff JR et al: Cystic masses of the knee: arthrographic and CT evaluation. AJR 148:329, 1987
112. Ogden JA, Tross RB, Murphy MJ: Fractures of the tibial tuberosity in adolescents. J Bone Joint Surg 62A:205, 1980
113. Ogden JA, Southwick WO: Osgood-Schlatter's disease and tibial tuberosity development. Clin Orthop 116:180, 1976
114. Ozonoff MB. Pediatric Orthopedic Radiology. WB Saunders, Philadelphia, 1979
115. Tindel NL, Nisonson B: The plica syndrome. Orthop Clin North Am 23:613, 1992
116. Kurosaka M, Yoshiya S, Yamada M, Hirohata K: Lateral synovial plica syndrome. Am J Sports Med 20:92, 1990
117. Yao L, Lee JK: Occult intraosseous fracture: detection with MR imaging. Radiology 167:749, 1988
118. Lynch TC, Crues JV III, Morgan FW et al: Bone abnormalities of the knee: significance and prevalence at MR imaging. Radiology 171:761, 1979
119. Mink JH, Deutsch AL: Occult cartilage and bone injuries of the knee: detection, classification and assessment with MR imaging. Radiology 170:823, 1989
120. Kosco A, Winalski CS: Evaluation of ankle and leg injuries. Postgrad Radiol 12:167, 1992
121. Solomon M, Gilula L, Oloff L et al: CT scanning of the foot and ankle: II. Clinical applications and review of the literature. AJR 146:1204, 1986
122. Maurice HD, Newman JF, Watt I: Bone scanning of the foot for unexplained pain. J Bone Joint Surg 69B:448, 1987
123. Karl RD, Hammes CS: Nuclear medicine imaging in podiatric disorders. Clin Podiatr Med Surg 5:909, 1988
124. Lawson JP, Ogden JA, Sella E et al: The painful accessory navicular. Skel Radiol 12:250, 1984
125. Matin P: Bone scintigraphy in the diagnosis and management of traumatic injury. Semin Nucl Med 13:104, 1983
126. Matin P: Bone scanning of trauma and benign conditions. In Freeman LM, Weissman HS (eds): Nuclear Medicine Annual—1982. Raven Press, New York, 1982
127. Helms CA: Magnetic resonance imaging of the foot and ankle. p. 1004 In Brant WE, Helms CA (eds): Fundamentals of Diagnostic Radiology. Williams & Wilkins, Baltimore, 1993
128. Wilson ES Jr, Catz FM: Stress fractures. An analysis of 250 consecutive cases. Radiology 92:481, 1969
129. Geslien GE, Thrall JH, Espinosa JL et al: Early detection of stress fractures using 99m Tc-polyphosphate. Radiology 121:683, 1976
130. Norfray JF, Schlachter L, Kernahan WT et al: Early confirmation of stress fractures in joggers. JAMA 243:1647, 1980
131. Pavlov H, Torg JS, Hersh A, Freiberger RH: The roentgen examination of runners' injuries. Radiographics 1:17, 1981
132. Torg JS, Pavlov J, Torg E: Overuse injuries in sports: the foot. Clin Podiatr Med Surg 4:939, 1987
133. McBryde AJ: Stress fractures in runners. Clin Sports Med 4:737, 1985
134. Pavlov H, Torg JS, Freiberger RH: Tarsal navicular stress fractures: roentgen evaluation. Radiology 148:641, 1983
135. Goergen TG, Venn-Watson EA, Rossmand J et al: Tarsal navicular stress fractures in runners. AJR 136:201, 1981
136. Graves J, Virtanen K: Osteochondrosis in athletes. Br J Sports Med 16:161, 1982
137. Brower AC: The osteochondroses. Orthop Clin North Am 14:99, 1983
138. Mandell GA, Harcke HT: Scintigraphic manifestations of infraction of the second metatarsal (Freiberg's disease). J Nucl Med 28:249, 1987
139. Yuh WTC, Corson JD, Baraniewski HM et al: Osteomyelitis of the foot in diabetic patients: evaluation with plain film, 99m-Tc-MDP bone scintigraphy, and MR imaging. AJR 152:795, 1989
140. Goldman AB, Pavlov H, Schneider R: Radionuclide bone scanning in subtalar coalitions: differential considerations. AJR 138:427, 1982
141. Cheung Y, Rosenberg ZS, Magee T, Chinitz L: Normal anatomy and pathologic conditions of ankle tendons: current imaging techniques. RadioGraphics 12:429, 1992
142. Quinn SF, Murray WT, Clark RA, Cochran CF: Achilles tendon: MR imaging at 1.5T. Radiology 164:767, 1987
143. Erickson SJ, Quinn SF, Kneeland JB et al: MR imaging of the tarsal tunnel and related spaces. AJR 155:323, 1990
144. Beltran J, Munchow AM, Khabiri H et al: Ligaments of the lateral aspect of the ankle and sinus tarsi: an MR imaging study. Radiology 177:455, 1990
145. Erickson SJ, Smith JW, Ruiz ME et al: MR imaging of the lateral collateral ligament of the ankle. AJR 156:131, 1991
146. Berkowitz JF, Kier R, Rudicel S: Plantar fascitis: MR imaging. Radiology 179:665, 1991
147. Keift GJ, Bloem JL, Rozing PM et al: Rotator cuff impingement syndrome. Radiology 166:211, 1988

148. Neer CS III: Impingement lesions. Clin Orthop 173:70, 1983
149. Bigliani LU, Morrison DS: The morphology of the acromion and its relationship to rotator cuff tears. Proceedings of the American Shoulder and Elbow Surgeons, New Orleans, 1986
150. Resnik CS, Deutsch AL, Resnick D et al: Arthrotomography of the shoulder. Radiographics 4:963, 1984
151. Seeger LL, Gold RH, Bassett LW et al: Shoulder impingement syndrome: MR findings in 53 shoulders. AJR 150:343, 1988
152. Farley TE, Neumann CH, Steinbach LS et al: Full-thickness tears of the rotator cuff of the shoulder: diagnosis with MR imaging. AJR 158:347, 1992
153. Raffi M, Firooznia H, Sherman O et al: Rotator cuff lesions: signal patterns at MR imaging. Radiology 177:817, 1990
154. Mack LA, Matsen FA, Kilcoyne RF et al: US evaluation of the rotator cuff. Radiology 157:205, 1985
155. Deutsch AL, Resnick D, Mink JH et al: Computed and conventional arthrotomography of the glenohumeral joint: normal anatomy and clinical experience. Radiology 153:603, 1984
156. Haynor DR, Shuman WP: Double contrast CT arthrography of the glenoid labrum and shoulder girdle. Radiographics 4:411, 1984
157. Shuman WP, Kilcoyne RF, Matsen FA et al: Double-contrast computed tomography of the glenoid labrum. AJR 141:581, 1983
158. Rafii M, Firooznia H, Golimbu C et al: CT arthrography of capsular structures of the shoulder. AJR 146:361, 1986
159. Bunnell DH, Fisher DA, Bassett LW et al: Elbow joint: normal anatomy on MR images. Radiology 165:527, 1987
160. Murphy BJ: MR imaging of the elbow. Radiology 184:525, 1992
161. Mirowitz SA, London SL: Ulnar collateral ligament injury in baseball pitchers: MR imaging evaluation. Radiology 184:525, 1992
162. Kaplan PA, Dussault RG: MR imaging of the elbow. p. 97–105. In Weissman BN (ed): Syllabus: A Categorical Course in Musculoskeletal Radiology. RSNA Publications, Oak Brook, IL, 1993
163. Wilson AJ, Mann FA, Gilula LA: Review article: imaging of the hand and wrist. J Hand Surg (Br) 15:153, 1990
164. Levinsohn EM: Imaging of the wrist. Radiol Clin North Am 28:905, 1990
165. Levinsohn EM: Evaluation of wrist pain. Radiol Rep 2:60, 1989
166. Hodge JC, Gilula LA, Yin Y et al: The wrist: specialized conventional radiography and CT techniques, indications and findings. In Weissman BN (ed): Syllabus: A Categorical Course in Musculoskeletal Radiology. RSNA Publications, Oak Brook, IL, 1993
167. Gumucio CA, Fernando B, Yound VL et al: Management of scaphoid fractures: a review and update. South Med J 82:1377, 1989
168. Linn MR, Mann FA, Gilula LA: Imaging the symptomatic wrist. Orthop Clin North Am 21:515, 1990
169. Pin PG, Young VL, Gilula LA et al: Wrist pain: a systematic approach to diagnosis. Plast Reconstr Surg 85:42, 1990
170. Stewart NR, Gilula LA: CT of the wrist: a tailored approach. Radiology 183:13, 1992
171. Levinsohn EM, Rosen ID, Palmer AK: Wrist arthrography: value of the three-compartment injection method. Radiology 179:231, 1991
172. Manaster BJ: The clinical efficacy of triple-injection wrist arthrography. Radiology 178:267, 1991
173. Manaster BJ, Mann RJ, Rubenstein S: Wrist pain: correlation of clinical and plain film findings with arthrographic results. J Hand Surg (Am) 14:466, 1989
174. Metz VM, Mann FA, Gilula L: Three-compartment wrist arthrography: correlation of pain site with location of uni- and bi-directional communications. AJR 160:819, 1993
175. Mesgarzadeh M, Schneck CD, Bonakdarpour A: Carpal tunnel: MR imaging I. Normal anatomy. Radiology 171:743, 1989
176. Zlatkin MB, Chao PC, Osterman AL et al: Chronic wrist pain: evaluation with high-resolution MR imaging. Radiology 173:723, 1989
177. Golimbu CN, Firooznia H, Melone CP Jr et al: Tears of the triangular fibrocartilage of the wrist: MR imaging. Radiology 173:731, 1989
178. Rominger MB, Bernreuter WK, Kenney PJ et al: MR imaging of anatomy and tears of wrist ligaments. RadioGraphics 13:1233, 1993
179. Gundry CR, Kursunoglu-Brahme S, Schwaighofer B et al: Is MR better than arthrography for evaluating the ligaments of the wrist: in vitro study. AJR 154:337, 1990
180. Mesgarzadeh M, Schneck CD, Bonakdarpour A et al: Carpal tunnel: MR imaging II. Carpal tunnel syndrome. Radiology 171:749, 1989
181. Reinus WR, Conway WF, Totty WG et al: Carpal avascular necrosis: MR imaging. Radiology 160:689, 1986
182. Sowa DT, Holder LE, Patt PG et al: Application of magnetic resonance imaging to ischemic necrosis of the lunate. J Hand Surg (Am) 14:1008, 1989
183. Trumble TE: Avascular necrosis after scaphoid fracture: a correlation of magnetic resonance imaging and histology. J Hand Surg 15A:557, 1990
184. Rominger MB, Bernreuter WK, Kenney PJ et al: MR imaging of the hands in early rheumatoid arthritis: preliminary results. RadioGraphics 13:37, 1993

185. Gilkeson G, Polisson R, Sinclair H et al: Early detection of carpal erosions in patients with rheumatoid arthritis: a pilot study of magnetic resonance imaging. J Rheumatol 166:1361, 1988
186. Foley Nolan D, Stack JP, Ryan M et al: Magnetic resonance imaging in the assessment of rheumatoid arthritis: a comparison with plain film radiographs. Br J Rheumatol 30:101, 1991
187. Gubler FM, Maas M, Dijkstra PF et al: Cystic rheumatoid arthritis: description of a nonerosive form. Radiology 177:829, 1990
188. Konig H, Sieper J, Wolf KJ: Rheumatoid arthritis: evaluation of hypervascular and fibrous pannus with dynamic MR imaging enhanced with Gd-DTPA. Radiology 176:473, 1990
189. Genant HK, Kosin F, Bekerman C et al: The reflex sympathetic dystrophy syndrome. A comprehensive analysis using fine-detailed radiography, photon absorptiometry, and bone and joint scintigraphy. Radiology 117:21, 1975
190. Kosin F, Soin JS, Ryan LM et al: Bone scintigraphy in the reflex sympathetic dystrophy syndrome. Radiology 138: 437, 1981
191. Holder LE, MacKinnon SE: Reflex sympathetic dystrophy in the hands: clinical and scintigraphic criteria. Radiology 152:517, 1984
192. Maurer AH, Holder LE, Espinola DA et al: Three phase radionuclide scintigraphy of the hand. Radiology 146: 761, 1983

SUGGESTED READINGS

Jette A: Diagnosis and classification by physical therapists. Phys Ther 69:967, 1989

Lippert FG III, Teitz CC: Diagnosing Musculoskeletal Problems: A Practical Guide. Williams & Wilkins, Baltimore, 1987

Wood R: Footprints. Phys Ther 69:975, 1989

Wolf SL: Clinical Decision Making in Physical Therapy. FA Davis, Philadelphia, 1985

I APPENDIX: EXAMINATION—REVIEW OF SYSTEMS SUMMARY

A. General health
   1. Unexplained weight change
   2. Fever, chills, sweats
   3. Malaise
   4. Weakness
   5. Medical history (illness, surgery, medication)
   6. Family medical history
   7. History of smoking
   8. Substance abuse
B. Skin
   1. Color
   2. Temperature
   3. Texture
   4. Dry/moist
   5. Masses, lumps
   6. Rash
   7. Hair
   8. Nails
C. Head
   1. Headache
   2. Head trauma
   3. Dizziness
   4. Lightheadedness
   5. Visual: problems/changes
   6. Nystagmus
   7. History of glaucoma, cataracts
   8. Hearing: problems/changes
   9. Tinnitus
   10. Vertigo
   11. Ear discharge
   12. History of ear infection, earache
   13. Nosebleeds
   14. Olfactory: problems/changes
   15. Nasal congestion
   16. History of hay fever, sinus trouble/infection
   17. Condition of teeth
   18. Condition of gums
   19. Bleeding gums
   20. Mouth sores
   21. Sensory changes associated with taste
   22. Difficulty with swallowing
D. Neck
   1. Lumps in the neck
   2. Swollen glands
   3. Goiter
   4. Pain and stiffness
E. Breasts
   1. Date of last self-examination
   2. Lumps, masses
   3. Dimpling of tissue
   4. Nipple discharge
F. Pulmonary system
   1. Dyspnea
   2. Wheezing

3. Stridor
4. Cough
5. Sputum
6. Hemoptysis
7. History of asthma, emphysema, pneumonia, tuberculosis, pleurisy, bronchitis

G. Cardiovascular system
1. Angina
2. Extremity intermittent claudication
3. Complaints of upper-quarter pressure or tightness sensations
4. Pain associated with sweating
5. Palpitations
6. Dyspnea
7. Orthopnea
8. Fatigue
9. Syncope
10. History of heart trouble, high blood pressure, rheumatic fever, heart attack, heart murmur

H. Gastrointestinal system
1. Difficulty with swallowing
2. Heartburn, indigestion
3. Specific food intolerance
4. Nausea
5. Vomiting
6. Change in appetite
7. Excessive belching or flatulence
8. Bowel habits (frequency, stool caliber and color)
9. History of liver, gallbladder, stomach problems; ulcers

I. Urinary system
1. Urinary frequency, including nocturia
2. Dysuria
3. Hematuria
4. Reduced caliber or force of urine stream
5. Incontinence
6. History of urinary, kidney infections

J. Genital reproductive system (male)
1. Hernia
2. Self-examination (sores, masses, lumps)
3. Urethral discharge
4. Pain with intercourse
5. Sexual dysfunction
6. History of venereal disease

K. Genital reproductive system (female)
1. Hernia
2. Change in menstruation (frequency and duration of cycle, dysmenorrhea, amount of bleeding)
3. Date of last period
4. Menopause
5. Vaginal discharge
6. Self-examination (lumps, masses, sores)
7. Number of pregnancies
8. Number of deliveries
9. Complications of pregnancy and delivery
10. Pain with intercourse
11. Sexual dysfunction
12. Birth control methods
13. History of venereal disease, infertility

L. Nervous system
1. Numbness/paresthesias
2. Weakness
3. Abnormal reflexes
4. Clonus/spasticity
5. Seizures
6. Syncope
7. Tremors

M. Hematologic system
1. Easy bruising
2. Easy bleeding
3. Anemia

N. Endocrine system
1. Excessive thirst
2. Excessive hunger
3. Polyuria
4. Excessive sweating
5. Heat or cold intolerance
6. Fatigue
7. Weakness
8. Paresthesia
9. History of diabetes, thyroid trouble

O. Psychiatric
1. Nervousness
2. Tension
3. History of depression, other psychological disorders.
4. History of abuse (physical, emotional, sexual)

SUGGESTED READINGS

Bates B: A Guide to Physical Examination and History Taking. 5th Ed. JB Lippincott, Philadelphia, 1991

Malasanos L, Barkauska V, Stoltenberg-Allen K: Health Assessment. 4th Ed. CV Mosby, St. Louis, 1990

II Appendix: Objective Examination—Upper-Quarter Screening Examination

A. Standing
   1. Posture
   2. Gait
B. Sitting
   1. General survey (vital signs, skin, hair, nails)
   2. Head
      a. Facial contour.
         i. Eyes (oculomotor n., ptosis; facial n., Bell's palsy)
         ii. Pupil size (oculomotor n.)
         iii. Mouth (facial n., Bell's palsy)
         iv. Cheeks (trigeminal n., masseter atrophy)
      b. Palpation
         i. Muscle
         ii. Bone
         iii. Lymph nodes (pre- and postauricular, submental, occipital, submandibular) (Fig. 1)
      c. Intraoral observation
         i. Tongue (hypoglossal n.)
         ii. Gums (inflamed, bleeding)
         iii. Teeth (absence, occlusive pattern)
   3. Neck
      a. Observation
         i. Surface anatomy contour
      b. Palpation
         i. Soft tissues
         ii. Bone
         iii. Lymph nodes (anterior and posterior cervical, supraclavicular) (Fig. 2)
         iv. Trachea
         v. Thyroid gland (Fig. 3)
   4. Head and neck
      a. Verticle compression and distraction
      b. Active movements, including overpressures (forward bending, rotation including vertebral artery test, side bending, backward bending)
      c. Resisted motions (forward bending, backward bending, side bending, rotation)
   5. Thorax, respiratory pattern
   6. Shoulder girdle
      a. Palpation soft tissues and bone
      b. Active motions (elevation, depression, protraction, retraction)
      c. Resisted elevation (spinal accessory n.)
   7. Upper extremity
      a. Palpation (bone soft tissues including lymph nodes; infraclavicular, axillary, epitrochlear) (Figs. 4 to 9)
      b. Pulses, including brachial, radial, ulnar (Figs. 10 to 12)
      c. Elbow active movements, including overpressure
         i. Flexion
         ii. Extension

d. Shoulder active movements, including overpressure
   i. Elevation (in the plane of the scapula)
   ii. External rotation
   iii. Internal rotation
e. Wrist active movements, including overpressures
   i. Extension
   ii. Flexion
f. Finger active movements, including overpressures
   i. Extension
   ii. Flexion

8. Neurologic examination
   a. Sensory (light touch, trigeminal n., C2–T6/T8)
   b. Motor
      i. Shoulder abduction (C5–6, axillary n.)
      ii. Elbow flexion (C5–6, musculocutaneous n.)
      iii. Elbow extension (C7, radial n.)
      iv. Wrist extension (C6, radial and ulnar n.)
      v. Thumb extension (C8, radial n.)
      vi. Finger abduction (T1, radial and median n.)
   c. Reflexes
      i. Deep tendon reflexes (biceps C5–6, brachioradialis C6, triceps C7)
      ii. Hoffman's reflex

C. Supine/prone: Any of the above if standing, sitting not tolerated
   1. Repeat any positive neurologic test noted in weight-bearing postures

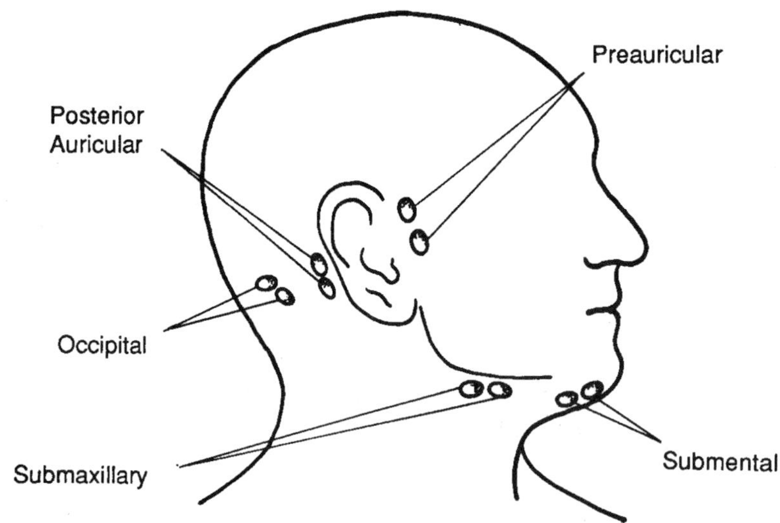

Fig. AII-1. Lymph nodes of the head and neck.

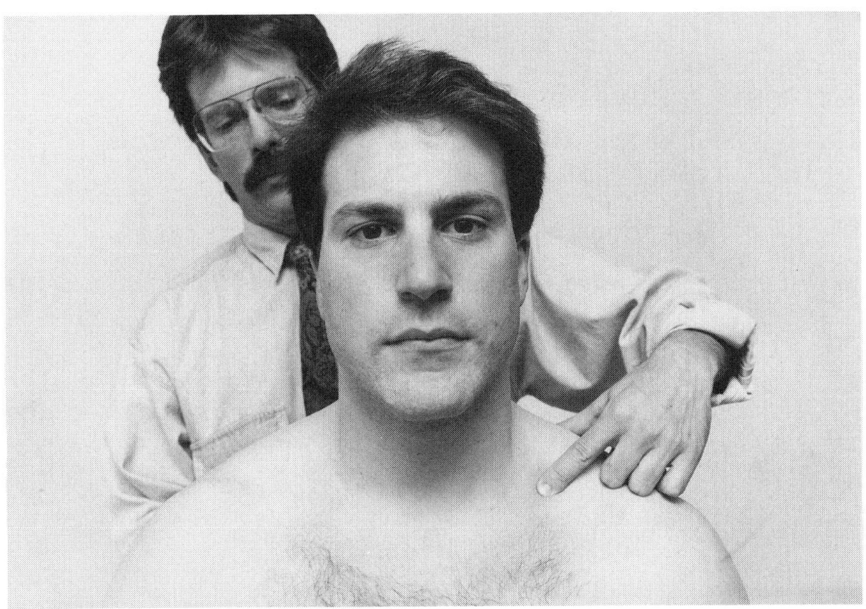

Fig. AII-2. Palpating for the supraclavicular lymph node lateral to the sternocleidomastoid attachment on the clavicle.

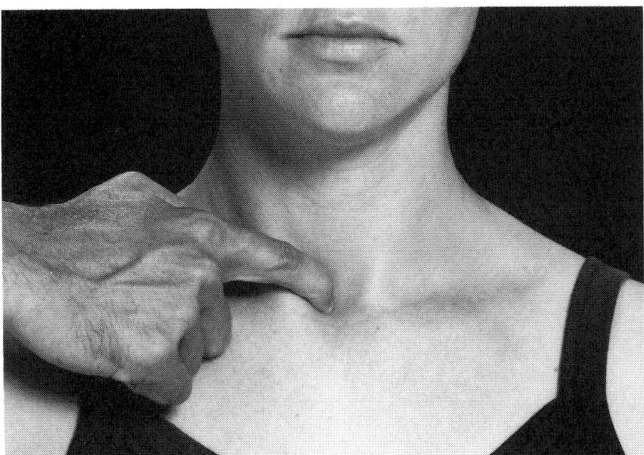

Fig. AII-3. Palpation of the thyroid gland. The examiner's finger is placed below the cricoid cartilage in the space just above the sternal notch and medial and posterior to the sternocleidomastoid muscle.

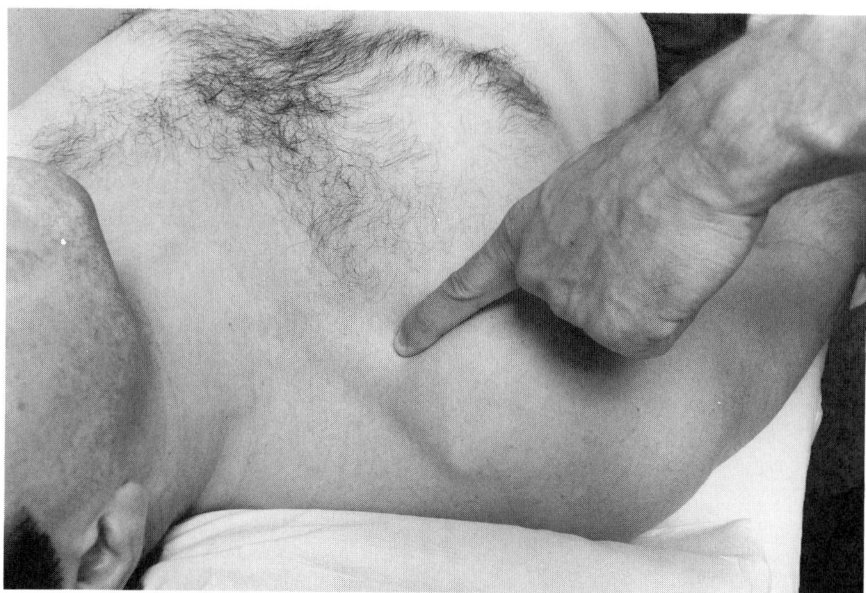

Fig. AII-4. Palpating for the infraclavicular lymph node between the deltoid and pectoralis major muscle.

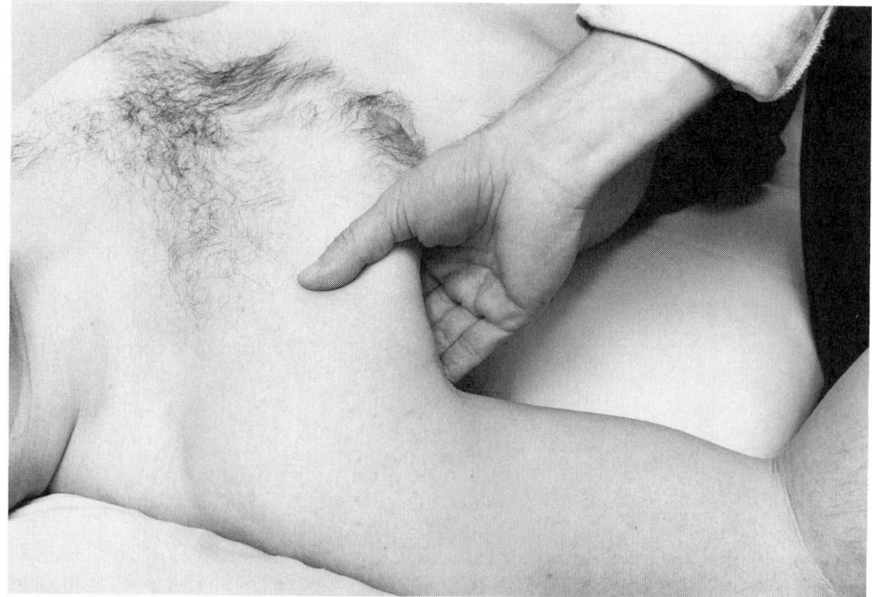

Fig. AII-5. Palpating for lymph nodes, anterior axillary wall, posterior surface of pectoralis major.

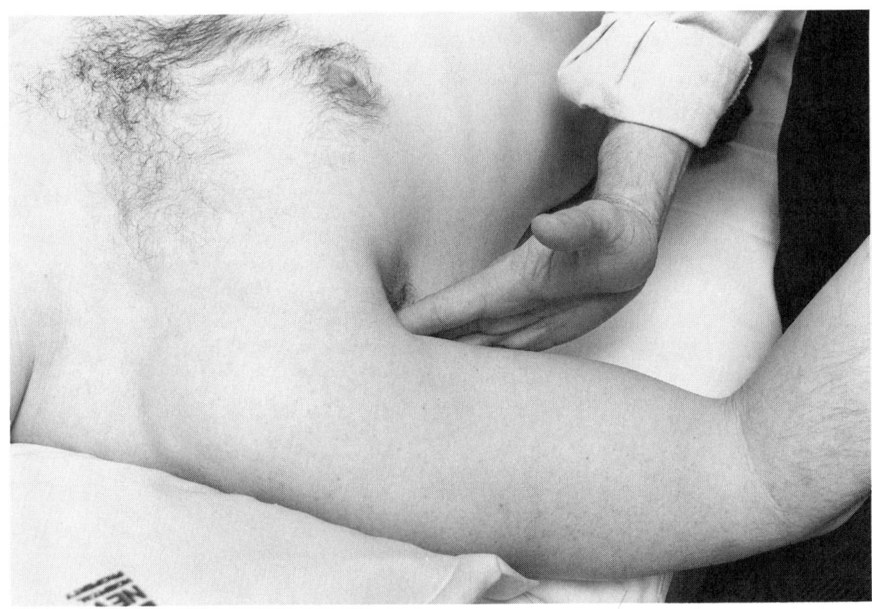

Fig. AII-6. Palpating for lymph nodes, lateral axillary wall, along shaft of upper humerus.

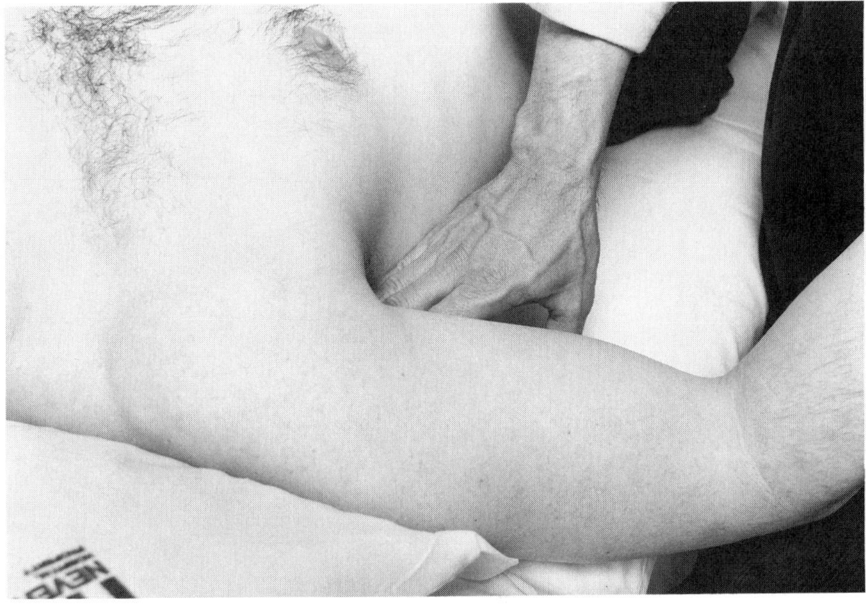

Fig. AII-7. Palpating for lymph nodes, posterior axillary wall, anterior surface of teres major, and latissimus dorsi.

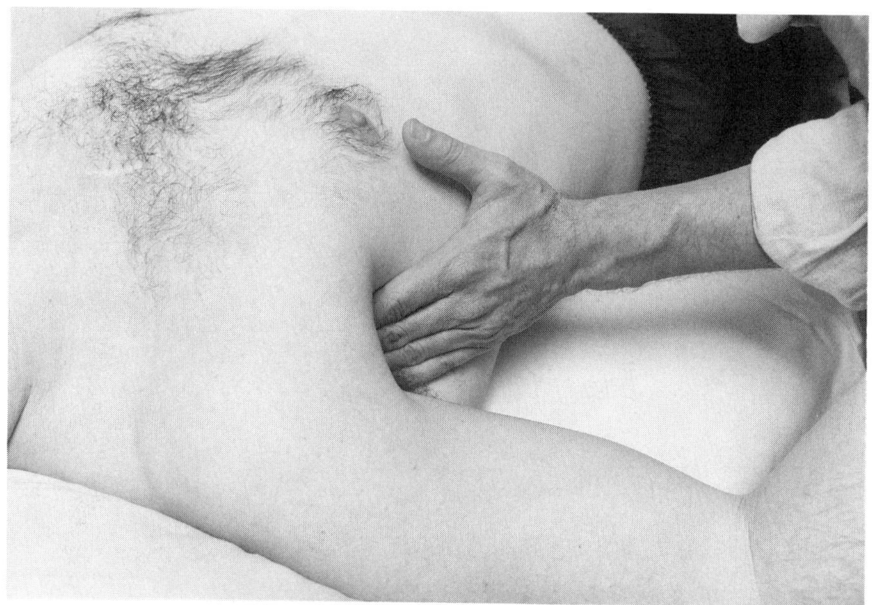

Fig. AII-8. Palpating for lymph nodes, medial axillary wall, along thorax.

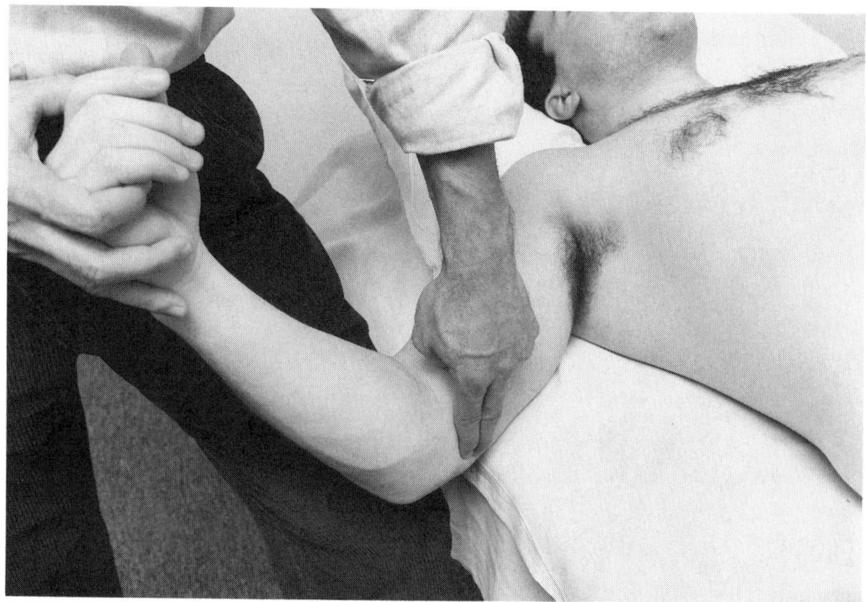

Fig. AII-9. Palpating for epitrochlear lymph nodes.

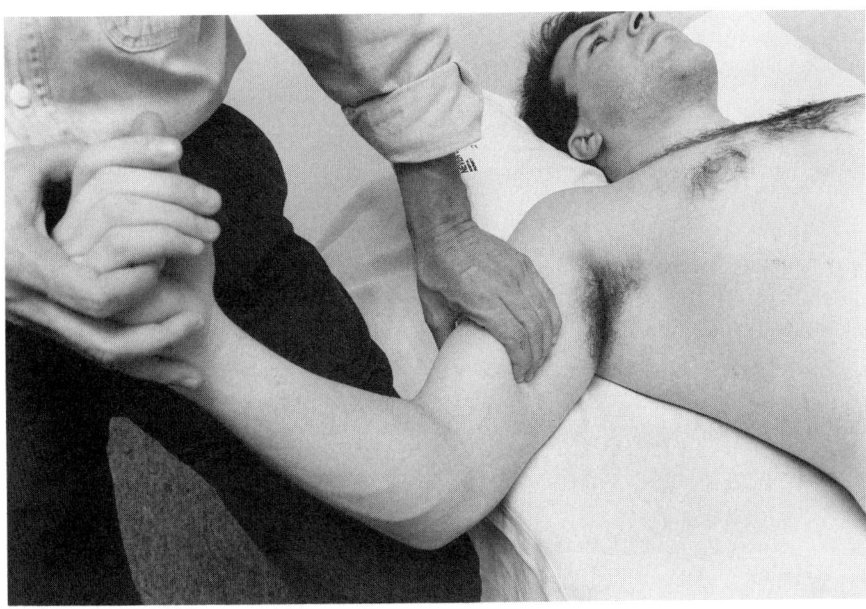

Fig. AII-10. Assessing pulse at the brachial artery, upper half of medial aspect of humerus.

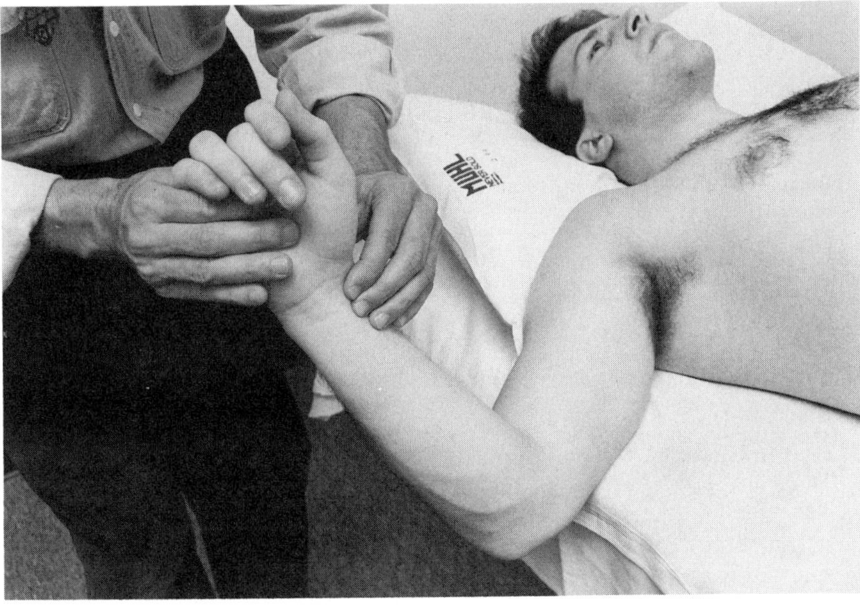

Fig. AII-11. Assessing pulse at the radial artery, just proximal to wrist joint.

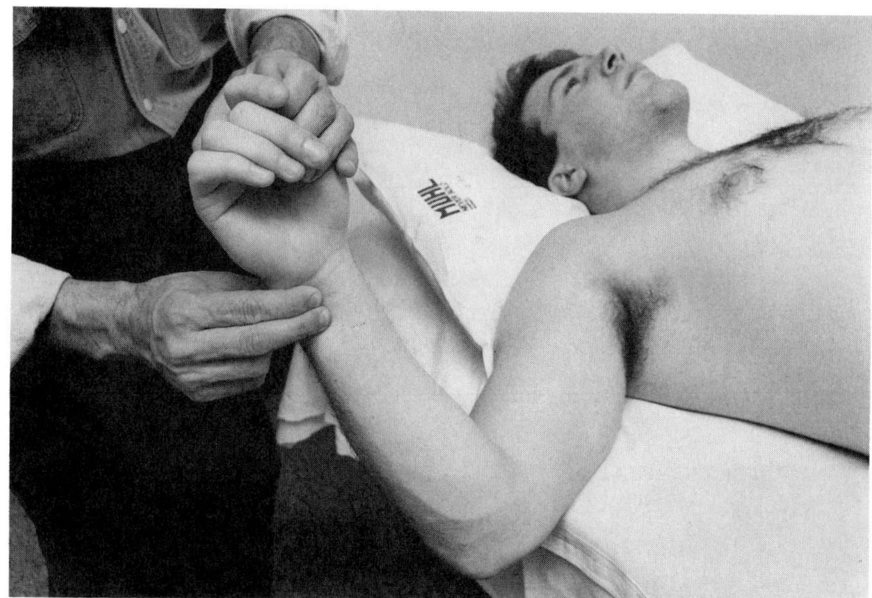

Fig. AII-12. Assessing pulse at the ulnar artery, just proximal to wrist joint.

III Appendix: Objective Examination—Lower-Quarter Screening Examination

A. Standing
   1. Posture
   2. Gait
   3. General survey, including vital signs, skin, hair, nails, surface anatomy contour
   4. Palpation, including tone, temperature, soft tissue, and bony landmarks
   5. Perform a squat for general screen of lumbar spine, hips, knees, ankles
   6. Verticle quick compression (heel bounce)
   7. Active trunk movements with overpressures
      a. Forward bending, including palpation of PSIS for iliosacral test
      b. Backward bending
      c. Side bending
      d. Rotation
   8. Neurologic examination
      a. Motor
         i. Heel raise tested unilaterally (S1, S2)
         ii. Toe raises (heal walking) (L4, L5)
      b. Sensory (light touch S1, S2)

B. Sitting
   1. Posture
   2. Thorax, respiratory pattern
   3. Verticle trunk compression/distraction
   4. Active trunk rotation, including overpressure if not tested in standing
   5. Trunk active forward bending while palpating PSIS for sacroiliac mobility test
   6. Resisted trunk forward, backward, and side bending and rotation
   7. Neurologic examination
      a. Sensory (light touch T7–S2)
      b. Motor
         i. Hip flexion (L1, L2, L3, femoral n.)
         ii. Knee extension (L2, L3, L4, femoral n.)
         iii. Ankle dorsiflexion (L4, deep peroneal nerve) if not tested in standing
         iv. Hallux extension (L5, deep peronea nerve)
         v. Knee flexion (L5, S1, S2, sciatic, tibial nerve) if heel raises not tested in standing
      c. Deep tendon reflexes
         i. Quadriceps (L2, 3, 4)
         ii. Hamstring (L5)
         iii. Achilles (S1, S2)
      d. Babinski (Fig. 1)

C. Supine
   1. Observation
      a. Surface anatomy contour
   2. Palpation
      a. Soft tissues, including abdomen, inguinal lymph nodes (Fig. 2)

b. Bony landmarks of thorax, pelvis, and lower extremities
c. Pulses, including aorta, femoral, popliteal, posterior tibial, dorsalis pedis (Figs. 3 to 6)
3. Neurologic examination, abdominal reflexes (T7–L1) (Figs. 8 and 9)
4. Sacroiliac joint gapping or ilial shear test
5. Knee active movements with overpressures
   a. Flexion
   b. Extension
6. Hip active movements with overpressures
   a. Flexion
   b. Internal rotation
   c. External rotation
7. Ankle/foot active movements with overpressures
   a. Dorsiflexion
   b. Plantarflexion
   c. Inversion
   d. Eversion
8. Toe active movements with overpressures
   a. Extension
   b. Flexion
9. Neurologic examination
   a. Repeat tests that were positive in weight-bearing positions
   b. Complete entire examination if unable to do in weight-bearing postures
   c. Dural tension tests (neck flexion, straight leg raise with/without neck flexion and ankle dorsiflexion)

D. Prone
1. Observation
   a. Surface anatomy contour
2. Palpation
   a. Soft tissues
   b. Bony landmarks
3. Hip active movement with overpressure
   a. Extension
4. Dural tension test, femoral n.

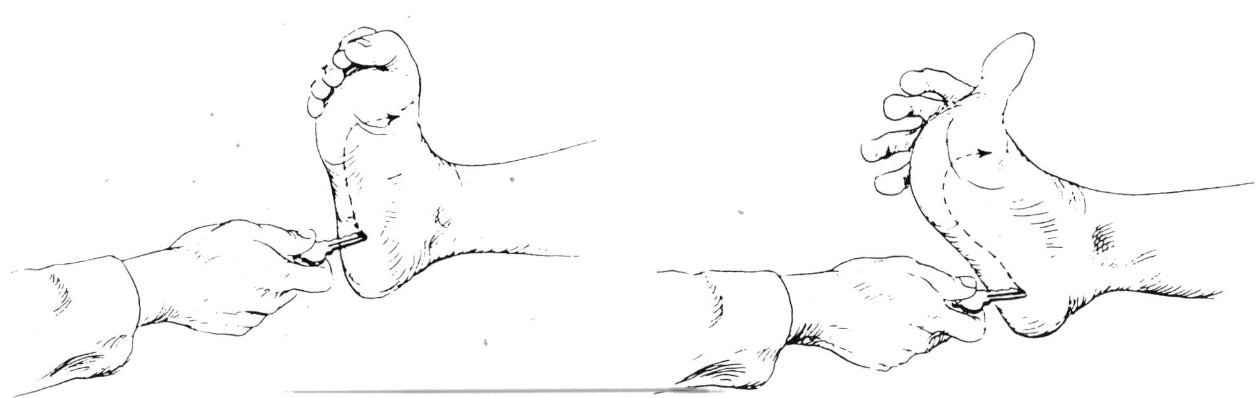

Fig. AIII-1. Babinski test. (From Hoppenfeld S: Physical Examination of the Spine and Extremities. Appleton and Lange, New York, 1976, with permission.)

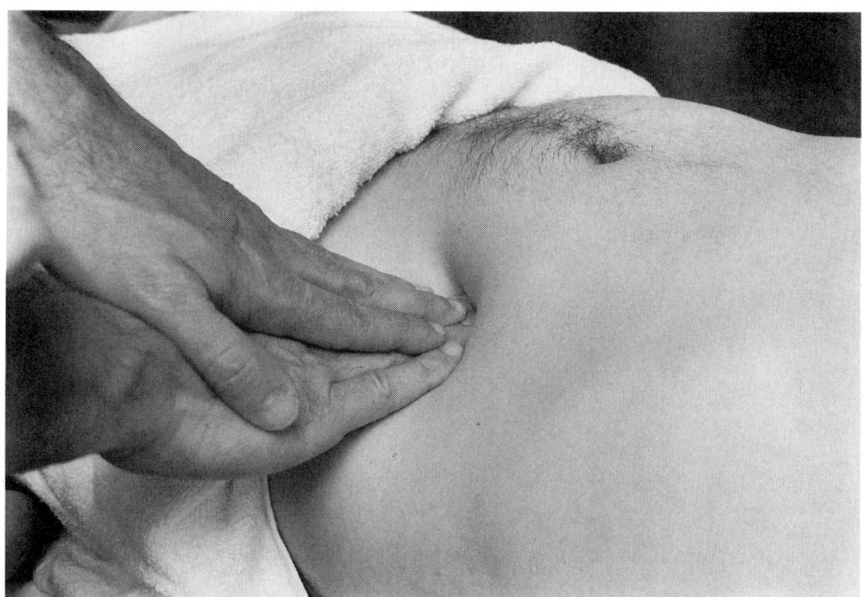

Fig. AIII-2. Palpating the abdomen for tone, provocation, dysfunction. All four abdominal quadrants should be assessed.

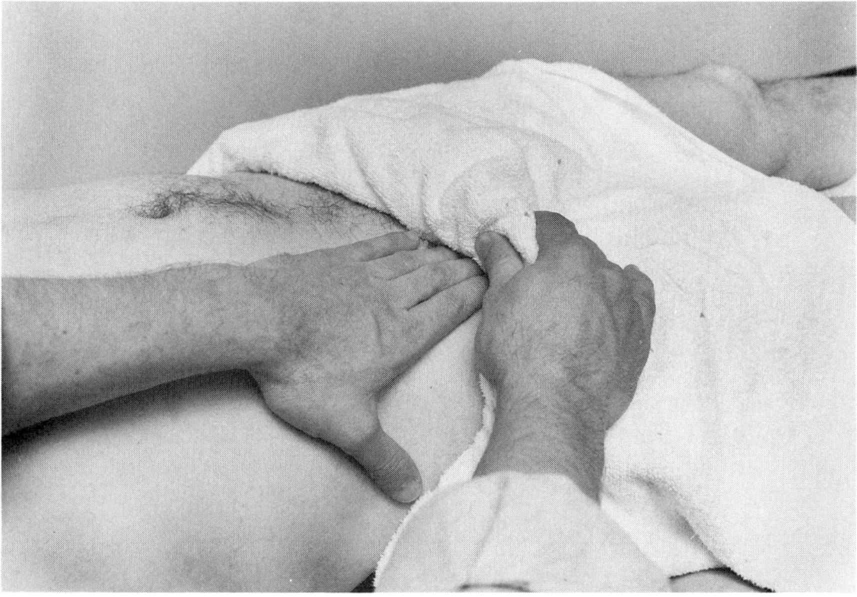

Fig. AIII-3. Palpating the inguinal lymph nodes, superficial to the inguinal ligament and then the femoral artery in the femoral triangle.

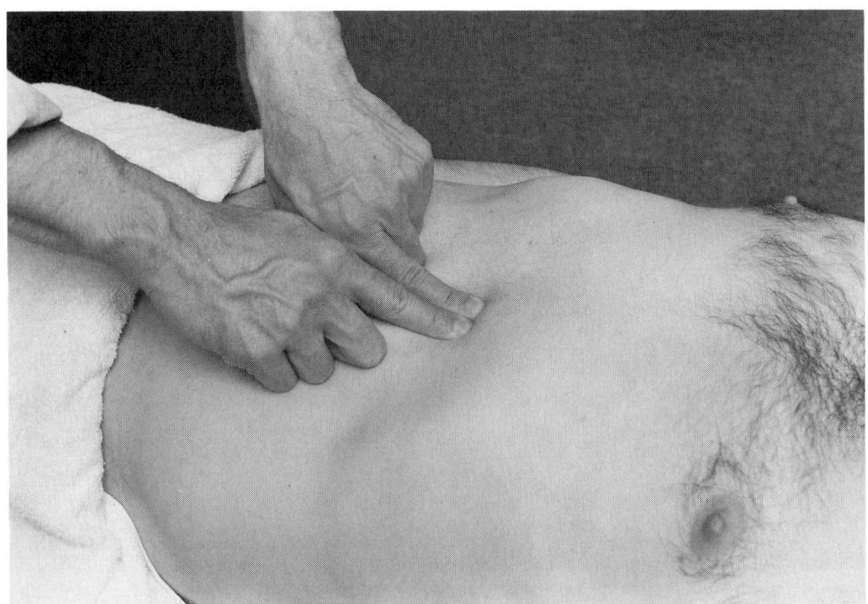

Fig. AIII-4. Assessing pulse at the aortic artery.

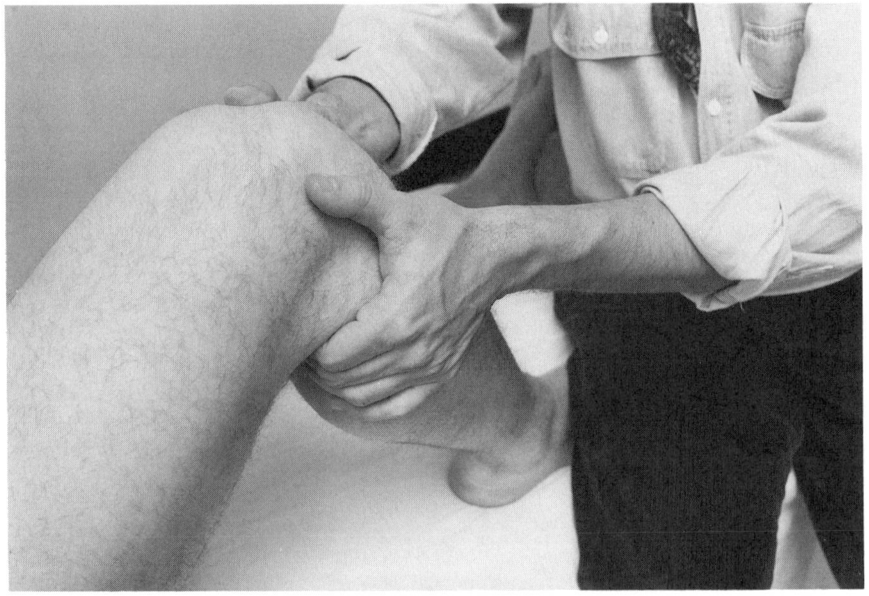

Fig. AIII-5. Assessing pulse at the popliteal artery in the popliteal fossa.

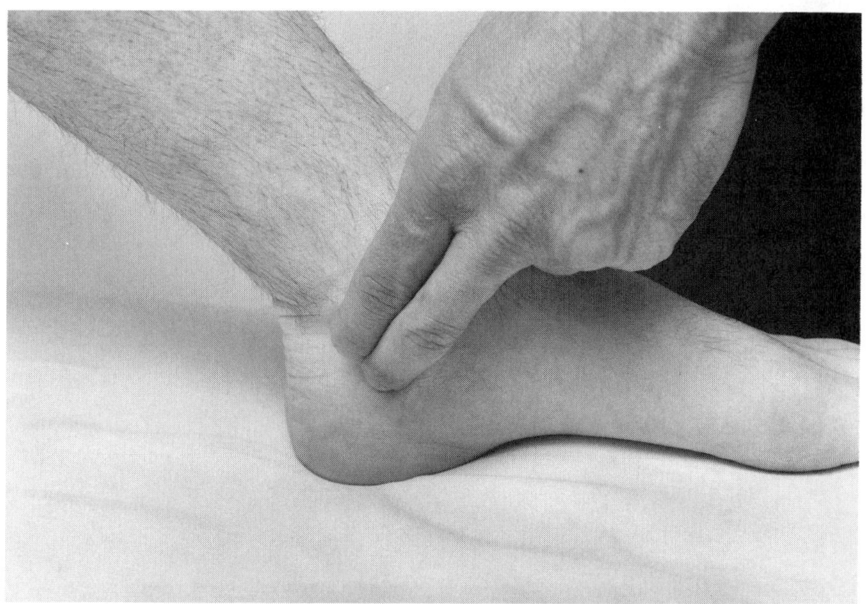

Fig. AIII-6. Assessing pulse at the posterior tibial artery, posterior to the medial malleolus.

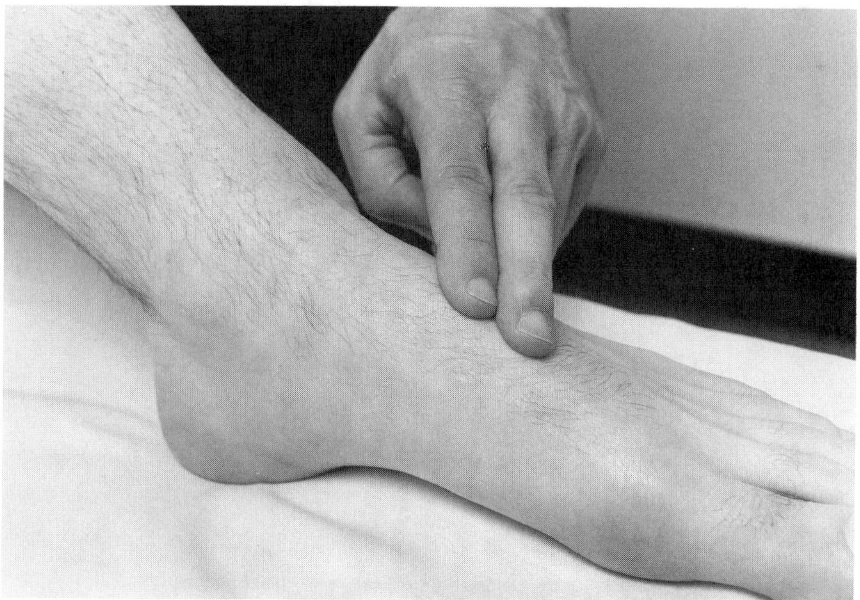

Fig. AIII-7. Assessing pulse at the dorsalis pedis artery between metatarsals I and II, proximal aspect.

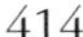

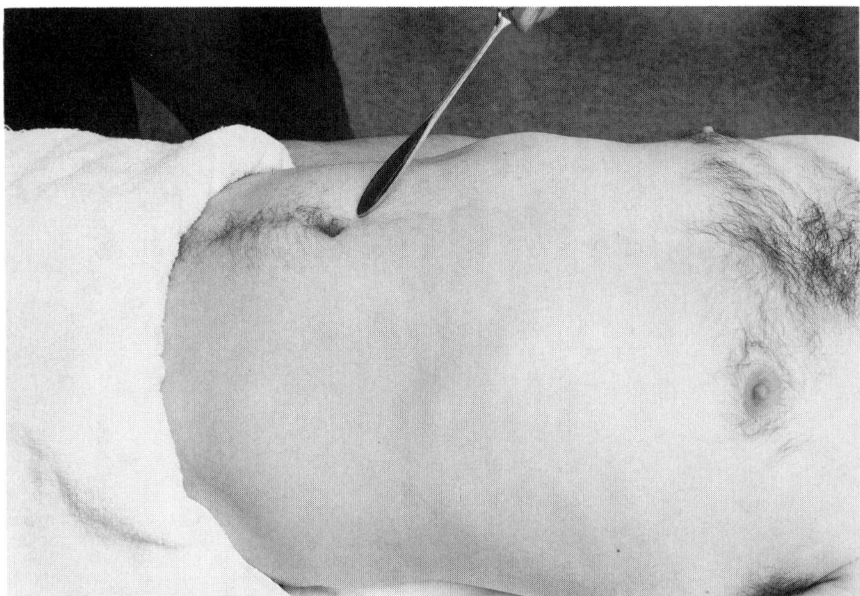

Fig. AIII-8. Assessing abdominal reflex, upper abdominal quadrant (T7–T10). Umbilicus should move toward the stimulus as the quadrant is stroked. Repeat for both left and right sides.

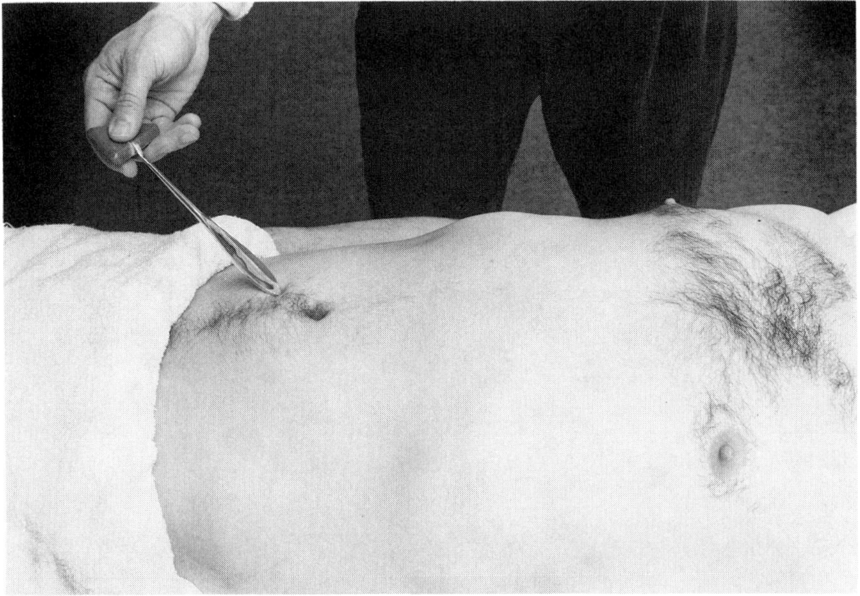

Fig. AIII-9. Assessing abdominal reflex, lower abdominal quadrant (T10–L1). Umbilicus should move toward stimulus as the quadrant is stroked. Repeat for both left and right sides.

IV Appendix: Glossary of Terms

Abscess: a focal collection of pus resulting from liquifactive necrosis of a tissue, usually caused by a pyogenic microorganism

Acetone: the simplistic ketone, formed by decarboxylation of acetoacetic acid and occurring in the blood and breath of persons with high concentrations of this acid in their blood

Acetylation: the introduction into a molecule of an acetyl group in replacement of a hydrogen atom

Acidosis: a disturbance of the acid–base state of the body toward the acid

Acinus: a rounded sac that opens into a small excretory duct in the terminal secretory portion of an exocrine gland

Acroparesthesia: paresthesia of the hands and feet

Acuity: sharpness, distinctness, acuteness

Adenohypophysis: the anterior lobe of the pituitary gland

Adenoma: a benign epithelial tumor of glandular structure; the cells may show evidence of glandular function, such as production of mucus and hormones

Adriamycin: a proprietary name for doxorubicin hydrochloride

Adventitia: the outermost layer of organs or structures that are not covered by a serous coat (e.g., the outermost layer of the three layers of an artery)

Agranulocytosis: the absence of granulocytes in the blood

Akathisia: the inability to sit down or remain seated because of motor restlessness and a sensation of muscular quivering that occurs as a side effect of neuroleptic drugs, especially phenothiazine; it is also an uncommon manifestation of Parkinson's disease

Akinesia: the inability to initiate movement

Amenorrhea: the absence of menstrual bleeding

Amyloid: starchlike

Amyloidosis: an incurable multisystemic disease process of uncertain etiology, characterized by the interstitial accumulation of amyloid fibrils; the affected tissues have a firm, waxy texture

Amyotrophy: muscular atrophy of neurogenic origin

Anabolic: any substance that increases the rate of metabolism in a cell or organism

Analgesic: causes loss of sensitivity to pain without loss of consciousness

Anaphylaxis: an acute or exaggerated allergic response in a sensitized host following injection of or exposure to a foreign protein or other substance

Anasarca: severe edema involving the entire body, including marked swelling of subcutaneous tissues and the accumulation of fluid in serous cavities

Anemia: an abnormal decrease in the concentration of erythrocytes, hemoglobin, or hematocrit, which may result from decreased production, increased loss, or destruction of erythrocytes; often accompanied by characteristic signs and symptoms including pallor, asthenia, and dyspnea

Anesthesia: partial or complete loss of all forms of sensation, such as cold, heat, pain, or touch, attributable to a lesion of the nervous system; conventionally the term *anesthesia* is often used to identify loss of touch sensation, while *analgesia* is more often used to identify loss of pain sensibility

Aneurysm: a saccular or fusiform outpouching of a layer or layers of an arterial wall, usually found in the elderly and thought to arise from a systemic collagen synthetic or structural defect

Angina: severe sore throat with implied quality of choking

Angina pectoris: a strangling sensation or heavy chest discomfort often radiating to the arms, especially the left, and usually precipitated by exertion; in current usage the term implies a cardiac ischemic origin

Angioma: a benign vascular tumor composed of blood or lymphatic vessels

Anhidrosis: a deficient production of sweat; also called *anaphoresis*

Ankylosis: stiffness or immobilization of a joint, resulting from injury, disease, or surgical intervention

Anorexia: a lack of appetite or desire for food

Anteflexion: a forward bend or curvature as in part of an organ; for example, a forward bending of the body of the uterus at its junction with the cervix

Anticholinergic: counteracting the action of acetylcholine, used especially with drugs that block conduction at cholinergic endings

Apnea: the absence or cessation of breathing

Arrhythmia: any variation from normal, regular rhythm, especially cardiac rhythm

Arthralgia: joint pain with objective findings of heat, redness, tenderness to touch, loss of motion, or swelling

Arthropathy: any joint disease

Ascites: the intraperitoneal accumulation of watery fluid in the nature of a transudate

Asthenia: a nonspecific symptom characterized by loss of energy and strength and a feeling of weakness; usually accompanies chronic debilitating conditions such as infectious diseases and cancer

Ataxia: unsteadiness, incoordination, or disorganization of movements in the absence of paralysis

Atelectasis: a state of airlessness and hence reduced volume, especially of the lung

Atheroma: a disorder of arterial walls characterized by degenerative changes, deposition of the lipid, proliferation of smooth muscle cells, and fibrosis

Basal: pertaining to or situated adjacent to the base of a structure or organ

Benign: relatively mild, likely to have a favorable outcome; not malignant, not having the potential for metastasis; describes a neoplasm

Bradycardia: a slow heart rate, usually defined as less than 60 beats per minute in adults

Bronchiectasis: abnormal dilatation of bronchi

Bronchophony: the auscultatory sound of the voice characteristically heard over an area of consolidation in the lung

Bruit: an auscultatory sound of murmur, especially when arising from the heart or vessels

Bruxism: a grinding or gnashing of the teeth in sleep

Buccal: relating to or in the direction of the cheek; in dentistry, used especially to describe the surface of a tooth facing the cheek or lips

Carcinoma: a spreading sore, ulcer, or cancer

Causalgia: a specific syndrome of severe, peculiar, unpleasant, and burning pain, often associated with smooth, shiny skin in the affected area; there may also be hypersensitivity to touch and temperature, following an incomplete lesion of a peripheral nerve

Cavitation: formation of a cavity or cavities

Chloasma: moth patch; melanoderm or melasma characterized by the occurrence of extensive brown patches of irregular shape and size on the skin of the face and elsewhere

Cholecystic: of or relating to the gallbladder

Cholecystitis: inflammation of the gallbladder

Cholinergic: denoting a synapse, nerve terminal, or aggragate of neurons for which the principle neurotransmitter is acetylcholine

Chondrogenic: giving rise to or forming cartilage

Chorea: a form of involuntary movement marked by fine, disorganized, and random movements of the extremities, usually affecting the hands and feet and involving the proximal limb and trunk muscles to a lesser extent

Choreiform: resembling the movements of chorea

Chronotropism: an alteration in the rate of a recurring phenomenon; for example, an alteration in heart rate

Claudication: lameness or limping, often associated with pain; cramplike pain and weakness in muscles, most often those of the calf with consequent lameness

Clonus: a repetitive rhythmical contraction and relaxation such as that which may occur in one phase of a convulsion, the similar phenomenon induced at a joint by stretching a muscle in a spastic limb, or one showing hyperreflexia

Coarctation: constriction or narrowing

Colic: relating to or associated with the colon, used primarily in anatomic terms; also, any of various conditions characterized by abdominal pain, especially paroxysmal pain occurring in a crescendo–decrescendo pattern, dependent upon visceral smooth muscle peristalsis

Constipation: the condition in which bowel movements are delayed or inadequate; undue retention of feces in the large intestine

Cyanosis: a bluish discoloration, particularly of the skin or mucous membranes, due to an excessive proportion of reduced hemoglobin in the blood, to stagnation of blood in capillaries of the skin or mucous membranes, or to the presence of methemoglobin, sulfhemoglobin, or other abnormal pigments

Cystitis: acute or chronic inflammation of the urinary bladder

Cystocele: a defect of the pelvic supporting structures causing a prolapse of the bladder into the vagina, clinically manifested by varying degrees of frequency, urgency, incontinence, dysuria, and mechanical discomfort

Cytotoxic: having the effect of poisoning or destroying cells, as a drug or infective organism

Dactylitis: inflammation or infection of a finger

Delirium: an organic brain syndrome characterized by clouding of consciousness, difficulty in sustaining attention, impaired orientation in memory, and perceptual disturbances leading to hallucinations

Dementia: a state in which there is a significant loss of intellectual capacity and cognitive functioning leading to impairment in social or occupational functioning, or both

Diaphoretic: an agent capable of inducing sweating

Diarrhea: abnormal fecal discharge characterized by frequent and/or watery stool

Diastole: the period of atrial and ventricular myocardial relaxation in the cardiac cycle

Diplopia: the seeing of a single object as double, usually resulting from misalignment of the two eyes, but sometimes due to optical faults such as variations of density and consequently of refractive index within the crystaline lens

Discoid: roughly disk shaped or characterized by disk-shaped lesions

Diuretic: inducing a state of increased urine flow

Diverticulum: a localized sac or pouch formed in the wall of a hollow viscus and opening into its lumen

Dysesthesia: abnormal spontaneous sensation, often with an unpleasant quality; for example, itching, pins and needles, burning, or sensation as of hot or cold water, or of an electric shock; these are symptoms of disease or dysfunction of sensory pathways

Dyskinesia: any abnormality of movement, such as incoordination, spasm, or irregular or ill-formed movements

Dysmenorrhea: painful menstruation; the colicky lower abdominal pain of ovulatory menstruation

Dyspareunia: coitus associated with recurrent, persistent genital pain

Dyspepsia: indigestion and upset stomach; a functional disturbance of the upper gastrointestinal tract characterized by abdominal discomfort, bloating, and, to a variable degree, nausea

Dysphagia: difficulty in swallowing; a sensation of food sticking in the esophagus

Dysphonia: abnormal phonation; an abnormal low-pitched, rough vocalization produced not by the vocal cords, but by the ventricular bands, often occurring when an attempt is made to disguise some underlying vocal cord disease

Dysphoria: a feeling of unpleasantness or discomfort

Dyspnea: shortness of breath; labored or difficult breathing; breathlessness

Dysrhythmia: disordered or abnormal rhythm

Dystonia: any abnormality of muscle tone

Dysuria: painful or difficult urination, generally caused by lower urinary tract disease such as cystitis, urethritis, urethral stricture, and prostatic disease

Ectopic: out of place, outside the usual range of locations or relationships, or abnormally exposed to view

Egophony: a vocal sound likened to the bleating of a goat, heard on auscultation of the chest over pleural effusion

Embolus: a thrombus formed within or a foreign material introduced into the vascular tree and carried by the bloodstream to a site where it lodges and obstructs further flow of blood

Empyema: the accumulation of pus in a cavity, especially in the thoracic cavity

Endocrine: secreting into the bloodstream; describes a gland that delivers a substance into the circulation, causing that substance to have an effect at a remote site

Endogenous: originating within an organism or resulting from causes within the organism

Enteric: of or relating to the intestine, especially the small intestine; intended to be dissolved or digested in the intestine but not in the stomach; describes capsules and pill coatings that protect their contents from the action of gastric juice

Enthesitis: traumatic disease occurring at the insertion of muscles where recurring concentration of muscle stress provokes inflammation, with a strong tendency toward fibrosis and calcification

Enuresis: incontinence of urine with full bladder emptying, after the age at which bladder control should have been attained

Epigastrium: the wall of the abdomen above the naval

Epiphenomenon: an incidental event or symptom occurring as an accompaniment of a disease, but not essentially or typically with it

Erythema: an increased redness of the skin that is caused by capillary dilation

Exocrine: secreting in the direction of the body surface, usually through a duct

Exogenous: produced or otherwise originating outside the organism

Extroversion: a personality trait that orients one toward external events, other people, and social interactions rather than toward inner feelings or thoughts

Fibrillation: spontaneous contraction of single muscle fibers that can be recorded electromyographically and that is usually a manifestation of denervation, with wallerian degeneration of at least some motor axons

Fugue: a condition in which the subject takes leave of usual activities and wanders about; typically, the individual suffers from amnesia for the period he is absent from his usual activities

Functional: of or relating to a function; specifically, serving to contribute to the operation of a bodily function; having no known organic cause as in *functional disorder*

Goiter: any diffuse or nodular enlargement or swelling of the thyroid gland, often visible as a prominence in the lower anterior neck

Gynecology: the branch of medicine devoted to the care and prevention of genital tract disorders in women that for the most part is not concerned with pregnancy

Gynecomastia: enlargement of the male breast, occurring sometimes in a mild form as a normal phenomenon of male puberty and as a sequela of various pathologic conditions

Hemarthrosis: a hemorrhage into a joint

Hematochezia: the passage of bright red, easily identifiable blood from the anus, usually a sign of fresh bleeding distal to the ileocecal valve

Hematoma: a localized accumulation of blood in a tissue or space

Hematuria: excretion of urine containing blood either gross or microscopic

Hemianesthesia: loss of sensation on one side of the body

Hemiballismus: a syndrome manifested by a sudden onset of violent, writhing, involuntary movements, often of wide excursion and confined to one-half of the body

Hemoptysis: the expectoration of blood

Hemothorax: a collection of blood within the pleural cavity

Hepatic: of or relating to the liver

Hirsutism: the growth of hair in a woman in the male sexual pattern

Hormone: any substance secreted by specialized cells in the endocrine glands, in clusters, or diffusely spread through the brain, lungs, and gastrointestinal tract; the substances act upon specific target tissues more or less remote from the site of secretion or upon the regulation of metabolic processes throughout the organism

Hydrocele: an accumulation of serous fluid in a body cavity, especially between the visceral and parietal layers of the tunica vaginalis in the scrotum

Hyperacusis: a condition in which sounds are perceived as unduly loud

Hyperalgesia: excessive sensitivity to painful stimuli

Hypercapnia: an elevated concentration of carbon dioxide in the blood

Hyperemia: increase in blood volume to a part or tissue owing to arterial or arteriolar dilatation

Hyperesthesia: exaggerated sensibility

Hyperparathyroidism: a condition resulting from excessive secretion of parathyroid hormone by the parathyroid glands

Hyperplasia: increase in the number of cells in a tissue or an organ with concomitant increase in the size of the structure involved

Hypertension: abnormally high tension or pressure; applied especially to the systemic arterial or pulmonary arterial blood pressure

Hyperthyroidism: excessive secretion of thyroxine and/or triiodothyronine from the thyroid gland, accompanied by increased rate of oxygen consumption, accelerated basal metabolic rate, thyroid enlargement, and systemic disturbances

Hypoesthesia: reduction in sensitivity

Hypokalemia: an abnormally low concentration of potassium in the blood or blood serum

Hypokinesia: a reduction in motor activity or in the range of motion of the body or limbs

Hyponychium: the part of the fingertip that extends from the distal end of the nail bed to the distal crease on the palmar aspect of the finger; corresponds to the pulp of the finger

Hypoparathyroidism: a condition resulting from subnormal or absent secretion of parathyroid hormone by the parathyroid glands

Hypophysis: an unpaired, ovoid body that lies below the hypothalamus in the pituitary fossa of the sella turcica; the pituitary gland

Hypothyroidism: deficient hormone secretion by the thyroid gland or the condition resulting from it

Hypoxemia: reduced oxygen concentration in arterial blood

Hypoxia: inadequate oxygen concentration in body tissues

Impotence: a dysfunction in which the male is unable to perform the sexual act

Incontinence: absence of voluntary control of an expiratory function, especially defecation or urination

Infarct: a discreet, usually wedge-shaped area of ischemic coagulative necrosis caused by interruption of blood flow

Inotropic: affecting the force of speed of muscular contraction by either enhancing or inhibiting it

Intima: an innermost layer

Introversion: the dynamic process in personality development by which the psychic energy of the individual is directed inwardly toward the self

Ischemia: inadequate blood flow to a part or organ

Isoelectric: possessing the same electric potential

Jaundice: yellow discoloration of the skin and membranes, resulting from hyperbilirubinemia and subsequent deposition of bile pigment in the involved structure

Ketoacidosis: a metabolic acidosis associated with an accumulation of ketone bodies that are characteristic of uncontrolled diabetes mellitus

Leukorrhea: a gynecologic disorder characterized by an abnormal, whitish, nonbloody discharge from the genital tract

Libido: the energy of the sexual drive in Freud's psychoanalytic psychology; often includes the energy of the aggressive drive as well

Lingula: a small structure or process shaped like or suggestive of a tongue

Lysis: any form of dissolution, particularly the breaking of membrane-bound structures such as cells

Malaise: a feeling of untoward weakness, lethargy, or discomfort as of impending illness

Malar: pertaining to the cheek

Malignant: tending to destroy, harm, or kill; as malignant tumor

Mania: a syndrome consisting of elated although unstable mood, hyperactivity, mental overactivity, and expressed garrulousness

Media: a middle layer

Melena: the passage of dark or blackish, tarlike stools stained with altered blood

Meningioma: a tumor of the cellular elements of the meninges; most often attached to the dura, especially where arachnoid villi are numerous

Menopause: the immediate postreproductive phase of a woman's life, when menstrual function ceases due to failure to form ovarian follicles and ova

Menorrhagia: excessive or prolonged menstruation

Metastasis: the transfer of a disease from one body site to another; said especially of cancers and infectious diseases

Metrorrhagia: uterine bleeding occurring at times other than the expected menses

Micturition: urination

Murmur: a prolonged or continuous auscultatory sound, particularly one deriving from the heart or cardiovascular system

Myalgia: pain in the muscles

Myelogenous: the development of bone marrow

Myeloma: a neoplastic proliferation of plasma cells, characterized by bone tumors and often complicated by pathologic fractures

Myopathy: any disease of skeletal or voluntary muscle

Myxedema: the condition that accompanies severe hypothyroidism, characterized by yellowish pallor and nonpitting edema, especially in the face with scanty hair in the eyebrows, periorbital puffiness, and thick lips

Myxoma: a benign but often infiltrating growth of unknown histogenesis

Narcissism: the stage and development of object relationships that follow the autoerotic or sematogenic stage

Necrosis: the morphologic changes that follow cell death, characterized most frequently by nuclear changes

Neoplasm: a benign or malignant expanding lesion composed of proliferating cells; a tumor

Neurohypophysis: the posterior lobe of the pituitary gland

Neurosis: any of various functional disorders of behavior characterized by excessive anxiety, by behavior distorted by an exaggerated use of avoidance behaviors, or by other recognized mechanisms for defending against anxiety

Neutropenia: a decreased number of neutrophils in the circulating blood

Nidus: a focus of origin, such as a collection of bacteria in infections or the point of precipitation in calculus formation

Nociception: pain sense

Nociceptive: responsiveness of sensitivity to noxious stimuli capable of eliciting pain

Nociperception: recognition by the nervous system or an organism of a traumatic or hurtful stimulus

Nocturia: urination during normal sleeping hours

Nosology: the science of the systematic classification of diseases

Nystagmus: spontaneous, rapid, rhythmic movement of the eyes, occurring either on fixation or on occular movement, and often due to faulty supranuclear or internuclear innervation

Obstetrics: the field of medicine dealing with the care of women during pregnancy, labor, delivery, and the postpartum period

Occult: not readily apparent or detectable; hidden or disguised, as an infection, presence of blood, or a tumor

Oculogyric: describing, pertaining to, or producing spontaneous or sustained occular movements, usually in an upward direction as in Parkinson's disease

Oligoarthritis: arthritis of a few joints

Onychia: an inflammation of the nail matrix, either following trauma or accompanying paronychia

Onycholysis: a separation of the nail plate from the nail bed

Opisthotonos: spasmodic contraction of the muscles of the neck and back with arching of the body; when severe, subjects may rest only on their head and heels

Orchitis: inflammation of the testes, manifested by swelling and tenderness and usually of infectious origin, as in tuberculosis, mumps, syphyllis, or certain fungal diseases

Organic: of or relating to an organ, structural in nature or origin as in organic defect

Orthopnea: shortness of breath experienced when lying down

Orthostatic: relating to the erect posture

Osteogenesis: the process by which bone tissue and the bones of the skeleton are formed, including all stages of bone formation, not just mineralization

Osteolysis: the resorption of bone, especially its mineralized component

Osteopenia: a reduction in bone mass that is caused by decreased osteoid formation and the presence of normal bone resorption; any decrease in bone density or mass below normal amounts

Osteoporosis: a reduction in the quantity and quality of bone by the loss of both bone marrow and protein content

Pallor: paleness due to lack of melanin or lack of blood in the skin

Palpitation: the sensation produced by rapid, forceful, or irregular beating of the heart

Papilloma: a benign tumor of skin, mucous membrane, and ducts, composed of epithelium covering a fibrous stalk

Paradoxical: possibly true, but appearing to contradict facts or confirmed opinion

Parenchyma: the characteristic or functional tissue or cells of a gland or an organ

Paresthesia: any sensation, such as pins and needles, burning, or prickling, that occurs spontaneously without external cause in disease or dysfunction of the central or peripheral nervous system

Paronychia: an inflammation of the proximal or lateral nail folds

Paroxysm: a sudden attack or sharp intensification

Pericarditis: inflammation of the pericardium

Perineum: the diamond-shaped area superficial to the inferior pelvic aperture

Peristalsis: successive waves of contraction passing for shorter or longer distances along tubular muscular organs such as the alimentary tract

Phobia: pathologic fear, dread, avoidance, or abhorrence

Photophobia: an abnormal intolerance of light, usually due to inflammation of the iris and ciliary body

Pneumothorax: the presence of air in the pleural cavity

Polyarthritis: arthritis of multiple joints

Polydipsia: the drinking of water in abnormally large quantities

Polymyositis: an inflammatory autoimmune disorder of muscle, related to other disorders of the collagen or connective tissue group

Polyneuropathy: any systemic infection of the peripheral nerves of toxic, metabolic, or unknown etiology

Polyp: any mass of tissue that protrudes outward from a surface, usually an epithelium

Polyuria: the formation of urine in abnormally large volume, reflected by frequency and by volume of urination

Premonitory: forewarning, give advance notice

Prognathism: the characteristic of having a projected jaw; an abnormally anterior anatomic position of the mandible

Proteinuria: urinary excretion of abnormal amounts of protein; normally, up to 150 mg of protein may be excreted per 24 hours

Psyche: the mind in contradistinction to the body

Psychogenic: of psychological or mental origin

Psychosis: a class of mental disorders that usually includes organic mental disorders, schizophrenias, major affect disorders, and certain paranoid states

Ptosis: the prolapse or downward displacement of an organ; commonly used to describe abnormal downward displacement of the upper eyelid, which can result from paralysis of the third cranial nerve

Purpura: a focal hemorrhage into the skin

Pyelography: roentgenography of the renal pelvis after the use of a contrast agent

Pyelonephritis: inflammation of the renal pelvis and parenchyma due to bacterial infection

Pyogenic: able to cause formation of purulent lesions in tissues

Pyuria: the presence of an abnormal number of leukocytes or pus in the urine, reflecting urinary tract inflammation such as that resulting from infection

Rale: an abnormal sound heard on auscultation of the chest during breathing, especially one that is caused or seems to be caused by air passing through fluid in the airways

Rhonchus: an abnormal sound heard on auscultation of the lungs, ranging from a wheeze to a snoring sound and due to air passing through a partially obstructed or narrowed airway

Roentgenogram: radiograph

Roentgenography: a special radiologic technique that demonstrates, on film, the details of structures in a predetermined plane of tissue while blurring the details of structures in other planes

Sarcoidosis: a disease of unknown cause characterized by noncaseating granulomas in many organs of the body; the most commonly involved tissues are those of the lungs, lymph nodes, and liver

Scintigraphy: a clinical diagnostic procedure consisting of an injection, usually intravenous, of a solution containing a radioactive agent with a specific affinity for an organ or tissue of interest, followed by the determination of the distribution of radioactivity

Sclerosis: a hardening of the interstitial connective tissue following damage to the parenchyma of an organ; hardening is due to increases in the amount of interstitial fiber connective tissue

Scotoma: a circumscribed area of blindness or reduced vision within the visual field

Sepsis: a syndrome resulting from overwhelming invasion of the circulation by pathogenic microorganisms or the toxins they produce

Septicemia: severe generalized infection resulting from hematogenous dissemination of pathogenic microorganisms and their toxins

Serotonin: a neurotransmitter with action on blood vessels; it also acts as a hormone and is formed by the decarboxylation of 5-hydroxytryptophan

Soma: all the body tissues except germ cells; the body as distinct from the mind or psyche

Somatic: relating to or involving the skeleton or skeletal muscle as distinct from the viscera of the body; also relating to or involving the body as distinct from the mind or psyche

Somnolence: unnatural sleepiness or drowsiness

Souffle: a soft, blowing murmur, especially an extracardiac murmur

Spermatogenesis: a series of stages and cellular differentiations resulting in the formation of spermatozoa

Splenomegally: enlargement of the spleen

Spondylitis: an inflammation of one or more vertebrae

Spondylolisthesis: a forward displacement of one vertebra upon the other, usually in the lower lumbar spine, due to either a traumatic or congenital weakness defect of the pars interarticularis

Spondylolysis: the breaking down of a vertebra

Spondylosis: a noninflammatory disease of the spine, usually osteoarthritis and/or degenerative disk disease

Squama: a scalelike or thin platelike structure

Stasis: a cessation or reduction of flow or movement

Stridor: a harsh, high-pitched noise on breathing, especially on inspiration, indicative of a degree of obstruction of the airway, especially of the larynx or trachea

Syncope: transient loss of consciousness due to generalized cerebral ischemia secondary to a global reduction in cerebral blood flow

Systole: the contraction phase of the atria or ventricles in a cardiac cycle

Tachycardia: a fast heart rate; term applied when adult heart rate exceeds 100 per minute

Tachypnea: rapid breathing

Tamponade: compression of the heart due to accumulation of fluid

Tardive: characterized by lateness or delay; said especially of a condition with late-emerging signs and symptoms

Tetany: a syndrome marked by a state of neuromuscular hyperexcitability, which may cause reversible muscular contractures, particularly in the extremities

Thrombus: a semisolid aggregate of blood cells enmeshed in fibrin and clumps of platelets that results from the rapid conversion of fibrinogen to fibrin, especially within a blood vessel

Thyrotoxicosis: a condition resulting from hyperthyroidism due to any cause

Tinnitus: any form of adventitious noise arising within the ears or head and audible to the subject; the nature of the noise may be whistling, ringing, clicking, or pulsating, and in some instances may be audible to others

Tomography: a radiologic examination in which a thin, collimated x-ray beam rotates about the patient with registration of photon exit doses on detectors; the exit doses then undergo manipulation by computer to produce an image of the slice of tissue examined

Trismus: spasm or contracture of the masticatory muscles, making it difficult to open the mouth

Trophic: having to do with nutrition; pertaining to that which stimulates growth and development or stimulates increased activity; pertaining to nutritional changes in skin and other tissues that may follow impairment of a nerve supply

Tumor: an expanding lesion due to progressive, apparently uncontrolled proliferation of cells; a neoplasm

Turgor: the condition of being swollen or extended

Tympany: a low-pitched, drumlike sound produced by percussion over an air-filled region, especially in the stomach and intestine or in the peritoneal and pleural cavities

Varix: a mass composed of enlarged and tortuous blood or lymphatic vessels

Vegetative: engaged in or relating to the process of nutrition or growth as distinct from reproduction; also pertaining to involuntary bodily functions or to the autonomic nervous system

Vertigo: a hallucination of movement, especially of rotation, of the subject or of his or her surroundings

Vesicle: a small sac, cyst, pouch, or follicle

Vesicular: designating a soft auscultatory breath sound presumably originating in the pulmonary vesicles and generally characteristic of the normal lung

Wheeze: a high-pitched, more or less musical nonvocal sound emitted during breathing, usually audible subjectively and without auscultation; it is usually produced by bronchial, tracheal, or laryngeal constriction or obstruction

Index

Note: Page numbers followed by *f* indicate figures; page numbers followed by *t* indicate tables.

A

Abdomen
  bloating of, in females, 147
  palpation of, 17, 411f
  percussion of, 17
Abdominal hernia, 109, 111–112
Abdominal reflexes, 18–19, 414f
Abducens nerve (cranial nerve V), testing of, 213–214, 216f
Abscesses
  epidural, 247
  pelvic, in females, 148
  perinephric, in males, 124
Accelerated junctional beats, 56
Accessory nerve (cranial nerve XI), testing of, 217
Acetaminophen, 328
Achilles tendon, rupture of, imaging of, 385f, 385–386
Acoustic neuromas, headache and, 182
Acromegaly, 158, 167–168
  subjective and objective changes in, 170t
Action potentials, cardiac, 35
Adaptive mechanisms, personality and, 279–280
Addison's disease, 167
  subjective and objective changes in, 170t
Adenohypophysis, 158
Adjustment, to disability, 290
Adjustment disorder, 290
Adrenal gland
  diseases of, 166–167
    Addison's disease, 167, 170t
    Cushing syndrome, 166, 167t, 170t
    metabolic bone disease and, 241
  hormones of, 157t
Adrenocortical hyperactivity, 166, 167t
  subjective and objective changes in, 170t
Adrenocortical insufficiency, 167
  subjective and objective changes in, 170t
Adult respiratory distress syndrome, 97
Adventitia, 33, 34f
Adventitious breath sounds, 76, 80–82. *See also* Rales.
  rhonchi, 51, 82, 94
  stridor, 82
Affective disorders, 283–287. *See also* Depression.
  bipolar disease, 283, 286t, 286–287
  clinical presentation of, 285–286, 286t
  diagnosis of, 284–285, 285t
  epidemiology of, 283
  etiology of, 283–284, 284t
  seasonal, 287
Afterload, 38
Aggressive patients, 358–359, 360t
Agitated patients, 358–359, 360t
Agitation-aggression rating scale, 359, 360t
β-Agonists, for asthma, 347, 347t
Airways obstruction, blood gases in, 87
Akinesia, in Parkinson's disease, 211
Alcohol abuse, 290–291
Alerting response, headache and, 180–181
"Allergic" headache, 184
Allergic reactions
  of skin, 310
  skin lesions due to, 309, 310
Alternate heel to knee and toe test, 219
Amantadine (Symmetrel), 342
Ambien (zolpidem), 340
Amiodarone, for arrhythmias, 338t, 338–339
Amoxapine, 341, 341t
Amygdala, 193
Amyotrophic lateral sclerosis (ALS), 202
Amyotrophy, diabetic, 160t, 161–162
Analgesics. *See* Nonsteroidal anti-inflammatory agents (NSAIAs); Opioids; Salicylates.
Aneurysms, 41, 50, 50f, 112
  aortic. *See* Aortic aneurysms.
  rupture of, headache caused by, 182–183
Angina pectoris, 39–40, 49
  in aortic stenosis, 60
  atypical, 39
  drug therapy for, 336–337, 338t
  exercise tolerance testing in, 56
  Prinzmetal, 40
  stable, 40
  typical, 39
  variant, 40
Angiotensin, 119
Angiotensin-converting enzyme (ACE) inhibitors
  for congestive heart failure, 336
  for hypertension, 333, 333t, 334
Ankles
  edema of, 48
  imaging of, 383–386, 384f
    in osteonecrosis, 384
    of soft tissue abnormalities, 385f, 385–386
    of stress fractures, 384
Ankylosing spondylitis (AS), 261, 263t, 264f
  back pain in, 263
  cervical spine in, 267
  cervical stenosis in, 266
Annular lesions of skin, 309
Annulus fibrosis, bulging, imaging of, 376
Antacids, for peptic ulcer disease, 344
Anterior compartment syndrome, 40
Anterior cord syndrome, 209
Anterior cruciate ligament (ACL) injuries, imaging of, 381
Anteroposterior (AP) film, 366

Antidepressants, 340–341
mechanism of action of, 340
monoamine oxidase inhibitors, 341, 341t
newer, 341, 341t
tricyclic, 340–341, 341t
Antidiuretic hormone (ADH). *See* Vasopressin.
Antiepileptic drugs (AEDs), 343–344, 344t
Antinuclear antibodies (ANA), in systemic lupus erythematosus, 258
Antisocial personality disorder, 282
Anxiety disorders, generalized, 287
Anxious personality disorders, 282–283
Aorta, 32, 32f
occlusive disease of, 61
Aortic aneurysms, 17, 39, 61
dissecting, 39, 61
rupture of, 61
Aortic artery pulse, palpation of, 412f
Aortic valve, 35
regurgitation of, 60
stenosis of, 39, 59–60
Aortitis, 61
Apical pulse, 49
Apnea, 95, 98
Apocrine glands, 305
Arrhythmias, 41–42, 43f, 49, 53, 56–57
drug therapy for, 338t, 338–339
Arterial insufficiency, 40
Arteries, 32, 33, 34f. *See also specific arteries.*
reactivity of, 41
Arteriovenous malformations, headache and, 183
Arthritis, 259–261
enteropathic, 261, 263t
joints commonly involved in, 260, 260f
osteoarthritis, 259–260, 260f
psoriatic, 261, 263t
reactive, 261, 263t
rheumatoid. *See* Rheumatoid arthritis (RA).
septic, acute, 270
spondyloarthropathies, 261, 263t, 264f
Arthropathy, crystalline, acute, 271
Aseptic necrosis. *See* Osteonecrosis.
Aspirin, 324, 325t, 325–326, 326t
Asthma, 94
drug therapy for, 347t, 347–348
Ataxic gait, cerebellar lesions and, 211
Atherosclerosis, 47–48, 54, 61
headache and, 183
Atlantoaxial subluxation, imaging of, 371
Atria, of heart, 32
Atrial systole, 33, 35
Atrial tachycardia, 56
Atrioventricular block. *See* Heart block.
Attenuation, 366
Auscultation, 17–18
apical, 42
in cardiovascular disease, 50–51
in gastrointestinal system disease, 110, 111f
of heart, 35–36, 37f
of lungs, 70–75, 72f, 73f. *See also* Breath sounds; Vocal sounds.
pleural friction rub and, 82
in pulmonary system disease, 90, 94, 96, 99
in thyroid disease, 162
Autonomic dysreflexia, 354
Autonomic nervous system (ANS), 194
Autonomic neuropathy, diabetic, 161
Avascular necrosis. *See* Osteonecrosis.
Avoidant personality disorder, 282

B

Babinski reflex, testing of, 220, 220f, 410f
Back pain
algorithm for evaluation of, 249, 250f
lumbar, imaging in, 375–376, 376, 376f
mechanical, 263
in osteomyelitis, 246–247
in osteoporosis, 241
patient case studies of, 22, 27–28, 28f
in rheumatic disease, 261, 263, 265–266
ankylosing spondylitis, 263
danger signs and, 263, 265
inflammatory back pain, 263
spinal stenosis and, 265f, 265–266
Baclofen, 332
Bacteremia, 246
Bacterial endocarditis, 60
Baker's cyst, imaging of, 382
Ballism, 211
"Bamboo spine," in ankylosing spondylitis, 261, 264f
Basal cell carcinoma, of skin, 16, 311
Basal ganglia
anatomy of, 202
calcification of, in hypoparathyroidism, 166
lesions of, 210–211
Beau's lines, 16
Beck Depression Inventory (BDI), 293
Behavioral assessment, 292
Behavioral rehabilitation programs, for chronic pain syndrome, 296
Benadryl (diphenhydramine), 342
Benign hypermobility syndrome, 269–270
Benzodiazepines, 339–340, 340t
Benztropine (Cogentin), 342
Bepridil, 335
Biliary tree, anatomy and physiology of, 105
Bipolar disease, 283, 286t, 286–287
drug therapy for, 342
Bladder
alteration of function of, 354–355
anatomy and physiology of, 117, 118f, 120f
cancer of, 126–127
infection of, in males, 125
Bleeding
abnormal, 149
vaginal, 146. *See also* Menstrual physiology.
Blisters, 310
α_1-Blockers, for hypertension, 333, 333t, 335
β-Blockers
for angina pectoris, 337
for hypertension, 333, 333t, 334
Blood gases, in pulmonary system disease, 87
Blood pH, in pulmonary system disease, 87
Blood pressure, 38, 38f, 50. *See also* Hypertension; Hypotension.
in cardiovascular disease, 51–52
diastolic, 38, 38f, 52
in dyspnea, 47
measurement of, 42
monitoring of, 55–56
in pregnancy, 143–144, 145
pulse, 38, 38f, 52
systolic, 38, 38f, 52
Blood vessels, in Cushing's syndrome, 166
Blue nevus, 311
Bone(s)
bowing of, in Paget's disease, 244, 245f
demineralization of. *See* Osteoporosis.
fractures of. *See* Fractures; pathologic fractures; Stress fractures.
metabolic disease of, 340–345
osteoporosis. *See* Osteoporosis.
Paget's disease, 244–245, 245f
physiology of, 241, 242f
tumors of, 224t, 224–226
age and, 225, 226t
benign and malignant, 224, 226t
chondrogenic, 228–231, 230f–233f
clinical features of, 225, 225f, 226t
metastatic, 234–235, 237–240
osteogenic, 227f, 227–228, 229f
patient referral for, 225–226
vertebrae. *See* Cervical spine; Lumbar spine; Spine; Thoracic spine.
Bone scans, 368–369, 372
Bony pelvis, female, anatomy and physiology of, 133–134, 134f, 135f
Borderline personality disorder, 282
Bowel function, alteration of, 354–355

Bowel sounds, 110
Brachial plexus lesions, 203, 206t, 207t, 208f
Brachial pulse, palpation of, 49, 50, 407f
Bradycardia, sinus, 53, 56
Bradykinesia, in Parkinson's disease, 211
Brain
anatomy of, 192–193
tumors of, 210
headache and, 181–182
Brain stem
anatomy of, 192
lesions of, 209
motor function of, 199
"Break" test, for motor neuron lesions, 218
Breasts
cancer of
skeletal metastases of, 238
treatment of, 238
fibrocystic disease of, 146–147
tenderness of, 146–147
Breathing. *See also* Respiration.
patterns of, in pulmonary system disease, 89–90
shortness of breath and. *See* Dyspnea.
Breathlessness. *See* Dyspnea.
Breath sounds, 70–75, 76–77, 78–82
adventitious. *See* Adventitious breath sounds; Rales.
in cardiovascular disease, 50–51
of left lung, 74–75
normal, 78–80
bronchial, 79, 83
bronchovesicular, 71–75, 80, 80f
diminished, 80
tracheal, 78
vesicular. *See* Vesicular breath sounds.
of right lung, 71–74, 72f, 73f
in ventilatory muscle dysfunction, 96
vesicular. *See* Vesicular breath sounds.
Bronchial breath sounds, 79, 83
Bronchodilators. *See also specific drugs.*
for asthma, 347t, 347–348
for pulmonary system disease, 85, 85t
Bronchophony, 77–78
Bronchopulmonary segments, 69–71, 70f, 71t, 72f, 73f
Bronchospasm, 94
Bronchovesicular breath sounds, 71–75, 80, 80f
Brown-Sequard syndrome, 208
Bruce treadmill protocol, 55–56
Bruits, 110
Bug bites, 311
Bulging annulus fibrosis, imaging of, 376
Bulla, 308f, 318
Bupropion, 341, 341t
Burrow, 319
Bursae
infections of, 247
pain in, in rheumatic disease, 258
Bypass tract conduction, 57

C

CAGE questionnaire, 291
Calcification, of basal ganglia, in hypoparathyroidism, 166
Calcific tendinitis, of shoulder, imaging of, 387
Calcium, osteoporosis and, 241, 244
Calcium channel blockers
for angina pectoris, 337
for congestive heart failure, 336, 337t
for hypertension, 333, 333t, 335
Calluses, 310
Calor, 245. *See also* Temperature.
Cancellous bone, 241
Cancer. *See also specific cancers and anatomic sites.*
back pain in, 263
metastatic. *See* Metastases.
screening for, 240
splenic enlargement and, 108
Capillaries, 32, 33
Carafate (sucralfate), for peptic ulcer disease, 344, 345
Carbamazepine (Tegretol), 343, 344t
Cardiac catheterization
in aortic stenosis, 60
in coronary artery disease, 55
in heart failure, 58
Cardiac cycle, mechanical events of, 35–36, 36f, 37f
Cardiac index (CI), 37
Cardiac output, 36–38
Cardiac shunt, 49
Cardiac tamponade, 61
Cardiomyopathy
hypertrophic, 39
ischemic, 57
restrictive, 57
Cardiovascular disorders, 39–65
angina. *See* Angina pectoris.
aortic, 61. *See also* Aortic aneurysm.
arrhythmias. *See* Arrhythmias.
in chronic renal failure, 129
coronary artery disease. *See* Coronary artery disease (CAD).
differentiation from musculoskeletal dysfunction, 31
drug therapy for, 335–336, 336t
electrocardiography in, 52–53
endocarditis, 60
heart failure. *See* Congestive heart failure (CHF).
history in, 47–48, 48t
hypertension. *See* Hypertension.
infection and, 272
oral contraceptives causing, 345–346
pathophysiology of, 53–61
patient case studies of, 62–65
pericardial, 61
physical examination in, 48–52, 67–68
auscultation in, 50–51
blood pressure in, 51–52
observation in, 48–49, 49f
palpation in, 49–50, 50f
signs and symptoms of, 39–47
cough, 46–47
dyspnea, 46, 47
fatigue, 45–46
irregular heartbeat, 41–42, 43f
lightheadedness, 42, 44
pain, 39–41
syncope, 44–45
valvular. *See* Heart valves; *specific valves.*
Cardiovascular system, 31–65
anatomy and histology of, 32f–34f, 32–33
disorders. *See* Cardiovascular disorders.
physiology of, 33–38
blood pressure, 38, 38f
cardiac output, 36–38
heartbeat, 33, 34f, 35
mechanical events of cardiac cycle, 35–36, 36f, 37f
oxygen consumption of heart, 38
Carotene, 305
Carotid artery
occlusion/emboli of, headache and, 183
stenosis of, headache and, 183
Carotid pulse, palpation of, 49, 50
Carotid sinus hypersensitivity, 45
Carpal tunnel syndrome
imaging in, 390–391
in pregnancy, 143, 145
in thyroid disease, 164
Cauda equina lesions, 209
Cauda equina syndrome, 354
Central cord syndrome, 208–209
Central nervous system (CNS). *See also* Brain; Spinal cord.
anatomy of, 191, 192f, 192–193
Cerebellum, 202
lesions of, 211
Cerebral artery, infarction of, 210
Cerebral cortex, 199, 201f
lesions of, 210
Cerebral hemispheres, 192–193

Cervical radiculopathy, 18–19
Cervical spine
in ankylosing spondylitis, 267
imaging of, 369–372
in nontraumatic disorders, 370f, 370–372, 371f
in traumatic injuries, 369–370
rheumatoid, 266f, 266–267, 267f
Cervical stenosis, 266
Cervical strain, headache and, 181
Cervix, of uterus, 134
cancer of, 149
Charcot's joint, 160
Chemical dependency, 290–291
Chest, barrel-shaped, 93
Chest pain. *See also* Angina pectoris.
differential diagnosis of, 356, 356t
Chief complaint, 6
Chills, 13
Chlamydia trachomatis, pelvic inflammatory disease caused by, 148
Chlorine gas exposure, 360
Chlorphenesin, 331
Chlorpromazine (Thorazine), 342, 342t
Chlorzoxazone, 332, 332t
Cholecystitis, 107
Cholesterol-lowering drugs, for angina pectoris, 337, 338t
Chondroblastoma, 226t, 229–230
Chronic obstructive pulmonary disease (COPD), 46. *See also* Pulmonary system disease, obstructive.
blood gases in, 87
pulmonary function tests in, 86
Chronic pain syndrome, 294–298
behavioral rehabilitation programs for, 296
cognitive rehabilitation programs for, 296–298
procedural pain clinics for, 295–296
Chronic renal failure, 127–129
Chvostek's sign, in hypoparathyroidism, 165
Circulation, 33, 34f
Claudication
intermittent, 40
neurogenic, in spinal stenosis, 265–266
"Claw" toes, in diabetes mellitus, 161
Clozapine (Clozaril), 342, 342t
Clubbing, of nails, 16, 49, 49f, 93, 93f, 98
Cluster headache, 183
Codeine, 330t, 330–331
Codfish vertebra, in osteoporosis, 241
Codman's angle, 228, 229f
Cogentin (benztropine), 342
Cognitive rehabilitation programs, for chronic pain syndrome, 296–298
Colon. *See* Large intestine.
Color, of skin. *See* Skin, color of.
Coma, 356–357, 357t
Combative patients, 358–359, 360t
Comedones, 319
Compartment syndromes, anterior, 40
Compliance, pulmonary, 95
Compression fractures
back pain and, 263, 265
imaging of, 372
Computed tomography (CT), 366–367
quantitative, 373
Computed tomography myelography, 371, 372
Conducting system, of heart, 33, 33f
Congestive heart failure (CHF), 46, 47, 48, 51, 57–58
drug therapy for, 335–336, 336t, 337t
left ventricular, 46
Consciousness, loss of, 356–357, 357t. *See also* Syncope.
Consolidation, 77
Consultation, 248–249
Contact dermatitis, 309, 310
Conversion disorder, 280–281
Convulsions. *See* Seizures.
Coordination, testing of, 219
Coping, with stress, 289–290
Coping Strategies Questionnaire (CSQ), 294
Cord compression, 203, 208
Corns, 310
Coronary angiography, in coronary artery disease, 55
Coronary arteries, 33, 34f
Coronary artery disease (CAD), 39–40, 54–56, 55f
history in, 47–48, 48t
Cor pulmonale, 46
Cortical bone, 241
Corticobulbar pathway, 199, 200f
Corticospinal pathway, 199, 200f
Corticospinal tract, ventral, 199, 201f
Corticosteroids, 328–330, 329t. *See also specific drugs*.
for asthma, 347, 347t
mechanism of action of, 329
for pulmonary system disease, 86, 86t
side effects of, 329–330
Corticotropin, 158
Cough, in cardiovascular disease, 46–47
Counseling, for chronic pain syndrome, 297
Crackles. *See* Rales.
Cranial infection, headache caused by, 184–185
Cranial nerves
activation of, 199
anatomy of, 194
brain stem lesions and, 209
diabetic lesions of, 161
testing of, 213f–218f, 213–214, 216–217
Crust, 318
Crystalline arthropathy, acute, 271
Cushing syndrome, 166, 167t
subjective and objective changes in, 170t
Cutaneous reflexes, testing of, 220, 220f
Cyanosis, 16, 305, 306t
of nail beds, 47
Cycle ergometry, 56
Cyclobenzaprine, 331–332, 332t
Cystic medial necrosis, 61
Cystitis, in males, 125

D

Dantrolene, 332
Deep knee bends, 19
Deep tendon reflexes (DTRs), 18–19
cerebellar lesions and, 211
testing of, 219–220
in thyroid disease, 163, 164
upper and lower motor neuron lesions and, 202
Deep vein thrombosis (DVT), 50
Delusional disorders, 288
Dental disease, headache caused by, 184
Depakene (valproate), 343, 344t
Depakote (valproate), 343, 344t
Dependent personality disorder, 282, 283
Depolarization, 35
Depression, 283
in bipolar disease, 283, 286t, 286–287
chronic pain and, 297
diagnosis of, 284–285, 285t, 285–286, 286t
drug therapy for. *See also* Antidepressants.
lithium in, 342
fatigue and, 45
pain and, 278
suicide risk in, 285–286, 286t
Dermatitis, contact, 309, 310
Dermatomes, 203, 208f
Dermis, 304
Dermopathy. *See* Skin.
Diabetes mellitus, 158–162
clinical features of, 159
corticosteroids causing, 329
drug therapy for, 348t, 348–349
insulin-dependent, 158, 162
neuropathy in, 159–162, 160t
amyotrophy, 160t, 161–162
autonomic, 160t, 161
cranial, 160t, 161
peripheral motor neuropathy, 160t, 161

peripheral sensory neuropathy, 160, 160t
proximal motor neuropathy, 160t, 161–162
trunk and limb, 160t, 161
noninsulin-dependent, 158, 159, 162
in pregnancy, 144
subjective and objective changes in, 170t
vascular disease in, 162
Diagnostic and Statistical Manual of Mental Disorders, 3rd edition, revised (DSM III-R), 280
Diaphragm
dyspnea and, 46
failure of, 96
Diastasis recti abdominis, 142f, 143
Diastole, 33
Diastolic pressure, 38, 38f, 52
Diazepam, 332
Diencephalon
anatomy of, 192
lesions of, 209–210
Digitalis preparations, for congestive heart failure, 336, 337t
Digoxin, 336, 337t
Dilantin (phenytoin), 343, 344t
Diltiazem, 333t, 335
for arrhythmias, 338t, 338–339
Diphenhydramine (Benadryl), 342
Disability, 278
adjustment to, 290
Disc extrusion, imaging of, 377
Discharge planning, for pulmonary system disease, 88
Disc herniation, lumbar, imaging in, 376–377, 377f, 378
Discography, 378
Disc prolapse, imaging of, 377
Discrimination, two-point, 219
Disopyramide, for arrhythmias, 338t, 338–339
Dissociative disorders, 288
Distress, 289
Diuretics
for congestive heart failure, 336, 337t
for hypertension, 333t, 333–334
Diverticulitis, 108, 111
Dizziness, 185
neurologic disorders and, 212
Documentation, of emergencies, 354
Dolor. *See* Pain.
Doppler probe, 41
Dorsal column-medial lemniscal pathway, 194, 197f, 198, 199
Dorsal column nuclei, 198
Dramatic personality disorders, 282
Drug(s), 321–349. *See also specific drugs and drug types.*
allergic reactions to, 311
for asthma, 347t, 347–348
for cardiovascular diseases, 333t, 333–339, 336t–338t
clinical examination and, 321–324, 322f
depression caused by, 283–284, 284t
for diabetes, 348t, 348–349
for epilepsy, 343–344, 344t
hyperventilation caused by, 99
lightheadedness caused by, 44
oral contraceptive agents, 345–346
for pain and inflammation, 324–332, 325t, 326t, 327f, 329t–332t
patient case studies of, 349
for peptic ulcer disease, 344t, 344–345
psychotropic, 339–343, 340t–342t
side effects of, 324. *See also specific drugs and drug types.*
Drug abuse, 290–291
Drug overdose, blood gases in, 87
Drug Use Education Tips (DUET), 321
Dual-energy radiographic absorptiometry (DRA), 243, 373
Dual-photon absorptiometry (DPA), 373
Duodenum
acid peptic disorders of, 106–107
anatomy and physiology of, 103f, 103–104
Dural headache, 175
Dysesthesias, in hyperparathyroidism, 165
Dysfunction, detection of, 15–16
Dyspareunia, 147
Dyspnea, 14, 357t, 357–358
in cardiovascular disease, 46, 47
on exertion (DOE), 46
in mitral stenosis, 59
in pregnancy, 144, 145
Dysthymia, 287
Dysuria, 14
in urogenital system disease, in males, 122, 125E

E

Eccentric personality disorders, 281–282
Eccrine glands, 304f, 305
Echocardiography
in aortic regurgitation, 60
in aortic stenosis, 60
in endocarditis, 60
Ectopic pregnancy, 149–150
Eczema, 311
Edema
of ankles, 48
of leg, 40
local, 50
pretibial, 98
pulmonary. *See* Pulmonary edema.
Egophony, 78
Ehlers-Danlos type III collagenosis, 269–270
Ejaculation, 120
Elbow
bursitis in, 247
imaging of, 387–389
in nontraumatic lesions, 389
in traumatic injuries, 387–398
Electrocardiography (ECG)
in aortic regurgitation, 60
in aortic stenosis, 60
in arrhythmias, 43f, 57
in cardiovascular disease, 52–53
in coronary artery disease, 54
PQRST pattern of, *34*, 35, 52–53
signal-averaged, 57
Electromyography (EMG), 294
Electrophysiologic studies (EPS), in arrhythmias, 57
Emergencies, 353–361
agitated/combative patients, 358–359, 360t
autonomic dysreflexia, 354
chest pain, 356, 356t
documentation of, 354
dyspnea, 357t, 357–358
falls, 355
loss of bowel or bladder control, 354–355
loss of consciousness, 356–357, 357t
nonbreathing, 357
pulselessness, 357
seizures, 358
shock, 357
suicide risk, 355
swelling of extremities, 355–356
in therapeutic pools, 360, 360t
training for handling, 354
Emotional abuse, 290
Encainide, for arrhythmias, 338t, 338–339
Encephalitis, headache caused by, 185
Enchondroma, 231, 233f
Endocarditis, 39
infective, 60, 272
Endocardium, 33
Endocrine system, 155–172. *See also* Hormones; *specific hormones.*
disease of, 158–172, 169f, 170t. *See also* Diabetes mellitus; *specific glands.*
brain tumors and, 210
in females, 149
patient case studies of, 168, 170–172
physiology of, 155–156, 156f, 157t, 158
Endometriosis, 147–148
Enteropathic arthritis, 261, 263t
Epicardium, 33

Epicondylitis, lateral, imaging in, 389
Epidermis, 303–304
Epididymis, anatomy and physiology of, 117, 118f
Epididymitis, 124
Epidural abscesses, 247
Epilepsy. *See* Seizures.
Epitrochlear lymph nodes, palpation of, 406f
Erosion, 308f
Erosive synovitis, cervical, 266
Erythropoietin, 119
Esophagus
  anatomy and physiology of, 101–102
  spasm of, 106
Estradiol, 346
Estrogens
  conjugated (Premarin), 346
  as contraceptives, 345–346
  lack of, 149
  menstrual cycle and, 136
Eustress, 289
Ewing sarcoma, 232–233, 236f–237f
  of bone, 226t
Excoriations, 318
Exercise
  osteoporosis and, 241
  for pregnancy-induced glucose intolerance and diabetes, 144
Exercise intolerance
  signs and symptoms of, 362
  in therapeutic pool, 360
Exercise prescription, 56
Exercise tolerance test (ETT)
  in coronary artery disease, 55–56
  in heart failure, 58
Exertional syncope, 45
Extroversion, suffering and, 279
Eye movement, testing of, 213–214, 216f

F

Facial features, in acromegaly, 168
Facial nerve (cranial nerve VII)
  paralysis of, in diabetes mellitus, 161
  testing of, 214
Facial pain. *See* Headache.
Fallopian tubes
  anatomy and physiology of, 134, 140f
  pregnancy in, 150
Falls, in therapy, 355
False aneurysm, 61
Family dynamics, pain and, 279
Fatigue
  in Addison's disease, 167
  in cardiovascular disease, 45–46
  in hyperparathyroidism, 165
  in pregnancy, 145
  in thyroid disease, 163, 164
Fatty streak, 54
Fearful Personality disorders, 282–283
Fecal incontinence, 354–355
Feet
  in diabetes mellitus, 160
  imaging of, 383–386, 384f
    in osteonecrosis, 384
    of soft tissue abnormalities, 385f, 385–386
    of stress fractures, 384
    of tarsal coalition, 385
Felbamate (Felbatol), 343–344, 344t
Felon, infection of, 248
Female urogenital system, 133–153
  anatomy and physiology of, 133–145, 134f–141f, 137t
    menstrual, 136–138, 141f
    in pregnancy. *See* Pregnancy.
  disease of. *See* Female urogenital system disease.
Female urogenital system disease, 151f
  ectopic pregnancy, 149–150
  endometriosis, 147–148
  evaluation in, 145–147
    abdominal tenderness/bloating in, 146–147
    bleeding in, 146
    dyspareunia in, 147
    nausea and vomiting in, 147
    pain in, 146
    urinary changes in, 147
    vaginal discharge or burning in, 146
  fibroids, 148
  hormonal dysfunction, 149
  neoplastic, 149
  patient case studies of, 150–153
  pelvic inflammatory disease, 148
  symptomatic pelvic relaxation, 149
Femoral pulse, palpation of, 40–41, 50
Fever, 13
Fibrocystic disease, of breasts, 146–147
Fibroids, 148
Fibromyalgia, 269, 269f
Fibrositis, 269, 269f
Fick principle, 37
Fight-or-flight response, 277
Finger opposition test, 219
Finger percussion, in pulmonary system disease, 90
Finger to nose test, 219
Finger to therapist's finger test, 219
Fissure, 309f, 318
Flecainide, for arrhythmias, 338t, 338–339
Fluoxetine, 341, 341t
Fluphenazine (Prolixin), 342, 342t
Foods, allergic reactions to, 311
Foot. *See* Feet.
Fractures
  compression. *See* Compression fractures.
  osteochondral, imaging of, 382
  pathologic. *See* Pathologic fractures.
  stress. *See* Stress fractures.
Frieberg's infractions, imaging of, 384
Functional pain, 293
Functional respiratory capacity assessment, 90–92
Fundus, of uterus, 134

G

Gabapentin, 344
Gait, ataxic, cerebellar lesions and, 211
Gallbladder
  anatomy and physiology of, 102f, 105
  disease of, 107
    estrogens causing, 346
Gallium 67 bone scans, 369
Gallstones, 107
Gangrene, 40, 41
Gastrointestinal disorders, salicylates causing, 325–326
Gastrointestinal system, 101–116, 102f
  anatomy and physiology of, 101–106, 103f, 104f
  disorders of. *See* Gastrointestinal system disorders.
  hormones of, 157t
Gastrointestinal system disorders, 106–116
  abdominal evaluation in, 109–112, 110f
    auscultation and percussion in, 110–111, 111f, 112f
    diagnosis and, 112
    history in, 109, 110f
    palpation in, 111–112
  abdominal hernia, 109
  acid peptic disorders. *See* Peptic ulcer disease.
  in Addison's disease, 167
  in chronic renal failure, 128
  of colon, 108
  diverticulitis, 108
  esophageal spasm, 106
  infectious, of mouth and throat, 106
  of liver and gallbladder, 107
  nonsteroidal anti-inflammatory agents causing, 328
  pancreatitis, 108
  patient case studies of, 113–116, 115f
  splenic enlargement, 108–109

General adaptation syndrome, 289
Generalized anxiety disorders, 287
Gestational diabetes, 144
Giant cell tumor, of bone, 226t, 230–231, 231f–232f
Glossopharyngeal nerve (cranial nerve IX), testing of, 216–217
Glucocorticoids, 329
Glucose intolerance, pregnancy-induced, 144
Goiter, nodular, hyperfunctioning, 163
Gonadotropins, 158
Gottron's papules, 267, 267f
Gout, 271
Graphesthesia, 219
Graves disease, 163
Grouped lesions of skin, 309
Growths, on skin, 310, 318
Guillain-Barré syndrome, 203

H

Hair, 304f, 304–305
  loss of, 40
  observation of, 16
Hair follicles, 304–305
Haloperidol (Haldol), 342, 342t
"Hammer" toes, in diabetes mellitus, 161
Hand and wrist, imaging of, 389–391
  in arthritis, 391
  in carpal tunnel syndrome, 390–391
  in ligamentous abnormalities, 390
  in nontraumatic lesions, 390
  in osteonecrosis, 391, 391f
  in reflex sympathetic dystrophy, 391
  in traumatic injuries, 390
H_2 antagonists, for peptic ulcer disease, 344t, 344–345
Hashimoto's thyroiditis, 164
Head, lymph nodes of, 402f
Headaches, 21, 175–188, 176f
  "allergic," 184
  brain tumors and, 210
  cluster, 183
  diseases and disorders causing, 179–185
    infection, 183–185, 184f
    tumors, 181–182
    vascular, 182–183
    vertigo, 185
  dural, 175
  estrogens causing, 346
  history in, 176–178, 177f, 177t
  lower-half, 183
  migraine, 180
  muscle contraction, 180–181
  nonsteroidal anti-inflammatory agents causing, 328
  in Paget's disease, 244
  patient case studies of, 21, 22f, 22–23, 24f, 25f, 185–188
  physical examination in, 178–179, 179f
  sinus, 183–184, 184f
  systems review in, 178, 178t
Hearing, testing of, 214, 216, 217f
Heart, 32f, 32–33
  auscultation of, 35–36, 37f
  conducting system of, 33, 33f
  hormone of, 157t
  innervation of, 33
  oxygen consumption of, 38
  pacemaker of, 33, 35f
Heartbeat, 33, 34f, 35
  irregular. *See* Arrhythmia.
  premature, 53
Heart block, 42, 56–57
Heart murmurs, 35–36, 37f
Heart sounds, 35, 42
  in cardiovascular disease, 50, 51
Heart valves, 32f, 32–33, 35. *See also specific valves.*
  incompetent, 35–36
  murmurs and, 35–36, 37f
  stenosis of, 35, 39
Heel on shin test, 219
Heel raising, 19
Heleobacterium pylori, 106
Hemarthrosis, 271
Hematomas, subdural, headache and, 182
Hematuria
  in kidney cancer, 125
  in urogenital disease, in males, 122
Hemianopsia, homonymous, 213, 215f
Hemoglobin, skin color and, 305
Hemorrhoids, in pregnancy, 144
Hepatic disease, 107
Hepatitis, 107
Hernias, abdominal, 109, 111–112
Herniation of central nucleus pulposus (HNP), imaging of, 376–377, 377f, 378
Herpes zoster infection, 39
Hiatal hernia, 109
Hip
  imaging of, 378–380
    in osteoarthritis, 378
    in osteonecrosis, 378–379, 379f
    of stress fractures, 380
    in traumatic injuries, 379, 380f
  osteoporosis of, in pregnancy, 144–145
Hippocampus, 193
History taking, 2–14, 3f, 19–20. *See also under specific diseases.*
  general patient profile in, 4
  medical, 8, 9f–11f, 12
  symptoms in, 4–8
    behavior of, 6–8
    history of, 8
    location and description of, 4–6, 5f, 6f
  systems review in, 12–14, 13f
Holter monitor, 57
Homonymous hemianopsia, 213, 215f
Hormones. *See also* Endocrine system.
  effects of, 156, 157t, 158
  gastric, 103
  menstrual cycle and, 136–138, 141f
  metabolic bone disease and, 241
  release of, 156
  renal, 119–120
  testicular, 120–121
Huntington's disease, 211
Hydralazine, for congestive heart failure, 336, 337t
Hydrocele, 127
Hydrocodone, 330t, 331
Hypercapnia, 95
Hyperglycemia, 46
Hyperlipidemia, drug therapy for, 337, 338t
Hyperparathyroidism, 164–165
  subjective and objective changes in, 170t
Hyperpigmentation
  in Addison's disease, 167
  of skin, 306t
Hypertension, 58
  in chronic renal failure, 129
  drug therapy for, 333t, 333–335
  monoamine oxidase inhibitors causing, 341, 341t
Hyperthyroidism, 45
  skin in, 312
  subjective and objective changes in, 170t
Hypertrophic cardiomyopathy (HCM), 39
Hypertrophic osteoarthropathy, 270
Hypertrophic scars, 318
Hyperventilation, 42, 99
Hypochondriasis, 281
Hypoglossal nerve (cranial nerve XII), testing of, 217
Hypoglycemia, 44
  recognition and treatment of, 363
Hypokalemic periodic paralysis, in thyroid disease, 163
Hypomania, 287
Hypoparathyroidism, 165–166
  subjective and objective changes in, 170t
Hypoperfusion, 57–58
Hypophysis. *See* Pituitary gland.
Hypopituitarism, metabolic bone disease and, 241
Hypotension, 50, 357

Hypotension *(Continued)*
postural, 44
antidepressants causing, 340–341
in pregnancy, 143–144, 145
Hypothalamus, 158
hormones of, 157t
lesions of, 209–210
Hypothyroidism, 45, 164, 164t
pulmonary manifestations of, 98
skin in, 312, 314
subjective and objective changes in, 170t
Hypotonia, cerebellar lesions and, 211
Hypoxia, 45–46, 47

I

Ileum, anatomy and physiology of, 104
Illness Behavior Questionnaire (IBQ), 293
Imaging, 365–392. *See also specific modalities, anatomic sites, and disorders.*
Impetigo, 310
Impotence, 129
Incontinence
fecal, 354–355
urinary, stress, 149
Indicator dilution technique, 37
Indium 111 bone scans, 369
Infections
cardiac, 39
headache caused by, 183–185, 184f
of musculoskeletal system, 245–248. *See also* Osteomyelitis.
of bursae and tendons, 247–248
pyogenic, 245–246
rheumatic syndromes associated with, 271t, 271–272
septic arthritis and, 270
skin lesions due to, 310
spinal cord lesions caused by, 209
of urogenital system, in males, 124–125
Infectious mononucleosis, 108
Infective endocarditis, 60, 272
Inferior vena cava, 32
Inflammation, 257. *See also* Arthritis; Rheumatic disease.
cardiac, 39
drug therapy for, 324–332, 325t, 326t, 327f, 329t–332t
of joints, in rheumatic disease, 258–259
skin lesions due to, 310
Inflammatory bowel disease, arthritis of, 261, 263t
Infraclavicular lymph node, palpation of, 404f
Inguinal lymph nodes, palpation of, 411f
Innominate bones, 133
Insect bites, 311
Inspection
in gastrointestinal system disease, 110, 111f
in pulmonary system disease, 93, 95, 96
Insulin, 158, 159
preparations of, 348, 348t
Intercourse, painful, 147
Intermittent claudication, 40
Intestine. *See* Bowel function; Large intestine; Small intestine.
Intima, 33, 34f
Intracranial pressure, increased
headache and, 181, 210
vomiting and, 210
Introversion, suffering and, 279
Ipratropium bromide, for asthma, 347, 347t
Ischemia
cerebral, 210
intermittent claudication and, 40
myocardial, 39–40
Ischemic necrosis. *See* Osteonecrosis.
Isometric contraction, 19
Isovolumic contraction, 35
Itching. See Pruritus.

J

Jaundice, 16
Jejunum, anatomy and physiology of, 104
Joints
bloody effusions in, 271
hypermobility of, 269–270
inflammation of, in rheumatic disease, 258–259
involved in arthritis, 260, 260f
pain in
in aseptic osteonecrosis, 270
in rheumatic disease, 258
swollen, 270
Jugular venous distention (JVD), 48, 49f

K

Karvonen equation, 56
Keloids, 318
Ketoacidosis, 99
Kidney(s)
anatomy and physiology of, 117, 118–120
disease of. *See* Kidney disease.
hormones of, 157t
vasopressin and, 156, 157t, 158
Kidney disease, 123f, 123–124
cancer, 125–127
skeletal metastases of, 239
treatment of, 239
chronic renal failure, 127–129
stones, 125
Kinesthesia, testing of, 219
Knee, imaging of, 380–383
of Baker's cyst, 382
in meniscal and ligamentous injuries, 381f, 381–382, 382f
of Osgood-Schlatter lesion, 382
of osteochondral fractures, 382
in osteochondritis dissecans, 382
in osteonecrosis, 382
of plicae, 383
Knee bends, deep, 19
Knee jerk, in amyotrophy, diabetic, 161
Kohler's disease, imaging of, 384
Korotkoff sounds, 42, 51
Kussmaul breathing, 99
Kyphosis
in osteoporosis, 241, 242f
in Paget's disease, 244

L

Laboratory reports, in pulmonary system disease, 87
Laboratory tests, in skin disorders, 314
Large intestine
anatomy and physiology of, 105
cancer of, 111
disorders of, 108
Lateral epicondylitis, imaging in, 389
Lateral view, 366
Left ventricular failure, 48
Left ventricular filling, 35
Left ventricular filling pressures, elevated, 58
Leg(s)
edema of, 40
pain in, in cardiovascular disease, 40–41
Legg-Calvé-Perthes disease, imaging in, 378–379, 379f
Leiomyomata uteri, 148
Lesions, 318. *See also specific anatomic locations.*
Leukorrhea, physiologic, 146
Lice, skin lesions due to, 311
Lichenification, 318
Ligamentous injuries
of knee, imaging of, 381
of wrist and hand, imaging of, 390
Lightheadedness
in cardiovascular disease, 42, 44
neurologic disorders and, 212
Limb mononeuropathy, in diabetes mellitus, 161

Linear lesions of skin, 309
Lipoma, 233–234
Lithium, 342
Liver
  anatomy and physiology of, 105
  disease of, 107
  hormone of, 157t
  percussion of, 110, 111f
Lobes, of lungs, 69–75, 70f, 71t, 72f, 73f
Lower back pain. *See* Back pain.
Lower-half headache, 183
Lower motor neuron lesions, 202–203
  testing for, 217–218
  upper motor neuron lesions versus, 202
Lower-quarter screening examination, 409–410, 410f–414f
Lumbar canal stenosis, 265
Lumbar spine
  imaging of, 375–378
    in acute pain, 375–376, 376f
    in chronic pain, 376
    in herniation of central nucleus pulposus, 376–378, 377f
    in neurologic disorders, 377, 377f, 378
    in spinal stenosis, 377, 377f
    in traumatic injuries, 375
  in osteoporosis, 241
Lungs. *See also* Pulmonary system disease; Pulmonary system.
  anatomy of, 69–71
    bronchopulmonary segments, 69–71, 70f, 71t, 72f, 73f
    left lung, 74–75
    pulmonary fissures, 69, 70f
    right lung, 71–74
Luteinizing hormone (LH), 120–121
Lyme disease, 272
Lymphatics, 32
  retroperitoneal, 127, 128f
Lymphedema, 50
Lymph nodes
  of head and neck, 402f
  palpable, 17
  palpation of, 403f, 404f–406f, 411f
    passive, 179, 179f

M

McGill Pain Questionnaire (MPQ), 294
Macroangiopathy, diabetic, 162
Macrophages, hormones of, 157t
Macule, 306f, 318
Magnetic resonance imaging (MRI), 367–368
Male urogenital system, 117–132
  anatomy and physiology of, 117–121, 118f–120f, 118t
  disease of. *See* Male urogenital system disease.
Male urogenital system disease, 121–132
  cancer, 125–127, 126f
    of bladder, 126–127
    of kidneys, 125–126
    of prostate, 127
    of testes, 127, 128f
  chronic renal failure, 127–129
  impotence, 129
  infectious, 124–125
  patient case histories of, 129–132
  signs and symptoms of, 121–124
    history of, 121–122, 122f, 123f
    physical examination and, 122–124, 123f
Malignant melanoma, of skin, 311
Malingering, 287
Mania, 283, 286t, 286–287
Maprotiline, 341, 341t
Marital dysfunction, pain and, 279
Maximum inspiratory force (MIF), 94
Maximum stress test, in dyspnea, 46
Mean pressure, 38, 38f
Mechanical pain, 280
Media, 33, 34f
Medical history, 8, 9f–11f, 12
Medications. *See* Drug(s); *specific drugs and drug types*.
Medroxyprogesterone (Provera), 346
Medulla, 192
Melanocytes, 305
Melanoma, 16
  malignant, of skin, 311
Mellaril (thioridazine), 342, 342t
Meningiomas, headache and, 181–182
Meningitis, headache caused by, 184–185
Meniscal injuries, imaging of, 381f, 381–382, 382f
Menopause, 146
  drug therapy for, 346
  premature, 149
Menstrual physiology, 136–138, 141f
Mental status examination, 213
Metabolic bone disease. *See* Bone(s); Osteoporosis.
Metastases
  to cervical spine, imaging of, 373–375, 374f
  definition of, 224
  skeletal, 234–235, 237–240
    clinical features of, 237–239
Metaxalone, 331
Methylxanthines. *See also specific drugs*.
  for pulmonary system disease, 85, 85t
Mexiletine, for arrhythmias, 338t, 338–339
Microangiopathy, diabetic, 162
Migraine headaches, 180
Milia, 319
Millon Behavioral Health Inventory (MBHI), 293
Mineralocorticoids, 329
Minipill, 345, 346
Minnesota Multiphasic Personality Inventory (MMPI), 292–293
Minute volume, 37
Mites, skin lesions due to, 311
Mitral valve, 32f, 32–33, 35
  prolapse of, 39, 59
  regurgitation of, 59
  stenosis of, 47, 59
Mittelschmerz, 146
Mobility, of skin lesions, 312
Moles, 312
  mobility of, 312
Monoamine oxidase inhibitors (MAOIs), 341, 341t
Monocytes, hormones of, 157t
Moricizine, for arrhythmias, 338t, 338–339
Morphine, 330, 330t
Motor assessment, 19
Motor system, 199–203, 200f
  basal ganglia, 202
  brain stem, 199
  cerebellum, 202
  cerebral cortex, 199, 201f
  lesions of, 202–203
    lower, 202–203
    upper, 203
    upper versus lower, 202
  spinal cord, 199
Mouth, infectious diseases of, 106
Movement
  decomposition of, cerebellar lesions and, 211
  testing of sensation for, 219
Mucolytics. *See also specific drugs*.
  for pulmonary system disease, 85t, 85–86
Multiple sclerosis (MS), 203
Murmurs, 35–36, 37f
Muscle(s)
  pain in, in rheumatic disease, 258
  pelvic, of females, 134, 139f, 144
  plexus injuries and, 203, 206t, 207t
  in polymyositis, 268
  resisted manual muscle testing of, 217–218
  rheumatism and, 267
  weakness of. *See* Weakness.
Muscle contraction headache, 180–181
Muscle guarding, 112
Musculoskeletal disorders, 223–252. *See also* Bone(s); Muscle(s).

Musculoskeletal disorders *(Continued)*
- in acromegaly, 167–168
- consultation and referral for, 248–249
- differentiation from cardiovascular disease, 31
- in hyperparathyroidism, 165
- infections, 245–247
  - of bone, 246–247
  - of bursae and tendons, 247–248
- neoplastic
  - of bone. *See* Bone.
  - dermatologic, 234
  - lipoma, 233–234
  - myelogenic, 231–233, 235f–237f
  - treatment of, 234
- patient case studies of, 249, 251–252
- in pregnancy, 140, 142–143

Myasthenia gravis, 268
Myelography, computed tomography, 371, 372
Myeloma, plasma cell, 226t, 231–232, 235f
Myocardial infarction (MI), in diabetes mellitus, 162
Myocardial ischemia, 39–40
- silent, 40

Myocarditis, 39
Myocardium, 33
- excitability states of, 52

Myopathy, in thyroid disease, 163
Myositis ossificans, imaging in, 389
Mysoline (primidone), 343, 344t

N

Nails, 305, 305f
- clubbing of, 16, 49, 49f, 93, 93f, 98
- cyanosis of nail beds and, 47
- observation of, 16, 312, 313f
- pitting of, 16
- spoon-shaped, 16

Narcissistic personality disorder, 282
Nausea, 13–14
- in pregnancy, 145
- in urogenital disease, in females, 147

Neck. *See also* Cervical spine.
- lymph nodes of, 402f

Neck pain
- inflammatory, 266f, 266–267, 267f
- in temporal arteritis, 268

Negative inspiratory force (NIF), 94, 95
Neisseria gonorrhea, pelvic inflammatory disease caused by, 148
Neoplastic disease. *See also* Cancer; Metastases; Tumors; *specific anatomic sites and diseases.*
- of cervical spine, imaging in, 373–375, 374f
- definition of, 224
- of female reproductive tract, 149

Nerve compression syndromes. *See* Carpal tunnel syndrome; Tarsal tunnel syndrome.
Nerve plexi, 194, 195f, 196f
Nervous system, 191–222. *See also* Central nervous system; Motor system; Peripheral nervous system; Somatosensory systems; *specific structures*.
- anatomy of, 191–194, 192f
- autonomic, 194
- disorders of. *See* Diabetes mellitus, neuropathy in; Neurologic disorders; Neuropathy.
- parasympathetic, 194
- sympathetic, 194

Neurofibromas, headache and, 182
Neurogenic claudication, in spinal stenosis, 265–266
Neurohypophysis, 158
Neuroleptic agents, 342t, 342–343, 343t
Neurologic disorders, 202–222. *See also* Diabetes mellitus, neuropathy in; Neuropathy.
- basal ganglia lesions, 210–211
- brachial plexus injuries, 203, 206t, 207t, 208f
- brain stem lesions, 209
- cerebellar lesions, 211
- cerebral cortex lesions, 210
- in chronic renal failure, 128–129
- diencephalon injuries, 209–210
- evaluation of, 211–212, 211–220, 212t
  - of coordination, 219
  - of cranial nerves, 213f–218f, 213–214, 216–217
  - history in, 212
  - of mental status, 213
  - of motor function, 217–218
  - of reflexes, 219–220, 220f
  - of sensory function, 218–219
- in hyperparathyroidism, 165
- lower motor neuron lesions, 202–203
  - testing for, 217–218
- nonsteroidal anti-inflammatory agents causing, 328
- patient case studies of, 220–222
- peripheral nerve lesions, 203, 204f–205f. *See also* Peripheral neuropathy.
- radicular nerve injuries, 203
- spinal cord lesions. *See* Spinal cord lesions.
- upper motor neuron lesions, 202, 203
  - testing for, 217–218

Neurologic examination, 18–19
- passive, 179

Neuromas, acoustic, headache and, 182
Neuropathic arthropathies, diabetic, 160
Neuropathy
- diabetic. *See* Diabetes mellitus, neuropathy in.
- peripheral, 40
- sympathetic, 40
- in thyroid disease, 164

Neurotic triad, 293
Nevi, 311
Nicardipine, 333t, 335
Nifedipine, 333t, 335
Night pain, 14
Nimodipine, 335
Nitrates
- for angina pectoris, 337, 338t
- for congestive heart failure, 336, 337t

Nociception, 278
Nocturia, in urogenital disease, in males, 121
Nodule, 307f, 318
Nonsteroidal anti-inflammatory agents (NSAIAs), 324, 326t, 326–328
- contraindications to, 328
- indications for, 327–328
- mechanism of action of, 327, 327f
- side effects of, 328

Nuchal rigidity, headache and, 182
Numbness, 14
Nurturance, for chronic pain syndrome, 297
Nystagmus
- cerebellar lesions and, 211
- in vertigo, 185

O

Obesity-hypoventilation syndrome, 95
Observation, 16
- in headaches, 178–179
- of pain behavior, 292
- of skin, 312, 313f

Obsessive-compulsive personality disorder, 282, 283
Oculomotor nerve (cranial nerve III), testing of, 213–214, 216f
Olecranon bursa, infection of, 247
Olfactory nerve (cranial nerve I), testing of, 213
Omeprazole (Prilosec), for peptic ulcer disease, 344, 345
"Ondine's curse," 98
Opioids, 330–3310t
- indications for, 330
- mechanism of action of, 330, 331t
- oral, 330–331

Optic nerve (cranial nerve II), testing of, 213, 213f, 214f
Oral contraceptive agents (OCAs), 345–346
  indications for, 346
  side effects of, 345–346
Oral hypoglycemic agents, 348t, 348–349
Orchitis, 124
Orphenadrine, 332, 332t
Orthopnea, 46
Orthostatic hypotension, 44
Orthostatic intolerance, 42
Osgood-Schlatter lesion, imaging of, 382
Osteitis deformans, 244–245, 245f
Osteitis fibrosa cystica, in hyperparathyroidism, 165
Osteoarthritis, 259–260, 260f
  imaging in, 378
Osteoarthropathy, hypertrophic, 270
Osteoblastoma, 226t, 227–228, 229f
Osteoblasts, 241
Osteochondral fractures, imaging of, 382
Osteochondritis dissecans, imaging of, 382
Osteochondroma, 226t, 228–229, 230f
Osteoclastoma, 230–231, 231f–232f
Osteoclasts, 241
Osteodystrophy, in chronic renal failure, 129
Osteoid osteoma, 226t, 227, 227f
Osteomalacia, 240–241
Osteomyelitis, 246–247
  acute, 246
  chronic, 246
  vertebral, 246–247
Osteonecrosis
  aseptic, 270
  of foot and ankle, imaging of, 384
  of hip, imaging in, 378–379, 379f
  of knee, imaging in, 382
  in pregnancy, 145
  of wrist, imaging in, 391, 391f
Osteopenia, 242–243, 243f
  of spine, with plasma cell myeloma, 232, 235f
Osteoporosis, 241–244
  back pain and, 263, 265
  bone physiology and, 241, 242f
  corticosteroids causing, 329
  in Cushing's syndrome, 166
  etiology of, 241–243, 243f
  of hip, in pregnancy, 144–145
  imaging in, 373
  physical activity and, 243, 244t
  in thyroid disease, 163
  treatment of, 244
Osteosarcoma, 226t
Outflow tract obstruction, 39
Ovaries
  anatomy and physiology of, 134, 140f
  hormones of, 157t
  tumors of, 149
Oviducts, anatomy and physiology of, 134, 140f
Ovulation, pain at, 146
Oximetry, 94, 95
Oxycodone, 330t, 331
Oxygen consumption, of heart, 38
Oxytocin, 158

P

Pacemaker, cardiac, 33, 35f
Paget's disease, 244–245, 245f
Pain
  acute versus chronic, 277–279
  in back. *See* Back pain.
  brain tumors and, 210
  in breasts, 146–147
  in bursitis, 247
  with cancer, 240
  in cardiovascular disease, 39–41
  in chest. *See* Angina pectoris; Chest pain.
  chronic. *See* Chronic pain syndrome.
  depression and, 278
  in diabetic neuropathies, 161
  drug therapy for, 324–332, 325t, 326t, 327f, 329t–332t
  in ectopic pregnancy, 150
  in endometriosis, 148
  in epidural abscess, 247
  estrogens causing, 346
  with Ewing sarcoma, 232
  facial. *See* Headache.
  fibroids and, 148
  following falls, 355
  functional, 293
  in gout, 271
  headache. *See* Headache.
  during intercourse, 147
  ischemic, 41
  in leg, in cardiovascular disease, 40–41
  mechanical, 280
  in musculoskeletal infections, 245
  in musculoskeletal neoplasms, 225
  in neck, in temporal arteritis, 268
  night, 14
  with osteoblastoma, 227, 228
  with osteoclastoma, 230–231
  with osteoid osteoma, 227
  in osteonecrosis, 379
  in osteoporosis of hip, in pregnancy, 145
  in Paget's disease, 244
  with plasma cell myeloma, 232
  in pregnancy, 145
  psychogenic, 280
  psychological disorders and. *See* Chronic pain syndrome; Psychological disorders, pain and.
  psychophysiology of, 288–289
  referred, 270
  in reflex sympathetic dystrophy syndrome, 270
  in rheumatic disease, 258
    management of, 260
  secondary gain and, 278
  with skeletal metastatic disease, 237
  stress and, 289–290
  in tenosynovitis, 248
  testing of sensation for, 218
  thoracic, differential diagnosis of, 39
  in thyroid disease, 162
  in tuberculosis, 247
  in urogenital system disease
    in females, 135, 137t, 146, 147
    in males, 121, 122f, 124, 125, 127
  visceral, 5, 6f, 16
Pain behavior, 278–279
  assessment of, 292
Pain Behavior Scale, 292
Pain clinics, procedural, for chronic pain syndrome, 295–296
Pain Distress Scale, 294, 295
Pallor, of skin, 16
Palpation, 16–17
  of abdomen, 411f
    fibroids and, 148
  in cancer screening, 240
  in cardiovascular disease, 49–50, 50f
  in gastrointestinal system disease, 111–112
  of lymph nodes, 403f, 404f–406f, 411f
    passive, 179, 179f
  in pulmonary system disease, 93–94, 96
  of pulses, 35, 40–41, 42, 49–50, 50f, 407f–408f, 412f–413f
  of skin, 312, 314
  of thyroid gland, 162, 162f, 403f
  in urogenital system disease, in males, 122–123
Palpitations, 41–42, 43f
Pancreas
  anatomy and physiology of, 105
  hormones of, 157t
Pancreatitis, 108
Papule, 307f, 318
Paradoxical pulse, 94
Paralysis, periodic, hypokalemic, in thyroid disease, 163
Paranoid disorders, 281–282, 288
Parasitic infestations, skin lesions due to, 311

Parasympathetic nervous system, 194
Parathyroid gland
  disease of, 164–166
    hyperparathyroidism, 164–165, 170t
    hypoparathyroidism, 165–166, 170t
  hormone of, 157t
Paraxetine, 341, 341t
Paresthesia, of upper extremities, in pregnancy, 142–143
Parkinson's disease, 210–211
Paronychia, infection of, 248
Paroxysmal nocturnal dyspnea (PND), 46
Passive-aggressive personality disorder, 282–283
Pathologic fractures
  back pain and, 263, 265
  enchondroma and, 231, 233f
  with Ewing sarcoma, 233
  with skeletal metastatic disease, 237
Patient profile, 4
Pedal pulse, palpation of, 41, 413f
Pelvic abscesses, in females, 148
Pelvic inflammatory disease (PID), 148
Pelvic relaxation, symptomatic, 149
Pelvis
  female
    anatomy and physiology of, 133–134, 134f, 135f
    muscles of, 134, 139f, 144
    nerves of, 135, 137t, 141f
  imaging of, 378–380
    in osteoarthritis, 378
    in osteonecrosis, 378–379, 379f
    of stress fractures, 380
    in traumatic injuries, 379, 380f
Pentazocine, 330, 330t, 331
Peptic ulcer disease, 106–107
  drug therapy for, 344t, 344–345
Percussion, 17
  finger, in pulmonary system disease, 90
  in gastrointestinal system disease, 110–111, 111f, 112f
  of musculoskeletal neoplasms, 225, 225f
  in pulmonary system disease, 99
  in urogenital system disease, in males, 123f, 123–124
Pericardial disease, 61. *See also specific disorders.*
Pericardial effusion, 61
Pericarditis, 39
  chronic, 47
  in chronic renal failure, 129
  constrictive, 57
Pericardium, 33
Perimenopause, 146
Perinephric abscesses, in males, 124
Peripheral nervous system (PNS)
  anatomy of, 191, 192f, 193f, 193–194, 195f, 196f
  sensory distribution of, 203, 204f–205f
Peripheral neuropathy, 40
  diabetic. *See* Diabetes mellitus, neuropathy in.
Peripheral vascular disease (PVD), 40, 41, 48
Personality, pain and, 279–280
Personality disorders, 281–283
  anxious, 282–283
  dramatic, 282
  eccentric, 281–282
  Fearful, 282–283
  self-defeating, 283
Petechia, 318
pH, of blood, in pulmonary system disease, 87
Phenobarbital, 343, 344t
Phenytoin (Dilantin), 343, 344t
Photosensitive reactions, 309
Physical abuse, 290
Physical examination, 14–19, 20f. *See also under specific diseases.*
  alteration of symptoms and, 15
  auscultation in. *See* Auscultation.
  detection of dysfunction in, 15–16
  neurologic examination in, 18–19
  observation in. *See* Observation.
  palpation in. *See* palpation.
  percussion in. *See* Percussion.
  principles of, 2–3, 3f
Physicians' Desk Reference (PDR), 321
Physiologic leukorrhea, 146
Physiologic variables, pain and, 294
Pigmented lesions, 309
Pineal gland, hormone of, 157t
Pituitary gland, 158
  disorders of, 158, 167–168
    corticosteroids causing, 329
    metabolic bone disease and, 241
    subjective and objective changes in, 170t
    tumors, headache and, 182
  hormones of, 157t, 158
Placenta, hormones of, 157t
Plaque, cutaneous, 318
Plasma cell myeloma, 226t, 231–232, 235f
Pleural friction rub, 82, 98
Pleurisy, 39, 98
Plexi, 194, 195f, 196f
Plexus injuries, 203, 206t, 207t, 208f
Plicae, imaging of, 383
Pneumothorax, 97
Poliomyelitis, 203
Polymyalgia rheumatica (PMR), 268–269
  headache and, 183
Polymyositis, 267f, 267–268, 268t
Popliteal pulse, palpation of, 41, 50, 412f
Position sense, testing of, 219
Posterior cord syndrome, 209
Posteroanterior (PA) film, 366
Postganglionic neuron, 194
Postpolio syndrome, 203
Post-rest gel
  management of, 260
  in rheumatic disease, 258
Post-traumatic stress disorder, 290
Postural hypotension, postural, SeeHypotension
Posture
  dysfunctional, abuse and, 290
  in neurologic examination, 19
PQRST method, 121
PQRST pattern, 34, 35, 52–53
Pre-excitation, 57
Preganglionic neuron, 194
Pregnancy, 138, 140, 142–145
  blood pressure in, 143–144
  diabetes in, 144
  diastasis recti abdominis in, 142f, 143
  drug therapy during, 326
  ectopic, 149–150
  osteonecrosis and osteoporosis in, 144–145
  respiration in, 144
  skin changes in, 143
  spine in, 138, 140, 142–143
  urinary tract in, 144
  vascular changes in, 143
  weight gain in, 143
Pregnancy-induced glucose intolerance, 144
Preload, 38
Premarin (conjugated estrogens), 346
Premature beats, 53, 56
Pretibial edema, 98
Prilosec (omeprazole), for peptic ulcer disease, 344, 345
Primidone (Mysoline), 343, 344t
Prinzmetal angina, 40
Procainamide, for arrhythmias, 338t, 338–339
Procedural pain clinics, for chronic pain syndrome, 295–296
Progesterone, menstrual cycle and, 136–137
Prolixin (fluphenazine), 342, 342t
Propafenone, for arrhythmias, 338t, 338–339
Propoxyphene, 330t, 331
Proprioceptive senses, testing of, 219
Prostate gland
  anatomy and physiology of, 117, 118f, 120f
  cancer of, 127

skeletal metastases of, 238–239
treatment of, 239
infection of, 124
Provera (medroxyprogesterone), 346
Pruritus, 310, 318
nonsteroidal anti-inflammatory agents causing, 328
Pseudogout, 271
Pseudotumor cerebri, headache and, 182
Psoriatic arthritis, 261, 263t
Psychogenic pain, 280
Psychological disorders, 277–300. *See also* Affective disorders; Personality disorders; Somatoform disorders.
chemical dependency, 290–291
delusional, 288
dissociative, 288
drug therapy for. *See* Psychotropic drugs.
evaluative algorithm for, 298, 299f
fatigue and, 45
generalized anxiety disorders, 287
malingering, 287
pain and. *See also* Chronic pain syndrome.
acute and chronic, 277–279
family dynamics and, 279
personality and, 279–280
psychophysiology of, 288–289
stress and, 289–290
patient case studies of, 298–300
physiologic assessment in, 294
psychological testing in. *See* Psychological testing.
schizophrenic, 288
Psychological testing, 291–294
Beck Depression Inventory, 293
behavioral assessment, 292
Coping Strategies Questionnaire, 294
Illness Behavior Questionnaire, 293
McGill Pain Questionnaire, 294
Millon Behavioral Health Inventory, 293
Minnesota Multiphasic Personality Inventory, 292–293
Pain Behavior Scale, 292
Pain Distress Scale, 294, 295
Sickness Impact Profile, 292
Symptom Checklist-90, 293
Visual Analogue Scale, 293
West Haven-Yale Multidimensional Pain Inventory, 294
Psychotropic drugs, 339–343
antidepressants. *See* Antidepressants.
benzodiazepines, 339–340, 340t
lithium, 342
neuroleptics, 342t, 342–343, 343t
Pulmonary edema, 46, 47, 51
Pulmonary embolism, 47
Pulmonary fissures, 69, 70f
Pulmonary function tests, 86–87, 98
Pulmonary shunt, 49
Pulmonary system, 69–100
anatomy of, 69–75, 70f, 71t, 72f, 73f
diseases of. *See* Pulmonary system disease.
Pulmonary system disease
auscultation in, 75–83, 90
hints for, 83
pleural friction rub and, 82
stethoscope and, 75–76, 76f
vocal and breath sounds and. *See* Adventitious breath sounds; Breath sounds; Rales; Vocal sounds.
breathing patterns in, 89–90
cancer, skeletal metastases of, 239
chart review in, 83t, 83–90
of blood gases, 87
of laboratory reports, 87
of medical history, 84
of medication history, 84–86
of psychosocial history, 84
of pulmonary function tests, 86–87
of radiographic results, 84
of work history, 88
cough in, 89
discharge planning for, 88
finger percussion in, 90
functional respiratory capacity assessment in, 90–91
history in, 88
obstructive, 92–95, 93f. *See also* Chronic obstructive pulmonary disease (COPD).
pulmonary function tests in, 86
of upper airways, 94–95
physical examination in, 88–89
restrictive, 95–97
invasive or space-occupying, 96–97
pulmonary function tests in, 86
thoracic cage abnormalities in, 95
ventilatory muscle dysfunction in, 96
signs and symptoms of, 91t, 91–92
vascular, 97–98
ventilatory regulation disorders, 98–99
Pulmonary valve, 35
Pulmonic valve, 32, 32f
Pulsatile masses, 41
Pulse(s), 35
absence of, 357
absent or diminished, 41
arterial, palpable, 17
lacking, 50
palpation of, 35, 40–41, 42, 49–50, 50f, 407f–408f, 412f–413f
paradoxical, 94
Pulse pressure, 38, 38f, 52
Pulsus paradoxus, 47, 98
Purpura, 318
Pustule, 308f, 318
Pyelonephritis, in males, 124

Q

Quadriceps muscle, assessment of, 19
Quantitative computed tomography (QCT), 373
Quinidine, for arrhythmias, 338t, 338–339

R

Radial pulse, palpation of, 49, 50, 407f
Radiculopathy, 203
cervical, 18–19
Radiographic reports, in pulmonary system disease, 84
Radiography, conventional, 365–366
in aortic regurgitation, 60
in aortic stenosis, 60
Radiologic assessment. *See* Imaging; *specific modalities*.
Radionuclide bone scans, 368–369, 372
Rales, 51, 80–82
coarse, 81–82
fine, 81
medium, 81
"velcro," 97, 98
Range of motion (ROM)
active, 15, 19
in headaches, 179
passive, 15
in headaches, 179
in rheumatic disease, 258
Ranitidine (Zantac), for peptic ulcer disease, 344t, 345
Rashes, 318–319
causes of, 310
chronology of, 310
in dermatomyositis, 267, 267f
location of, 309
in Lyme disease, 272
nonsteroidal anti-inflammatory agents causing, 328
Rate pressure product (RPP), 51–52
in angina, 56
Raynaud's disease, 312
Raynaud's phenomenon, 312
Reactive arthritis, 261, 263t
Reactive hyperemia test, 41
Rebound tenderness, 112

Re-entry, 57
Referral, for musculoskeletal disorders, 248–249
Referred pain, 270
Reflexes
abdominal, 18–19, 414f
Reflexes *(Continued)*
cutaneous, 410f
testing of, 220, 220f
deep tendon. *See* Deep tendon reflexes (DTRs).
Reflex sympathetic dystrophy, 270
imaging in, 391
Rehabilitation programs, for chronic pain syndrome. *See* Chronic pain syndrome.
Reiter syndrome, 261, 263t
Relaxin, menstrual cycle and, 137
Renal arteries, 118, 119f
Renal cell carcinoma, 125
Renal disease. *See* Kidney disease.
Renal failure, chronic, 127–129
Reproductive system. *See* Female urogenital system; Female urogenital system disease; Male urogenital system; Male urogenital system disease; *specific organs*.
Resisted manual muscle testing, 217–218
Respiration. *See also* Breathing.
absence of, 357
in pregnancy, 144
Respiratory distress, 97
signs of, 91, 91t
Reticular formation, 192
Retrolisthesis, imaging in, 376
Retroperitoneal lymphatics, 127, 128f
Rheumatic disease, 257–274, 273f. *See also* Arthritis.
infection and, 271t, 271–272
patient case studies of, 272, 274
signs and symptoms of, 257–271
in aseptic osteonecrosis, 270
back pain. *See* Back pain.
in benign hypermobility syndrome, 269–270
in fibromyalgia, 269, 269f
in gout, 271
in hemarthrosis, 271
in hypertrophic osteoarthropathy, 270
local tissue assessment and, 258–259, 259f
in muscular rheumatism, 267
in myasthenia gravis, 268
neck pain, 266f, 266–267, 267f
in polymyalgia rheumatica, 268–269
in polymyositis, 267f, 267–268, 268t
in pseudogout, 271
referred pain, 270
in reflex sympathetic dystrophy syndrome, 270
in systemic lupus erythematosus, 258, 258t
in temporal arteritis, 268–269
Rheumatic fever, 271, 271t
valvular disease and, 59
Rheumatism, muscular, 267
Rheumatoid arthritis (RA), 260–261, 262f
cervical stenosis in, 266
imaging in, 391
Rheumatoid factor, 261
Rhonchi, 51, 82, 94
Rickets, 240
Right ventricular filling pressures, elevated, 58
Right ventricular heave, 93–94
Rigidity, in Parkinson's disease, 211
Rotator cuff disease, imaging in, 386–387, 388f
Rubor, 245

S

Sacroiliitis, 261
Sacrum, anatomy and physiology of, 133–134, 134f, 135f
Salicylates, 324–326, 325t
contraindications to, 326
excess of, 99
mechanism of action of, 325
side effects of, 325–326, 326t
Scabs, 319
Scale, 308f, 319
Scars, 319
hypertrophic, 318
Schizoid personality disorder, 281
Schizophrenic disorders, 288
Scoliosis, imaging in, 372–373
Scrotum, masses in, 124
Scurvy, 240
Seasonal affective disorder, 287
Secondary gain, pain and, 278
Seizures, 358
brain tumors and, 210
drug therapy for, 343–344, 344t
headache following, 183
syncope and, 44–45
in therapeutic pool, 360
Self-defeating personality disorder, 283
Self-observation, of pain behavior, 292
Seminal vesicles, anatomy and physiology of, 117, 118f, 120f
Sensory testing, 19, 218–219
Septic arthritis, acute, 270
Serpiginous lesions, 309
Sertraline, 341, 341t
Sexual abuse, 290
Sexual function
disorders of, 14, 354
in urogenital disease, in males, 122
Sexual intercourse, painful, 147
Sexually transmitted diseases (STDs), in females, 148
Shin splints, 40
Shock, 357
Shoulder
imaging of, 386–387
in calcific tendinitis, 387
in rotator cuff disease and shoulder impingement syndrome, 386–387, 388f
in traumatic injuries, 387, 389f
pain in, patient case studies of, 23–27, 26f
Shoulder abduction weakness, 19
Shoulder impingement syndrome, imaging in, 386–387, 388f
Sickle cell disease, 109
Sickness Impact Profile (SIP), 292
Signal-averaged electrocardiography, 57
Single-photon absorptiometry (SPA), 373
Sinus bradycardia, 53, 56
Sinus headache, 183–184, 184f
Sinus node, 33, 35f
Sinus tachycardia, 53, 56
Sinus tarsi syndrome, imaging of, 386
Sjögren syndrome, 261
Skeletal muscle relaxants, 331–332, 332t
side effects of, 331–332
Skeletal scintigraphy, 368–369, 372
Skin, 303–316, 304f
brachial plexus injuries and, 203, 208f
color of, 305
changes in, 305, 306t
hyperpigmentation, 167, 306t
of lesions, 309
in dermatomyositis, 267, 267f
layers of, 303–304
observation of, 16
osteoblastoma and, 228
in pregnancy, 143
sweat glands of, 304f, 305
temperature of, 16–17, 41, 50, 312, 314
in thyroid disease, 163
trophic changes of, 40
Skin disorders, 305–316, 314t
color changes associated with, 305, 306t
examination in, 311–314
history in, 311
laboratory tests in, 314
observation in, 312, 313f
palpation in, 312, 314
physical examination in, 311–312

lesions and, 234, 306–311
causes of, 310–311
chronology of, 310
classification of, 306, 306f–309f
configuration of, 309
location of, 309–310
primary, 306, 318
secondary, 306, 318–319
special, 306, 319
patient case studies of, 314–316
rashes. *See* Rashes.
Skopit's ring of diagnosis for, 303, 304f
tumors, 234, 311, 318
Sleep disorders, in fibromyalgia, 269
Small intestine
acid peptic disorders of, 106–107
anatomy and physiology of, 103f, 103–104
Somatization disorder, 281
Somatoform disorders, 280–281
conversion disorder, 280–281
hypochondriasis, 281
somatization disorder, 281
somatoform pain disorder, 281
Somatoform pain disorder, 281
Somatosensory systems, 194, 198–199
dorsal column-medial lemniscal pathway, 194, 197f, 198, 199
spinothalamic pathway, 198f, 198–199
Sotalol, for arrhythmias, 338t, 338–339
Spermatocele, 127
Spermatogenesis, 120
Spermatozoa, 120
Sphygmomanometer, 41
Spinal cord
anatomy of, 192
lesions of. *See* Spinal cord lesions.
motor function of, 199
Spinal cord lesions, 203, 208–209
autonomic dysreflexia and, 354
incomplete syndromes and, 208–209
nontraumatic, 209
traumatic, 203, 208
Spinal nerve root compression, 18–19
Spinal stenosis, 265f, 265–266
cervical, 266
imaging of, 377, 377f, 378
Spine. *See also* Back pain.
"bamboo," in ankylosing spondylitis, 261, 264f
cervical. *See* Cervical spine.
lumbar. *See* Lumbar spine.
osteomyelitis of, 246–247
osteopenia of, with plasma cell myeloma, 232, 235f
in Paget's disease, 244
percussion of, 17
in pregnancy, 138, 140, 142–143
thoracic. *See* Thoracic spine.
Spinothalamic pathway, 198f, 198–199
Spleen
anatomy and physiology of, 105–106
enlargement of, 108–109
percussion of, 110–111, 112f
rupture of, 108
Spondylitis, 261
Spondyloarthropathies, 261, 263t, 264f
Spondylolisthesis, imaging in, 376, 376f
Spondylolysis, imaging in, 376
Spondylosis, imaging in, 376
Squamous cell carcinoma, of skin, 311
Standing tests, of coordination, 219
Staphylococcus aureus
osteomyelitis caused by, 246
tenosynovitis caused by, 247–248
Status asthmaticus, 94
Stereognosis, 194, 219
Stethoscope, 75–86, 76f. *See also* Auscultation.
Stomach
acid peptic disorders of, 106–107
anatomy and physiology of, 102–103, 103f, 104f
Strangulated hernia, 109
Stress, pain and, 289–290
Stress fractures
of foot and ankle, imaging of, 384
of hip, imaging of, 380
Stress urinary incontinence, 149
Stridor, 82
Stroke volume, 37
Subcutis layer of skin, 304
Subdeltoid bursa, infection of, 247
Subdural hematomas, headache and, 182
Substance abuse, 290–291
Sucralfate (Carafate), for peptic ulcer disease, 344, 345
Suffering
definition of, 278
introversion-extroversion and, 279
Suicide
depression and, 285–286, 286t
risk of, 355
Supination/pronation test, 219
Supine hypotension, in pregnancy, 145
Supine position, in pregnancy, 143–144
Supraspinatus muscle lesions, 19
Supraspinatus tendon, tears of, imaging of, 387, 388f
Supraventricular tachycardia, 56
Swallowing, 101
testing of, 216–217
Sweat(s), 13
Sweat glands, 304f, 305
Swelling. *See also* Edema.
with Ewing sarcoma, 232
of joints, 270
in musculoskeletal infections, 245
with musculoskeletal neoplasms, 225
painful, of extremities, 355–356
with skeletal metastatic disease, 238
Symmetrel (amantidine), 342
Sympathetic nervous system, 194
Sympathetic neuropathy, 40
Sympathomimetics. *See also specific drugs*.
for pulmonary system disease, 84–85, 85t
Symptom(s). *See also specific disorders*.
alteration of, 15
behavior of, 6–8
history of, 8
location and description of, 4–6, 5f, 6f
visceral, 7
Symptom Checklist-90 (SCL), 293
Syncope, 42, 356–357, 357t
in cardiovascular disease, 44–45
Synovitis, erosive, cervical, 266
Systemic lupus erythematosus (SLE), 258, 258t
Systems review, 12–14, 13f, 399–400
in headaches, 178, 178t
Systole
atrial, 33, 35
ventricular, 33, 35
Systolic pressure, 38, 38f, 52

T

Tachycardia
sinus, 53, 56
supraventricular, 56
ventricular, 56
Tactile localization, 219
Tardive dyskinesia
basal ganglia lesions and, 211
neuroleptics causing, 342–343
Tarsal coalition, imaging of, 385
Tarsal tunnel syndrome, imaging in, 386
Technetium skeletal imaging, 368–369
Tegretol (carbamazepine), 343, 344t
Telangiectasia, 319
Temperature
of skin, 16–17, 41, 50, 312, 314
testing of sensation for, 218
Temporal arteritis, 268–269
headache and, 183
Tenderness
abdominal, 112
of breasts, 146–147
in hypertrophic osteoarthropathy, 270
rebound, 112

Tenderness *(Continued)*
in reflex sympathetic dystrophy syndrome, 270
with skeletal metastatic disease, 238
in thyroid disease, 162
Tender points, in fibromyalgia, 269, 269f
Tendinitis
calcific, of shoulder, imaging of, 387
in foot, imaging of, 385
Tendinous injuries
of Achilles tendon, imaging of, 385f, 385–386
of supraspinatus tendon, imaging of, 387, 388f
Tendons
infections of, 247–248
pain in, in rheumatic disease, 258
Tennis elbow, imaging in, 389
Tenosynovitis, 247–248
in foot, imaging of, 385
Tensilon test, 268
Terazosin, for hypertension, 333, 333t, 335
Testes
anatomy and physiology of, 117, 118f, 120–121
cancer of, 127, 128f
change in size of, 124
hormones of, 157t
infection of, 124
torsion of, 124
Testosterone, 120–121
Tetany, in hypoparathyroidism, 165–166, 166f
Thalamus, lesions of, 209
Theophylline, for asthma, 347t, 3470348
Therapeutic pool emergencies, 360, 360t
Thermography, 41
Thioridazine (Mellaril), 342, 342t
Thoracic cage, abnormalities of, in restrictive pulmonary disease, 95
Thoracic outlet syndrome, in pregnancy, 143, 145
Thoracic spine, imaging of, 372–375
in neoplastic disease, 373–375, 374f
in nontraumatic thoracic pain, 372
in osteoporosis, 373
in scoliosis, 372–373
in traumatic injuries, 372
Thoracoabdominal dyssynchrony, 93
Thorazine (chlorpromazine), 342, 342t
Throat, infectious diseases of, 106
Thromboembolism, pulmonary, 97–98
Thrombophlebitis, 40, 50
Thymus gland, hormone of, 157t
Thyroid gland
disease of. *See* Thyroid gland disease.
hormones of, 157t
palpation of, 403f
Thyroid gland disease, 162f, 162–164. *See also* Hyperthyroidism; Hypothyroidism.
auscultation in, 162
cancer, skeletal metastases of, 239
metabolic bone disease and, 241
palpation in, 162, 162f
thyrotoxicosis, 163, 163t
Thyrotoxicosis, 163, 163t
subjective and objective changes in, 170t
Thyrotropin, 158
Tibial pulse, 50
palpation of, 41, 413f
Ticks, skin lesions due to, 311
Tinnitus
salicylates causing, 326
vestibulocochlear nerve lesions and, 214
Titubation, cerebellar lesions and, 211
Tocainide, for arrhythmias, 338t, 338–339
Tooth disease, headache caused by, 184
"Touch-me-not" syndrome, 287, 290
Touch sensation, testing of, 219
Trabecular bone, 241
Tracheal breath sounds, 78
Training, for handling emergencies, 354
Transient ischemic attack (TIA), 42
Trauma. *See specific anatomic site*.
Trazodone, 341, 341t
Treatment response, 21
Tremor
cerebellar lesions and, 211
neurologic disorders and, 212
in Parkinson's disease, 211
Trendelenburg position, 356
Tricuspid valve, 32, 32f, 35
Tricyclic antidepressants (TCAs), 340–341, 341t
Trigeminal nerve (cranial nerve VI), testing of, 214, 216f
Trochlear nerve (cranial nerve IV), testing of, 213–214, 216f
Trousseau's sign, in hypoparathyroidism, 165, 166f
Truncal mononeuropathy, in diabetes mellitus, 161
T1/T2, 368
Tuberculosis, 247
Tumor (swelling). *See* Swelling.
Tumors. *See also* Cancer; Metastases; Neoplastic disease; *specific anatomic sites and tumors*.
definition of, 224
headache and, 181–182
intracranial, 210
palpating, 17
pulmonary system disease and, 97
in scrotum, 124
of skin, 311, 318
of spinal cord, 209
Turgor, of skin, 314
Two-point discrimination, 219

U

Ulcers
of feet, in diabetes mellitus, 160
peptic. *See* Peptic ulcer disease.
of skin, 310, 319
venous stasis, 40, 41
Ulnar pulse, palpation of, 408f
Ultrasound, 369
Unconsciousness, 356–357, 357t. *See also* Syncope.
Upper motor neuron lesions, 202–203
deep tendon reflexes in, 220
lower motor neuron lesions versus, 202
testing for, 217
Upper-quarter screening examination, 401–402, 402f–408f
Ureters
anatomy and physiology of, 117, 118f
infection of, in males, 125
Urethra, infection of, in males, 125
Urinary bladder. *See* Bladder.
Urinary incontinence, stress, 149
Urinary tract infection
in females, 147
in males, 124
Urination
frequency and urgency of, 14
in pregnancy, 144, 145
in urogenital disease, in males, 121
in urogenital system disease, in males, 124, 125
in urogenital disease, in males, 121–122
Urogenital system. *See* Female urogenital system; Female urogenital system disease; Male urogenital system; Male urogenital system disease.
Uterus
anatomy and physiology of, 134, 140f
cancer of, 149
fibroids in, 148
prolapse of, 149

V

Vagina, anatomy and physiology of, 134–135
Vaginal burning, 146
Vaginal discharge, 146
Vaginal dryness, 146

Vagus nerve (cranial nerve X), testing of, 216–217
Valproate (Depakene, Depakote), 343, 344t
Varicose veins, in pregnancy, 144
Vascular disease
  diabetic, 162
  headache caused by, 182–183
  peripheral, 40, 41, 48
  pulmonary, 97–98
Vascular system, in pregnancy, 143
Vasculitis, in polymyalgia rheumatica, 268–269
Vas deferens, anatomy and physiology of, 117, 118f
Vasodilators, for congestive heart failure, 336, 337t
Vasopressin, 156, 157t, 158
Vasovagal syncope, 44
Vegetations, 60
Veins, 32, 33
  varicose, in pregnancy, 144
Venlafaxine, 341, 341t
Venous insufficiency, 40
Venous stasis ulcers, 40, 41
Ventilator settings, 93
Ventilatory muscle dysfunction, 96
Ventilatory regulation disorders, 98
Ventral corticospinal tract, 199, 201f
Ventral horns, 192
Ventricles, of heart, 32, 35
Ventricular arrhythmias, 41–42
Ventricular ectopic activity (VEA), 42, 44
Ventricular ejection, 35
Ventricular systole, 33, 35
Ventricular tachycardia, 56
Verapamil, 333t, 335
  for arrhythmias, 338t, 338–339
Vertebra. *See* Spine.
Vertebrae. *See* Cervical spine; Lumbar spine; Thoracic spine.
Vertebral artery, stenosis of, 183
Vertigo, 185
  neurologic disorders and, 212
Vesicle, 307f, 318
Vesicular breath sounds, 71–75, 79f, 79–80, 83
  in pulmonary system disease, 94
Vestibulocochlear nerve (cranial nerve VIII), testing of, 214, 216, 217f
Vibration, testing of sensation for, 219
Violent patients, 358–359, 360t
Vision, testing of, 213, 213f, 214f
Vocal sounds, 76–78
  abnormal, 77–78
    bronchophony, 77–78
    egophony, 78
    whispered pectoriloquy, 78
  normal, 77
Vomiting, 13–14
  increased intracranial pressure and, 210
  in pregnancy, 145
  in urogenital disease, in females, 147
Vulva, cancer of, 149

W

Weakness, 14, 19
  in adrenal gland disease, 166, 167
  in chronic renal failure, 128
  in diabetic neuropathies, 161–162
  in hyperparathyroidism, 165
  neurologic disorders and, 212
  in peripheral motor neuropathy, diabetic, 161
  in thyroid disease, 163, 164
  of upper extremities, in pregnancy, 142–143
Weapons, 359
Weber's test, 216
Weight change, unexplained, 13
Weight gain, in pregnancy, 143
West Haven-Yale Multidimensional Pain Inventory (WHYMPI), 294
Wheal, 307f, 318
Wheezes. *See* Rhonchi.
Whispered pectoriloquy, 78
Wolff-Parkinson-White syndrome, 57
Wrist. *See* hand and wrist.

Z

Zantac (ranitidine), for peptic ulcer disease, 344t, 345
Zolpidem (Ambien), 340